CONSULTANT WRITERS

ADRIENNE ARDIGO, R.N., B.S.

Instructor, Department of Health Occupations and Nursing
Los Angeles Trade Technical Community College
Los Angeles, California

INICE CHIRCO, R.N., M.A., M.S.

Chairman, Allied Health Programs
Rio Hondo College
Whittier, California

JANE M. KAHN, R.N., M.N.

Director of Nursing
Hollywood Presbyterian Hospital
Hollywood, California

MYDA MAGARIAN, R.N., M.N.

Director of Medical Nursing
St. Vincent's Hospital
Los Angeles, California

LINDA NEWELL, R.N., B.S.

Formerly, Assistant Superintendent
The Neuropsychiatric Institute
Los Angeles, California

BEVERLY RAMBO, R.N., M.A., M.N.

Assistant Professor, School of Nursing
Mt. St. Mary's College
Los Angeles, California

VIRGINIA STOPERA, R.N., M.N.

Director, Staff Development
Center for Health Sciences, University of California
Los Angeles, California

Nursing Skills for Allied Health Services

Volume 3

LUCILE A. WOOD, R.N., M.S.

Formerly Associate Director for the Nursing Occupations
U.C.L.A. Allied Health Professions Project
Los Angeles, California

Presently Director of Nursing
Bay Area Hospital
Coos Bay, Oregon

W. B. Saunders Company
PHILADELPHIA • LONDON • TORONTO

W. B. Saunders Company, Publisher: West Washington Square
                                      Philadelphia, Pa. 19105

                                      12 Dyott Street
                                      London, WC1A 1DB

                                      833 Oxford Street
                                      Toronto, Ontario M8Z 5T9, Canada

---

Library of Congress Cataloging in Publication Data (Revised)

Wood, Lucile A

Nursing Skills for allied health services.

Page 768, blank for "Notes."

1. Nurses and nursing
    I. Title.   [DNLM: 1. Nursing care. WY150 N974]
RT41.W84   610.73   79-186957
ISBN 0-7216-9602-3 (v. 3)

The project presented or reported herein was performed pursuant to a grant from the U.S. Office of Education, Department of Health, Education, and Welfare. The opinions expressed herein, however, do not necessarily reflect the position of the policy of the U.S. Office of Education, and no official endorsement by the U.S. Office of Education should be inferred.

Nursing Skills for Allied Health Services   VOLUME ONE–ISBN   0-7216-9600-7
                                                   VOLUME TWO–ISBN   0-7216-9601-5
                                                   VOLUME THREE–ISBN 0-7216-9602-3

Library of Congress Catalog card number 79-186957.

Printed by W. B. Saunders Company

Print No.:   9   8   7   6   5   4   3   2

To

Hi

and My Parents

ALLIED HEALTH PROFESSIONS PROJECTS NURSING NATIONAL TECHNICAL ADVISORY COMMITTEE

J. P. Myles Black, M.D.
Clinical Instructor, College of Medicine
University of Southern California
Los Angeles, California

Mary Bruton, R.N., M.S., Assistant Professor
St. Anselms College
Manchester, New Hampshire

Terry Crowley, Educational Consultant
National Federation of Licensed Practical Nurses
New York, New York

Bernice Dixon, R.N., M.S., Director
School of Nursing, Grady Memorial Hospital
Atlanta, Georgia

Phyllis Drennan, R.N., M.S., Coordinator
Associate Degree Nursing Program
Kirkwood Community College
Cedar Rapids, Iowa
(Official Representative of the National League for Nursing)

Elizabeth J. Haglund
Regional Nursing Consultant for the Division of Nursing
Bureau of Health Professions Manpower Training
Department of Health, Education, and Welfare, Region IX
San Francisco, California

William F. Hartnett, R.N., M.S.
Assistant Administrator, Nursing Services
Riverside Methodist Hospital
Columbus, Ohio

Nannette Turner, L.V.N.
Past Executive Director
California Licensed Vocational Nurses Association
Los Angeles, California
(Official Representative of National Federation of Licensed Practical Nurses)

Captain Ouida Upchurch, Captain, NC, USN
Special Assistant for Education and Training R and D
Department of the Navy
Bureau of Medicine and Surgery
Washington, D.C.

George Wells, Associate Director
Health Insurance Council
Chicago, Illinois

Gerry White, R.N., M.S., Director
Allied Health Careers Institute
El Centro College of Dallas County
Dallas, Texas

Lucie Young, R.N., Ph.D., Chairman
Nursing Department of California State College, Los Angeles
Los Angeles, California
(Official Representative of the American Nurses Association)

NATIONAL ADVISORY COMMITTEE ALLIED HEALTH PROFESSIONS PROJECTS

Phillip L. Williams, Vice-President, Chairman
The Times Mirror Company
Los Angeles, California

Lowell Burkett, Executive Director
American Vocational Association
Washington, D.C.

L. M. Detmer, Director
Bureau of Manpower and Education
American Hospital Association
Chicago, Illinois

Dale Garrell, M.D., Director
Adolescent Unit, Children's Hospital
Los Angeles, California

John F. Henning, Executive Secretary-Treasurer
California Federation of Labor
San Francisco, California

Joseph Kadish, Ph.D., Acting Chief
Education Program Development Branch
National Institutes of Health
Department of Health, Education, and Welfare
Washington, D.C.

Bernard Kamins, Public Relations Consultant
Beverly Hills, California

Ralph C. Kuhli, Director
Department of Allied Medical Professions and Services
American Medical Association
Chicago, Illinois

Leon Lewis, Chief
Division of Occupational Analysis and Employer Services
Manpower Administration, Department of Labor
Washington, D.C.

Walter J. McNerney, President
Blue Cross Association
Chicago, Illinois

Peter G. Meek, Executive Director
National Health Council
New York, New York

NATIONAL ADVISORY COMMITTEE ALLIED HEALTH PROFESSIONS PROJECTS

Marc J. Musser, M.D., Chief Medical Officer
Department of Medicine and Surgery, Veterans Administration
Washington, D.C.

Leroy Pesch, M.D.
Deputy Assistant Secretary for Health Manpower
Department of Health, Education, and Welfare
Washington, D.C.

Helen K. Powers, R.N., Program Officer
Health Occupations
U.S. Office of Education
Washington, D.C.

William M. Samuels, Executive Director
Association of Schools of Allied Health Professions
Washington, D.C.

William Shannon, Ph.D., Acting Executive Director
American Association of Junior Colleges
Washington, D.C.

Elizabeth Simpson, Ph.D.
Instructional Materials and Practices Branch
Division of Comprehensive and Vocational Education
Bureau of Research, U.S. Office of Education
Washington, D.C.

John D. Twiname, Commissioner
Social and Rehabilitation Services
Department of Health, Education, and Welfare
Washington, D.C.

C. Gordon Watson, D.D.S., Executive Director
American Dental Association
Chicago, Illinois

Richard S. Wilbur, M.D.
Assistant Secretary of Defense
Department of Defense
Washington, D.C..

FOREWORD

The Division of Vocational Education, University of California, is an administrative unit of the University concerned with responsibilities for research, teacher education, and public service in the broad area of vocational and technical education. During 1968 the Division entered into an agreement with the U.S. Office of Education, Department of Health, Education and Welfare, to prepare occupational analyses, curricula, and instructional materials for a variety of allied health occupations. For the most part, these materials are related to pre-service and in-service instruction for educational programs ranging from on-the-job training through the associate degree level.

This third instructional manual in the series entitled *Nursing Skills for Allied Health Services* completes the work undertaken in the nursing field which started with a task inventory, followed by an occupational analysis *(A Study of Nursing Occupations)*, and a curriculum guide *(A Career Model for the Nurse Practitioner)*. In order to implement the curriculum, instructional materials were developed, culminating in the publication of three volumes that cover the tasks delineated in the occupational analysis and curriculum guide.

The educational philosophy exemplified in these materials is task-oriented instruction in which the emphasis is on helping the student learn to perform the tasks of the occupation and to use the basic scientific and technical knowledge related to them. This approach is designed to shorten the learning process, so that the goal of "more learning in less time with greater retention" can be achieved. If these materials make a significant contribution toward accomplishing this goal, they will help to solve the health manpower problem, and the members of the staff of the Allied Health Professions Project will feel that the endless hours they have labored on the development of these manuals were not in vain.

We want especially to thank the staff of the W. B. Saunders Company for their willingness to publish the manuals without a copyright, and for their enthusiastic cooperation in producing these books. Without their help, we could not have completed the job.

MELVIN L. BARLOW, Ed. D.
Professor of Education and
Director, Division of Vocational Education
University of California, Los Angeles

MILES H. ANDERSON, Ed.D.
Director, Allied Health
Professions Project
University of California, Los Angeles

PREFACE

From the time of their initial publication, *Nursing Skills for Allied Health Services*, Volumes 1 and 2, have been utilized as the basic texts for nursing skills in countless nursing education and allied health programs in this country and abroad. Moreover, they are being used increasingly in hospitals, nursing homes, and other health care agencies as procedure books.

This volume of the series covers the remaining nursing skills as identified in the Allied Health Professions Projects (AHPP) research survey as being performed by the LPN (LVN) and RN. The only exceptions are:

1. Those tasks dealing with respiratory therapy, which are planned for a companion volume that is in preparation.

2. Those skills dealing with the reading of cardiac monitors, because there are already so many excellent resources on this subject.

3. Teaching skills per se, since they can be learned in various short-term programs.

4. Management techniques, which can be learned from numerous texts and courses now being offered.

This volume continues the development of the more complex nursing skills as identified in the original AHPP research survey. During the intervening years since that survey was completed, the LPN's duties have rapidly incorporated most of the remaining skills originally designated as "... entirely within the realm of the RN." This trend gives further impetus to the development of a nursing curriculum that will train the basic practitioner for the nursing profession by combining the present curricula of LPN (LVN), associate degree, and diploma nursing into a single instructional program.

LUCILE A. WOOD

PREFACE TO VOLUMES ONE AND TWO

Nursing, like all other health professions, has been undergoing monumental change since 1965, when major health legislation was begun at the federal and state levels of government.

In order to meet the growing health needs of our citizens, the nursing profession is taking some positive steps to make sure that care from competent and concerned health personnel is provided whenever and wherever the need arises.

As a Director of Nursing Service in a large suburban hospital, it was my responsibility and desire to employ nurses whose first concern was for people, and who were also skillful and knowledgeable when administering nursing care to patients. Nursing administrators generally agree that many graduates of recent nursing programs are not able to give such direct bedside care. Hence, when these new nurses are first employed, they face not only the frustrations of evolving from a student to a graduate nurse, but they must also simultaneously develop their clinical competence.

Therefore, when the opportunity presented itself to develop a nursing curriculum based on national occupational statistics for the U.C.L.A. Allied Health Professions Projects, I was eager to accept the challenge.

The Allied Health Professions Projects (AHPP) is a national curriculum research and development program funded in August 1968 as a four-year grant by the U.S. Office of Education. The core curriculum concept and career mobility patterns in allied health were two of its primary considerations.

The instructional materials in this textbook are built around the 184 activities designated in the AHPP national survey as those which are accomplished by all levels of nursing—N.A., L.P.N. (L.V.N.), AND R.N. These activities were incorporated into the 36 instructional units which comprise this text.

Because AHPP was attempting something new in media methodology, the process of developing the materials was a difficult one. Initially, the activities defined in the national survey were outlined in a job breakdown (i.e., subdivided into a logical, orderly sequence which was designated as "Important Steps"). Then, each Important Step was supported by practical content under the heading "Key Points," giving related theory which clarified this step. This included factors that make or break the successful attainment of a skill, e.g., safety precautions; suggestions for making the step easier to do (special timing, handling, positioning, or sequencing); related biological concepts or principles of microbiology where applicable; communication and human relations skills required to assure successful completion of the activity; and pertinent ethical or legal concepts.

The sequence of units was established on the premise of progression from the general and simple to the more specific and complex subjects. It should be noted here that all nursing personnel, regardless of their final exit point on the nursing career ladder, should be well-grounded in the theory and practice of these basic nursing skills before moving on to more advanced responsibilities. Successful completion of this text should assure a competent practitioner who can interrupt the nursing educational process to work as a nursing assistant (entry-level practitioner). It should also provide a sound basis for moving on to the complex skills and theoretical knowledge required in the succeeding levels of nursing practice.

These materials represent an example of media methodology which, on the one hand, permits the student to move at his own rate of speed through the background information and procedural skills and, on the other hand, permits the instructor to be released from the need to repeat information to each incoming student. This allows the instructor additional time that can be spent more productively and creatively in the practice and clinical laboratories, assisting the students to polish their performance, expand their interests and comprehension, and to apply the knowledge and skills related to the care of their patients in the clinical assignments.

PREFACE TO VOLUMES ONE AND TWO

The materials are adaptable to a variety of teaching settings; they can be used for on-the-job training through the Associate degree in nursing as well as for adult education and staff development programs for nursing personnel and other allied health professionals who require these skills.

LUCILE A. WOOD

ACKNOWLEDGMENTS

Credit is due to many people for their assistance in developing and in completing this textbook.

The students and faculty members of the following test sites have given their suggestions: Black Hills Area Vocational Technical School of Practical Nursing, Rapid City, South Dakota; Community College of Denver (North Campus), Denver, Colorado; Dalton Vocational School of Practical Nursing, Dalton, Georgia; Coosa Valley Vocational Technical School, Rome, Georgia; School of Practical Nursing, Southwest Oregon Community College, Coos Bay, Oregon.

The writer-consultants provided basic content for the development of many chapters. Many thanks go also to the members of the National Advisory Committee for Nursing and the UCLA Allied Health Professions Projects, as well as the individual members of the Project staff. In particular, I wish to thank Melanie Herrick, my secretary on the staff, and Marian McCready, who did the typing for the final chapters of the book. The Project administrators, Dr. Miles Anderson and Dr. Melvin Barlow, gave me substantial assistance in the development of the final chapters; their support and aid are gratefully acknowledged.

Thanks also are extended to friends who critically reviewed various chapters: Ruth Higgs, Marian Watanabe, Alice Rodriquez, Eleanor Finlayson, Pat Downer, Glenys Pare, Dr. Joseph Morgan, Dr. Carl Grossman, Dr. Michael McKeown, Louise Thomas, and Thelma Bushnell. As always, a vital link in the production of any text is the editor: Seba Kolb is genuinely commended for her usually fine job. Sylva Grossman, also an AHPP editor, pinch-hit when Seba was tied up with other priorities. Sylva's efforts and fresh viewpoints were most appreciated. The artwork in this volume was done by Sharon Lee Belkin, of the UCLA Media Center Staff. Sharon has done an outstanding rendition for which I am most grateful.

Of course, this text could not have been completed without the help, encouragement, and understanding of my husband, Hi, as well as the same from my fellow staff members at the Bay Area Hospital, Coos Bay, Oregon.

And to Robert Wright, Nursing Editor, and Helen Dietz, Associate Nursing Editor, both of the W. B. Saunders Company, my thanks not only for assistance and counsel, but also for welcome friendship.

L.A.W.

CONTENTS

Volume 3

Unit 1.	ASEPTIC TECHNIQUE	1
Unit 2.	PREPARATION AND ADMINISTRATION OF MEDICATIONS	63
Unit 3.	PREPARING FOR AND ASSISTING WITH EXAMINATIONS	135
Unit 4.	IRRIGATIONS AND INSTILLATIONS	156
Unit 5.	URINARY CATHETERIZATION	206
Unit 6.	APPLICATION OF HOT AND COLD COMPRESSES, PACKS AND SOAKS	227
Unit 7.	PHARYNGEAL SUCTIONING	246
Unit 8.	TRACHEOSTOMY CARE	262
Unit 9.	APPLICATION OF TOURNIQUETS	284
Unit 10.	INSERTION OF NASOGASTRIC AND GAVAGE TUBES	307
Unit 11.	SMEARS AND CULTURES	325
Unit 12.	SKIN TESTS, IMMUNIZATIONS AND OTHER PROPHYLACTIC AGENTS	348
Unit 13.	ASSISTING WITH SOMATIC PSYCHIATRIC THERAPIES	375
Unit 14.	TECHNIQUES OF FETAL AND MATERNAL MONITORING	401
	INDEX	433

Unit 1
ASEPTIC TECHNIQUE

I. DIRECTIONS TO THE STUDENT

Study the entire unit, take the written post-test, and be ready to demonstrate your proficiency in the surgical and obstetrical scrub techniques, opening sterile packages, handling sterile instruments, putting on sterile gown and gloves, pouring sterile solutions, and changing or applying sterile dressings.

II. GENERAL PERFORMANCE OBJECTIVE

Upon completion of this unit, you will correctly employ aseptic technique to protect yourself, the patient, and others from contamination and infection.

III. SPECIFIC PERFORMANCE OBJECTIVES

When you have finished this unit, you will be able to carry out the following activities correctly:

1. Perform a surgical or obstetric scrub.
2. Use aseptic technique to put on a sterile gown and gloves.
3. Use aseptic technique to change sterile dressings.
4. Use aseptic technique to pour sterile solutions and handle sterile instruments.
5. Open sterile packages without contaminating the contents.
6. Discuss at least four principles for maintaining aseptic technique.
7. Discuss four of the six broad classes of microorganisms, and be able to identify at least two common diseases which are caused by these organisms.

IV. VOCABULARY

Read the definitions of the terms listed below. Do not attempt to memorize them before proceeding with the lesson. Each term will be explained or defined again in the text. On completion of the lesson, however, you should know the correct definition of each term.

antibody—a protein substance in the body that develops an immunity in the body to a specific pathogen.
body resistance—the body's ability to oppose an infection (does not imply immunity).
body tract—a group of organs or parts that form a continuous pathway; e.g., respiratory tract, alimentary tract.
capillaries—minute blood vessels that connect the smallest arteries (arterioles) and the smallest veins (venules) to form the capillary system.
conductive shoe covers—paper or cloth covering worn over shoes to prevent static electricity.
contagion—the communication of a disease from one person to another by direct or indirect contact.
disinfect—to reduce the numbers of pathogenic microorganisms, usually by germicides or boiling water.

endogenous—originating inside an organism or cell.
endotoxin—bacterial toxin confined within the body of the bacterium; it is freed when the bacterium disintegrates.
excoriation—an abrasion of the outer skin (epidermis) or the coating of an organ by trauma, chemicals, burns, or other causes.
exogenous—originating outside of an organ or a part.
exotoxin—a toxin excreted by a microorganism into its surrounding medium (exotoxins are produced by the diphtheria and tetanus organisms).
flagellum (plural flagella)—a hairlike, mobile whip-like process on the extremity of a bacterium or protozoan.
fomites (singular fomes)—any objects (books, clothing) that are not themselves corrupted but can harbor and transmit infectious organisms.
forceps (tongs)—an instrument used to grasp, pull and extract objects; there are many types, varying according to their usage.
gangrene—death (necrosis) of tissue.
gaping wound—a wound with an opening or a break; an interruption in continuity.
germicide—a chemical substance that destroys bacteria.
hair follicle—small cavity or invagination of the epidermis from which hair grows and which holds the rest of the hair shaft.
hexachlorophene—a bactericidal or bacteriostatic substance contained in certain soaps.
host—animal or plant upon which a parasite lives (gains its nourishment).
incision—a surgical cut made with a knife.
infection—a condition in which the body or part of it is invaded by a pathogenic agent that under favorable conditions multiplies and produces injurious effects.
leukocytosis—increased number of leukocytes in the blood, generally caused by infection.
malaise—discomfort, uneasiness, often indicative of infection.
microbiologist—one who studies microbes (minute forms of life not visible to the naked eye).
parasite—organism that lives on or within another living organism.
pathogen—microorganism capable of producing disease.
pathogenic—capable of producing disease.
pH range—a symbol used in chemistry to express acidity and alkalinity.
purulent (suppurative)—forming or containing pus.
pus—a liquid product of inflammation made up of tissue debris, bacteria, leukocytes, and serum.
scrub suit—clothing made of cotton or special disposable paper, worn in aseptic areas; may be a gown, or pants with a separate top.
sebaceous gland—an oil-secreting gland of the skin.
sedimentation rate—a laboratory test of the speed at which red cells (erythrocytes) settle when an anticoagulant is added to the blood; used as a diagnostic tool for identifying different diseases.
spore—a reproductive cell produced by plants and some protozoans that has a thick wall enabling it to withstand unfavorable environments.
toxin—a poisonous substance of plant or animal origin.
transmission—the transfer from one individual to another e.g., of a disease or hereditary characteristic.
turban—a special type of cap used for covering the hair while in aseptic areas.
virulence—relative power or strength of a pathogen to produce disease.

V. INTRODUCTION

Not all authorities agree about the sources, incidence, and nature of infections, but most concur that postoperative infections are classified either as "endogenous" or "exogenous" in nature.

Many factors influence the development of endogenous infections: advanced age and debility of the patient; surgical operations on major body tracts; active remote infections; duration of preoperative hospitalization; and influence of preoperative antibiotic therapy.

ASEPTIC TECHNIQUE

Sterile technique is an attempt to control sources of infection by carrying out a procedure to destroy all microorganisms (non-pathogenic and pathogenic) and to use special handling for sterile supplies. Lack of knowledge of how bacteria spread from person to person or via the environment is often the cause of major outbreaks of infection and even legal problems.

Legal difficulties may arise from negligence and the failure to meet special standards of practice. Some of these are listed below:

1. Violation of sterile technique.

2. Use of malfunctioning equipment, with resultant injury to the patient.

3. Wrong medication.

4. Injury or harm to patient due to lack of safety standards; e.g., failure to strap a dizzy, semi-sedated patient to a stretcher, operating-room table, or recovery-bed cart.

Medical asepsis should be distinguished from surgical asepsis. *Medical asepsis* is an attempt to prevent the transfer of microorganisms by confining them within the source or to a particular area. Microorganisms cannot move about by themselves; they move only when someone or something transports them. (Refer to the unit on Isolation Technique in Volume 2.)

Surgical asepsis is a method of holding to an absolute minimum the chance of infection or entrance of microorganisms into a wound. Freshly cut living tissue can be easily infected; it is therefore essential for all members of the health team to know the common microorganisms and the means by which they can reach the sterile field and contaminate it. The warning, "Asepsis is a chain which is as strong as its weakest link," has been handed down for generations. In other words, every member must carry out aseptic technique. Failure of just one person to carry out the correct aseptic procedure breaks the "chain" that prevents transmission of microorganisms to susceptible persons. Bacteria, which the tissues cannot destroy, may be brought to an open wound if the health worker violates the principles of sterile (aseptic) technique. The patient may consequently spend extra days in the hospital, or his life may even be at stake! Antibiotics cannot supplant sterile techniques.

Controlling the spread of pathogenic and non-pathogenic microorganisms is essential. Transmission of pathogens and the multitude of microorganisms grossly classified as bacteria, viruses, rickettsiae, yeasts, molds, and protozoa can be prevented. This unit discusses the opening of sterile packages, handling of equipment, and pouring of sterile solutions as essentials of the many methods of infection prevention.

INFECTION AND pH

Infection is the response of the body to injury by microorganisms. When microorganisms are permitted access to tissue not covered by intact skin or mucous membrane, they are capable of multiplying and producing injury to tissue. Normal body tissue provides all the requirements for growth and reproduction of the microorganisms. This includes moisture, food, oxygen, proper temperature, and suitable pH.

pH indicates the acidity or alkalinity of the body or body part; it is a chemistry symbol or mathematical expression in which the letter p stands for power and the letter H for hydrogen ion. Bacteria and other microbes are sensitive to changes in pH for growth or destruction. Most pathogens need a medium between pH 5.0 and pH 8.0 for optimum growth. The pH range is 0 to 14 with 7 as a neutral point; e.g., pH 1 indicates a strongly acid condition and pH 14 indicates a strongly alkaline condition. A state of illness affects the normal pH and thus lowers the body's resistance to bacterial growth.

pH SCALE

0 (Acid)   7 (Neutral)   14 (Alkaline)

The skin, respiratory passage, alimentary tract, and vagina normally have some bacteria present. When the unbroken skin or mucous membrane is intact, the pH is between 5.0 and 8.0, and the bacteria can live in harmony with the host without excessive growth. However, if the skin or mucous membrane is broken and/or the normal pH is not maintained, bacteria grow rapidly. Also, prolonged illnesses may upset the delicate pH balance.

TYPES OF INFECTION

An infection may be *acute* and run a rapid course, or it may be *chronic* and run a slow course extending over a period of time. An infection may be *primary*, which means that the patient is the first to have the infection, or that it is located in the first tissue affected; or it may be *secondary*, which means that the microorganism is passed on to another person or another tissue. An infection may be *latent* and lie dormant (or hidden) for a long period of time. There may even be a *mixed infection*, which is one caused by more than one kind of organism.

Thus, course of infection depends upon these three major factors: the *number* of *focal*, which means that it once was confined and localized but has traveled to another part of the body, e.g., a tooth abscess which has spread to the heart or joints. A *generalized (systemic)* infection is an infection involving the whole body.

COURSE OF INFECTION

A typical course of an acute infection occurs as follows: first comes the *incubation period*, or the time between the microorganism's entry into the body and the onset of symptoms. This time will vary according to the type and virulence of the causative organism and the resistance of the individual. Next comes the *prodromal period*, which is short. It may last only a day or two. At this time the patient is mildly aware of discomfort. Third comes the *acute period*, or actual illness, the duration of which depends on the exact organism causing the illness and the treatment that is instituted. Fourth, the *convalescent period* begins with the decline of fever and acute symptoms, and lasts until the patient regains normal function.

Thus, course of infection depends upon these three major factors: the *number* of microorganisms entering the body, the *virulence* of the organism, and the *resistance* of the patient's body.

BODY REACTIONS TO INFECTIOUS AGENTS

Body reactions vary. There may be a reaction to a mechanical injury causing the blood vessels to be blocked in the tissue, or an actual destruction of body cells and tissues can occur. Air sacs in the lungs may be blocked owing to an acute inflammatory process in the lungs.

Resistance to microorganisms varies among individuals. The body has an inborn power to defend itself against invasion by infectious organisms, but other factors are also important. Age and stress, as well as exposure to heat and cold, may also have pronounced detrimental effects on the body's resistance to infection.

Another factor that influences the process of infection is the *virulence* of the organism. Virulence, or strength, depends on the structure of the organism, its invasiveness, and the toxins which it produces. An encapsulated microorganism (one that has a covering) is more difficult to detroy because it is protected from the body's defenses. Some microorganisms are not affected by the defense mechanisms of the body and they invade healthy tissue, i.e., toxins of the pathogens, whether endotoxins or exotoxins, increase the virulence of the organisms.

Body tissue reaction to infection can be described by these *symptoms*: redness (rubor), heat (calor), swelling (tumor), pain (dolor), and possibly the loss of function of a part. The

ASEPTIC TECHNIQUE

patient may also manifest other symptoms such as malaise, tachycardia, fever, chills, leukocytosis, and may have an increased blood sedimentation rate.

Microorganisms are classified in six broad categories that relate to the inflammatory (infectious) process within the body:

1. Bacteria
2. Fungi
3. Protozoa
4. Metazoa
5. Viruses
6. Rickettsiae

Bacteria and viruses are responsible for most of man's diseases. More is understood about the anatomy and physiology of bacteria than of viruses because some of the minute viruses simply pass through the microbiologist's present-day "filters" and therefore complete study of their life cycle has been impossible.

CLASSIFICATION OF MICROORGANISMS

Bacteria are classified under many subdivisions, each of which is responsible for a distinctive type of disease:

Cocci. The chief members of this group are:

1. Staphylococci which cause infection and inflammation; these produce a thick yellow or white pus.
2. Streptococci, which may cause infection and inflammation throughout the body.
3. Gonococci, which may cause infection and inflammation in the genital tract, eyes, joints, and elsewhere; these produce pus.

Bacilli. Belonging to this group are:

1. *Escherichia coli*, the normal inhabitant of the intestinal tract, responsible for causing urinary and abdominal infections.
2. *Pseudomonas aeruginosa (pyocyanea)*, which causes infection and inflammation; it is characterized by greenish pus and musty odor (seen in infant diarrhea, otitis media, suppurative lesions).
3. *Mycobacterium tuberculosis*, which attacks bones, joints, lungs, and the abdominal cavity.
4. *Clostridium tetani*, which causes tetanus (commonly called lockjaw); it cannot live in the presence of air (is *anaerobic*); it enters through a small skin opening such as a puncture wound made by a nail or needle, etc., and attacks deep tissue.
5. *Clostridium welchii*, which infects dead or dying tissue and forms a gas in the tissue; the common name for the condition is "gas gangrene."

Viruses are the smallest of all microorganisms, and have many strains and modifications. They are more resistant to chemical disinfection than bacteria and are not destroyed by such drugs as sulfa and penicillin. They may be classified according to the part of the body affected:

Skin: smallpox, measles (rubella and rubeola), chickenpox, cold sores (herpes simplex) and shingles (herpes zoster).

Respiratory tract: influenza, common cold, mononucleosis, mumps.

Neurosensory organs: rabies, encephalitis.

Internal organs: yellow fever, infectious hepatitis, serum hepatitis.

Intestinal tract: acute anterior poliomyelitis—if mild is limited to respiratory and gastrointestinal symptom; if it progresses to a major illness, there is involvement of muscles and reflexes. The polio virus may also invade the central nervous system (anterior horn cells of the spinal cord and cells of the brain), producing death or dysfunction of the nerve cells that supply the motor nerves. Although polio immunizations have decreased the incidence of poliomyelitis dramatically, major impairment may still occur.

Fungi. Fungi are commonly called *yeasts* and *molds*; some are disease-producing.

Yeasts: Candida albicans (Monilia) causes thrush (an infection of the throat and mouth) and vaginal infections.

Molds: Molds cause coccidioidomycosis (valley fever, San Joaquin Valley fever), histoplasmosis, ringworm, athlete's foot, jungle rot, and fungus infections of the nails.

Metazoa: These cause such conditions as trichinosis in pork, hookworms, pinworms, and tapeworms.

Protozoa: These cause such diseases as malaria, amoebic dysentery, and trichomonas infections of the vagina.

METHODS OF TRANSMISSION

COMMON MODES OF TRANSMISSION

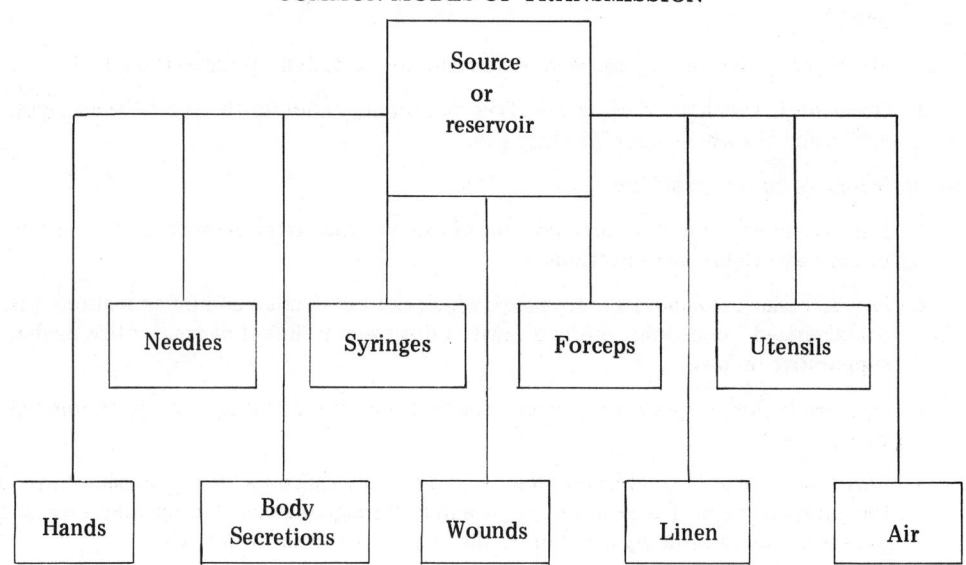

Source or reservoir → Needles, Syringes, Forceps, Utensils, Hands, Body Secretions, Wounds, Linen, Air

Health Workers Can Protect Patients

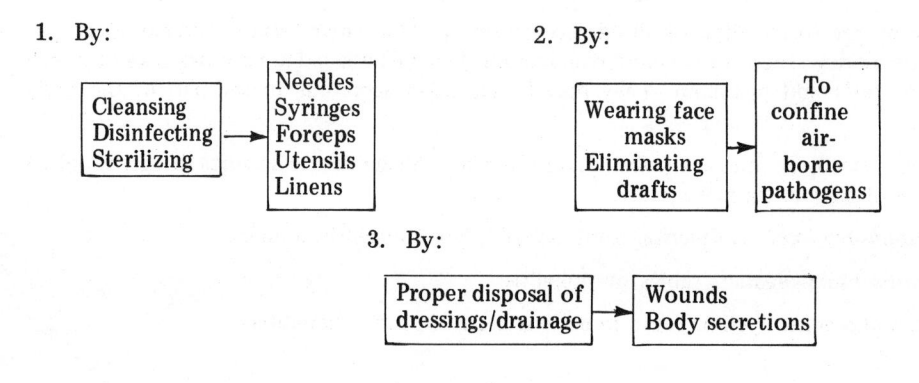

1. By: Cleansing / Disinfecting / Sterilizing → Needles, Syringes, Forceps, Utensils, Linens

2. By: Wearing face masks / Eliminating drafts → To confine airborne pathogens

3. By: Proper disposal of dressings/drainage → Wounds, Body secretions

ASEPTIC TECHNIQUE

The above microorganisms may be transmitted either directly or indirectly. When *direct transmission* occurs the microorganism passes from the host to the exposed person. No time elapses from the moment the microorganism leaves the first host until it enters the second host. A minute prick of the finger may be sufficient for direct transfer of pathogenic organisms from a contaminated source. Likewise, incomplete surgical asepsis may result in infection of the patient.

Microorganisms are transferred *indirectly* by way of articles handled by the infected person or an intermediate host such as food, water, animal, insect, or other carrier. The hospital worker, for example, may be an innocent carrier.

The most common method of indirect transfer of microorganisms is by *fomites* (articles to which microorganisms may cling). Improperly sterilized equipment, improper scrubbing, or glove and gown that have been handled improperly may serve as fomites.

Some microbiologists now say there is no group of strictly pathogenic microorganisms and no group which is strictly non-pathogenic. The fact is that any microorganism, given the right conditions in the host, will cause disease. However, it is true that in usual circumstances certain microorganisms will produce disease in man and are therefore considered to be pathogenic, and certain other microorganisms do not produce disease in man and are considered to be non-pathogenic.

Some facts which are commonly known to the microbiologist help us to develop methods to prevent the transmission of microorganisms. They are listed on page 6.

Bacteria:	Viruses:
1. Are unicellular.	1. Are not cellular.
2. Are microscopic.	2. Are visible only with electron microscope.
3. Are composed of two parts: a cell wall and a cell body.	3. Are composed of two parts: an outer protein shell and a central nucleic acid core of either DNA or RNA.
4. Are destroyed by heat and chemicals.	4. Are destroyed by heat; resistant to chemicals.
5. Reproduce by splitting.	5. Multiply within living cells; viruses are incapable of independent life.
6. Are classified by form as round (cocci) spiral, or rod-shaped.	6. Are classified by part of body affected as respiratory, neurological, intestinal, or skin.

Coccal

Spiral

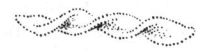

Rod-shaped

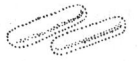

7. May produce spores.
8. Produce toxins.
9. May have "flagella" for locomotion.

7. Do *not* produce spores.
8. Do *not* produce toxins.
9. Do *not* have "flagella."

Flagellated

The greater the quantity of bacteria and viruses, the more difficult they are to destroy, and the longer must the sterilization time be. Also, unprotected microorganisms are easier to kill than those protected by the body excreta.

The "barrier technique" must be employed to protect patients and health workers from becoming victims of microorganism transmission. This technique consists of observation and prevention of any possible transmission of microorganisms.

Pathogenic microorganisms are opportunists that are always present in the environment, looking for a host. With a host and suitable conditions, infection develops. The manner in which organisms are transmitted are as follows:

1. They enter the body via the:

   —gastrointestinal tract.

   —respiratory tract.

   —open wounds of skin.

   —open wounds of mucous membrane.

   —urinary tract.

2. They leave the body via the

   —gastrointestinal tract

   —respiratory tract

   —open wounds

   —blood

3. They are transferred to a body via

   —a *vector* (carrier), which may be human, animal or insect

   —*direct contact* through a person or contaminated instruments or equipment

   —*fomites* (anything which absorbs and transmits microorganisms, such as food, clothing, excreta)

   —*air* such as in forced-air ventilation (filters may be a source of microorganism spread)

In *medical asepsis* (practices which keep microorganisms within a given area) and *surgical asepsis* (practices which keep an area free from microorganisms), suitable disinfectants and antiseptics must be used. Zephiran chloride or Ceepryn chloride are commonly used as antiseptics or surface-active germicides. Disinfectants frequently used are *mercurials*, such as bichloride and cyanide; *phenolics* such as Staphene, Tergisyl, Ves-phene, Amphyl, and O-syl; *chloride compounds*, intended for use on floors; *iodine* and *iodophors* which are bactericidal, tuberculocidal, virucidal and fungicidal; *alcohols*, which are antiseptic as well as germicidal; and *formaldehyde*, an excellent disinfectant which also kills spores. Hexachlorophene preparations were used in the past with success; however, recent research studies have pointed to some serious brain complications in rats subjected to high dosage and prolonged usage. The hexachlorophene preparations are now used in limited, carefully supervised instances.

The following criteria should be considered in choosing a disinfectant:

1. It should kill the pathogen within a reasonable time.

2. It should not be readily neutralized by proteins, soaps, or detergents.

3. It should not be harmful to the material or surface on which it is used.

4. It should not be harmful to human skin.

5. It should be stable in solution.

ASEPTIC TECHNIQUE

Sterilization may be done by one of several methods: 1) steam under pressure (autoclave); 2) dry heat; 3) boiling; 4) the use of chemicals; and 5) gas (such as ethylene oxide).

When handling sterile packages, instruments, solutions, or equipment, care must be exercised to check that the sterilization process was complete. This may be done by timing (clock records) or the inclusion of chemically treated strips of paper that change color when fully sterilized.

Four rules of asepsis are important. They are:

1. Know what is sterile;
2. Know what is *not* sterile;
3. Separate sterile from unsterile;
4. Remedy contamination *immediately.*

Know what is sterile. Sterile supplies and equipment may be purchased prepackaged or they may be cleaned, packaged, wrapped, labeled, sterilized, and stored by the individual health agency. Equipment, instruments, linen, and other items are sterilized according to the accepted procedure of each health agency. Models of sterilizers vary, but the principles remain the same. Sterile items are designated by coding used in each agency (such as color-coded tapes). Simplicity should characterize the procedures and activities used in carrying out aseptic technique. Standardized equipment and supplies must be used to avoid waste and spoilage caused by lack of familiarity with new articles. There are three types of drapes and wrappers in use today:

1. Cloth or linen (must be used in double thickness).
2. Disposable paper (usually single thickness is sufficient).
3. Disposable polyethylene drapes (used in single thickness).

Know what is not sterile. People cannot be sterilized; nor can certain equipment and furniture. These must therefore be covered with sterile drapes (or clothing) when being used as a "sterile field." A sterile field is a work surface area prepared with sterile drapes to hold sterile instruments and linens during a surgical procedure.

Keep sterile and nonsterile objects apart to avoid contamination. Sterile and nonsterile items must be stored separately. Since it is impossible to determine with the naked eye what is sterile or not sterile, one must rely on the indicators of sterility: packaging, color coding, and labeling. If sterile and nonsterile items are separated, there is less danger of using an unsterile object when a sterile object is required.

Remedy contamination immediately. Contamination is the act of introducing microorganisms to a sterile object. It can be done accidentally by touching a sterile object with an unsterile one, or by accidentally dropping a sterile item on the floor. Contamination can be remedied by:

1. Removing the contaminated object from the sterile field at once;
2. Covering the contaminated area with extra sterile towels or with drapes;
3. Replacing the "setup" for the sterile field. (Setup refers to the particular pieces of equipment and supplies needed for a specific procedure, e.g., dressing tray for a dressing change.) After a sterile setup is prepared, it must not be left unattended and exposed to the risk of accidental contamination.

Follow these simple principles of sterile technique:

1. If in doubt about the sterility of anything, consider that it is *not* sterile.
2. "Sterile persons" should not lean against an unsterile area. (Sterile persons are those who have gone through the surgical or obstetric scrub procedure and are wearing a cap and mask, sterile gown and gloves.)
3. Do not allow a nonsterile person to reach above or across a sterile field.

4. The sterile zone *ends at the level of the table*, or at waist height. Any item that falls below this level or touches anything below table level or waist level is considered contaminated. This includes the sterile gown, drapes, and other objects.

5. Gowns are considered sterile only from the waist to the shoulder level in front, including the sleeves. The back and the fabric below the waist are considered unsterile.

6. The edges of anything that encloses sterile contents are not sterile. This includes edges of wrappers on sterile packages, caps on solutions, test-tube covers, etc. They must never be touched by the person who is wearing sterile gloves. They can only be handled by the unsterile person.

7. Sterile persons must keep well within the sterile area.

8. A sterile person stands back at a safe distance while the patient is being draped.

9. Persons dressed in sterile gown and gloves must pass each other "back-to-back" (unsterile to unsterile).

10. A sterile person turns his back to a nonsterile person or area when passing, i.e., a sterile person *faces* a sterile area when passing.

11. A sterile person asks a nonsterile person to step aside, instead of trying to crowd past.

12. A sterile person does not wander around the room but remains close to the sterile zone.

13. A sterile person touches only what is sterile.

14. Keep sterile materials dry. Moisture permits contamination by allowing microorganisms from an unsterile surface to seep through the linen.

15. Sterile packages are stored in dry areas. If they become damp, they must be resterilized or discarded.

16. Wet ampules from a bactericidal solution to be used in a sterile area are placed on a dry sterile towel which absorbs moisture, or in a metal basin. Discard towel if it becomes soaked.

17. If a solution soaks through a sterile field to a nonsterile one, the wet area may be covered with another sterile drape, or discarded and redraped.

18. Hands that are wearing sterile gloves should be kept in sight or above waist level. Remember: anything below waist level is considered unsterile.

19. Be constantly aware of the need for clean surroundings. This is a mandate of nursing care to which every patient has a right.

20. Take floor cultures periodically to determine success of cleaning methods.

21. Air-conditioning units may be a source of bacteria. Filters should be changed frequently. Cultures of the air should be taken at prescribed intervals (i.e., one month to three months).

22. Mops and dust cloths must be washed and sterilized daily (usually by members of the housekeeping staff).

23. All flat surfaces and furniture must be washed frequently (i.e., between cases) with a germicide.

ASEPTIC TECHNIQUE

ITEM 1: SURGICAL SCRUB

The surgical scrub is an extension of the medical asepsis handwashing technique. It precedes the donning of the sterile gown and sterile gloves.

Important Steps	Key Points

1. Select the following to correspond with your body size:
  a. Scrub dress or suit
  b. Turban or surgical cap
  c. Conductive shoes (or covers)
	At the beginning of the tour of duty, street clothes are exchanged for a scrub uniform, hair covering, and conductive shoes in the dressing room. Remove your street clothes and place them on hangers in the space provided in your locker or closet. Use a clean scrub dress or surgical suit each day, or whenever it becomes soiled during the day.

2. Remove all jewelry.	Jewelry harbors bacteria that cannot be removed by surgical scrub and thus becomes a safety hazard. *Note:* Pin jewelry to undergarments. If items are pinned to the scrub uniform, you may forget them at the end of the day and discard them with the soiled uniform in the laundry. Male personnel usually conceal rings and wallets in the top of one of their socks.
3. Put on scrub attire.	

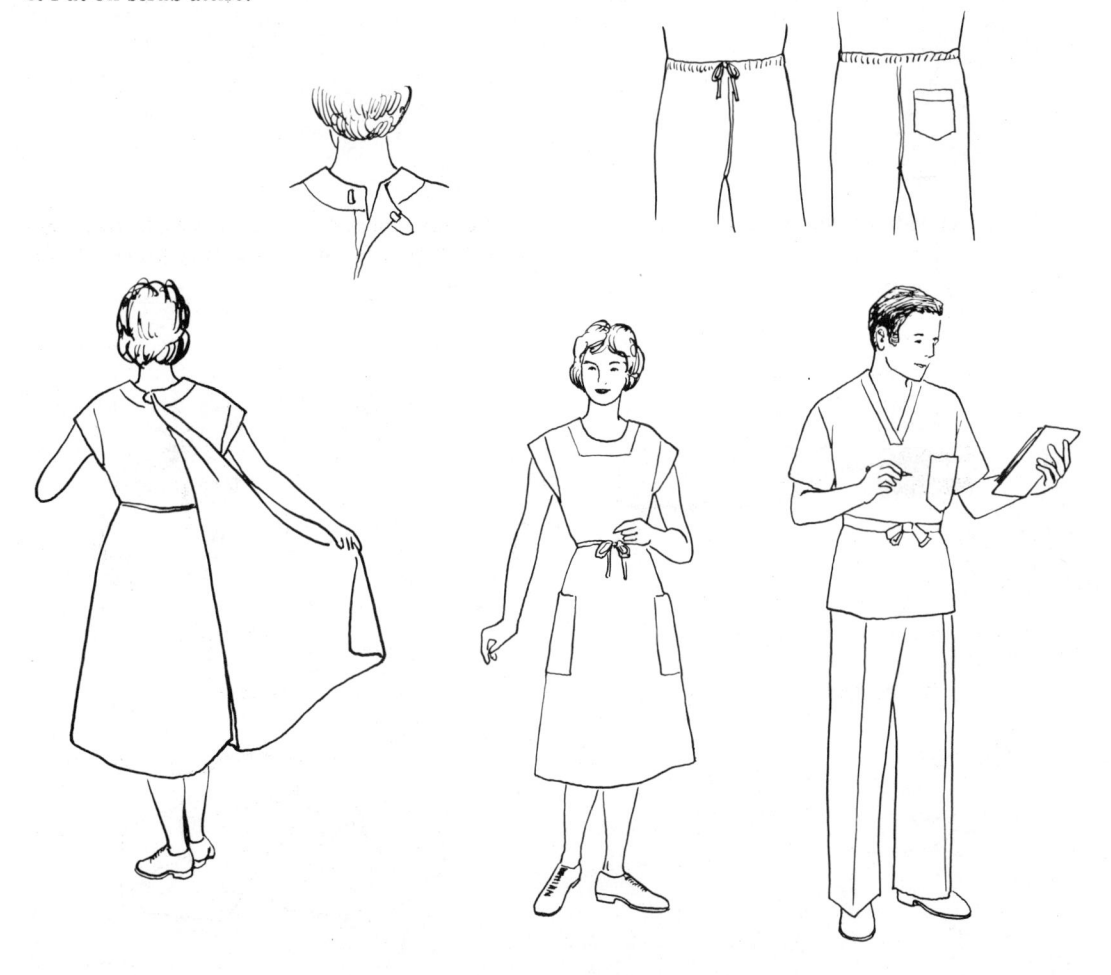

ASEPTIC TECHNIQUE

Important Steps	Key Points
4. Place turban on head.	Cover hair completely to prevent contamination and static electricity sparks. Tie securely so that hair does not fall and contaminate the working area.
5. Put on conductive shoes or shoe covering.	These are special shoes, of which there are several types; follow your agency procedure for putting them on.

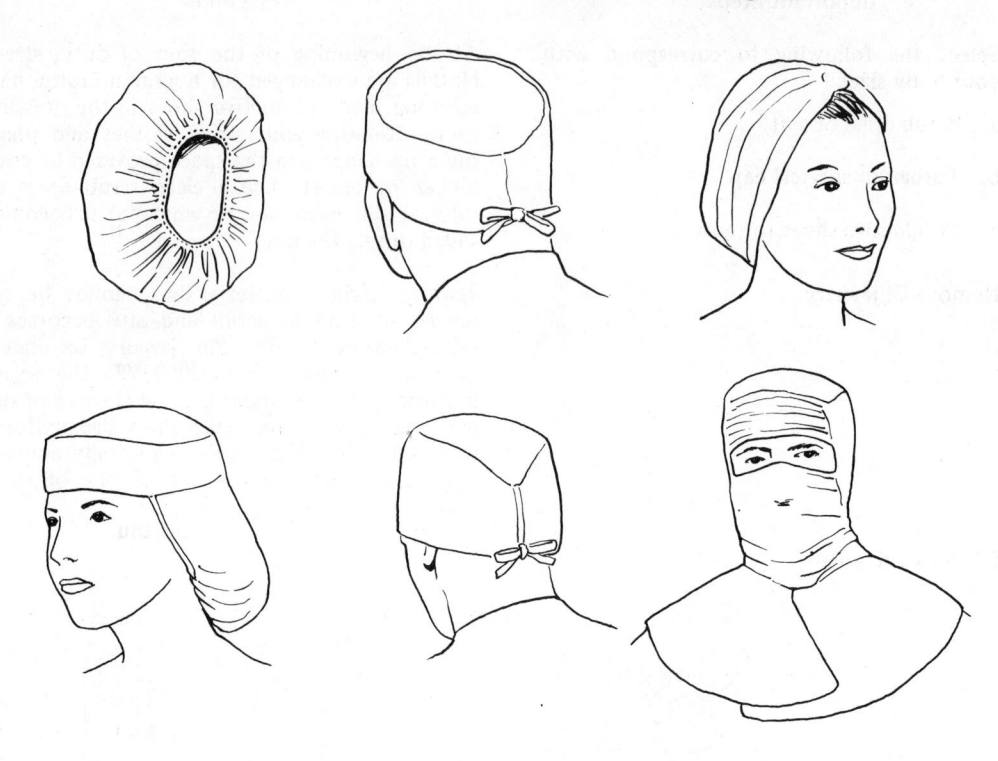

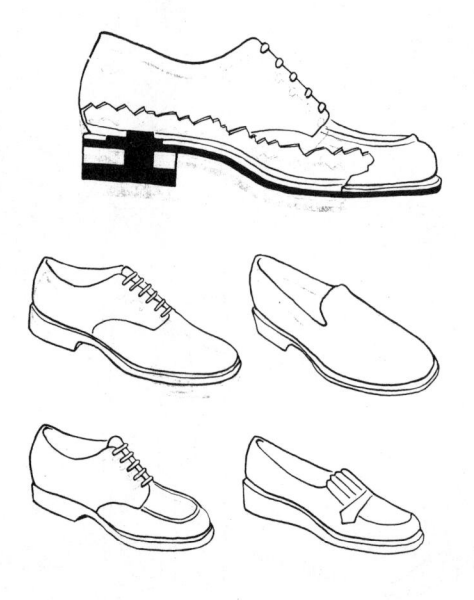

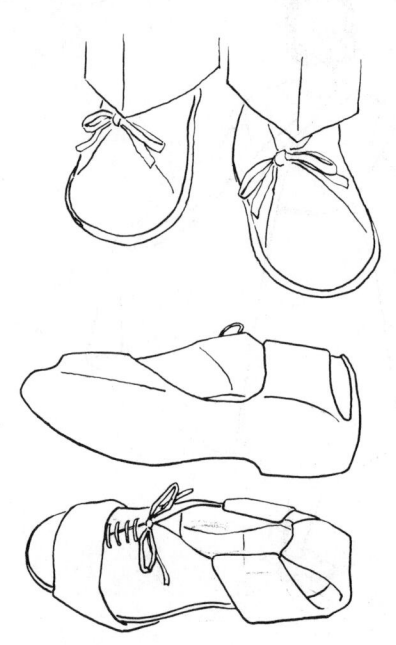

ASEPTIC TECHNIQUE

Important Steps	Key Points
6. Test for conductivity.	You will test the conductivity of the shoes by stepping on a test meter. If the needle on the meter moves to the *green* (safe) area or the green light flashes, your shoes are *conductive*, and you may proceed with the scrubbing procedure. If the needle on the meter moves to the *red* (unsafe) area, your shoes are *not conductive*, and you should report immediately to the charge nurse. You may be reassigned or given another pair of conductive shoes, which will then need to be tested for conductivity.
7. Put on a mask.	Cover both your nose and mouth. Tie snugly.

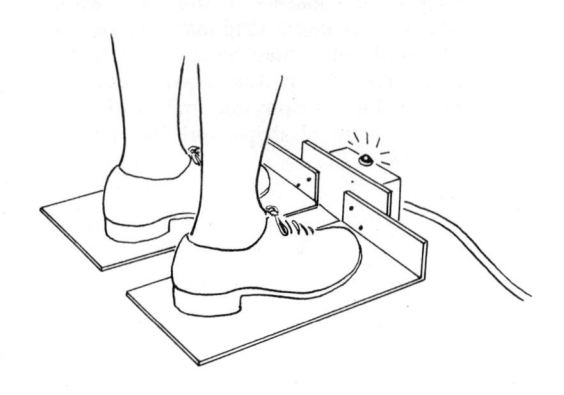

    a. Handle mask by its ties.

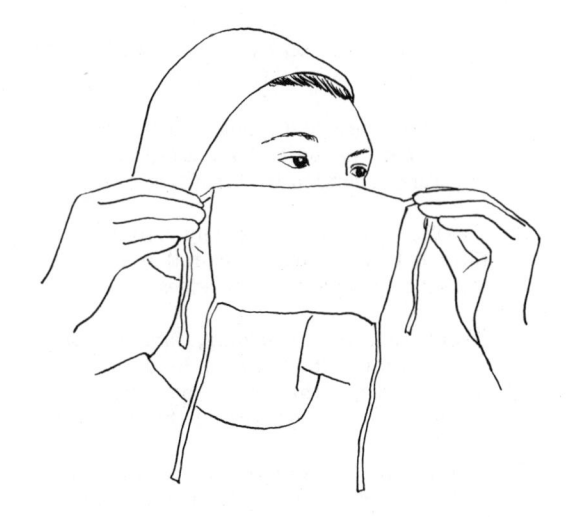

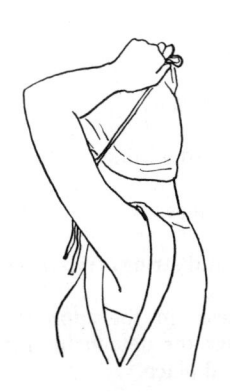

    b. Tie the uppermost strings over the top of your head.

ASEPTIC TECHNIQUE

Important Steps   **Key Points**

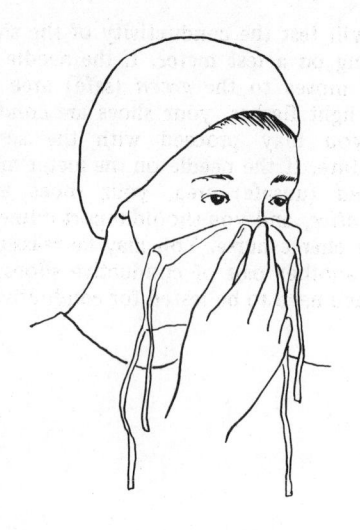

c. Mold the metal strip over the bridge of your nose. This strip provides a firm fit over the nose bridge and prevents fogging of eye-glasses if they are worn. NOTE: The metal strip may be a part of the mask, or it may be an insert that is removable when the mask has been used. Many disposable masks do not have the metal strips, but the mask is molded to fit.

d. Tie the lower strings at the nape of the neck.

Remember!

1. The mask is put on by all personnel *before* beginning the surgical scrub.

2. Both your nose and mouth must be covered to prevent bacteria from escaping in the moisture generated by breathing or talking.

3. Tie the mask strings snugly. Air must be filtered through the mask rather than permitted to escape from the edges.

4. Avoid sneezing, coughing, and excessive conversation, all of which load the mask with bacteria that may be forced out through the material with further breathing.

5. Change the mask between cases. A moist mask acts as a "wick" for bacteria to pass through; moistness also lessens the effectiveness of disposable masks. (Some new types of masks are being developed that absorb moisture.)

To remove the mask:

1. Untie the lower strings.

2. Hold the mask at the bridge of the nose.

3. Untie the top strings.

4. Pull the mask and strings free of your face.

5. Discard the mask in the appropriate container, and place the detachable metal strip in the designated place.

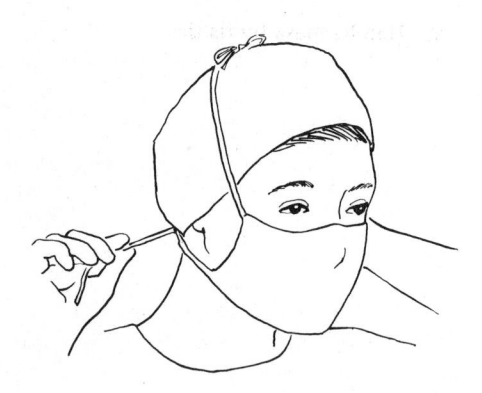

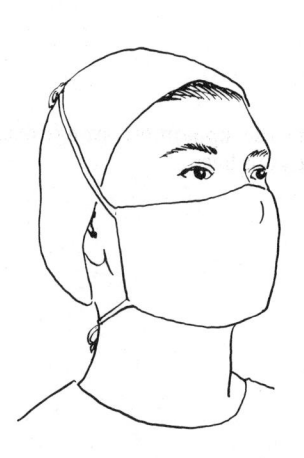

ASEPTIC TECHNIQUE

Important Steps	Key Points
8. Prepare for the scrub.	Roll the sleeves of the surgical attire approximately 4 inches above your elbows, and approach the sink. This prevents the sleeves from becoming wet. Adjust the water to a comfortable temperature, and let it run during the entire procedure. Neither the faucet handles nor any other object can be touched after beginning the surgical scrub.
9. Wet your hands and apply the detergent.	Spread an amount of surgical soap about the size of a quarter over the hands. Add enough water to make a lather. Wash to about 3 inches above the elbows, following the handwashing procedure you learned in Handwashing Technique for Medical Asepsis.
10. Rinse your forearms and hands under the running water.	Remember to run the water from the clean fingertips to the elbows. Hold your hands up and away from your face and uniform. (This is the opposite direction from the one you learned in the Handwashing for Medical Asepsis.) Run water from the clean to the unclean area.
11. Clean the fingernails.	The hands are now moist and the sediment under the nails can generally be removed with ease. Fingernails are cleaned at the beginning of the tour of duty and whenever necessary during the remainder of the tour. Use an orange stick or fingernail file (usually kept in a container on the scrub sink).

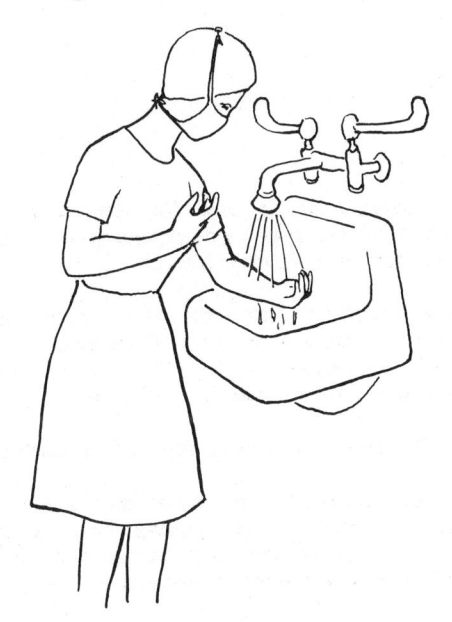

ASEPTIC TECHNIQUE

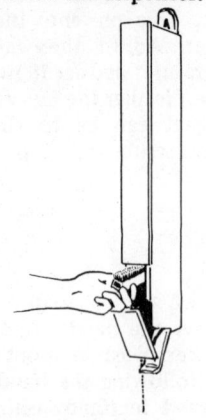

Important Steps	Key Points
12. Take the disposable sponge pad or sterile brush from the dispenser.	The dispenser is arranged to permit removal of brush or pad without gross contamination.
13. Apply the soap (detergent) to the brush or pad.	Add enough water to make a good lather. (*Note:* some disposable pads have detergent impregnated in them.) Scrub with *firm rotary motions*.
14. Scrub your hands and arms. Follow the same system as in Handwashing for Medical Asepsis, except that you use a brush or pad.	The actual time needed for the scrub will depend on the type of detergent used and the frequency with which you scrub. Daily scrubbing: first scrub of day *5 minutes*; successive scrubs *2 minutes*. Occasional scrubbing: first scrub of day *10 minutes*; then successive scrubs *5 minutes* on that day.
15. Rinse your hands and discard the brush in basin provided.	Rinsing floats away suds and surface bacteria. NOTE: Scrubbing time is measured by actual time in brushing, not rinsing time. (Some hospitals measure this time by the number of strokes. Follow agency procedures.)

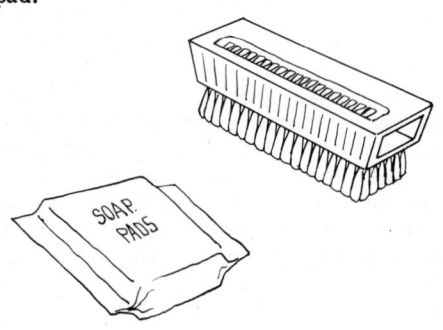

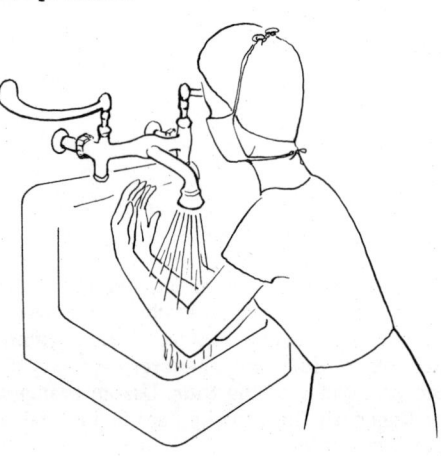

ASEPTIC TECHNIQUE

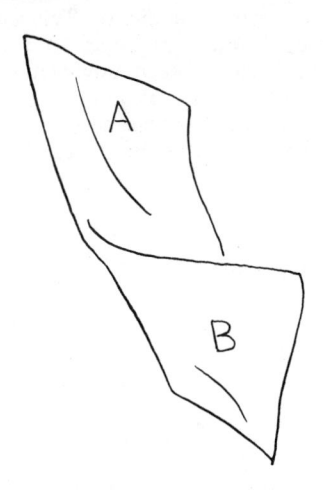

Important Steps	Key Points
16. Pick up a sterile towel and dry your hands and arms.	Open the towel full-length and take care that it does not touch your nonsterile scrub dress (suit) while you are unfolding it. Hold the towel out in front of you, waist-high.
17. Dry both hands.	Dry one arm with an end of the towel; use the other end of the towel for the other arm. (Electric dryer may be provided.) See that water does not drip onto a sterile area.

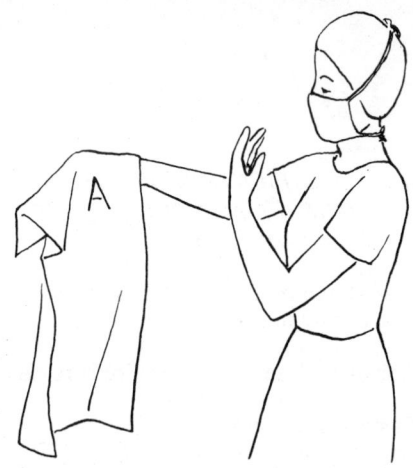

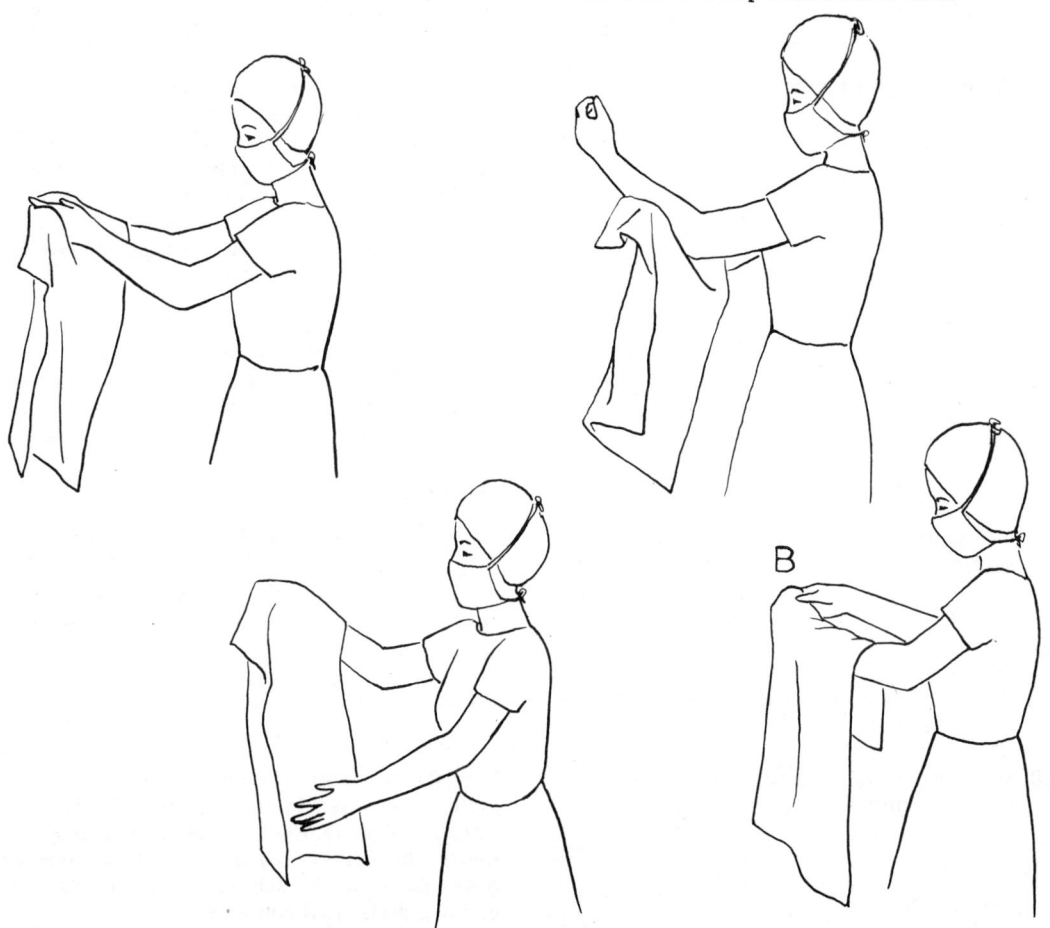

ASEPTIC TECHNIQUE

Modification of Surgical Scrub

1. Short scrub—3 minute scrub.

    This scrub follows a clean case if hands have not contaiminated. Be careful that your hands or arms do not touch the unsterile gown. Develop a surgical conscience. This short scrub may be used when preparing to carry out a sterile procedure or when moving directly from one sterile case to another, e.g., dressing change, spinal tap, thoracentesis, and the like. Follow Steps 1 through 10 of the previous procedure.

ITEM 2: MODIFICATION OF SURGICAL SCRUB FOR CARE OF THE MOTHER AND CHILD (SOMETIMES CALLED THE OB OR OBSTETRIC SCRUB.)

1. Remove your street clothes and place them on a hanger in the space provided.

2. Obtain a clean scrub dress or surgical suit.

3. Remove all jewelry.

    In some hospitals a plain wedding band is allowed.

4. Put on the scrub dress or suit.

5. Cover your hair with a turban or cap.

    Do not allow any hair to slip out lest debris drop from it and contaminate the working area. Tie the turban (cap) securely in place.

6. Put on a mask (if indicated).

    A mask is worn in the delivery room, where sterile technique is always required. It is usually not required in the nursery unless the worker has a cold. (Some hospitals do not allow a worker who has a cold to enter a nursery even with a mask.) If a mask is required, cover both your nose and mouth. Tie it snugly in place (as in the previous procedure).

7. Prepare for the scrub.

    Roll your sleeves about 4 inches above the elbows; adjust the water to a comfortable temperature, and let it run during the entire scrub. Faucet handles and other objects around the scrub sink may not be touched during the scrub. They are considered unclean or contaminated.

8. Wet your hands and spread liquid soap or detergent.

    The soap or detergent has a germicidal action. It may leave thin film on the skin and continues to inhibit bacteria growth even after the wash. Use the washing preparation designated by your agency.

9. Take a sterile brush or sponge pad from the sterile dispenser.

    Add a few drops of soap to the brush.

10. Scrub your nails; then scrub each hand for a half minute.

    Use strong friction-action. Follow the same system described in Handwashing for Medical Asepsis. This removes bacteria that may be under the nails or clinging to the cuticle or other parts of the skin. Discard the brush or pad in a designated container.

ASEPTIC TECHNIQUE

11. Take a nail file (or orange stick) and clean the nails.

    Discard the file in the designated container after cleaning your nails.

12. Rinse your hands.

    Rinse well, allowing the water to drain *from the fingertips to the elbows.* Marginal water will drip off your elbows and not contaminate your hands.

13. Take a second brush (sponge pad) from the sterile dispenser.

    Do not touch anything else; touching an unsterile object means that you must start the scrub all over again.

14. Scrub your nails and hands again with the brush, a half-minute for each hand.

    Most of the remaining bacteria will be removed by this second scrub.

15. Rinse your hands finally.

    Discard the brush in the basin provided.

16. Pick up a sterile towel and dry your hands and arms, following the same procedure as in Item 1, Steps 16 and 17.

ITEM 3: SELF-GOWNING TECHNIQUE

Before you scrubbed, you or your assistant opened the sterile gown package to make it easy to take out the gown without contamination after scrubbing. The sterile gown may be made of specially prepared disposable paper or linen; use whichever is available at your agency.

Important Steps	Key Points

1. Dry your hands and arms.

   Drying your hands and arms thoroughly is mandatory so that dampening of your gown sleeves does not occur. The damp gown sleeves would allow microorganisms from the skin to move through the gown (wick effect), thereby contaminating your gown.

2. Discard the towel in a designated container.

3. Pick up a sterile gown.

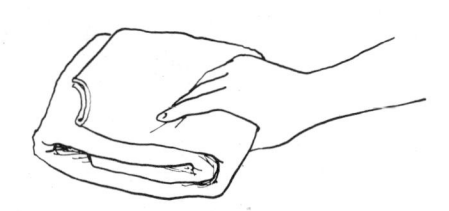

   Stand at least 12 inches from the sterile package. Take hold of the gown by the folded edge. Grasp it securely at both top and bottom. Lift it directly upward off the wrapper to avoid touching the wrapper to the edges of the gown. If you are dressing from a linen pack that has other sterile items, be sure not to touch any other article or object with your ungloved hand. If you do touch another item, the gown must be discarded and replaced.

4. Step back away from the sterile pack.

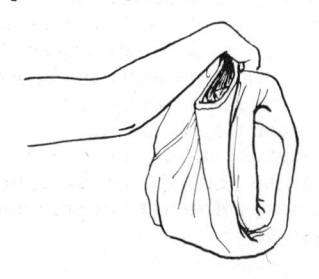

   This will permit a margin of safety for you so that you can unfold the gown safely without contaminating it. If the gown is held below the waist, discard it and take another. Remember, in a sterile field, items below the waistline are considered contaminated.

Important Steps	Key Points
5. Grasp the folded gown at its neckband.	Holding the gown at arm's length in front of you, let it unfold downward (gowns are usually folded inside out in thirds or fourths for easy storage). The *inside* of the gown front will be toward you. (The gown is full-length so that it covers your scrub dress or suit.)
6. Hold the open gown by the shoulder seams.	Gently shake it downward so that it opens freely. Be careful not to touch any objects with the gown during this activity. If you touch something or somebody, the gown must be discarded and you must take another.
7. Slip your arms into the armholes. Remain still.	Hold your hands upward near shoulder height while slipping your arms into the gown. *Another worker (unsterile)* will stand behind you and reach with both hands inside the one armhole, grasping at the lower and upper seams and pulling the sleeve gently, firmly, up and over your hand (open method). The closed method consists of pulling the sleeves up on the hand so that the fingertips are just visible. The *unsterile worker* will repeat this procedure with the other sleeve.

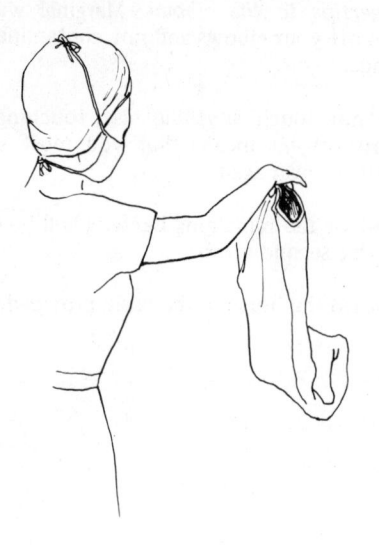

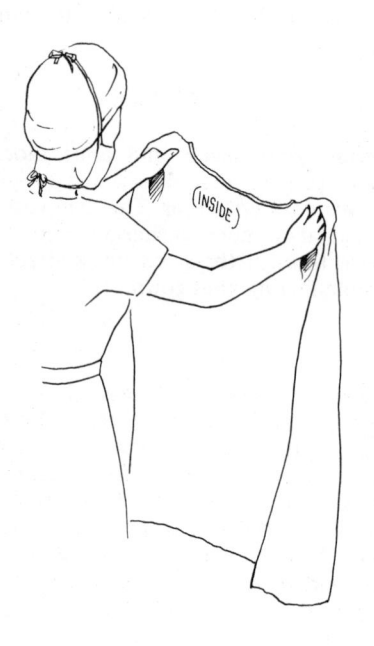

ASEPTIC TECHNIQUE 21

Important Steps	Key Points
8. Pull the gown over the shoulders.	The *unsterile worker* adjusts the gown on your shoulders—always working from the *inside* of the gown.
9. Fasten the neckline of the gown.	The *unsterile worker* secures the gown at the back of the neckline with ties or fasteners.

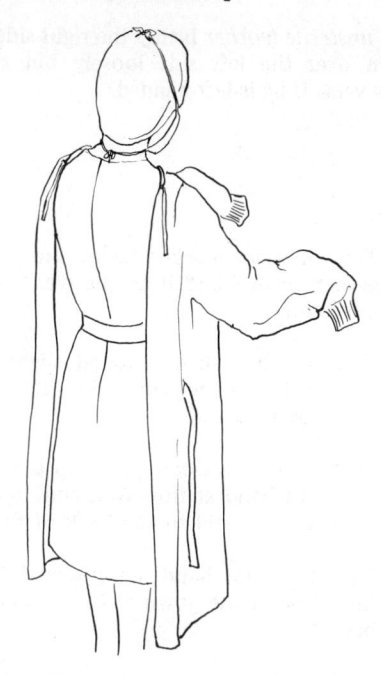

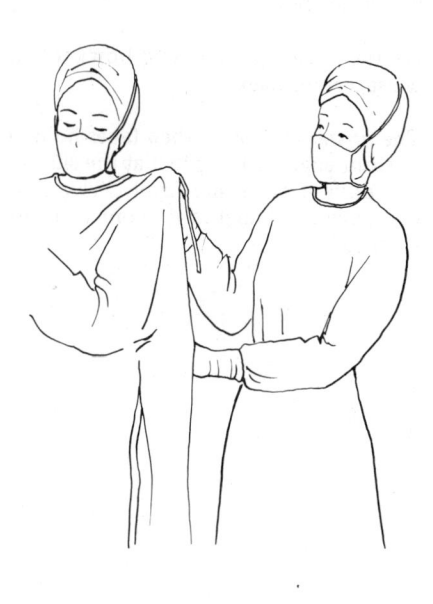

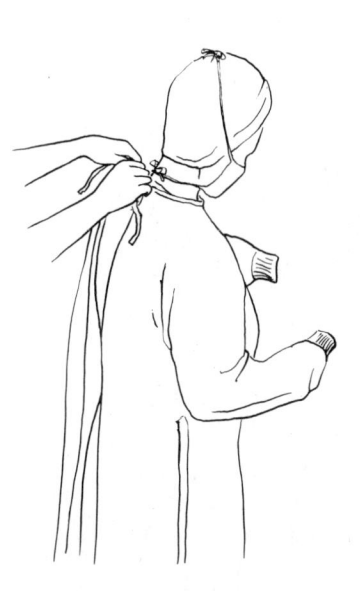

ASEPTIC TECHNIQUE

Important Steps	Key Points
10. Draw the edges of the gown together.	The *unsterile worker* brings the right side of the gown over the left side loosely but securely (vice versa if he is left-handed).
11. Fasten the waist-ties.	a. The *unsterile worker* keeps the gown together by holding it at the waist with his left hand. b. You will be asked to bend slightly from your waist to the right front. This permits the waist tie to fall free. c. The *unsterile worker* picks up the tie with the right hand at the distal end, and draws it up and around to the back of the gown. d. With the right hand, he grasps the tie and the back of the gown at the middle of the back. e. You are then to again bend slightly at the waist to let the tie fall free. The *unsterile worker* draws the left tip up and around to the center of the back. f. With his left hand he picks up the left tie at the distal end. g. He ties a secure and snug bowknot at the waist, center back. h. The *unsterile worker* then takes hold of the bottom edge of the gown at the side seams, and pulls straight and firmly. This smooths the gown and makes it more comfortable for you.

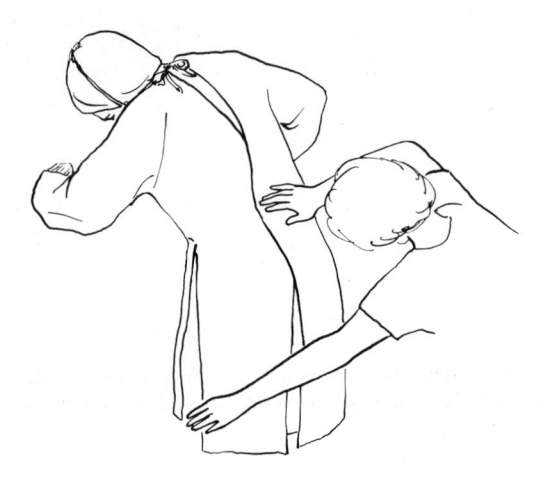

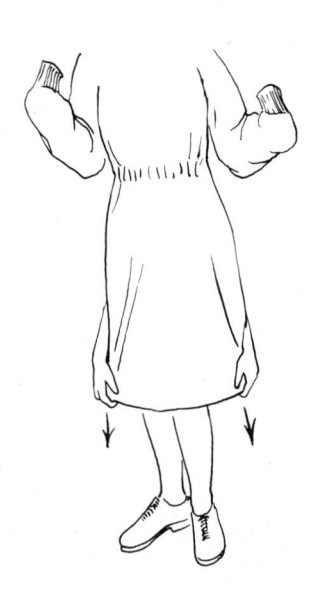

ASEPTIC TECHNIQUE

Some disposable gowns are now made so that one entire back panel overlaps the other back panel. This permits the sterile person to have a sterile back as well as a sterile front. These gowns have the belt ties attached either on the sides or on the front of the gown so that the sterile person can tie the waist belt in the front of the gown, thereby keeping the back portion of the gown sterile.

ITEM 4: SELF-GLOVING (CLOSED TECHNIQUE)

The glove wrapper will be opened before you scrub, and the gloves placed on the packet. After drying your hands as in Item 3, put on your gown. However, put your hands and arms into the sleeve only so far that the fingertips barely reach the distal edge of the ribbed cuffs. The closed method is the preferred method of gloving for several reasons: 1) it greatly reduces the possibility of contamination during gloving because the bare hands are covered by the gown sleeves; 2) it saves time; and 3) it decreases strain on gloves so that you do not have to pull strenuously to get the gloves on your bare hands.

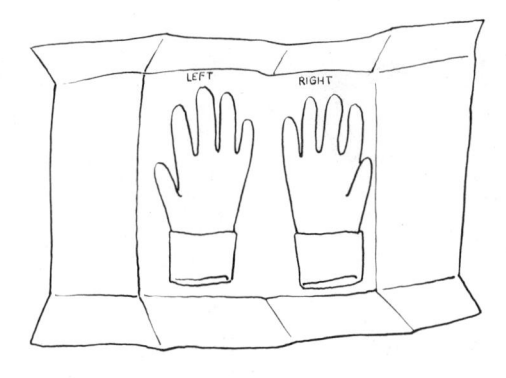

Important steps	Key Points
1. Approach the glove packet.	Make sure your hands are well-covered by the ribbed cuffs of the gown.
2. Pick up the right glove with your gown-covered left hand.	Reverse hand positions if you are left-handed.

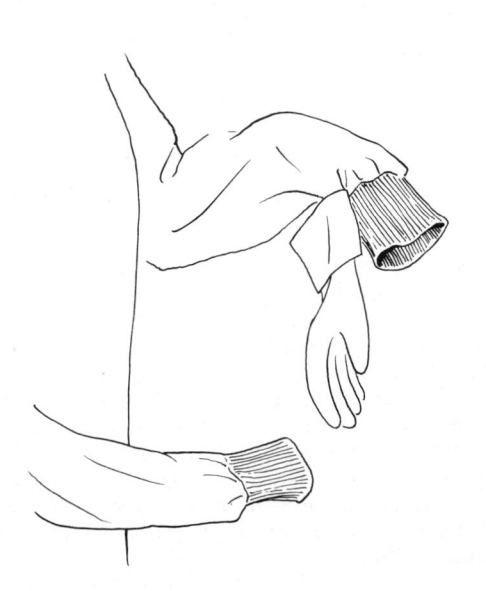

Important Steps	Key Points
3. Place the palm of the right glove against the palm of your right hand (palm to palm).	The open edge of the right glove will be parellel at the right fingertips. Therefore the glove fingers are pointing toward your elbow; the glove cuff lies directly over the ribbed cuff of the gown; and the thumb of the glove is directly over your right thumb.
4. Close the gown-covered fingers of your right hand over the glove cuff edge that is directly over the gown cuff.	Be sure that your fingers and thumbs are aligned to match the glove.
5. With your covered left hand, grasp the top edge of the glove cuff.	Draw the cuff forward over the end of your right sleeve and continue pulling up over the posterior gown cuff while holding the cuff securely. Cover the posterior ribbing completely with the glove. As you draw the glove over the ribbing, straighten and slightly spread your fingers in order to get into the glove more easily. Pull the glove completely over the ribbing by moving your left hand medially to the anterior of the glove. Now the glove covers the right ribbed cuff, and your left hand is still inside the left gown sleeve.
6. Grasp the proximal edge of the glove and ribbed cuff.	With your left gowned hand, firmly hold the glove and the gown cuff.
7. Pull the sleeve and glove on your hand simultaneously.	Still grasping securely as above, adjust the fingers of the right glove using your gown-covered left hand. Be sure that the right glove completely covers the ribbed cuff on your gown. You will need to stretch the cuffs of the glove to do this, but if you pull too vigorously, you may tear a hole in the glove. (If that happens, have the glove removed and start over again at Step 2.)

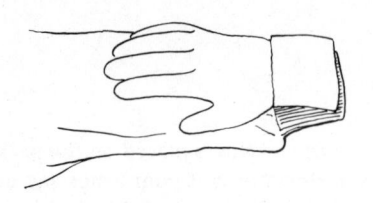

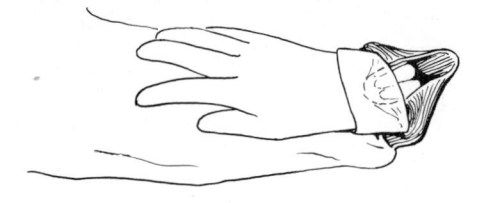

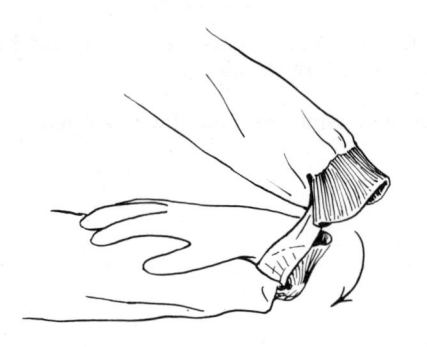

ASEPTIC TECHNIQUE

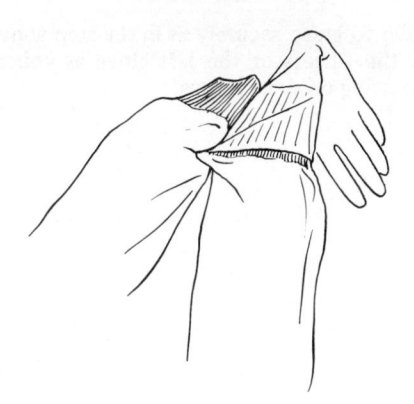

Important Steps   **Key Points**

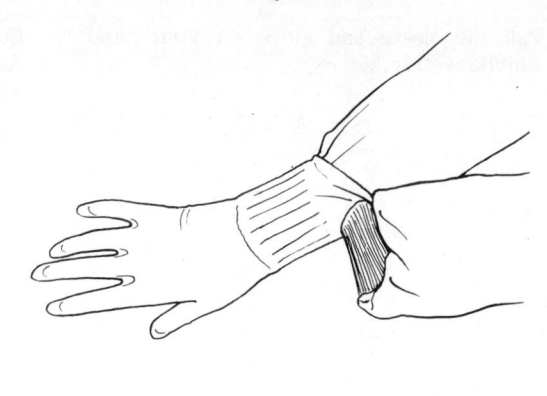

8. Pick up the left glove with your gloved right hand.

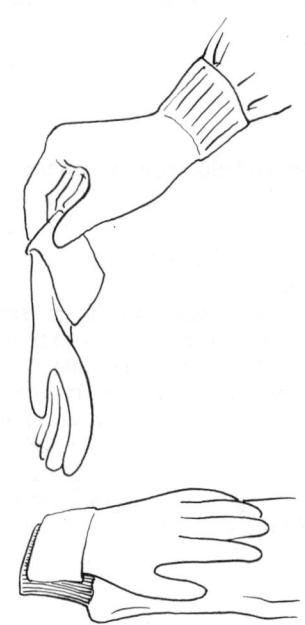

    Place the palm of the left glove against the palm of your left hand (thumbs will be directly above one another). The glove cuff lies directly over the cuff of the gown. Remember! The open edge of the glove is parallel to the fingertips, with glove fingers pointing toward your elbow.

9. Close the left gown-covered fingers over the edge of the glove cuff.

    Hold the glove securely.

10. Grasp the back side of the glove cuff.

    With your gloved right hand, draw the left cuff forward and over the edge of the sleeve and continue pulling it back up over your posterior gown cuff. Cover the cuff ribbing *completely* with the glove. As you draw the glove up over the ribbing, straighten and slightly spread your fingers apart to get into the glove more easily. Arrange the right glove around the sleeve so that the entire glove cuff is covering the entire gown cuff.

11. Grasp the proximal edge of the left glove and ribbed cuff.

ASEPTIC TECHNIQUE

Important Steps	Key Points
12. Pull the sleeve and glove on your hand simultaneously.	Continue to grasp securely as in the step above. Adjust the fingers of the left glove as you do when putting on dress gloves.
13. Keep your hands held upward above your waist.	Do not touch your face or any other unsterile object.

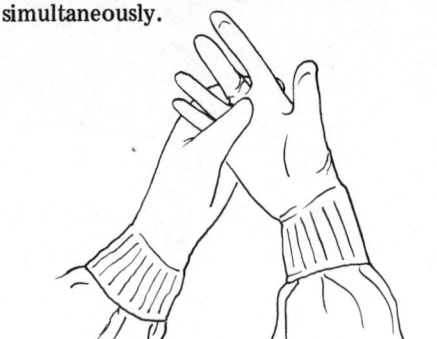

ITEM 5: SELF-GLOVING (OPEN TECHNIQUE)

The glove wrapper must be unwrapped before you scrub, and gloves placed on top of the glove packet. Put on your sterile gloves after you have gowned.

Important Steps	Key Points
1. Pick up the right-hand glove with your left hand.	Take the cuff edge, lift it up and off the wrapper, being careful to avoid touching an unsterile object. Since the folded cuff of the glove will be against the skin, it is contaminated as soon as it is touched. Be sure not to touch the *outside* of the glove with your ungloved hand. NOTE: Most gloves are now prepowdered for ease in donning. Additional powder is usually unnecessary.
2. Pull on the right glove.	Keep the fingers of your left hand extended and slightly apart while you pull the glove up on the hand with the cuff. Use the same motion as when you don dress gloves. Keep the cuff of the glove folded back on itself.

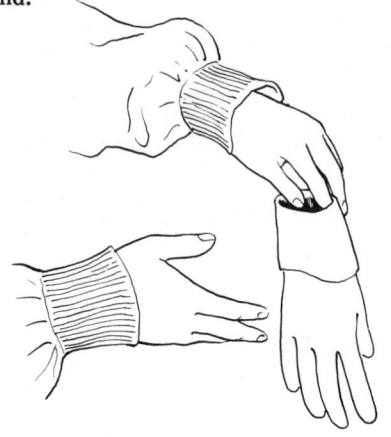

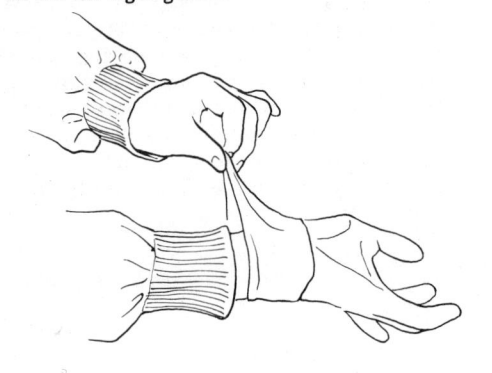

ASEPTIC TECHNIQUE

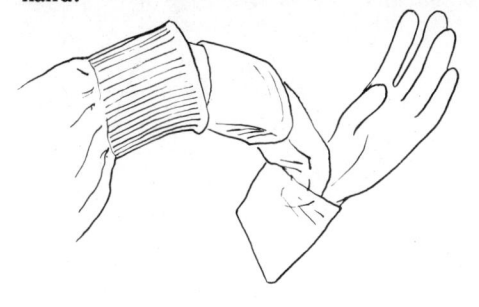

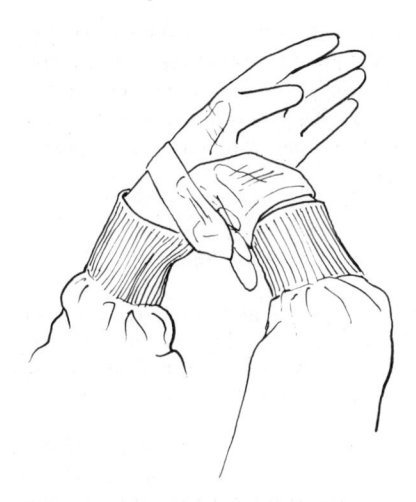

Important Steps	Key Points
3. Pick up the left glove with your right gloved hand.	This time, since you have a sterile glove on, pick up the other glove by placing the right sterile fingers *under* the cuff of the left sterile glove. Be sure that the fingers and thumb of your gloved hand do not inadvertently touch your skin. (Reverse hand positions in Steps 1 through 3 if you are left-handed.)
4. Pull the left glove on with your right hand.	Do not touch the outside of the glove with your bare hand. Keep your fingers straight and slightly apart while pulling the glove on. Continue pulling firmly and steadily. (Sometimes it is easier if you rest your thumb at the cuff of your gown.)
5. Continue pulling the left glove cuff up over the ribbed cuff of your gown.	The glove is now securely on your left hand. NOTE: If you touched your skin with the right sterile glove as you were pulling the left cuff over the gown cuff, discard and start with a new sterile glove package.
6. Pull the right glove up over the ribbed cuff of your gown.	Now that the left glove is in place, reach under the anterior cuff of the right glove with your gloved left hand. Rotate your right hand medially, pulling out and upward over the left ribbed cuff of the gown. To make sure you get the glove up over the ribbing, it is sometimes helpful to rest the right thumb at the top of the ribbing to serve as an anchor. Again be careful not to touch the skin with your sterile gloves.
7. Adjust the fingers of the gloves as necessary.	If your fingers were not held straight while the glove was being put on, and one or more fingers did not penetrate deep into the fingers of the glove, pull the glove fingers out with the opposite hand to straighten or knead them as you would dress gloves.

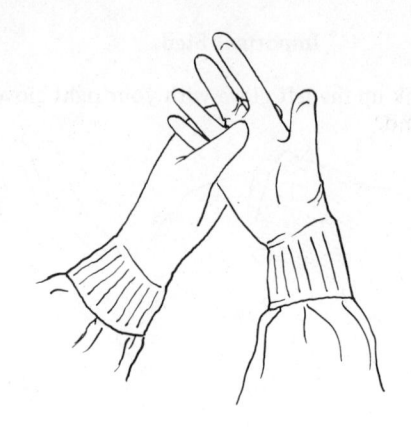

ITEM 6: GOWNING AND GLOVING TECHNIQUE FOR SOMEONE ELSE

In a sterile field, it may be your responsibility to gown and glove someone else (e.g., a physician) after you have put on your own sterile gown and gloves. In this case you are now sterile and must take special precautions against contaminating yourself. Remember to stand away from objects and others while you are gowning and gloving yourself and others. Avoid touching the outside of sterile wrappers. Again, all the sterile packs (linen, gowns, gloves, etc.) are opened before you start your scrubbing procedure.

Important Steps	Key Points
1. Pick up a sterile towel and hand it to the gownee.	Unfold the towel and lay it on the gownee's right palm. He will dry his arms in the same manner as in Steps 1, 2, and 3 of the previous procedure.
2. Begin with Step 5 of the previous procedure.	Grasp the gown at its neckband. Hold it at arm's length in front of you at shoulder height and let it unfold downward. Hold the gown by the shoulder seams so that the *outside* of the gown front is toward you.
3. Protect your gloved hands.	Do this by placing your hands under the back panel of the gown at the top shoulder seam, making a cuff to protect your gloves. The interior armholes will be facing the person you are gowning.

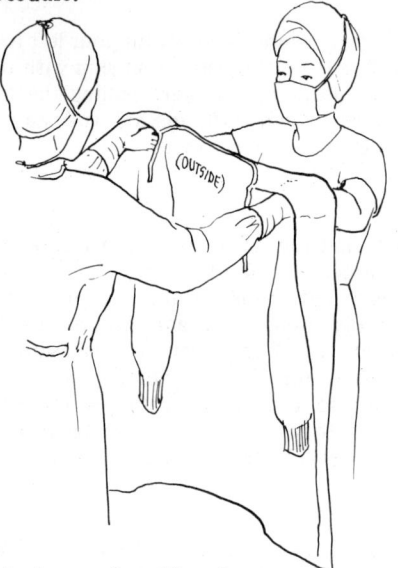

ASEPTIC TECHNIQUE

Important Steps	Key Points
4. Have the gownee slip his arms into the sleeves.	Ask him to put his hands and arms into the sleeves in a smooth, forceful, downward motion until his hands emerge from the sleeve openings. You must be careful that his unsterile hands are at arm's length and do not touch your gown front. As soon as his arms are entirely in the sleeves, he should bend them at the elbows and keep them upright in front at waist height.
5. Settle the gown on his shoulders.	With your cuffed hands continue to pull his gown up on his arms and shoulders. Hold the gown *firmly* at the shoulder seams.
6. Secure the gown at neck and waist.	This will be done by an *unsterile worker* as in Steps 8 through 11 of Item 3. The gownee himself will not be able to do anything until he is wearing sterile gloves.
7. Stand facing the gownee and pick up right glove.	Grasp cuff of gownee's glove at the lateral edges. Point the thumb of the glove toward the gownee. Hold cuff *firmly* and pull glove opening apart laterally. Be sure your thumbs are held out of the way so that they do not touch the gownee's bare hand as his hand goes into the glove.

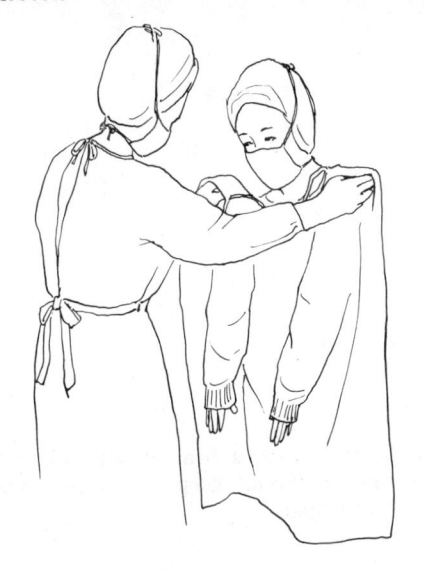

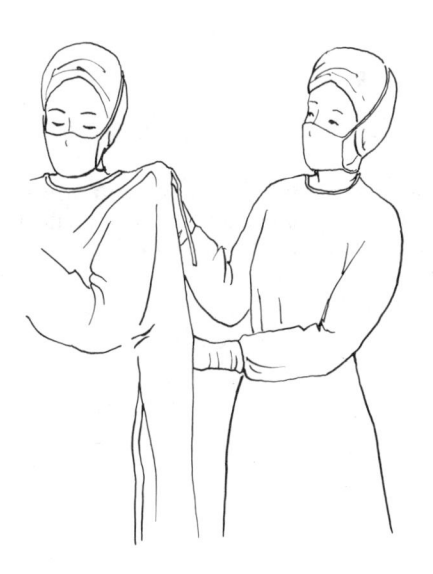

ASEPTIC TECHNIQUE

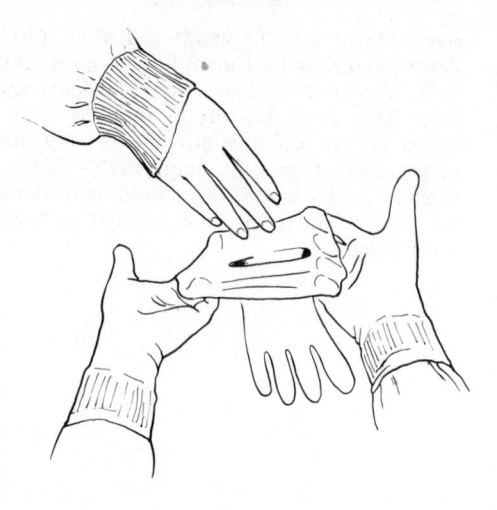

Important Steps   **Key Points**

8. Gownee inserts right hand into glove.

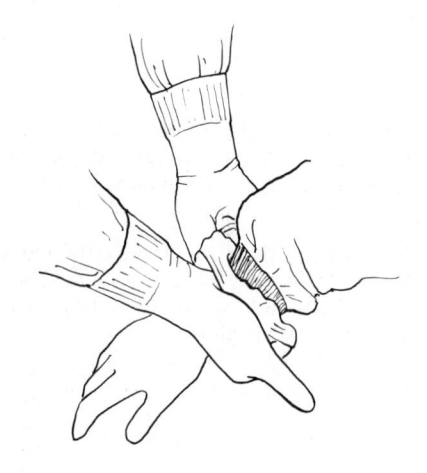

This is done with a firm, downward motion. The gownee should keep the fingers straight and slightly apart.

9. Pull glove up over gownee's cuff.

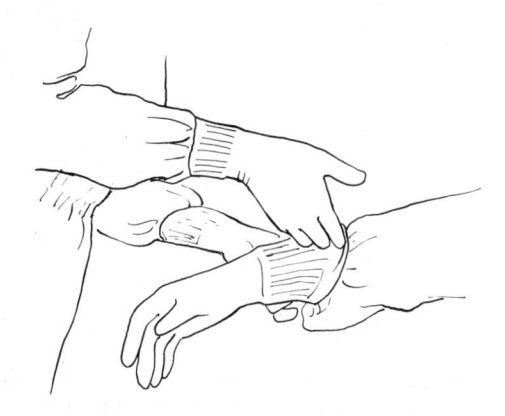

Continue holding the glove cuff spread apart with a strong lateral stretch as you pull glove up on the hand and over the gown cuff.

10. Pick up left glove.

Firmly grasp cuff of left glove and spread opening apart laterally. Be sure to keep your sterile gloves *away* from gownee's ungloved hand to avoid contamination.

ASEPTIC TECHNIQUE 31

Important Steps	Key Points
11. The gownee inserts his hand into the left glove.	He must keep his fingers straight and slightly apart for ease of insertion. His hand goes into the glove with a firm downward motion. Hold onto the gownee's glove *firmly*.
12. Pull gownee's left glove up over his gown cuff.	Continue to keep his glove cuff spread apart with a strong lateral stretch while pulling the glove upward over his hand and gown cuff.
13. Adjust the fingers of the gownee's gloves.	If necessary, pull the fingers of his gloves straight out to let his fingers slide in easily. He may have to knead on the fingers as you do with dress gloves.
14. Hand a sterile towel to the gownee.	This covers his hands like a muff and keeps them from becoming contaminated until the procedure begins. Then discard the towel in an appropriate container.

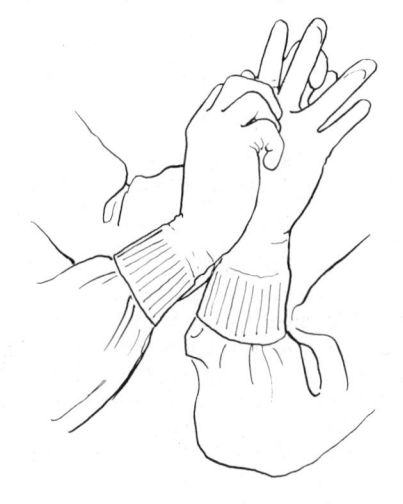

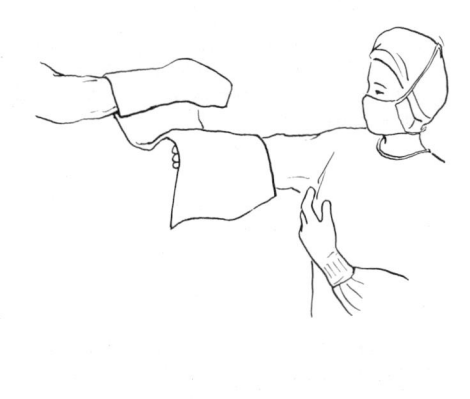

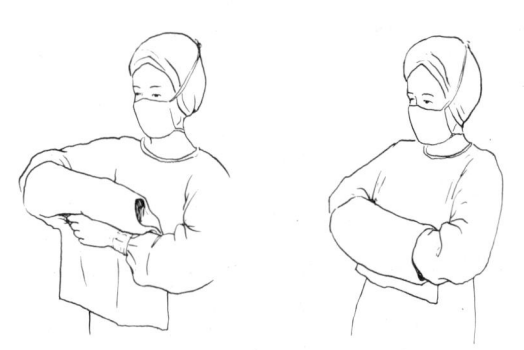

ITEM 7: OPENING STERILE PACKAGES

Packages are wrapped in linen of double thickness or specially prepared paper. This provides a strong shield to prevent microorganisms from entering the sterile package. If a sterile item becomes wet from spilled liquids or from being placed on a wet surface, it must be discarded as contaminated. As described earlier, moisture would make the wrapper serve as a wick that would attract organisms from the outside and thus contaminate the contents.

The correct procedure for opening sterile packages is as follows:

a. Wash hands.
b. Open sterile packages *away* from the body.
c. Touch only the outside of the wrapper.
d. Do not reach across a sterile field.
e. Always face the sterile field; go around the sterile field, if necessary.
f. Allow sufficient space between your body and the sterile field.
g. Keep sterile gloved hands in sight and under sufficient cuff to maintain sterility of the gloves when handling sterile linen.

Important Steps	Key Points
1. Obtain the sterile package containing the required item or items.	Get the package from the storage unit or department and take it to the area where it is to be used (patient's room, treatment room, or whatever).
2. Pick up the wrapped package (linen, gloves, instruments, utensils, suture sets, etc.).	Sterile items are wrapped in a special way so that the package can be opened easily without contaminating the contents. If the item is small, it can be held in the hand while being unwrapped. If the item is large, it should be placed on a table or flat surface for support and stability while being unwrapped. Place the package on the surface so that the wrapped edges are visible or uppermost. NOTE: Check package indicator for date and sterility of the package. Chemically treated indicators change color when sterilized.
3. Loosen the wrapper fastener (tape, string).	Move firmly, slowly, and cautiously while opening the fastener so as to avoid contaminating the contents. Discard the fastener in an appropriate container.
4. Open the distal flap (1) of the wrapper.	With your right hand, lift the distal flap up and toward the back, away from the package. Let the distal flap drop gently over the back of the table (or over your left hand if you are holding the sterile package). It is important to open the distal flap first so that your unsterile arm *does not* reach across the sterile contents. Unsterile objects (hair and dirt) could fall from your arm onto the sterile contents and contaminate them. In other words, begin unwrapping the package by opening the flap away from you. Hold the package away from your uniform, or if the item is on a table, stand at least 12 inches away to avoid contaminating the contents.

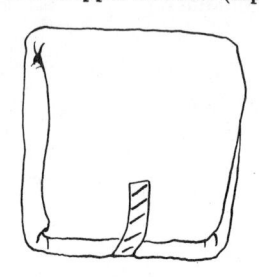

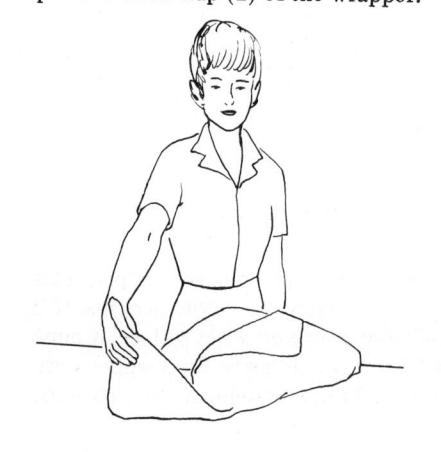

Important Steps	Key Points
5. Open the left flap (2).	With your left hand, move the flap up and laterally away from the package.
6. Open the right flap (3).	
7. Open the proximal flap (4).	Lift the flap up and toward you, dropping it gently over the front of the table or your hand. Remember to keep your fingers off the sterile contents and handle only the outside of the wrapper or you will contaminate it.

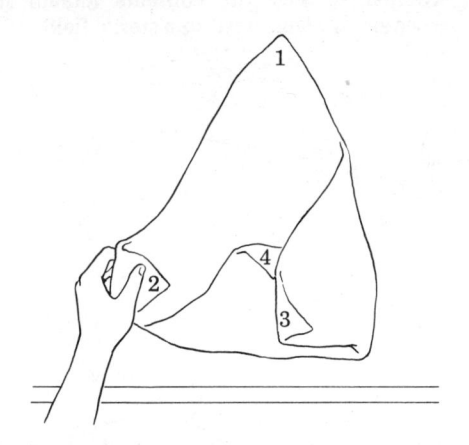

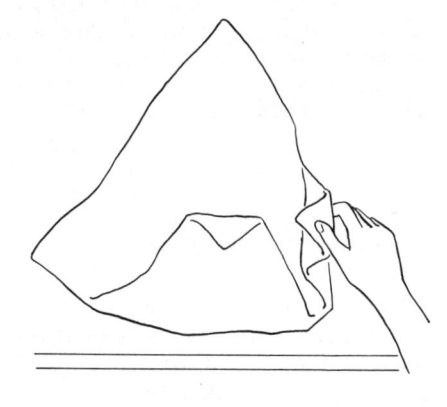

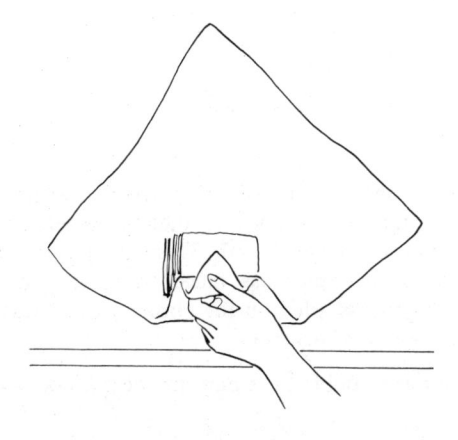

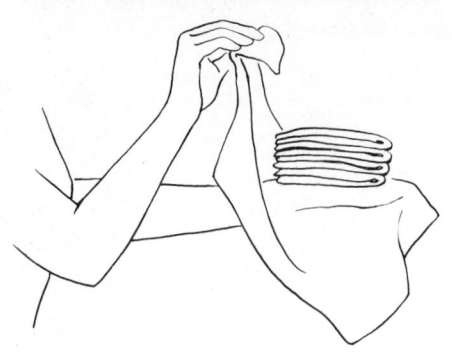

Important Steps	Key Points
8. Place the sterile item on a sterile field.	Be sure your hand is underneath the sterile wrapper so that the contents remain sterile when being transferred to a sterile field.
9. Or hand the item to someone in the sterile field.	Again, keep your hands under the sterile wrapper. Stand away from the sterile person and extend your arms. Be sure that the wrapper edges do not touch the sterile field. You may simply leave the sterile item resting on the sterile wrapper; you would then either don sterile gloves to handle the sterile item, or you would lift it with sterile "pickup forceps," as discussed in item 8, below.

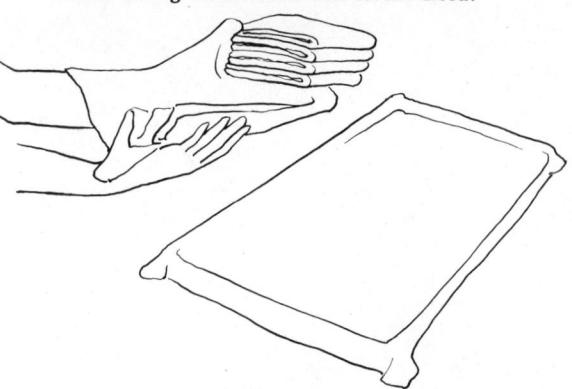

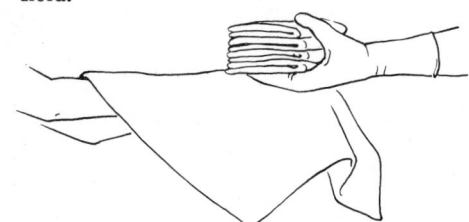

ITEM 8: STERILE HANDLING WITH FORCEPS (PICKUP OR SPONGE)

Sterile forceps are wrapped and sterilized individually if they are used. The recommended technique for transferring the contents of the sterile package to a sterile field is to open the sterile package and drop the contents directly on the sterile field.

Transfer forceps are no longer kept in germicidal solutions. If they are still utilized in your agency the following requirements must be met:

a. Start with clean or gloved hands.

b. Handle sterile equipment with sterile forceps or gloves only.

c. Establish a sterile field (area) for receiving all sterile equipment and supplies.

d. Keep the field sterile.

e. Keep the tip of the forceps down.

f. Carry the forceps high and in sight; never swing them at your side.

g. Drop objects from the forceps onto a sterile field.

h. To remove utensils from a sterile wrapper, observe the following procedure: first, open the corner fold away from you; then open the corner side folds to the left and right; and finally open the remaining corner (toward you). This eliminates the necessity of reaching over a sterile field. If a corner has failed to remain in a turned-back position during the sterilizing process, pick up the corner part at least two inches from the edge to allow for a margin of safety.

i. Never shake linen as you place it on a sterile field. Lint may provide a taxi for microorganisms.

ASEPTIC TECHNIQUE

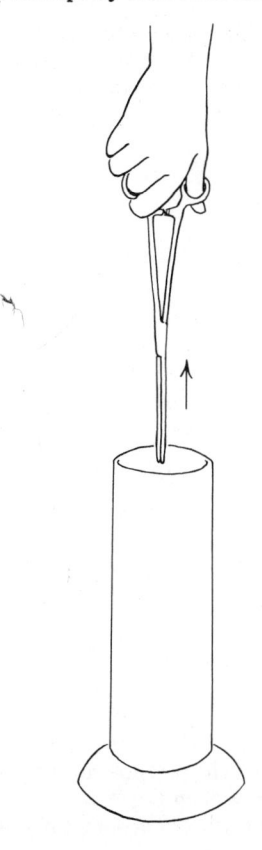

Commonly Used Handling Forceps

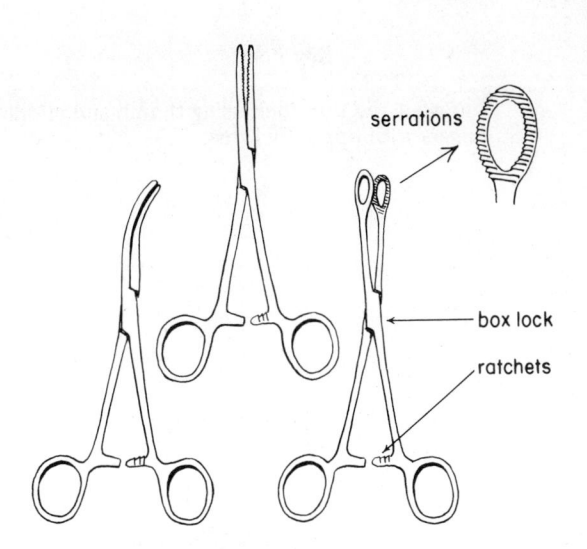

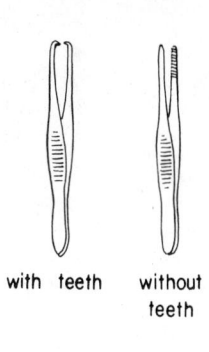

Procedure for Use of Handling Forceps

Important Steps	Key Points
1. Obtain forceps.	Get them from the storage area or department. As stated before, they are individually wrapped.
2. Carry the sterile packages to the work area (e.g., patient's room, treatment room, etc.).	
3. Grasp forceps by their handles.	Hemostats or other forceps may be used as lifting instruments. Lift vertically, keeping tips of forceps downward. The forceps is no longer sterile if it touches an unsterile object, or is exposed in an open room for more than a few hours (8 hours). The sterility of the forceps is assured only when the person handling the forceps maintains strict aseptic technique.

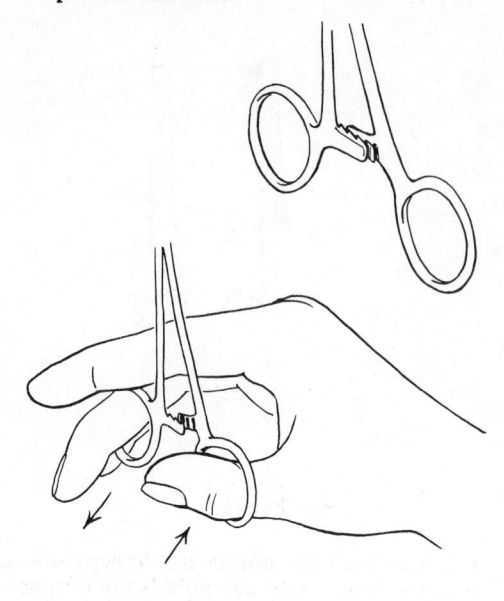

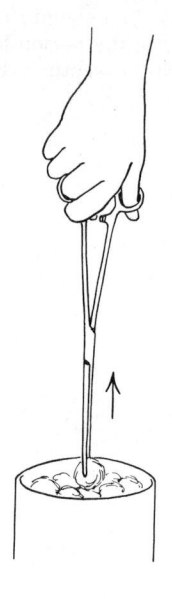

Important Steps	Key Points
4. Open the ratchets.	Unfasten the box lock using thumb and middle fingers with opposing force.
5. Lift up without touching the unsterile edges of the wrapper or container.	
6. Remove the supply you need from the sterile wrapper or container.	Close the ratchets again when you have picked up an object. Lift the forceps vertically. Avoid touching the sides of the container.
7. Remove the sterile item from its wrapper (linens, dressing, etc.).	Lift it vertically—do not drag it laterally. Work above a sterile field (wrapper or drape). Then if you accidentally drop the item, it will fall on a sterile field and will not be contaminated.

ASEPTIC TECHNIQUE

Important Steps	Key Points
8. Remove the sterile forceps from the tray.	Take hold of the forceps at the box lock and lift straight up.

| 9. Use two forceps to remove Vaseline gauze from a sterile container. | Take hold of each end of the gauze and lift upward. This provides a peeling action as each piece of gauze separates from the remainder. Release gauze before the forceps come in direct contact with the skin. Forceps will need to be cleaned and resterilized before being used again. |

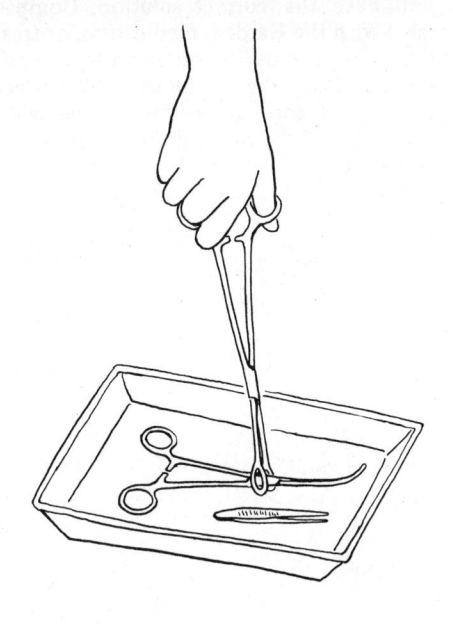

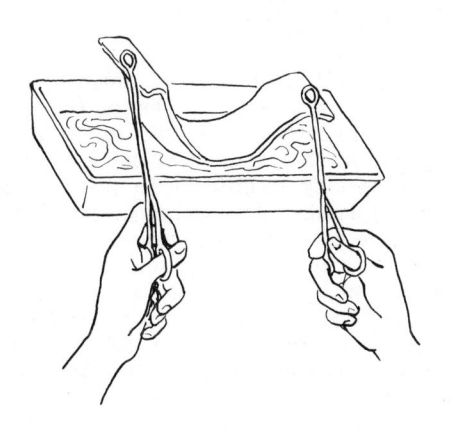

10. Replace the forceps on the sterile wrapper.

ITEM 10: POURING STERILE SOLUTIONS

Frequently you will need to pour a sterile solution from one container to another. Although you will not be sterile, you must use aseptic technique to prevent contaminating the solution.

ASEPTIC TECHNIQUE

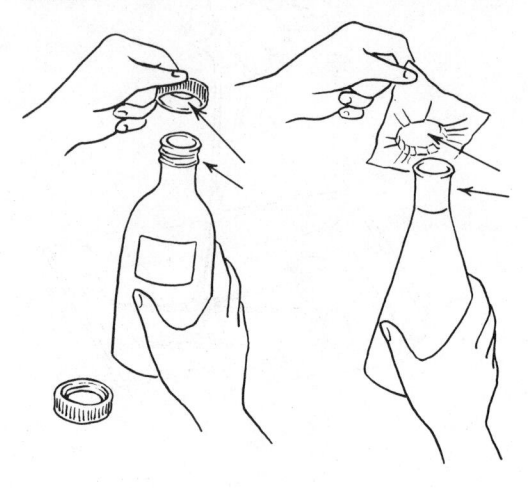

Important Steps	Key Points
1. Obtain the solution containers and remove the cap or cover.	Check the label on the container to be sure that you have the correct solution. Compare the label with the Kardex, medication, or treatment card. Touch only the outer unsterile surface of the cap. Place the cap on the table surface with the top of the cap resting on the table. The inner part of the rim and the cap are considered sterile.
2. Unwrap the sterile basin.	Follow procedure as described in previous item.
3. Pour the solution from the bottle into a basin.	Pour a small amount of solution into a waste container to cleanse the lip of the solution bottle. Hold the bottle with the label facing upward so that liquid will not spill over the label, making it difficult to read. To avoid undue splashing, pour from a height of about 6 inches to prevent contamination of the sterile basin with the outside of the bottle (or less if pouring small amounts of solution, e.g., 2 to 10 cc). Handles (or tongs) may be used to pour from hot bottles. These are specially prepared units, commonly used in the operating or delivery rooms.

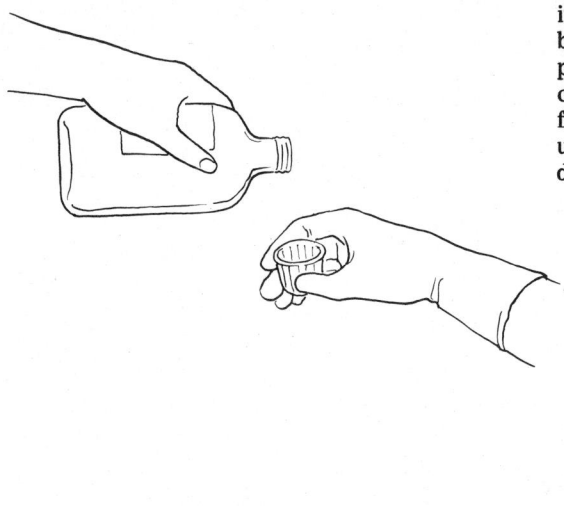

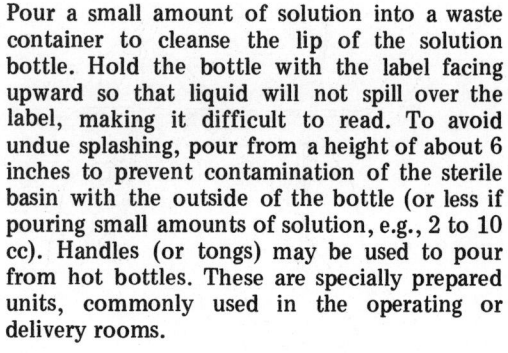

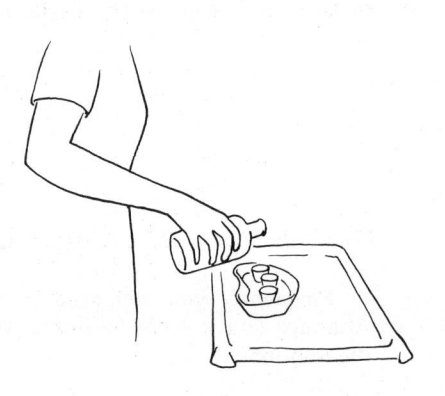

ASEPTIC TECHNIQUE

Important Steps	Key Points
4. Return the solution container to the designated area.	If it has a screw top, pick it up and replace it on the bottle. Carefully screw the cap on securely, without touching the inside of the cap or the rim. The cover may not be replaced if the entire contents have been used or if the cover is contaminated.

ITEM 11: HOLDING VIAL SO THAT SOLUTION CAN BE WITHDRAWN

This procedure is frequently performed in various sterile procedures, during minor surgery when a local anesthetic (such as Novocain) is used, or when a sterile liquid medication is to be introduced into an open wound.

Important Steps	Key Points
1. Obtain the correct vial of solution.	This is done by the unsterile worker. Check the label for name, dosage, and route to be used.
2. Verify the label.	Ask the sterile worker to verify that your solution is correct. Have the label read out loud (type, dosage, route).
3. Cleanse the vial stopper.	Use an alcohol pledget.
4. Hold the vial firmly, with label up.	The sterile person (with gloved hands) will attach the sterile needle to the sterile syringe, pull the plunger of the syringe back to the amount of solution to be withdrawn, and insert the needle and syringe into the stopper.

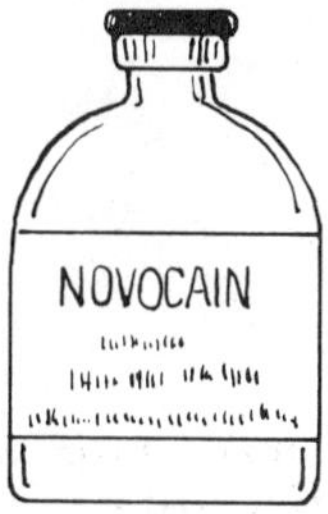

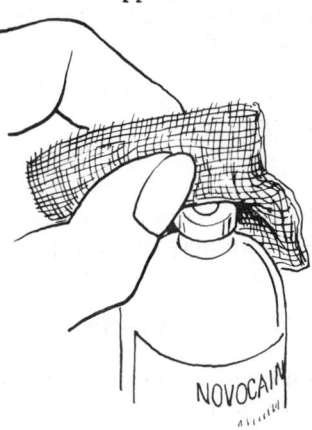

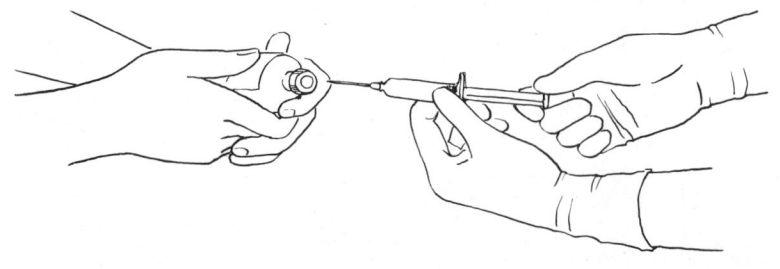

ASEPTIC TECHNIQUE

Important Steps	Key Points
5. The solution is drawn into the syringe by the sterile worker.	The unsterile person will continue to hold the vial firmly as the sterile person pushes the plunger into the syringe. This increases air pressure inside the vial so that the solution can then easily be drawn out by pulling back on the plunger.
6. Withdraw the needle from the vial stopper.	Sterile worker pulls firmly, quickly and straight back, away from the vial, being careful not to touch the needle against the outside of the unsterile vial.
7. Place the filled needle and syringe on a sterile surface.	This will make them ready for use by the doctor, when needed.
8. The unsterile worker then replaces the vial in appropriate storage area nearby.	The vial may be discarded if entire amount of solution was used.

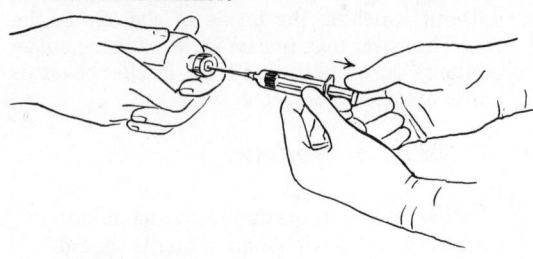

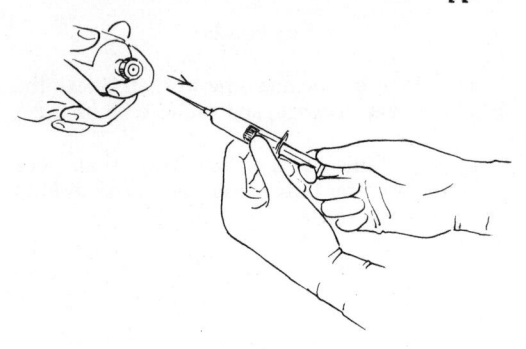

ITEM 12: OPENING A COMMERCIALLY PREPARED STERILE PACKAGE

Since there are a variety of commercially prepared sterile packages on the market, you should carefully read the directions on the wrapper before opening the package to avoid contaminating the contents.

Important Steps	Key Points
1. Grasp the package by the slightly extended edges provided.	Bring both your hands together and grasp the edges of the package.
2. Peel along the sealed edge.	Turn your hands outward to separate the sealed, sterile package. Peel in a downward motion. Note that your hands do not touch the inside of the wrapper.

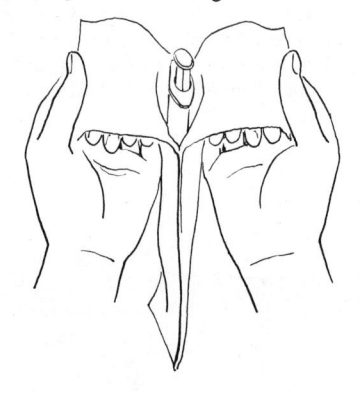

ASEPTIC TECHNIQUE

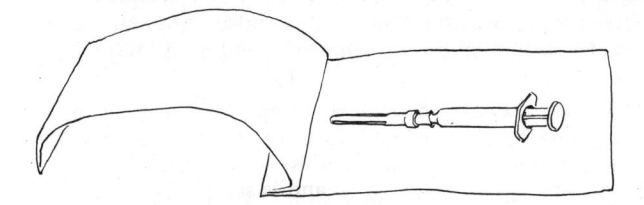

Important Steps	Key Points
3. Place the package on a flat surface, or	The inside area of the wrapper is sterile and may be used as a sterile field until the contents are used.
4. Hand the article to a sterile person, or	Keep your fingers away from the edges. The sterile person then picks up the sterile item.
5. Lift the sterile item from the wrapper by using sterile forceps.	

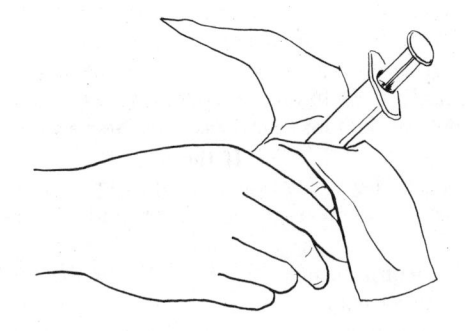

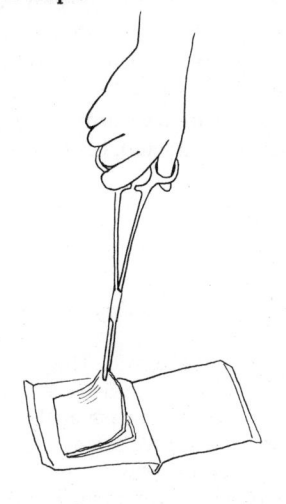

ITEM 13: CHANGING STERILE DRESSINGS

The dressing is a protective covering placed over a wound. It may be used to absorb drainage, to keep the wound sealed so that microorganisms are prevented from entering or escaping, to apply pressure for controlling hemorrhage, to assist a skin graft's adherence to the graft site, or to prevent injury to the wound. A description of the types of dressing materials appears in the enrichment section of this Unit.

Wounds are classified according to the presence or absence of microorganisms. A wound is clean if there are no pathogenic microorganisms present; it is infected when pathogenic microorganisms give rise to the infectious process. A wound that is acquired by accident is considered contaminated until it is proved that no pathogenic microorganisms are present. (Further information on wounds will be found in the enrichment section, Additional Information for Enrichment on p. 49.)

When you change a dressing, you have an excellent opportunity to observe the status of the healing process and to note the condition of the wound and surrounding tissue. Observe carefully, because it will be necessary for you to chart your observations.

Wounds heal in two ways. Healing by *first intention* is the process by which a wound heals without an infection. The wound edges heal accurately and closely and therefore with a minimal scar. This type of healing usually occurs when a wound has been sutured under aseptic technique.

When skin edges cannot be drawn closely together, the wound heals by *granulation* or *second intention*. Granulation is an outgrowth of new capillaries and is supported in cells which become fibrous scar tissue. Granulation brings a rich blood supply to the healing wound. Granulation tissue appears red and bumpy; you have probably observed this in yourself when a cut is wide and gaping. Healing by second intention takes place over a longer period of time.

Excessive growth of scar tissue is called a *keloid*. Negroes are prone to this type of scar, although under certain circumstances anyone can develop a keloid. The keloid may be excised surgically for cosmetic reasons.

When a wound does not heal, it frequently becomes *necrotic*. If the necrotic material becomes infected with microorganisms, *gangrene* can develop.

There are other results of improper healing that you should be informed about; e.g., an *abscess* is a localized infection in which there is an accumulation of pus. You will recall that pus is a liquid accumulation of phagocytes (leukocytes). The liquid may be white, yellow, pink, or green, depending on the infecting microorganism. *Cellulitis* is an inflammation of the cellular tissue surrounding the initial wound. *Empyema* is the collection of pus in an already existing cavity (i.e., gallbladder or lung). A *fistula* is an abnormal passage or communication usually formed between two internal organs, or leading from an internal organ to the surface of the body. A fistula may result from an infection or it may have a congenital origin. Common postoperative fistulas are designated according to the organs or parts with which they communicate, such as rectovaginal, fecal, anal, biliary, and the like. A *sinus* is a canal or passageway leading to an abscess.

Procedure for Changing Sterile Dressings

Important Steps	Key Points
1. Collect the required supplies.	They must be sterile. They may include hemostats, scissors, thumb forceps, drapes, dressings. NOTE: These items may be available in your agency as a suture set or dressing tray. Use the kind of sterile gloves and antiseptic solution preferred by your agency. Solutions vary from time to time because improvements are constantly being made through research efforts; therefore, no specific solution is indicated. Use current agency antiseptic for cleansing around the wound. Use a waxed paper bag for disposal of dressing.

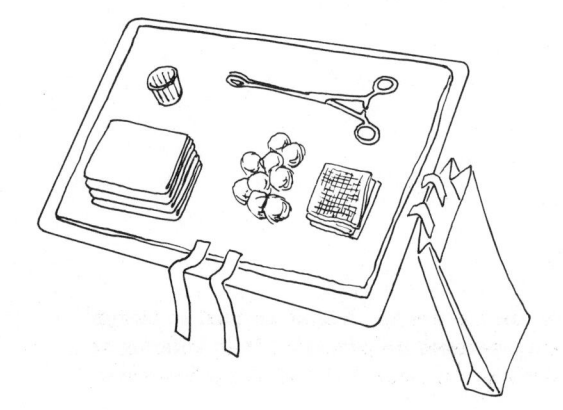

ASEPTIC TECHNIQUE

Important Steps	Key Points
2. Prepare the environment.	Close all windows and doors in the area to prevent drafts and to limit the dust and lint in the air which could carry microorganisms into the wound. Draw curtains around the bed for patient privacy. Clear a work surface so that you can place the dressing change supplies and equipment within easy reach.

Correct

Incorrect

Assemble the unsterile supplies nearby. Pour antiseptic solutions into sterile containers as indicated for cleansing purposes. Take care not to spill solution on sterile drapes (Remember! The wick action of the liquid transports microorganisms from the unsterile surface up through the sterile surface, dressings, drains, etc.). Open the sterile supplies.

Make ready for the dressing change. Tear off the amount of tape you will need to secure the dressing when you have finished the procedure; place the piece of tape on the edge of the table for easy access when applying it. To tear the tape, grasp tape with thumb nails together at the upper edge of the adhesive. Pull apart by using a smooth even pull. Do not pull apart by moving thumbs in opposite directions. Place a waxed paper bag nearby so that the soiled dressing can be dropped into it. Wash your hands.

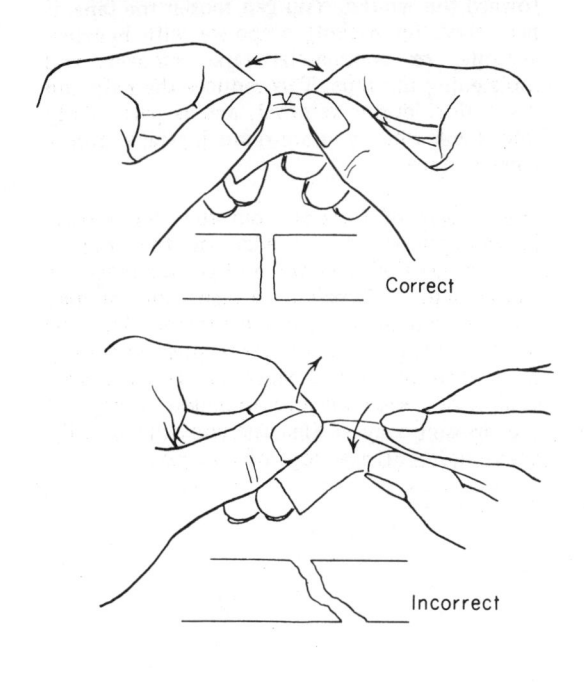

3. Prepare the patient.

Identify him by checking his Identaband. Maintaining proper body alignment for yourself and your patient, position him comfortably so that the wound site is easily accessible (usually in a dorsal recumbent position). Cover him with a bath blanket if indicated.

Expose the wound site by folding the bed linens away from the area and removing the patient's gown or pajamas (if they cover the site). Explain what you are going to do; answer questions promptly and simply; if you are unable to do so, tell him you will find out for him, or ask him to discuss the matter with his doctor.

Reassure the patient that there will be limited discomfort during the procedure. (If, on the other hand, the particular dressing change will be painful, tell him so, and assure him it will be done as quickly and gently as possible. Tell him to relax and stay as quiet as possible and that you will let him know what you are going to do throughout the procedure. Remind him not to talk during the procedure because the droplets of moisture can carry microorganisms into the wound. Also, ask him to keep his hands quietly on the bed and not to touch the open wound. (Soiled fingers harbor germs and can cause infection.)

ASEPTIC TECHNIQUE

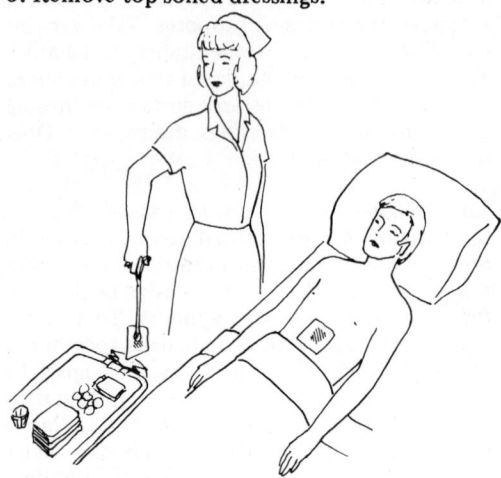

Important Steps	Key Points
4. Loosen binder or tapes.	If there is a binder, unpin it; if tape, pull toward the wound. You can loosen the tape, if necessary, by soaking a sponge with benzine, acetone, or commercial tape remover, and moistening the tape. This reduces the pain and discomfort during removal, and is particularly important when you are removing tape from a hairy surface.
5. Remove top soiled dressings.	Use a pair of forceps from the sterile trays usually placed at the edge of the tray or wrapper so that you will not contaminate the sterile field. This pair of forceps may or may not be held in a forceps container. With the forceps, pick up the top dressings and drop them into the waxed-paper bag you prepared earlier. Set aside the contaminated forceps on the dressing tray so that the contaminated tip is extending off the edge of the tray.
6. Inspect the wound.	Note the degree of healing, the presence and amount of infection, pus, necrosis, any putrid odor, the color, the odor of drainage, and the condition of the sutures or drains, if present.
7. Put on sterile gloves (usually disposable).	Put on a mask before gloving, if indicated by your agency procedure (see item 1). Take care not to contaminate the sterile gloves. You are putting them on to keep your hands as clean as possible and also to prevent introducing other germs you may be carrying on your hands into the wound.
8. Cleanse the area around the wound.	Use a prepared antiseptic pledget or antiseptic-soaked cotton ball. Pick up the pledget or cotton ball with your gloved hand. Hold securely between your thumb and index finger (or with forceps if used). Tell the patient, "This may be cool and it may sting a little because it is an antiseptic." Cleanse around the wound area using a circular motion, away from the wound in an ever-widening circle. Do not go back over the cleaned area. Discard the pledget or cotton ball, and repeat the process with a fresh pledget.

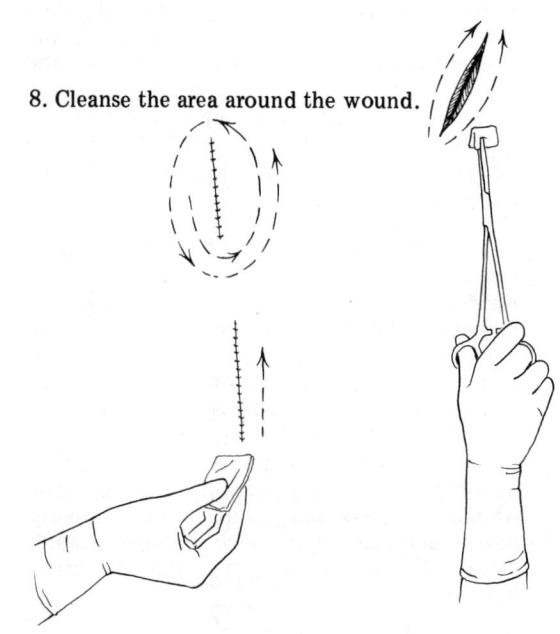

ASEPTIC TECHNIQUE

Important Steps	Key Points
	Do not cleanse directly over the wound unless there is a great amount of drainage and if it is agency policy. In that case, use a clean pledget, and with one stroke from top to bottom, cleanse the wound. The cleanest part of the wound is at the top. Discard the pledget. Repeat the cleansing process directly over the wound, using a fresh pledget for each single swipe until the wound is cleaned to your satisfaction. Allow the skin surface to dry, then observe the skin for excoriation, etc.
9. Drape the wound site.	This may be done by picking up sterile drapes with your gloved hands. (If forceps are also used, pick up the sterile drapes and arrange them properly). When applying a four-towel drape: put the first towel on the side of the wound furthest from you. Drop the proximal edge close to the wound (1 to 2 inches). The second towel is placed at the proximal side of the wound close to it. Lay the third towel near the left side of the wound edge and the fourth towel near the right wound edge. Now the entire area should be covered with sterile drapes, keeping only the wound area itself exposed.
	Single drape: Some dressing sets have a single drape that has a hole in the center. This type of drape is dropped from the proximal side toward the distal side, centering the opening directly over the wound site.
10. Apply ointment or powder.	This may be ordered by the physician, or it may be agency procedure. If so, apply it directly to the wound or around the wound (as ordered). Use applicators, discarding each after one swipe. Powder (such as sulfa powder) can be shaken directly onto the wound.
11. Apply the dressing.	Lift the dressing from the tray and drop it lightly, centering it over the wound area. Reinforce the dressing with additional layers of dressing as indicated by the type of wound or incision.
12. Discard the forceps and gloves.	Put them in the appropriate container. If they are disposable, they can go into a container to be incinerated. If they are reusable, place them in the container on the tray and return them to the processing room for cleaning and reprocessing. Remove the gloves by taking hold of the inside cuff and pulling the gloves off your hands (thus turning the gloves inside out). Discard in the container.

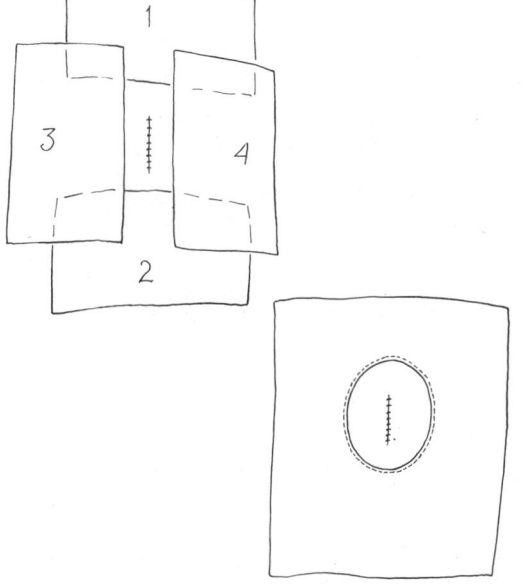

ASEPTIC TECHNIQUE

Important Steps	Key Points
13. Apply a dressing retainer.	Use tape, ties, or binders. (See the accompanying sketches for proper placement of retainers.) Some common problems encountered in applying dressings:

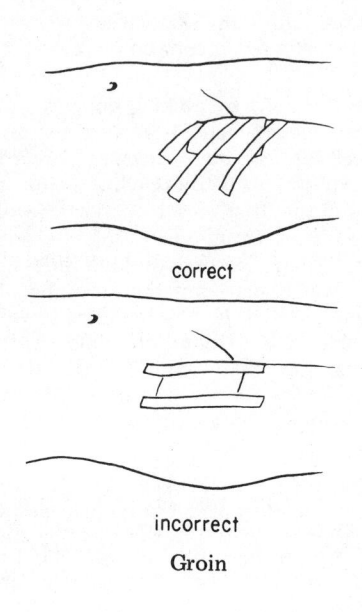

a. Adhesive running opposite from body action:

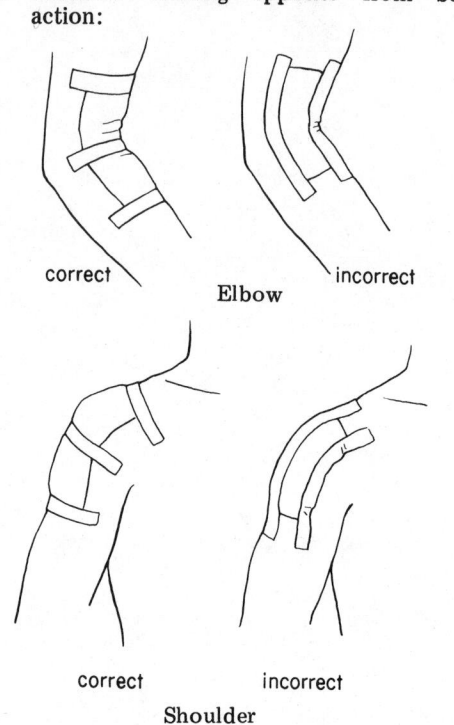

correct / incorrect
Elbow

correct / incorrect
Shoulder

correct
incorrect
Groin

b. Improper spacing of tape:

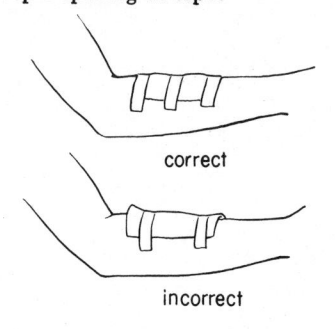

correct

incorrect

c. Adhesive too long or too short:

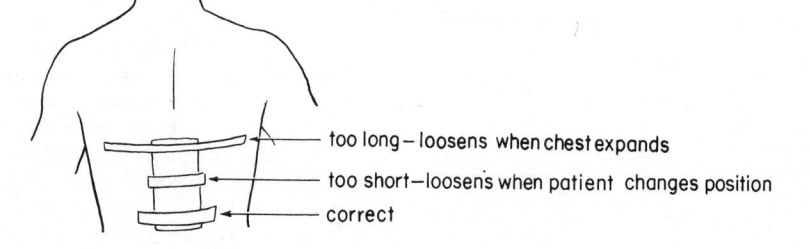

too long — loosens when chest expands
too short — loosens when patient changes position
correct

Important Steps	Key Points
	d. Tape too narrow:

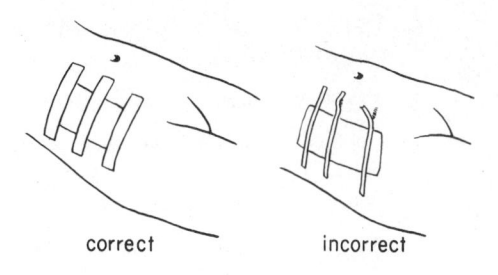

correct   incorrect

Remove the used items, discard the disposable items, return the reusable ones to the designated reprocessing room. Rearrange furniture within the patient's reach (bedside stand with fresh water and personal items). Attach the call light within his reach; adjust the bed and linen for comfort. Adjust the siderails for patient's needs. Ask if there is anything else you can do and tell him when you plan to return. Leave the room neat; pleasant surroundings assist in returning the patient to health.

14. Wash your hands.

15. Chart the procedure.

Charting example:

Record the dressing change promptly on the chart. Report any unusual signs to the charge nurse (drainage, inflammation, putrid odor, pus, evisceration, excoriation, or the like); e.g., 10:30 a.m. Abdominal dressing changed. Suture site cleansed with alcohol 70%. Wound looks clean, is healing well. No complaints of tenderness or pain.

L. Domer, R.N.

SUMMARY OF PRINCIPLES OF ASEPTIC TECHNIQUE APPLIED TO DRESSING CHANGE

1. Keep sterile dressings and equipment on a sterile field.
2. Open sterile packages away from your body to avoid touching your uniform or other contaminated objects.
3. Touch only the *outside* of a sterile wrapper.
4. Do not reach with bare arms across a sterile field or a wound (this eliminates the possibility of debris from your arm dropping into the wound or onto the sterile field).
5. Assemble all supplies and equipment needed *before* beginning the dressing change.
6. Minimize talk during the dressing change to prevent droplets of moisture from falling into the wound or onto the sterile field.
7. Clean the wound from top to bottom and from wound edge laterally.
8. Secure dressings firmly to protect wound and minimize contamination.

VI. ADDITIONAL INFORMATION FOR ENRICHMENT

Historical Background

Sepsis was prevalent in the early practice of medicine, although historical accounts reveal hints of asepsis as far back as Hippocrates. While the ancient practice of medicine and patient care appears crude today, it must be recognized that those methods were devised by the ablest minds of that time.

Hippocrates (460 B.C.), called the Father of Medicine, showed some understanding of asepsis as indicated by the use of boiled water or wine to irrigate wounds.

Galen (131-210 A.D.), a famous Greek physician, demonstrated greater understanding of asepsis by boiling instruments used in the care of wounded gladiators.

Andreas Vesalius (16th century) was known as the founder of modern anatomy, but he also wrote about suppuration (pus formation) as a part of the healing process and advocated the use of ligatures to tie off bleeding blood vessels.

Ignaz Semmelweis (1818-65) was a Viennese doctor who established the cause of puerperal fever (pathogenic microorganisms entering the body during child delivery and causing a morbid condition). His ideas were not understood and his writings created controversy.

Dr. Oliver Wendell Holmes, a Harvard Medical School graduate, wrote of the contagious nature of puerperal fever in 1843. He stated the belief that it was carried from patient to patient by nurses and doctors because they did not wash their hands properly after seeing each patient.

Louis Pasteur was a French chemist (19th century) who found that he could halt the growth of minute organisms by the use of heat. He pointed out the role of bacteria in causing disease and thus provided the basis for the study of bacteriology as we know it today. His demonstration that fermentation could be prevented by heat sterilization was the forerunner of the pasteurization process.

Robert Koch, a bacteriologist in the mid-1800's, proved that many different kinds of microorganisms cause infection. He developed the theory of specific infectious diseases, and is remembered especially for his discovery of the cause of tuberculosis in 1862.

Joseph Lister (1827-1912) had heard of Pasteur's work and searched for a chemical to destroy or combat bacteria. The English surgeon discovered that wound infections were caused by microorganisms, and he began to use carbolic acid on dressings to kill the microorganisms. It was Lister who introduced antiseptic technique in the operating room, which lead to a remarkable reduction in infectious complications.

ASEPTIC TECHNIQUE

Sterilization by boiling was initiated about 1880, and in 1886 sterilization by steam under pressure was devised by Charles Chamberland, a French bacteriologist (1851-1908). Modern aseptic techniques thereafter supplanted the earlier antiseptic methods. When rubber gloves first came into use, they were employed to protect delicate hands from the harsh antiseptics. Dr. William Stewart Halstead of Johns Hopkins Hospital and Dr. Bloodgood began using rubber gloves in the 1890's, and gradually they became accepted as a protection against patient contamination. Masks appeared about the turn of the century, and sterile technique as we now know it gradually evolved thereafter.

Wound Healing

Primary wound healing (or healing by first intention) is desired. The wound heals rapidly without post-operative swelling, infection, or discharge. There is no separation of the edges of the wound and the scar is minimal. In secondary wound healing (or healing by second intention) there usually is infection, healing is delayed, and the wound may break to form a hernia later with excessive scarring.

Delayed healing of a wound may be caused by infection, poor approximation of parts to each other (as in bone fracture), pronounced anemia, and general debilitating diseases such as cancer and diabetes. In these cases, scar tissue may form and the wound may break down later. Infection is the most common cause of delayed wound healing. Infections are generally preventable; strict adherence to aseptic technique by the health team must therefore be carried out at all times.

Complications of Wound Healing

1. *Hemorrhage*

This is a surgical emergency; it is evidenced by visible bleeding, or symptoms of concealed internal bleeding. It may be caused by the slipping of a ligature or a vessel that was not tied at the time of operation. Symptoms of hemorrhage include:

—Falling blood pressure

—Cold, clammy skin

—Pulse weak in volume, but increased in rate

—Respiration rapid and deep

—Restlessness and apprehension

—Thirst

2. *Wound Disruption*

This is described as *dehiscence* or a splitting open or gaping of a wound. If internal organs of the abdomen protrude through an abdominal incision, it is called evisceration. Symptoms of wound disruption may be:

—Abnormal serosanguineous (blood-colored fluid) discharge.

—A sudden pulling pain which the patient describes as "feeling something give."

In the normal healing process the body shows a remarkable ability to recover. New cells are formed at the base of the wound, and if aseptic conditions are maintained, healing proceeds at a maximal rate. A film of blood and lymph fills the space of the wound, and the fibrin and fibrils in the blood aid the clotting process of gluing the wound together. Serum and leukocytes are also present and the fibroblasts all multiply to fill in the gap. The capillary ends unite to provide blood supply and new collagen fibrils form. By the fourth day, a thin line of granulation (or scab and thin scar tissue) is present at the edges of the wound. Eventually this granulation resembles normal skin, and appears as a thin line of scar tissue.

ASEPTIC TECHNIQUE

Anatomy and Physiology

The skin has two layers. The *epidermis* (outer layer) sheds constantly. The *dermis* (inner layer) contains the blood vessels, sweat glands, sebaceous glands, nerves, and hair follicles.

Body cells require an internal chemical environment of pH 7.4 for normal functioning. Surface cells can resist a pH that is slightly acidic, and the pH may drop to 5.5 when the body sweats. However, bacteria prefer a slightly alkaline environment, and they live and multiply when the pH exceeds 7.4.

Transient bacteria cling to the surface of the skin and resident bacteria inhabit sebaceous glands and hair follicles which are deep in the skin. This makes the surgical scrub an important factor in preventing and controlling disease and infection.

Chemistry

The skin cannot be sterilized, but the use of antiseptics and germicidal soaps and solutions can reduce the bacterial count on the skin. Anti-bacterial agents may be added to soaps to reduce the bacterial count of the skin. Examples are Septisol and Germanedica. These continue to inhibit growth of bacteria on the skin even after the scrub has been performed.

Slight cuts or small open areas on the skin should have an antiseptic agent such as 70 per cent alcohol applied (for bacteriostatic effects) before a bandage is put on.

Benzine or one of its derivatives acts as a solvent to remove adhesive that remains on the skin after the tape is removed.

Microbiology

The skin (if unbroken) protects the body from disease-producing microorganisms. Outer skin is relatively dry, but with excessive dryness it may break open and permit an entry for infection.

Mucous membranes are normally moist, and if excessive dryness develops (particularly of the respiratory passages), the normal flushing action of protective mucus (which helps keep the surfaces free from colonizing microorganisms) is lost.

Dressings are used to help protect a wound from contamination. Aseptic technique is necessary when changing dressings; hands must be washed thoroughly before beginning the sterile dressing. Contaminated dressings should be discarded carefully for destruction in the incinerator.

Pharmacology

Antiseptics are useful in inhibiting microorganisms of the skin when cleaning around a wound. Such agents as alcohol 70 per cent, zephiran chloride 1:750, or Merthiolate may be used.

Protective ointments such as zinc oxide may be used on the skin when a dressing is being changed. (The physician may order others.)

Penicillin powder or other antibiotic preparations may be used as ordered by the physician to prevent the growth of bacteria.

Physics

The number of bacteria in the air depends on the amount of dust in the air. Dust from floors and other places is wafted into the air from currents of air. Microorganisms use dust particles and other movable objects as taxis. Bacteria can enter a wound from the air, a wet dressing, fingers, or instruments.

Gauze fibers absorb drainage by capillary action or attraction. Bandages, when correctly applied, support the body part. However, roller bandage has no elasticity, and edema of the injured part may constrict circulation. Useless turns of roller bandage increase pressure on the wound.

ASEPTIC TECHNIQUE

Psychology

Clean dressings are more acceptable to the patient, and dry dressings are more comfortable. For these reasons, dressings should be changed as indicated.

Soiled dressings should be removed from the patient's sight as soon as possible. Placing them in a waxed paper bag prevents the patient from seeing them and also prevents bacterial spread.

Dressings that are too tight should be removed and properly adjusted. A pull on the skin can produce irritation both physically and psychologically.

Sociology

The patient or members of the patient's family may have to learn how to change a dressing. The health worker is expected to teach the patient how to do so properly, and how to apply a bandage if needed.

Common Dressing Materials

1. Sterile folded gauze, sometimes called "flats." Some have a radiopaque marking so that they can be easily found with X-ray if inadvertently left in a wound.

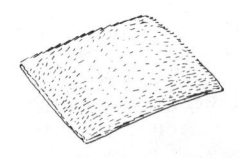

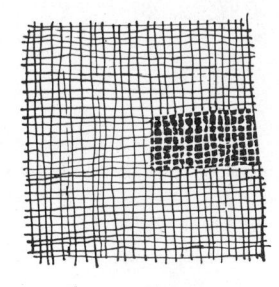

2. Sterile gauze fluffs are loosely folded large squares of gauze used to collect large amounts of drainage or to pack an opening. These, too, may have radiopaque markings.

3. ABD pads (for *abdominal*) are large, thick, absorbent gauze pads of various sizes, e.g., 10 X 10, 13 X 13 inches.

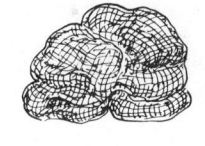

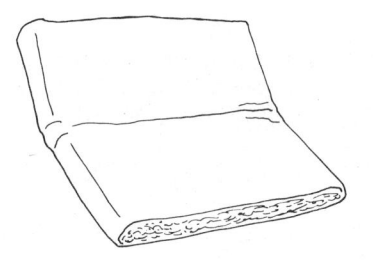

4. Telfa is a plastic-like coating on one side of a gauze dressing which prevents the dressing from adhering to the wound.

5. Adhesive bandages come in various sizes from the well-known 1/2 and 1/4 inch to 4 X 4 inch and 4 X 8 inch sizes.

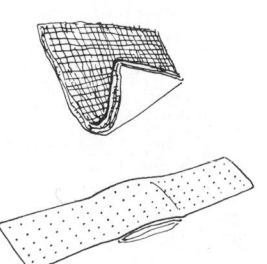

6. Spray-on dressing, when sprayed on a wound, forms a transparent protective film which allows for close observation of incision site. Spray-on dressings are non-toxic and mildly bacteriostatic.

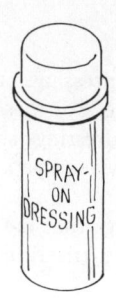

7. Petrolatum (Vaseline) gauze prevents the bandage from sticking to the wound.

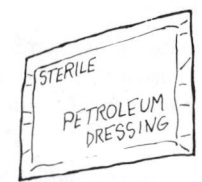

8. Roller gauze bandage is available in various sizes from 1 to 4 inches wide (5 yards long); it may be used as a base for additional gauze sponges or fluffs.

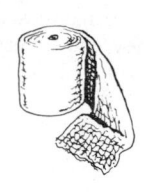

9. Adhesive tape comes in various sizes from 1/4 to 4 inches wide (5 yards long) and also as an elastic tape in sizes 2 to 6 inches wide (5 yards long).

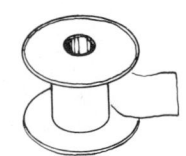

10. Paper or plastic tapes are anti-allergenic.

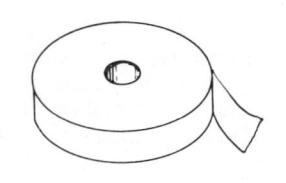

11. Liquid adhesive (creamy white substance supplied in tubes) is used for small dressings where bandaging is difficult.

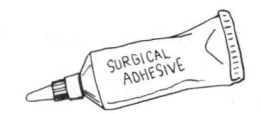

12. Montgomery tape (adhesive ties, butterfly ties) is used to tie across large or bulky dressings and eliminates the need for repeated removals of the tape and outer bandages. It is particularly useful in large, profusely draining abdominal or chest wounds.

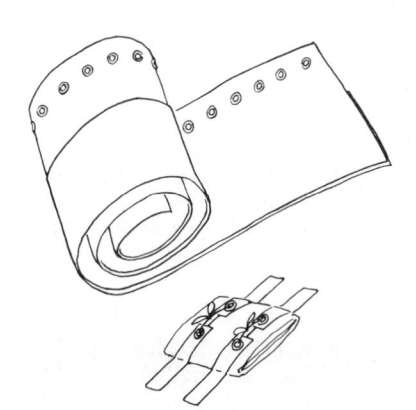

ASEPTIC TECHNIQUE

13. Various drains may also be used, such as the T-tube, Penrose tubes, or various catheters. Refer to Volume 2, Unit 25, Care of the Patient with Gastrointestinal Tubes, if you have forgotten about these.

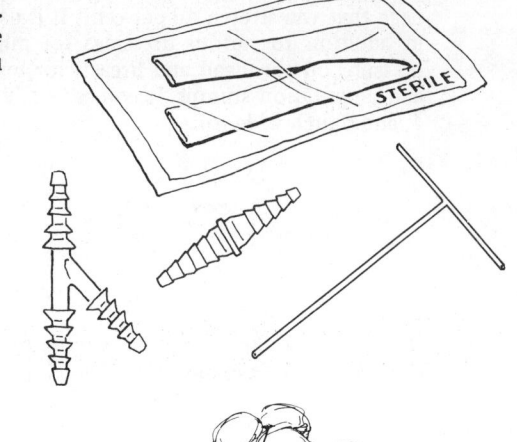

14. Cotton balls are ball-shaped masses of cotton that come in sizes from small to large. Some cotton balls also have a radiopaque marking that shows up in X-ray. Some cotton balls are covered with gauze to avoid having the cotton stick to a wound.

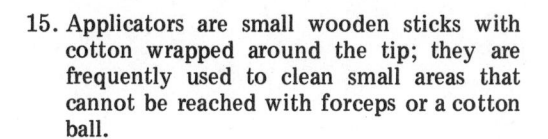

15. Applicators are small wooden sticks with cotton wrapped around the tip; they are frequently used to clean small areas that cannot be reached with forceps or a cotton ball.

16. Moleskin (a thick soft-napped cotton-back cloth) is intended for orthopedic use as cushioning. It comes in 12-inch wide 5-yard rolls, or 10-inch wide 4-yard rolls.

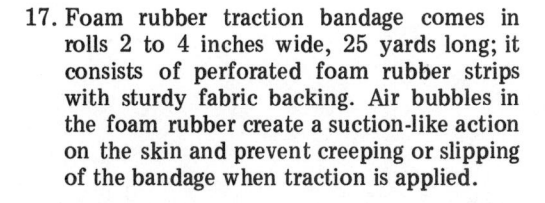

17. Foam rubber traction bandage comes in rolls 2 to 4 inches wide, 25 yards long; it consists of perforated foam rubber strips with sturdy fabric backing. Air bubbles in the foam rubber create a suction-like action on the skin and prevent creeping or slipping of the bandage when traction is applied.

18. Steripak (non-adhering sterile dressing) is a complete dressing that has eight layers of absorbent cellulose covered with a non-adhering perforated plastic film that is secured to a vented adhesive tape. It is useful for small-incision wounds, abrasions. Sizes are 4 × 8, 4 × 4, 2 × 4-1/2 inches.

19. Aseptic non-adhering dressing is an absorbent rayon that has sidewise stretchability, which allows it to mold to body contours without wrinkling (3 × 3, 3 × 8, 3 × 16 inches; also in 1/2-, 1-, and 2-inch wide rolls of 4 yards).

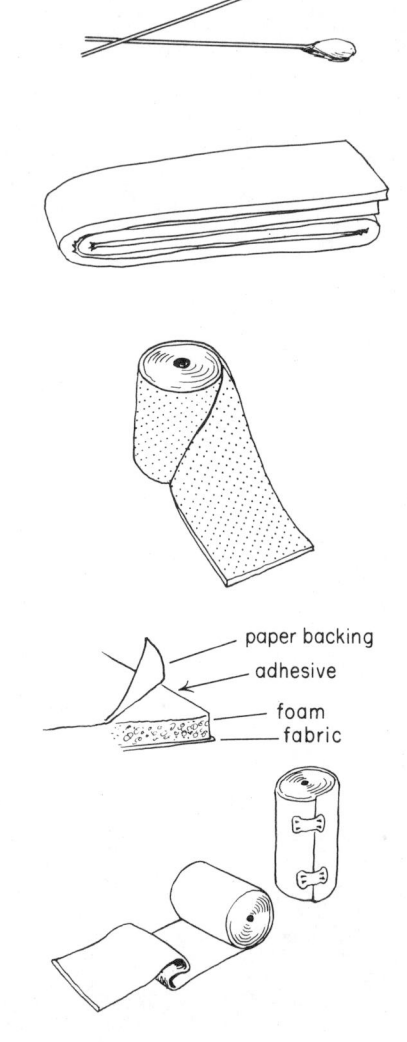

20. Kling bandage is a self-adhering gauze bandage that can stretch 40 per cent. It is used, in addition to various dressings for minor pressure on the head and breast, for burns and amputation stumps. It comes in 1, 2, 3, 4, and 6-inch wide rolls.

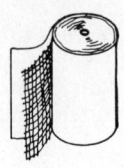

If you would like additional reading or experience with Aseptic Technique, confer with your instructor for assistance in following your own special area of interest.

ASEPTIC TECHNIQUE

POST-TEST

Select the one best answer:

1. The term that describes destruction of pathogenic microorganisms is
   a. antiseptic
   b. germicidal ✓
   c. conduction
   d. disinfect

2. A person who harbors a pathogenic organism and may show no symptoms is called a
   a. fomite
   b. carrier ✓
   c. host
   d. parasite

3. The layer of skin that sheds constantly and is a refuge for bacteria is called the
   a. dermis
   b. epidermis ✓
   c. sebaceous
   d. follicles

Circle "T" if the statement below is true and circle "F" if it is false.

T F 4. Cover the hair completely to prevent infection-contamination while in the surgical suite.

T F 5. Persons with colds are never admitted to the surgical suite.

T **F** 6. After the use of the brush in the surgical scrub, place the brush on the edge of the sink, clean the fingernails with a nail file, and then scrub the fingernails and hands again.

T F 7. Green soap with an alcohol rinse is considered as safe as pHisoHex for an effective surgical scrub.

T **F** 8. Rinse hands and arms allowing water to run *to* fingers *from* elbows.

T **F** 9. The 3-minute short scrub is used during a sterile procedure in the surgical suite if the hands have not been contaminated.

T F 10. The sterile towel used for drying the hands and arms is kept from touching the unsterile dress.

T **F** 11. The time in minutes needed for the *Surgical Suite* scrub and *Care of the Mother and Child* is the same.

Place the correct letter in the space provided:

_____ 12. The following factors must be considered in disinfection of microorganisms:

(1) concentration of chemical agent to be used.

(2) time needed for distruction of the organism.

(3) kind of material on which the microorganism is located.

(4) kind of organism to be destroyed.

(5) time of day at which disinfection takes place.

   a. all of the above
   b. none of the above
   c. (1) and (2)
   d. (1), (2), (3), and (4)

ASEPTIC TECHNIQUE

_____ 13. The method most often used to sterilize is:
   a. chemical treatments.   d. heat.
   b. radiation.   e. sunlight.
   c. cold.   f. open air.

_____ 14. Antiseptics:
   a. are germicidal.   c. prevent multiplication of bacteria.
   b. are bactericidal.   d. destroy all bacteria.

_____ 15. Transfer of infection occurs by indirect modes with the exeption of:
   a. moisture from mouth or nose.
   b. fomites.

_____ 16. The word *sterile* means
   a. without infection.
   b. free from pathogenic organisms.
   c. free from all living organisms.
   d. surgically clean.

_____ 17. In the open glove technique, the first step is to
   a. pick up the glove by placing the finger under the cuff.
   b. pick up the glove by the palm of the glove.
   c. pick up the glove by the folded edge of the cuff.

_____ 18. Select the *wrong* answer from the open glove techniques:
   a. Put on gloves without touching the outside of them with your bare hands.
   b. Avoid touching the side of the wrapper.
   c. Stay away from unsterile objects and the sterile table when putting on gloves.
   d. Hold the gloves slightly below your waistline to put on.

_____ 19. In putting on your sterile gown with surgical asepsis
   a. put the gown on and wait for someone to tie the back.
   b. hold the gown with your hands placed at shoulders inside the gown and wait for someone to pull the gown on.
   c. hold the gown by the neck ties and wait for someone to pull the gown over your shoulders.

_____ 20. Handle sterile articles with:
   a. sterile wrapper and gloves.   c. sterile gown and gloves.
   b. sterile forceps and gloves.   d. sterile nurse and gloves.

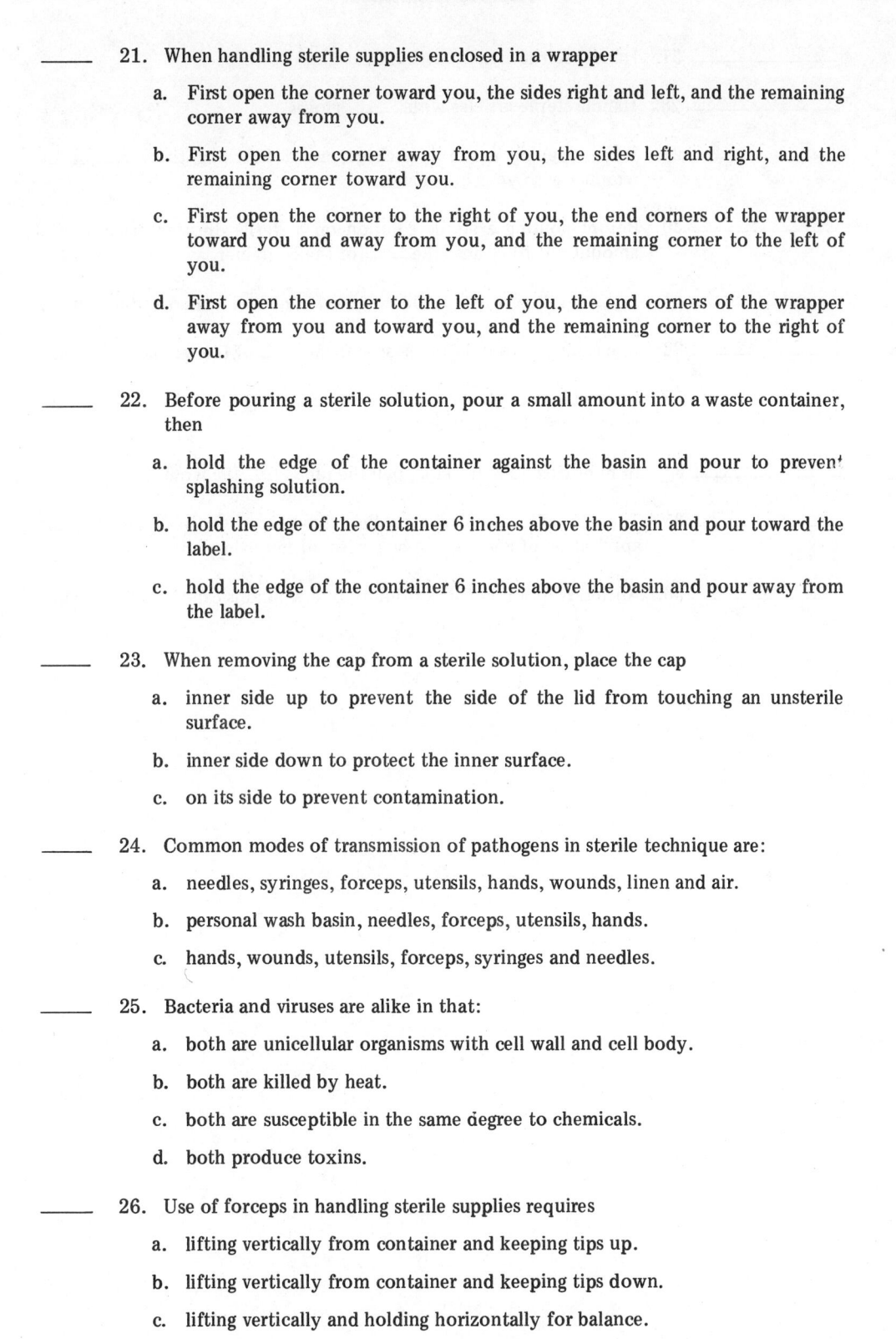

ASEPTIC TECHNIQUE

_____ 21. When handling sterile supplies enclosed in a wrapper

　　a. First open the corner toward you, the sides right and left, and the remaining corner away from you.

　　b. First open the corner away from you, the sides left and right, and the remaining corner toward you.

　　c. First open the corner to the right of you, the end corners of the wrapper toward you and away from you, and the remaining corner to the left of you.

　　d. First open the corner to the left of you, the end corners of the wrapper away from you and toward you, and the remaining corner to the right of you.

_____ 22. Before pouring a sterile solution, pour a small amount into a waste container, then

　　a. hold the edge of the container against the basin and pour to prevent splashing solution.

　　b. hold the edge of the container 6 inches above the basin and pour toward the label.

　　c. hold the edge of the container 6 inches above the basin and pour away from the label.

_____ 23. When removing the cap from a sterile solution, place the cap

　　a. inner side up to prevent the side of the lid from touching an unsterile surface.

　　b. inner side down to protect the inner surface.

　　c. on its side to prevent contamination.

_____ 24. Common modes of transmission of pathogens in sterile technique are:

　　a. needles, syringes, forceps, utensils, hands, wounds, linen and air.

　　b. personal wash basin, needles, forceps, utensils, hands.

　　c. hands, wounds, utensils, forceps, syringes and needles.

_____ 25. Bacteria and viruses are alike in that:

　　a. both are unicellular organisms with cell wall and cell body.

　　b. both are killed by heat.

　　c. both are susceptible in the same degree to chemicals.

　　d. both produce toxins.

_____ 26. Use of forceps in handling sterile supplies requires

　　a. lifting vertically from container and keeping tips up.

　　b. lifting vertically from container and keeping tips down.

　　c. lifting vertically and holding horizontally for balance.

ASEPTIC TECHNIQUE

_____ 27. Handle sterile articles with _____ transfer forceps or

_____ 28. Handle sterile articles with _____ gloves.

_____ 29. When opening a sterile package, avoid touching the _____ of the wrapper with your bare hands.

_____ 30. Before pouring a sterile solution on a sterile dressing, pour a small amount out to cleanse the _____ of the container.

_____ 31. _____ develops when a microorganism enters a wound and multiplies.

_____ 32. In cleaning a wound first cleanse from _____ of the wound downward.

_____ 33. Following the above cleansing process, begin at the _____ of the wound and clean outward.

_____ 34. In removing adhesive tape, pull the tape _____ the wound.

_____ 35. The use of _____ straps or ties allows removal of a dressing and application of another dressing without removing tape.

_____ 36. An interruption in the continuity of a wound is called a _____ wound.

ASEPTIC TECHNIQUE

POST-TEST ANNOTATED ANSWER SHEET

1. b, pp. 2-8.
2. b, p. 7.
3. b, p. 50.
4. T, p. 40.
5. T, p. 14.
6. F, p. 15.
7. T, p. 50.
8. F, p. 15.
9. F, p. 16
10. T, p. 16.
11. F, pp. 16, 18.
12. d, p. 9.
13. d, p. 9.
14. c, p. 50.
15. a, p. 7.
16. c, p. 3.
17. c, p. 17.
18. d, p. 10.

19. b, p. 20.
20. b, p. 34.
21. b, pp. 32, 33.
22. c, p. 38.
23. a, p. 38.
24. a, p. 3.
25. b, p. 7.
26. b, p. 38.
27. sterile, p. 34.
28. sterile, p. 34.
29. inside, p. 31.
30. lip or rim, p. 38.
31. Infection, p. 49.
32. top, p. 44.
33. edge, p. 44.
34. toward, p. 44.
35. Montgomery, p. 52.
36. gaping p. 49.

PERFORMANCE TEST

1. In the skill laboratory you will perform a surgical or OB scrub. You will put on and remove a sterile gown and gloves or you will gown a partner while you are wearing your sterile gown and gloves.

2. You will demonstrate opening a sterile package using pickup forceps and pouring a sterile solution from a bottle, and changing a sterile dressing.

3. At the completion of your demonstration activities, you should be able to discuss with your instructor at least four of the general priciples of aseptic technique, and at least four of the six classes of microorganisms and give examples of diseases that they cause.

PERFORMANCE CHECKLIST

SURGICAL SCRUB

1. Select and put on scrub suit.
2. Remove jewelry.
3. Test conductivity of shoes.
4. Put on mask and cover nose and mouth.
5. Prepare for scrub; roll up sleeves, adjust water temperature and flow.
6. Wet hands and apply detergent.
7. Wash hands and arms to 3 inches above elbows.
8. Rinse arms (fingertips to elbows with hands held upward away from uniform).
9. Clean fingernails.
10. Obtain sterile brush (pad) and apply detergent.
11. Scrub hands and arms 2 to 5 minutes.
12. Rinse arms and hands; hold upward away from uniform.
13. Discuss modification for OB or short scrub.

SELF-GOWNING TECHNIQUE

1. Dry hands and arms without contaminating hands.
2. Select and unfold sterile gown.
3. Open gown by holding at shoulder seam.
4. Slip arms into armholes. Keep arms held upward away from face.
5. Partner then pulls on gown and ties strings without contamination.
6. Partner straightens gown.

SELF-GLOVING (OPEN TECHNIQUE)

1. Pick up right glove with cuff edge.
2. Pull on glove.
3. Pick up left glove, insert right gloved fingers under cuff of sterile glove.
4. Pull left glove up over hand and gown cuff.
5. Pull right glove up over cuff of gown.
6. Adjust fingers of gloves.

CLOSED TECHNIQUE

1. Pick up right glove.
2. Place palm of right glove against palm of right hand, glove fingers pointing toward elbow.

ASEPTIC TECHNIQUE

3. Draw reverse side of glove back over end of sleeve, over gown cuff.
4. Pull on right glove and gown cuff simultaneously.
5. Adjust fingers in right glove with gowned left hand.
6. Pick up left glove with right hand.
7. Place left glove directly over left gown cuff, glove fingers pointing to elbow.
8. Draw glove back over end of sleeve and up over gown cuff.
9. Pull glove and ribbed gown cuff on hand simultaneously.
10. Hold hands upward away from face.

GOWNING AND GLOVING SOMEONE ELSE

1. Select sterile towel and hand to gownee. Towel is unfolded and laid in gownee's right palm.
2. Select and unfold gown.
3. Hold gown by shoulder seams, outside of gown toward self, armholes facing gownee.
4. Gownee puts arms in armholes with forceful downward motion.
5. Settle gown on gownee's shoulders without contaminating gloves.
6. Gownee's gown secured by unsterile person.
7. Pick up gownee's right glove, hold glove by cuff, with thumb of glove facing gownee. Hold your fingers away from gownee's unsterile hand.
8. Hold glove cuff firmly, waist high.
9. Gownee inserts right hand into glove.
10. Pull glove over cuff of gownee's gown.
11. Pick up left glove, thumb facing toward gownee.
12. Hold glove firmly, waist high, and spread cuff open laterally.
13. Gownee inserts left hand into glove.
14. Pull left glove onto hand and up over gown cuff.
15. Adjust fingers of gownee.
16. Hand sterile towel to gownee to cover gloves until procedure starts.

OPENING STERILE PACKAGE

1. Obtain sterile item.
2. Loosen wrapper fastener and discard.
3. Open distal flap, then left flap, then right flap, and finally proximal flap. Do not reach across sterile field; handle outside of wrapper only.
4. Place item on sterile wrapper, avoiding contamination.
5. Hand item to someone in sterile field.

ASEPTIC TECHNIQUE

STERILE HANDLING WITH PICKUP FORCEPS

1. Grasp forceps by handles, lift vertically, tip downward (do not touch sides of container), open ratchets.
2. Pick up sterile items and place on sterile wrapper or surface.
3. Replace forceps in container, avoiding contamination.

POURING STERILE SOLUTIONS

1. Remove cap and cover from container and place cap upside down on table.
2. Unwrap sterile basin.
3. Pour solution into basin, label up, from 6 inch height. Do not splash.
4. Replace cover without contamination, and return container to storage.

HOLDING VIAL TO WITHDRAW STERILE SOLUTION

1. Obtain vial and check labels with doctor's order.
2. Clean vial stopper with alcohol pledget.
3. Hold vial firmly, label up.
4. Sterile person inserts sterile needle into vial stopper, inserts air and withdraws solution into syringe.
5. Sterile person withdraws vial.
6. Vial is replaced in storage, or discarded, as indicated.

CHANGING STERILE DRESSING

1. Collect supplies and prepare patient and environment.
2. Loosen binder or tape.
3. Remove soiled dressing and discard.
4. Inspect wound.
5. Put on sterile gloves, if appropriate, or use sterile forceps.
6. Drape wound.
7. Cleanse around wound with antiseptic. Cleanse with circular motion.
8. Apply ointment or powder, if indicated.
9. Apply dressing.
10. Discard gloves or forceps.
11. Apply dressing retainer.
12. Leave patient comfortable and return items to storage.
13. Record procedure.

Unit 2

PREPARATION AND ADMINISTRATION OF MEDICATIONS

(Oral, Subcutaneous, Intramuscular, Intravenous, Intradermal, Topical, Inhalant)

I. DIRECTIONS TO THE STUDENT

You are to proceed through this Unit using the workbook as your guide. You will need to practice the skill for giving medications by using the appropriate equipment found in the skills laboratory. After you have completed the lesson and your practice of the procedures, arrange with your instructor to take the performance test. For this unit you will need the following items:

1. This workbook.
2. Patient medicine card.
3. Patient medications for oral, injectable, suppository, topical and inhalation drugs.
4. Souffle cup, if medicine is in solid form.
5. Graduated medicine droppers, minim glass, medicine glass (plastic or glass), graduated cylinder and syringe if the medicine is in liquid form.
6. Doctor's order sheet and Kardex card.
7. Medicine tray.

Please read the following paragraphs carefully. They will tell you what you will be expected to know and how you will be expected to set up and give medications, in order to care for the patient. If you feel that you have the necessary skills and would be wasting your time studying this material, discuss this with your instructor, and arrange to take the performance test. All students must demonstrate their skills in setting up and giving medications safely and efficiently to the patient.

II. GENERAL PERFORMANCE OBJECTIVE

Upon completion of this Unit, you will be able to prepare and give medications to the patient accurately, efficiently and safely.

III. SPECIFIC PERFORMANCE OBJECTIVES

When you have finished this lesson, you will be able to:

1. Prepare and give oral medications to the patient in an accurate, efficient, and safe manner that will not cause apprehension or injury to the patient.

2. Prepare and give subcutaneous, intramuscular, and intradermal injection medications to the patient in an accurate, efficient, and safe manner that will not cause apprehension or injury to the patient.

3. Prepare and give intravenous medications in an accurate, efficient, and safe manner that will not cause apprehension or injury to the patient.

4. Prepare and place inhalation medications in the inhalation equipment in an accurate, efficient, and safe manner that will not cause apprehension or injury to the patient.

5. Apply topical medications to the patient in an accurate, efficient, and safe manner that will not cause apprehension or injury to the patient.

6. Prepare and give rectal medications to the patient in an accurate, efficient, and safe manner that will not cause apprehension or injury to the patient.

IV. VOCABULARY

Read the definitions of the terms listed below. Do not attempt to memorize these definitions before proceeding with the lesson. Each term will be explained or defined again in the text. On completion of the lesson, however, you should know the correct definitions.

ampule (ampoule)—glass capsule containing a sterile solution of a drug, used for intravenous (IV), intramuscular (IM), or hypodermic (H) injection.

analgesic—drug used to relieve pain.

anaphylactic shock—intense reaction to an injection of a protein substance to which the patient is sensitized. Symptoms of shock result, which may be immediate or delayed, slight, severe or fatal.

anesthetic—drug that produces insensibility to pain.

anodyne—drug used to relieve pain (milder than an analgesic).

anthelmintic (vermifuge)—drug that destroys or expels worms.

antidote—preparation that neutralizes the effects of a poison.

antipruritic—drug that relieves itching.

antipyretic—drug that reduces fever.

antispasmodic—drug that lessens contraction of muscles and convulsions.

apothecary measure—the series of units of liquid measure (such as the gallon, pint, fluid ounce, minim).

astringent (styptic, hemostat)—agent or substance that checks secretions from wounds or mucous membranes, stops bleeding, lessens peristalsis or hardens tissue.

bitters—herb tonic that increases the appetite and flow of gastric juices.

capsule—medication enclosed in a gelatinous container that disguises the taste of the enclosed substance.

caustic—chemical that burns or destroys tissue.

circadian rhythm—cyclical variation occurring within a 24-hour period (e.g., sleeping, eating, or resting).

colloid—substance that is suspended and undissolved and is not diffusible through animal membrane (e.g., gelatin, albumin).

confection—medicinal preparation made with syrup, sugar or honey to disguise bad-tasting substances.

convulsant—a drug or agent that causes convulsions.

crude drug—unrefined (unprocessed) drug.

deodorant—agent that destroys or neutralizes foul odors.

depressant—agent that temporarily decreases a body function (e.g., cardiac, respiratory).

diaphoresis—profuse perspiration.

diaphoretic—drug that produces diaphoresis.

dilute—to diminish the strength of a mixture by admixture.

diuretic—drug that increases urine flow.

elixir—drug dissolved in sweetened or flavored alcohol and water.

emetic—agent that induces vomiting.

emollient—product that softens or soothes.
emulsion—mixture of oil and water having a milky appearance and consistency.
expectorant—drug that increases bronchial secretions and expectoration.
extract—a product (such as an essence or concentrate) prepared by extracting a soluble substance with alcohol. The remaining sediment (the extract) is usually several times stronger than the crude drug itself, e.g., cascara tablets used as a laxative.
fluid extract—concentrated fluid preparation of a drug, always 100 per cent in strength (1 gm. of drug to 1 cc. solution).
generic name—family name of a drug derived from the source of the drug.
hemostatic—drug that checks bleeding.
hypnotic—drug that produces sleep.
hypodermic—medication adapted for use in, or administered by injection beneath, the skin; hypodermics may be given subcutaneously, intramuscularly, intraspinally, or intravenously.
hypodermoclysis—injection of fluids into the subcutaneous tissues to supply the body quickly with large amounts of fluid. This method is used when other medication routes are unavailable because of the patient's condition.
inunction—act of anointing or applying an ointment with friction.
laxative (purgative, cathartic)—drug that produces a cleansing evacuation of the bowels.
liniment—liquid or soft preparation of a drug that is applied by rubbing on the skin.
lotion—liquid medicinal preparation for local, external application to a body part, e.g., calamine lotion.
lozenge (troche)—flat disc of a drug combined with sugar or other soothing agent and held in the mouth until it dissolves; e.g., cough drop.
metric—decimal system of weights and measures based on the meter (1 meter equals 39.37 inches).
miotic—drug used to contract the pupil of the eye.
mydriatic—drug used to dilate the pupil of the eye.
ointment (salve, unguent)—preparation consisting of a fatty substance (Vaseline, lard, lanolin) and a medicament. When applied to skin or mucous membrane, it is melted by the body heat and absorbed, e.g., A and D ointment, various antibiotic ointments.
oxytoxic—drug used to increase uterine contractions.
pill—globe-shaped solid form of drug that can be swallowed comfortably.
powders—two or more drugs ground up into a powder and thoroughly mixed.
proprietary name—name or trademark given to a drug by the manufacturer. For example, several manufacturers produce tetracycline (generic name); the manufacturers call it variously Achromycin, Panamycin, Tetracyn, Terramycin, etc.
pure drug—drug which has been refined (processed) to remove all impurities.
seasonal rhythm—cyclical variation from one season to another or year to year.
sedative—drug that lessens the activity of an organ of the body, or decreases nervous excitation.
solubility—ability to be dissolved.
solute—substance dissolved in a liquid.
solution—solvent containing a dissolved drug.
solvent—producing a solution; a liquid holding another substantial solution.
spirits—alcohol solutions of easily vaporized drugs.
stimulant—drug that temporarily increases functional activity, e.g., cardiac stimulant or respiratory stimulant.
stock supply—large supply of a drug, which may be kept in the pharmacy, on the unit in a medication storage area, and also can be the filled volume prescription for an individual patient.
suppository—cone-shaped or cylindrical medicament made with cocoa butter; when inserted into a body cavity (rectum, vagina, urethra), the suppository is dissolved and its components absorbed.
syrup—solution of sugar, water and flavoring in which drugs can be dissolved.
tablets—small discs of different sizes and thicknesses containing compressed, dried, powdered drugs.

tincture—diluted alcoholic solution, generally a nonvolatile substance in varying strengths from 10 per cent to 20 per cent (10 per cent being the most common standard, e.g., tincture of benzoin).

tonic—agent or drug that invigorates, restores, refreshes, or stimulates.

unit-dose—system for dispensing premeasured, prepackaged, prelabeled portions of drugs for an individual patient.

vasoconstrictor—drug that constricts the blood vessel.

vasodilator—drug that dilates the blood vessels; it helps to reduce the blood pressure by relaxing the muscles in the blood vessels.

vescettes—effervescent salts compressed into a tablet, e.g., Alka-Seltzer.

vesicant—agent or drug that produces blisters.

volatile—evaporating readily at a relatively low temperature.

Z track—a method of giving a deep intramuscular injection for certain iron preparations.

V. INTRODUCTION

Drug therapy as a method for treating diseases is a vitally important function that is carried out by the nurse. This Unit will teach you the procedure for giving medications via the various routes: oral, intramuscular, subcutaneous, intradermal, intravenous, inhalation, inunction. (You learned how to give rectal suppositories in Unit 22, Bowel Elimination.)

The pharmacologic action of specific drugs will be learned as you care for specific patients; it will not be discussed in this Unit. However, there is some general background information about drugs that you should know.

Standardization of drugs ensures uniformity of preparation and strength. In the early nineteenth century a committee of physicians and pharmacists was appointed in each country to determine the standards of acceptable preparation and strength of drugs. The official pronouncement of the standards is published in a book which is known as the Pharmacopeia. Drugs which conform to the standards set by the U. S. Committee are listed as U.S.P. (*The United States Pharmacopeia*). Other countries have similar designations, e.g., B.P. (*British Pharmacopoeia*). Some preparations that are official in one country may not be official in other countries. However, there are efforts to standardize drugs throughout the world. The *Pharmacopeia Internationalis*, the World Health Organization's publication, attempts to standardize drugs on a worldwide basis. The Pharmacopeia is revised regularly, with supplements printed between revisions to keep it up to date. Your pharmacists should have the current listing.

The *National Formulary* (N.F.), published frequently by the American Pharmaceutical Association, lists drugs and their methods of preparation which are not included in the Pharmacopeia. It is the official book for pharmacists.

According to the Federal Food, Drug, and Cosmetic Act of 1938, both the U.S.P. and the N.F. are legal standard books for drugs. The Act is amended periodically. It protects the physician and the public by providing controls for assuring the purity, standards, and composition of foods, drugs, and cosmetics. The first federal drug legislation began with the Pure Food Act of 1906, subsequently replaced by the Federal Food, Drug, and Cosmetic Act of 1938. The Act is implemented by the Food and Drug Administration (FDA), a department within the Department of Health, Education, and Welfare (HEW). The National Academy of Sciences-National Research Council (NAS-NRC) has been contracted to survey the effectiveness of drugs.

Another book that lists new drugs is put out annually by the American Medical Association; it is entitled, *New and Nonofficial Remedies* (N.N.R.).

The Dispensatory of the United States of America is a nonofficial, general reference book containing information on the ingredients, preparation and methods of compounding medications.

The Physicians' Desk Reference (P.D.R.), an annual reference publication that describes various pharmaceuticals and biologicals, is a common reference tool used by health workers.

The *trade name* (or proprietary name) is the manufacturer's name for a drug, used because it is generally easier to spell, pronounce or remember than the official (generic) name; e.g., Demerol is Winthrop Laboratories' brand name for the drug meperidine (generic name).

The development and usage of drugs are regulated not only by the FDA, but by various other federal and state laws as well.

The *Harrison Narcotic Act* went into effect in 1917 and has had many subsequent amendments. It regulates the manufacturing, dispensing, selling or prescription of narcotic drugs that produce stupor or sleep. The drugs in this group include opium as well as its compounds and derivatives, all of which are habit-forming. Strict records must be kept by the manufacturers, dispensers, sellers and prescribers of narcotic drugs. These records must be available at any time to the Department of Internal Revenue and must be kept for at least a two-year period. Another strict regulation regarding narcotics requires that they be kept in a locked drawer or cabinet. ANY UNAUTHORIZED INDIVIDUAL WHO HAS ANY OF THESE NARCOTIC DRUGS IN HIS POSSESSION IS SUBJECT TO A STIFF FINE AND/OR LENGTHY IMPRISONMENT!

Every agency that administers narcotics (whether hospital, clinic, or whatever) is legally obliged to keep a special book to record issuance of every drug, dose, date, name of person to whom it is given, and the signature of the individual giving the medication. The records are similar in all agencies and must be kept by the nurse and the pharmacist.

There are some exemptions to the narcotic regulations, e.g., when the drug meets certain small quanity requirements, such as less than one grain of codeine in a common cough medicine, such as elixir of terpin hydrate. Laws change, however, and your pharmacist can tell you about the current rulings.

States also have various laws regulating the manufacture and sale of barbiturates (drugs that are used as sedatives or hypnotics to produce sleep, but do not relieve pain). Barbiturates are synthetic compounds of barbital.

Each agency that you work in will have its own policies and procedures which serve to supplement and comply with state and federal regulations. It is your responsibility to learn these guidelines when you accept employment.

Under the various laws and regulations regarding medications:

—physicians *prescribe* medications;

—some nurses in extended roles prescribe designated medicines;

—pharmacists *compound*, *prepare*, *furnish*, or *issue* medications for immediate or future administration;

—registered nurses, licensed practical nurses, licensed vocational nurses, student nurses, and specified staff members such as respiratory therapy technicians (therapists), certain medical laboratory technicians (technologists), pharmacy technicians and the like, *administer* immediate, individual doses of medications.

Although licensed nursing personnel and other designated technicians still prepare and administer doses of medications to individual patients, within the last decade a new pharmacy distribution system known as *unit-dose* has become widely accepted. It should be stressed that the unit-dose system is a total agency or company system (for use by physicians, pharmacists, administrators, nurses, and other designated technicians). Thus it could be used not only within a large medical center or clinic, but also by satellite health agencies or a chain of health agencies, to effect uniform standards of safety, economy, and efficiency in a medication system.

The unit-dose medication system provides a premeasured, prepackaged, prelabeled individual portion of medication for patients. All medications, capsules, tablets, liquids, barbiturates, narcotics, suppositories, lotions, prefilled syringes for injections, etc., can be handled via the unit-dose system. Floor stock and emergency drugs are also available in this system.

The unit-dose system offers a high degree of accuracy, safety, speed, and convenience for those who prepare and administer the medications. In spite of these advantages, however, nurses who learned to administer according to the old rule, "*never* give a medication prepared by someone else", are frequently apprehensive and obstinate about trusting the unit-dose system; because of their earlier training, they believe that "the patient's safety is endangered." Notwithstanding this attitude, various unit-dose research studies in the last decade documented by the American Society of Hospital Pharmacists (ASHP) have recognized the benefits of the system, e.g.:

1. *Dramatic savings of time* (which would otherwise have been required to transcribe a medication order) result. In the unit-dose system, a copy of the original order (usually a carbon copy) is sent directly to the pharmacist for interpretation and filling. The only transcription needed by nursing is the transfer of the order to the medication record (Kardex). This also prevents frequent medication transcription errors. Various forms of nursing medication records are being used, but the most efficient current methods eliminate the need for medication cards. The medication order is transcribed directly on the medication Kardex which in turn is used to give and record the medication. Thus, the patient's medication record is current at all times, and becomes a permanent part of his or her chart.

   NOTE: One difficulty has arisen in this practice. Since the medication record is a part of the unit Kardex System, the individual patient's medication record does not appear on the patient's chart until the time of discharge, causing a continuing problem for the nurses and physicians. It is solved in a variety of ways: making duplicate medication records, one of which can be kept on the patient's chart for daily use by the physician; daily photocopying of the medication record, and placing it in the patient's chart; keeping the medication record on a flip-chart at the patient's bedside. Variations of these routines continue to evolve; no single system seems to fit all situations.

2. *Refill drug orders are handled entirely by the pharmacists* from their Patient Profile Record. This record is initiated by the pharmacist when the original order is received and it eliminates the need for a nurse to check all the orders and prepare refill prescriptions. The Patient Profile Record not only provides an accounting mechanism, listing charges for medications actually used, but it also supplies essential drug information data (such as age, weight, sex, allergies, diagnosis) so that the pharmacist can monitor drug therapy.

3. *The pharmacy delivers all medications* at designated times to the nursing unit, and therefore nursing personnel are no longer required to pick up medications at the pharmacy.

4. *Proof-of-use forms for sedatives and hypnotics are eliminated* on the nursing units, and thus the familiar intershift counting of sedatives and hypnotics is no longer required. Control of sedatives and hypnotics is handled entirely by the pharmacist. The nurse's time is further saved because she no longer has to record on proof-of-use forms, although these forms must still be maintained for narcotics in many agencies. As a result of increased efficiency and control mechanisms in the unit-dose system, perhaps proof-of-use forms will entirely disappear from the nursing units and the control mechanism for narcotics, sedatives and hypnotics will also be in the hands of the pharmacist, thus assuring even more time for nurses to give direct care to the patient.

5. *Credit processing for unused drugs is eliminated* by the unit-dose system. The unused drugs are returned to the pharmacy, where they are promptly removed from the pharmacy record and no charge is made for them. The pharmacy charge system for unit-dose drugs requires charging only when the medication is actually used.

6. *Preparation of injectables by the pharmacy could save as much as 12 hours a day or more* for the nurses giving injectables on a busy unit. This time could better be used recording and observing the patient's medication reactions; e.g., Was the pain or nausea eliminated? Did the diarrhea or bleeding cease?

PREPARATION AND ADMINISTRATION OF MEDICATIONS

7. *Floor stocks could be decreased*, thereby reducing the cost of medications held in stand-by status on the clinical unit.

8. *Savings on materials result*, since narcotic proof-of-use forms, medication cards, credit vouchers, medication cups, and the like are almost entirely eliminated.

It can be seen from the foregoing that the nurse's role in the medication scheme is changing. She may continue to prepare and administer medications, or another technician (such as in the pharmacy, medical laboratory, respiratory therapy unit, etc.) may do so. However, in either case, several vital responsibilities remain with the nurse:

1. The nurse continues to be responsible for *insuring safe patient care*. In other words, she must see that aseptic technique is carried out and that administering of medication (oral, IM, IV, etc.) is correct.

2. The nurse continues to be responsible for *observing the effect of medication* on the patient's physical or mental status. (Is the response immediate or delayed? Is the general condition improving or disintegrating? Is the response acceptable according to the age and diagnosis?) Some of these observations are primarily for the nurse's benefit as she plans the nursing care program for the patient. Some observations are important for the physician, pharmacist, radiologist, or other members of the health team as they develop their continuing patient care plans.

3. The nurse *maintains open communication channels* for reporting patient response to the drug therapy to co-workers on the health care team (such as the physician, pharmacist, various technicians).

4. The nurse is required to *record the patient's response* to the drug therapy.

5. The nurse is responsible for *using her pharmacologic knowledge* about drugs to develop continuity of care plans with other members of the health team.

6. The nurse must *teach the patient* about his drugs when he is ready for discharge.

7. The nurse is obligated to *assess the patient's request for various PRN medications* based on scientific principles of chemistry, physiology and psychology. She should try appropriate nursing measures before resorting to giving (or having administered) the medication. For example, she may offer a backrub and straighten the linens for the restless patient who can't sleep, rather than give the PRN sedative. Thus the nurse can contribute to decreasing drug dependence, a positive health concept.

The greatest benefit of the unit-dose distribution system is the near freedom from medication error. The second most important benefit of the system is the speed with which it is carried out, allowing the nursing personnel valuable time to give direct nursing care. More time is also available to pharmacy personnel to become directly involved in patient and staff contact, and to assist in managing improved drug therapy programs. Beyond this, the need for large stock supplies of seldom-used drugs is eliminated, or at least strictly controlled.

Safety precautions that must be taken by the individual who is administering medications, regardless of the route of administration, are as follows:

1. Give the *right drug* by checking the label on the medication with the medication order (Kardex or medicine card).

2. Give the *right dose* by again checking the medication order with the label on the medication. If a dosage is ordered that differs from the label on the medication, there is reason to verify the dosage calculation. You will learn how to calculate various dosages from a variety of stock amounts. Since the need for calculating drug dosages that vary from the ordered dosage is rare today, it is wise to have someone else check your calculations to assure that the correct dosage has been determined. (With the unit-dose system, this would be the responsibility of the pharmacist.)

3. Give the drug to the *right patient* by checking the name on the medication order, the Kardex, and the patient's identification. Do not call the patient by name; patients tend to answer to any name, even if it is not their own. Follow your agency procedure for checking your patient's identity.

4. Give the drug by the *right method* by again checking the medication order with the medication that you receive. Many drugs come in various forms, such as oral, IM, IV. Thus you must be sure that you give the drug in the form that is ordered for the patient; e.g., if a patient is vomiting, it would be unreasonable to give the oral preparation. However, the same medication may be available in an injectable form.

5. Give the drug at the *right time*, once more by comparing the medication order with the medication. The effects of drugs differ when given at different times. Often a sustained level of medication in the blood stream is critically important to the drug regime (e.g., in the use of antibiotics, or anticoagulants), and therefore rigid adherence to a prescribed time schedule is mandatory.

6. *Avoid distractions or interruptions* when preparing or administering drugs. In other words, keep your mind on the important and serious duty that you are performing.

7. Do not give *outdated drugs*, or ones which have changed color.

All of these safety factors are minimized by utilizing the unit-dose system, which is likely to be adopted by everyone in the foreseeable future.

ITEM 1: ORAL MEDICATIONS

A. *Preparation of Solid and Liquid Medications*

Important Steps	Key Points
1. Obtain the patient's medication record.	There are many settings and systems for preparing medicines; the term "medication record" is used here to mean medicine card, medication Kardex, or patient's chart (frequently used in clinics and homes).
	Medication cards are stored in hourly packets in the medication rack in the medicine room or on the medication cart.
	The medication Kardex may be kept in the medicine room, at the nurses' station, or on the medication cart.
2. Compare the medication record with the physician's order.	NOTE: With the changing role of the nurse, some nurse specialists or practitioners are permitted to write certain drug orders. Follow your agency procedure for this.
	Compare the medication record and the original order for accuracy of patient's name, identification number (if used; it may not be in a physician's office, the home, or industrial plant); name of the drug; the dosage; the time schedule, if it is given; the route of administration—oral (O), hypodermic (H), intramuscular (IM), intravenous (IV), etc.

PREPARATION AND ADMINISTRATION OF MEDICATIONS 71

Important Steps	Key Points
3. Wash your hands.	Use the nearest lavatory—in the medicine room, treatment room, patient's room.

Some agencies keep the patient's medication in a two-way cupboard in the patient's room called a "Nurseserver". |
| 4. Assemble the equipment. | Clear the medicine tray or cart; obtain paper souffle cups for solids and calibrated medicine cups (glass, plastic, paper) for liquids.

When handling the cups, handle only the *outside* of the cup. NEVER put your fingers on the inside of the cup. Even though your hands have been washed, they may still harbor some pathogens. If you touch the inside of the cup, the medicine will come in contact with pathogens that will then be ingested by the patient. In his already weakened condition he is vulnerable and would be exposed unnecessarily to disease. Therefore, if you accidentally touch the inside of the cup, discard it and obtain a new one.

NOTE: Unit-dose liquid laxatives come in disposable, premeasured cups. The patient drinks directly from the cup. |
| 5. Select the medication from the shelf or drawer. | Remove the bottle or prepackaged individual dose.

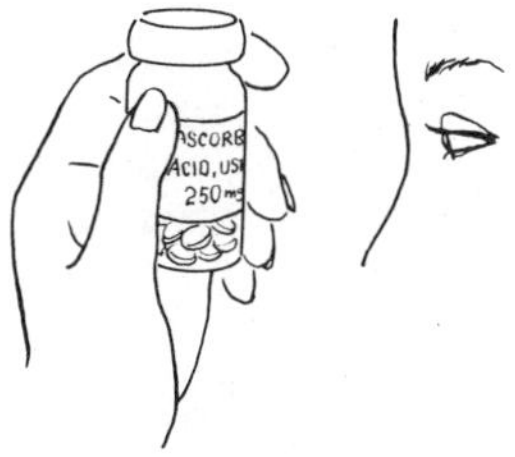

When you take the medication from its storage space, raise it to eye level and read the label as you:

(a) *remove* it from storage;

(b) *pour* the medication into the medicine cup;

(c) *return* the bottle to the shelf.

Obviously, if you are using a prepackaged unit (single-dose) steps (b) and (c) above would be omitted.

Read the label for patient's name, ID number (if indicated), room number (if indicated), name of drug, and dosage. |
| 6. Compare the medication record with the label on the medication bottle. | If it is easier to pick up the medicine card and hold it next to the medicine bottle, do so. However, if you are using the Kardex or chart, it may be easier to have it lying open on a nearby surface with the medicine bottle close by.

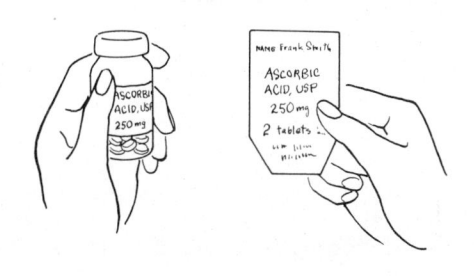

Place the medication card on the tray; set the medicine bottle down. |

PREPARATION AND ADMINISTRATION OF MEDICATIONS

Important Steps	Key Points
7. Calculate correct dosage of drug to be given.	If the medication record says: Tetrax 500 mgm BID, and the medicine in the bottle is Tetrax 250 mgm, then from your knowledge of ratios you know that you will give two 250 mgm capsules to provide the 500 mgm dose. (This step is omitted if the unit-dose system is used.)
8. Remove the bottle cap (lid).	Pick up the medicine bottle and lift off the cap, or unscrew the lid, as required.
9. Pour the medication.	For the pill or capsule: pour the desired number of tablets or capsules into the lid of the container, set the container aside, then transfer the tablets or capsules into the medicine cup.
	Pouring the medicine into the lid first prevents the possibility of putting the wrong amount in the patient's medicine cup; any excess would be wasted because <u>medicines ARE NEVER returned to the stock container.</u>
	NOTE: In the unit-dose system, the unused medication can be returned to the pharmacy stock since the package is individually wrapped and the medication and dosage are clearly labeled on each dose.
	Some children, geriatric patients, or confused patients may have difficulty swallowing a pill; for such people, the pill should be crushed in the medicine cup by using a spoon (available in the medication preparation area).
	CAUTION FOR LIQUID: place the lid *upside down* on a nearby flat surface so that the inside of the lid is not contaminated. Hold the bottle so that the label is uppermost to keep the liquid from soiling the label.
	Pour the desired amount of liquid into the calibrated medicine cup. Hold the medicine cup at eye level so that you can easily see what you are doing. Rotate the cup until you can clearly read the calibration scale. Use your thumbnail to mark the level on the calibration scale to which you will pour the medicine.
	Use the *lowest point of the meniscus* for reading the dose. (When a liquid is poured into a medicine cup, capillary action causes the portion of the fluid that is in contact with the glass to draw upward, making the surface of the liquid hollow and concave.)
10. Verify the poured medication with the medicine order.	Compare the label or stock container with the drug order. Read: patient's name, room number, drug, dosage, route, time of administration.

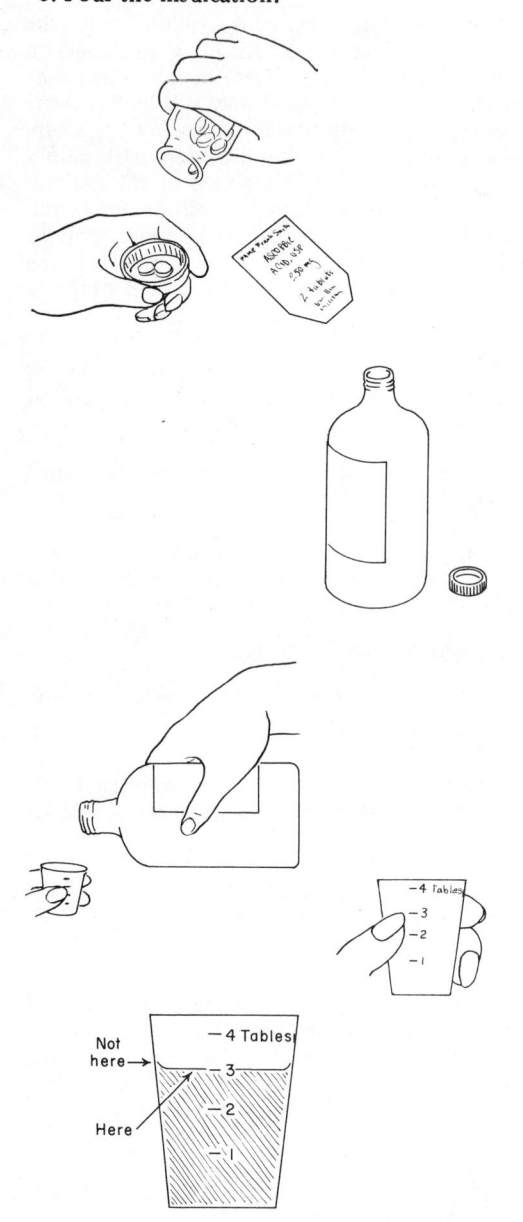

PREPARATION AND ADMINISTRATION OF MEDICATIONS 73

Important Steps	Key Points
11. Place the poured medicine on the tray.	Exact placement on the medication tray will depend upon the system that your agency utilizes: (a) Individual tray, using medication card (b) Trays for multiple drugs using medicine cards (c) Medication cart system with medicine cards (d) Medication cart and unit-dose system. NOTE: If you are using the medication card sytem *always* keep the medication card and the poured medicine *together.*
12. Return the stock bottle.	Securely replace the lid on the container and place the bottle on the medicine shelf or in the drawer. NOTE: If you are returning a bottle of liquid medicine on which some of the liquid has soiled the outside of the bottle, wipe it clean with a paper towel before returning it to storage.

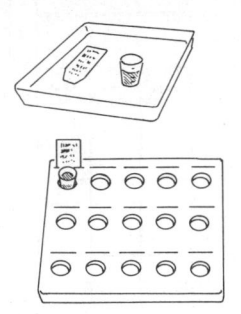

B. *Preparation of Oral Narcotic from Narcotic Dispenser*

   Utilization of a Controlled Dispenser for Preparing Tablets or Capsules for Distribution. Most agencies use a controlled dispensing system for distributing narcotics and hypnotics. With the advent of the unit-dose system, this procedure may become obsolete. Controlled dispensers are either reusable or disposable. You must follow agency procedure. Generally, pills or capsules are prepared by the pharmacist (or the pharmaceutical firm in the case of disposable containers), in plastic sectioned containers, usually with 25 compartments that are clearly marked on top of the container as #1, #2, #3, and so forth. The top surface of the container is movable, so that when the small opening in the top cover is centered over one of the compartments, the container can be inverted over the medicine cup and the pill or capsule falls into the cup without being handled. The dial proceeds counterclockwise in the ceramic dispenser from #25, to #24, to #23, and so on. The plastic cover on the box can be moved from distal compartment #25 to the proximal compartment #1 by pulling the lid toward you to uncover the next compartment, permitting you to drop that pill or capsule into the medicine cup. Thus you have an accurate count of the numbers of pills (capsules) left in the container after each use. The number can quickly be verified at the time each staff shift counts the narcotics before handing over the narcotic keys to the next shift.

   As soon as you have poured the medicine, verify the label on the dispenser with the patient's medication record. Replace the dispenser. Record the medication on the medication record form as seen in the following examples. When you have recorded the medications, proceed to the patient's room as described in Item 1,C, below.

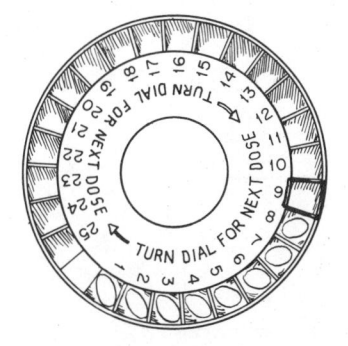

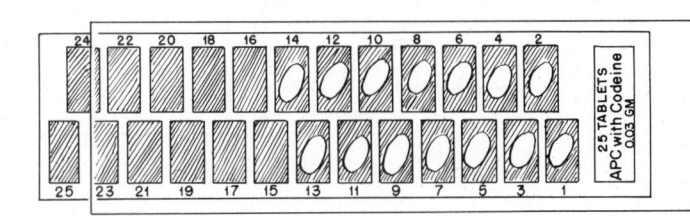

PREPARATION AND ADMINISTRATION OF MEDICATIONS

UCLA HOSPITALS & CLINICS
NARCOTIC ADMINISTRATION & INVENTORY RECORD

EACH SHIFT NARCOTIC INVENTORY REQUIRES TWO SIGNATURES. IF INITIALS ARE USED, PLEASE SIGN FULL SIGNATURE ON REVERSE SIDE OF THIS CARD.

Pharm. _____ Rn. _____ CART LOCATION: _____ DATE: _____

Name of Patient	DATE	TIME	RN	Name of Patient	DATE	TIME	RN
30				15			
29				14			
28				13			
27				12			
26				11			
25				10			
24				9			
23				8			
22				7			
21				6			
20				5			
19				4			
18				3			
17				2			
16				1			

NAME OF MEDICATION: _____

FORM 186 (REV AUG 72)

RECEIPT OF DELIVERY N⁰ 92806

Date Issued _____
Received of the Pharmacy _____
for _____
Signed _____
Ret'd Unused _____
Date Sheet Ret'd _____

Date Sheet Ret'd _____

UNIVERSITY OF CALIFORNIA HOSPITALS N⁰ 92806
CONTROLLED SUBSTANCE RECORD

To the Pharmacy
The following is an accurate record of _____
as used on _____

Record each tablet on separate line. Record losses under "Remarks," including responsibility.

Date	Time	No.	Patient	Room	Physician	Drug and Amount	Volume	Issued to	Bal.
		25							
		24							
		23							
		22							
		21							
		20							
		9							
		8							
		7							
		6							
		5							
		4							
		3							
		2							
		1							

Remarks: _____

Signed: _____ Resident   Signed: _____ Head Nurse

Series 6122—L 72, 73

PREPARATION AND ADMINISTRATION OF MEDICATIONS

C. *Administration of Oral Medication*

Important Steps	Key Points
1. Wash your hands.	
2. Take the medication to the patient.	Grasp the medication tray securely so that you do not drop it while moving along the hallways and into the patient rooms. Be sure that medicine cups or unit-dose medicines do not become separated from their patient identification (card, Kardex, or special unit-dose drawer).
3. Approach, identify, and explain the procedure to the patient.	Greet the patient warmly and verify his name (Identaband, or patient record if working in a clinic, office, or home setting). Explain that you are going to give him his medicine. In many agencies the physicians want their patients to know what medications they are receiving and for what reason. For example: "Mr. Johns, I'm going to give you some Demerol to relieve the pain. I will check back with you in 15 minutes to see if you are beginning to get some relief." In some agencies, nurses are still not permitted to discuss medicines with their patients. Follow your agency procedure. However, the fact that varying new health delivery systems are being tried will eventually lead to patients who are more knowledgeable about the exact treatment they are receiving, as well as the indications for therapy.
4. Hand the medicine to the patient.	If the patient's arms are restrained for any reason, you may have to place the medicine cup to his lips and assist him in taking the medicine. NOTE: If you are using the unit-dose system, open the package and drop the medicine into the patient's hand or mouth. Discard the wrapper in the designated container.
5. Hand a glass of water to the patient.	Pour a glass of fresh water for the patient. Assist him in drinking, if necessary. NOTE: _Water is not given following the administration of cough syrup._
6. Observe the patient closely.	Be sure that he swallows the medication. Sometimes a patient is crafty; he may hold the medicine in his mouth until you leave the room, and then will spit it out. Other patients will stockpile their medicines in order to take an overdose later on. If the patient has trouble swallowing a pill or capsule, have him put it as far back on his tongue as possible before taking the water and swallowing.

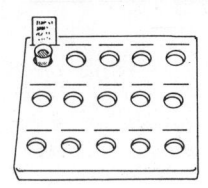

PREPARATION AND ADMINISTRATION OF MEDICATIONS

Important Steps	Key Points
	If the medicine has an unpleasant taste, it can be mixed with a fruit juice or bite of food to disguise the taste; or you can offer some ice chips to suck on immediately before taking the medicine. (Ice seems to deaden the taste buds in the tongue.)
	Observe the patient's initial reactions for recording later on his chart. For example, change of color, rate of respiration or pulse, tremors, or whatever, according to the expected reaction for the drug that is administered.
7. Discard the medicine cup after the patient has swallowed the medicine.	If disposable, discard the cup in a designated container. If reusable, place it on the tray to be reprocessed.
	NOTE: If a liquid was given in a reusable glass, rinse the glass in water in the lavatory in the patient's room. This makes it easier to reprocess.
	NOTE: If the patient is not ready to take his medicine when you are there to give it to him, return it to the medication area and dispose of it according to agency procedure. Do not return the medicine to a stock supply. This practice points up one more advantage of the unit-dose system; because the individual unit-dose is wrapped and labelled with the patient's name, the medication *can* be returned to the medications storage area (in the medication cart or room) until it is unwrapped and given.
	Medications are never left at the patient's bedside except in some special instances, for which you must have a written order stating that medications may be kept at the bedside.
	Medicines that are commonly left at the bedside include hourly antacids for gastric ulcer patients and nitroglycerin tablets for angina pectoris patients. Of course, these would be left by the bedside only if the patient is mentally responsible, regardless of the order.
8. Record the medication.	If you are using a Kardex system, make the notation on the Kardex while you are still in the patient's room. If you are using the medicine card system, you will record the administration of medication on the patient's chart as soon as you return to the charting area. Since there are various places to keep the chart (patient's room, nurses' station, nurses' substation, on the medication cart), you will have to follow your agency procedure.
	Your entry on the record should include the name of the medication, the dosage, the route (if other than oral), the time of administration, and your signature and designation. Usually,

PREPARATION AND ADMINISTRATION OF MEDICATIONS

Important Steps	Key Points
	only the initials are given on a Kardex system, while your first initial, last name and designation are required on patient's records. (NOTE: Recent regulations require your full signature on the Kardex at least once during your shift. Initials may then be used for the hourly designation when a drug is administered.)
9. Leave the patient safe and comfortable.	Position him for comfort; leave the bedside stand and call signal within easy reach. Ask if there is anything else you can do, then tell him when you expect to return.
10. Proceed to the next patient or return to the medication area.	If you are distributing medicines for an entire group of patients, you may be prepared to continue giving all the medicines, and when you have finished, return to the medication area.
	If you are giving a single dose, return to the medication area immediately.
11. Replace the supplies.	Put them in the designated areas. Wipe the tray clean with an alcohol sponge or damp paper towel. Discard the tray in the appropriate container. Return the medicine card to the designated storage locator.
	Leave the medication work area neat and clean for the next preparation time.

ITEM 2: PARENTERAL MEDICATIONS

Parenteral introduction of medications into the body tissues or fluids is accomplished through use of a needle. The injection method is used:

1. To obtain a more rapid action;

2. When the patient cannot take medications by mouth;

3. When the digestive juices would counteract the effect of the drug;

4. To act as a local anesthetic for minor operative procedures; or

5. To concentrate the medication in a specific area of the body.

A. Methods of Medication Administration

1. *Subcutaneous* (subq or sub q). The needle is inserted at an angle of 45° into the subcutaneous layer under the skin. A short needle (5/8 inch) with a tiny lumen is used. The absorption of medications given by this method is at a moderate rate of speed. It takes at least 30 minutes for maximal effect.

PREPARATION AND ADMINISTRATION OF MEDICATIONS

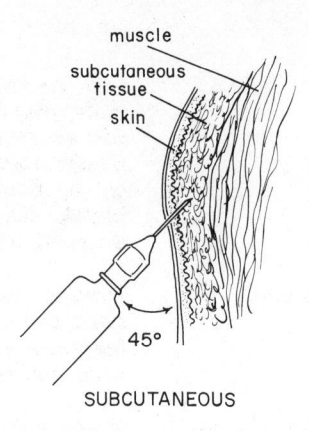

muscle
subcutaneous tissue
skin
45°
SUBCUTANEOUS

2. *Intramuscular (IM)*. The needle is inserted at a 90° angle into the muscular layer below the skin. Various sized needles are used for this injection depending on the size of the patient; however, for the usual adult patient, a needle 1½ to 3 inches long with a gauge of 16 to 20 (indicating the size of the lumen) is preferred. <u>The smaller the gauge size, the larger the lumen.</u>

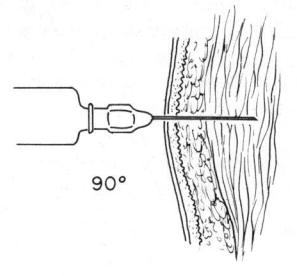

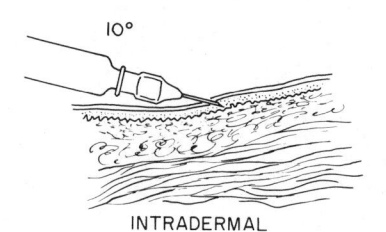

90°
INTRAMUSCULAR

10°
INTRADERMAL

3. *Intradermal*. The needle is inserted at an angle between the layers of the skin (see illustration). The needles are short (1/4 to 5/8 inch) with a fine gauge of 25 or 27. This method is most often used diagnostically for determining allergies, sensitivities to drugs, and presence of disease. Intradermal injections are used in the tuberculin test, commonly employed to assist in diagnosing tuberculosis; in the Schick test, to determine susceptibility to diphtheria; in the Dick test, used to determine susceptibility to scarlet fever. The intradermal skin test is also used to test sensitivity to dust, allergens, tetanus toxoid or tetanus antitoxin, among other uses. This type of injection has the longest absorption period.

4. *Intravenous* (IV). The needle is inserted into the specified vein at a 20° to 30° angle. The IV injection has the quickest absorption rate; effects can be seen within 30 seconds.

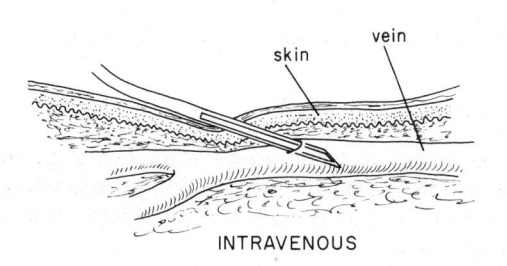

skin *vein*
INTRAVENOUS

PREPARATION AND ADMINISTRATION OF MEDICATIONS

5. *Hypodermoclysis* (clysis). The needle is injected into the subcutaneous layer below the skin at an angle nearly parallel to the skin; the needle is usually attached to tubing similar to IV tubing which is secured to a bottle of sterile IV fluid (such as NaCl, 2 to 5 per cent glucose in distilled water).

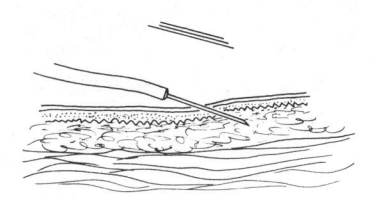

HYPODERMOCLYSIS

The solutions are given slowly over a prescribed period of time (e.g., 1,000 cc over 1 hour for a 150-pound adult). If the patient is dehydrated or has a circulatory disturbance, the absorption rate will be decreased. Thin persons absorb solutions more quickly than fat persons.

A hypodermoclysis may be given to an infant by using a needle and syringe (20 to 50 cc). The needle size will depend on the size of the infant.

6. *Intraspinal* (spinal, caudal). The long spinal needle (3½ inches), 20, 22 to 25 gauge, is introduced at a 90° angle into the selected spinal interspace. This will vary according to the kind of puncture to be done, whether caudal, lumbar, or the subarachnoid space. This injection is used for spinal anesthesias, or to obtain a spinal fluid specimen for laboratory examination to aid in making a diagnosis. Since this procedure is usually done by physicians, it will not be discussed further.

B. Needles

Needles come in various standard sizes and lengths from 1½ inches to 6 inches with various gauges from 13 to 27. The lumen size is indicated on the hub of reusable needles. Both size and length of needles are written on the outside of the prepackaged sterile wrapper. Some wrappers are also color-coded for easier and quicker identification. Because the products vary somewhat among manufacturers, the following drawings merely serve as an example.

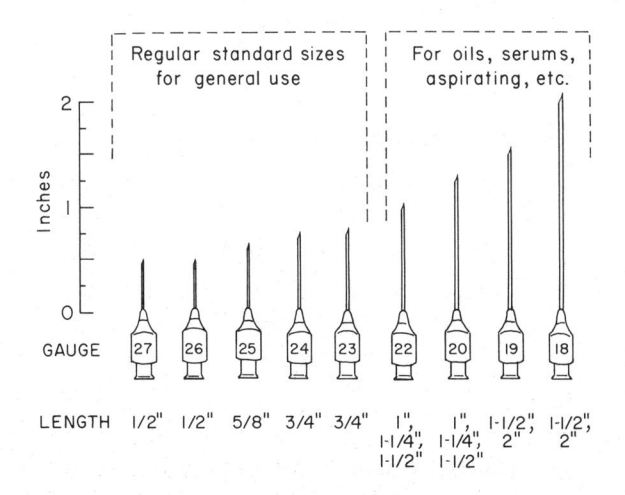

	Regular standard sizes for general use	For oils, serums, aspirating, etc.
GAUGE	27, 26, 25, 24, 23	22, 20, 19, 18
LENGTH	1/2", 1/2", 5/8", 3/4", 3/4"	1", 1-1/4", 1-1/2"; 1", 1-1/4", 1-1/2"; 1-1/2", 2"; 1-1/2", 2"

You should become familiar with the part of the needle: point, cannula, hub. See the examples below:

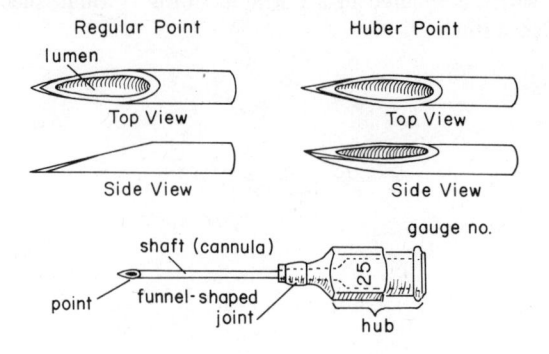

Regular Point (Top View, Side View) — lumen

Huber Point (Top View, Side View)

point — shaft (cannula) — funnel-shaped joint — hub — gauge no.

The length of the needle is determined by the measurement from the tip of the point to the junction of the cannula and the hub.

The outside diameter of the cannula wall must be selected according to the size of the patient, his condition, and the site of the injection. The thickness of the wall of the cannula must also be chosen according to the purpose for which the needle is being used (e.g., when intradermal injections are painful, and when solutions are watery, a thin cannula wall is required, whereas needles used to take bone marrow samples are thick-walled, with large lumens).

Needles may be disposable and used only once, or they may be the reusable type.

C. Syringes

Syringes come in several standard sizes and shapes. It is essential for you to become familiar with the barrel, the plunger, various types of tips (bevel, Luer-Lok, etc.), as well as the markings on the syringe.

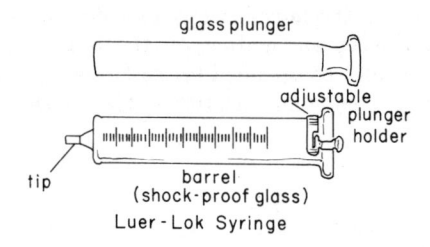

glass plunger — adjustable plunger holder — tip — barrel (shock-proof glass) — Luer-Lok Syringe

Luer-Lok glass syringe (2cc, 5, 10, 20)

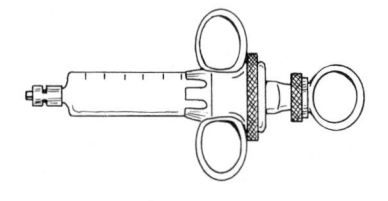

Luer-Lok syringe with control handles

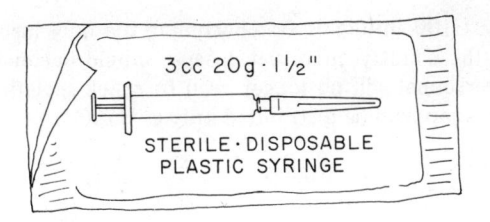

PREPARATION AND ADMINISTRATION OF MEDICATIONS

Disposable syringe in paper wrapper

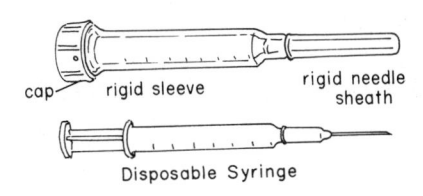

Disposable syringe in rigid plastic container
(e.g., Monoject by Sherwood Medical Industries)

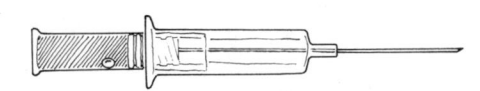

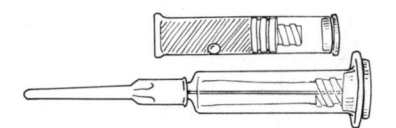

Disposable syringe unit-dose system (Vari-ject
System by CIBA Pharmaceutical Company)

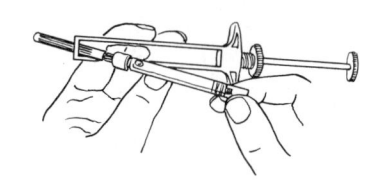

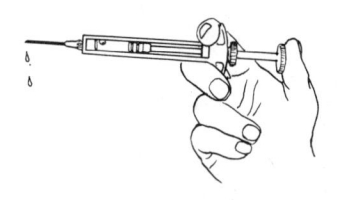

Carpuject Plastic Syringe for use with disposable
needle—cartridge unit (Winthrop Laboratories)

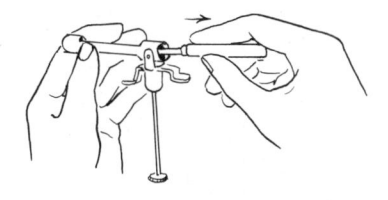

Tubex metal syringe for use with disposable needle-cartridge
unit (Wyeth Laboratories)

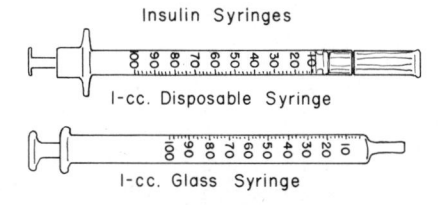

Insulin syringes (disposable or reusable) — U40,
U80, U100 (Becton-Dickinson Co.)

NOTE: The new U100 insulin is fast becoming the only insulin syringe in use. When accepted throughout the country, incorrect dosages should become nearly impossible, since patients and health personnel will no longer need to check specific types of insulin to use. (All insulin, hopefully soon, will be distributed only as U100.)

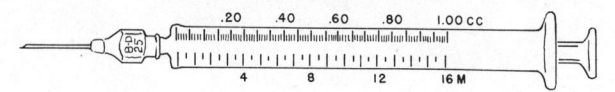

Tuberculin syringe

D. Containers

Various containers of sterile solutions will be used for different injection methods.

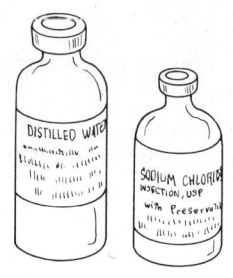

Vials (20 cc, 30, 50)

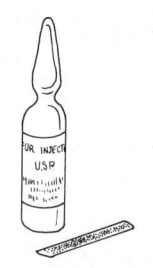

Ampule with file

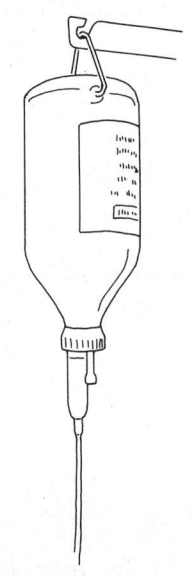

Vacoliters (250 cc, 500, 1,000)

E. *Tissue Structure and Site Selection*

The dermis is the layer directly below the epidermis; it is called the true skin. This layer contains the hair follicles (which are embedded in the smooth muscle), sweat glands, sebaceous (oil) glands, blood vessels and nerve endings.

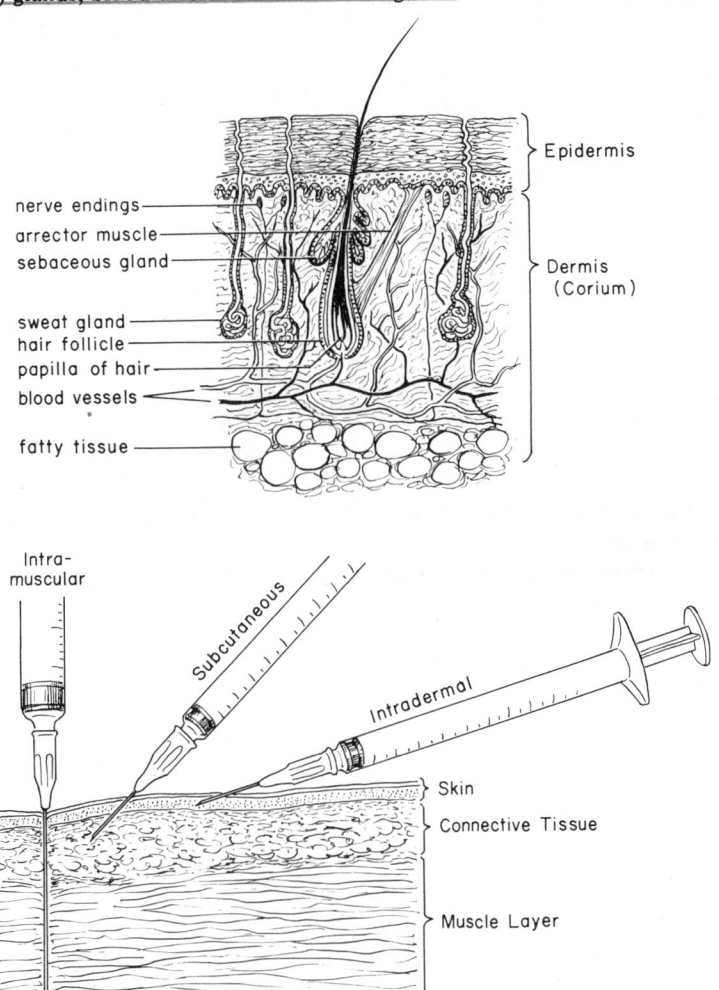

You will note from the above drawing that directly below the dermis (hypodermis or subcutaneous) there is a layer of connective tissue that contains varying amounts of fat cells. This is the layer that binds the skin to the deep tissues, fascia, muscles, or periosteum.

Extensive capillary and lymphatic systems are found in the skin. The capillary system plays a major role in the absorption of medications by the physiologic process of diffusion. The actual absorption rate is dependent on several factors, such as type of solution injected (e.g., hypotonic, hypertonic, isotonic), capillary permeability, blood flow, injection pressure, condition or lesions of the skin (e.g., inflammation, fibrosis, fat deposits), and chemical properties within the tissue layer which either inhibit or enhance drug absorption (e.g., the presence of histamine in the tissue retards absorption while the enzyme hyaluronidase breaks down hyaluronic acid in tissue and speeds up absorption).

Although the skin does have some elasticity or "stretchability" (as evident in edematous or pregnant patients), the amount of solution injected via the subcutaneous method should not be more than 2 cc. Because the skin varies in thickness over the body, various lengths of needles must be selected in accordance with the patient's size and the site of the injection.

PREPARATION AND ADMINISTRATION OF MEDICATIONS

Careful choice of injection sites is essential to assure optimal absorption and to prevent skin reactions that could lead to pain or disfigurement. The following illustrations show common sites for subcutaneous injections. If your patient receives repeated medications, you should use a rotation plan to avoid fibrosing the tissue, which could cause pain and disfigurement.

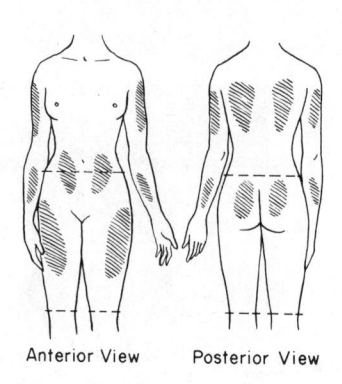

Anterior View   Posterior View

The preferred sites are the lateral surfaces of the upper arm or the back, and lateral aspects of the thigh.

For self-administration sites, areas of the abdomen and fronts of the thighs are recommended because they are easily reached.

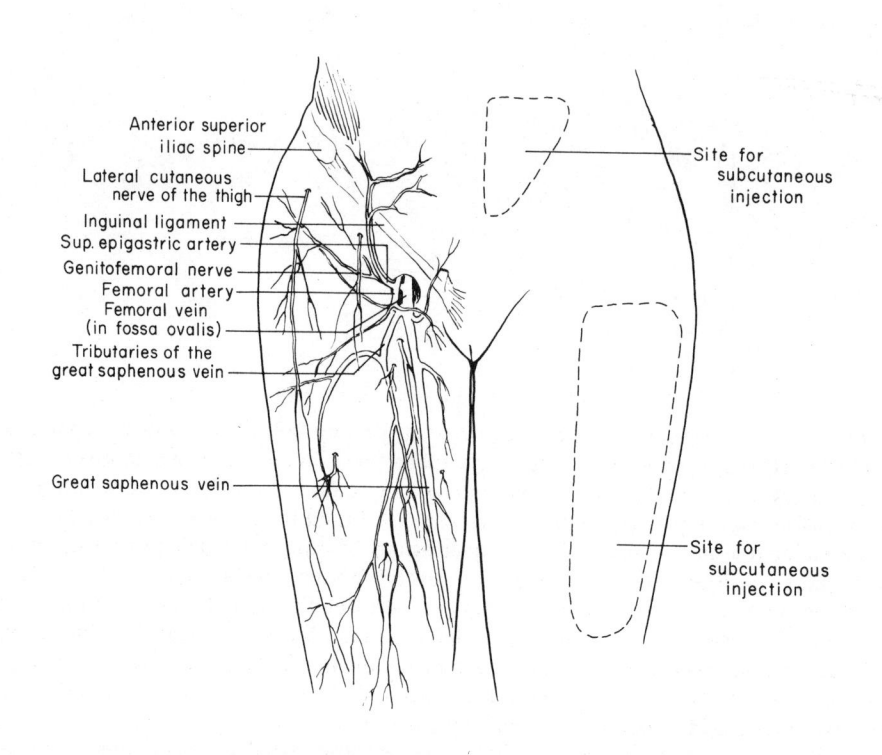

Anterior View Showing
Major Vessels and Nerves

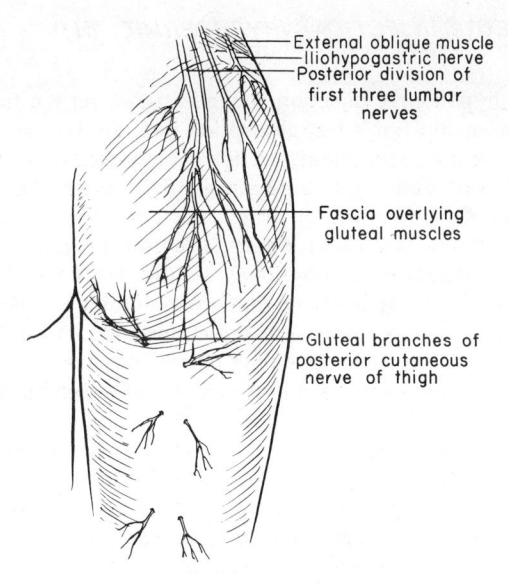

PREPARATION AND ADMINISTRATION OF MEDICATIONS

Posterior View Showing
Major Vessels and Nerves

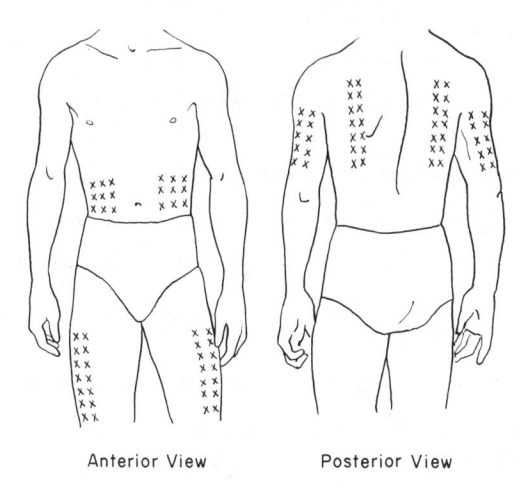

Anterior View   Posterior View

The above illustrations show rotation plans for injection sites in the diabetic patient. Obviously, the anterior sites can be used for self-administration, whereas the posterior sites can be reached only by someone else in administering injections to the patient.

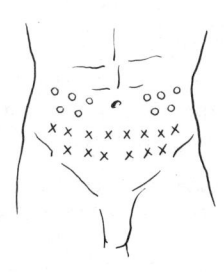

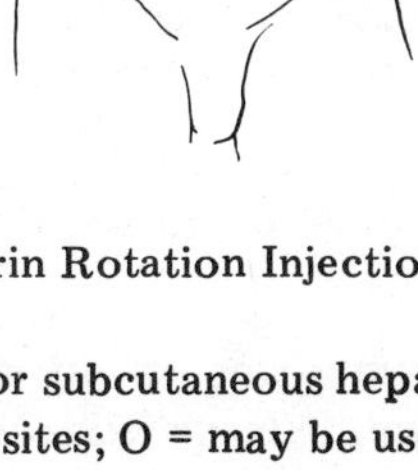

Heparin Rotation Injection Sites

Chart showing rotation sites for subcutaneous heparin injections on the abdomen.
X = preferred sites; O = may be used if necessary.

ITEM 3: SUBCUTANEOUS INJECTIONS (HYPODERMIC, "H")

The most common hypodermic injection is administered via the subcutaneous method, generally because of the medication's fast absorption rate and the fact that it is frequently the best route for injecting the unconscious, irrational, nauseated or vomiting patient.

Subcutaneous injections have been used since 1855, when Dr. Alexander Wood of Edinburgh published the first accounts of drugs injected subcutaneously via a needle and syringe. Subsequent techniques have changed very little over the years.

A brief review of the anatomy and physiology of the skin will be helpful here. You will recall from your study of Unit 13: Special Skin Care in Volume 1 that the skin is the largest organ of the body. A protective covering over the entire body, it acts as a barrier between the individual and his environment by shielding against physical attack on the underlying tissues; while intact, it prevents microorganisms and other foreign objects from entering the body.

The outer layer of the skin is known as the *epidermis*, often called the false skin. This layer constantly sheds dead cells and serves as the protective barrier for the skin.

The *dermis* is the layer directly below the epidermis; it is called the true skin. This layer contains the hair follicles, which are embedded in the smooth muscle, sweat glands, sebaceous (oil) glands, blood vessels, and nerve endings.

A. Hazards of Faulty Injection Technique

1. Irreparable damage to a major nerve or other structure, due to improper selection of injection sites.

2. Introduction of an infection through the needle hole in the skin.

3. Damage to tissues due to improper technique or dull needle.

4. Entrance into the wrong tissue, thereby creating a health hazard for the patient.

5. Introduction of foreign particles into body tissues, which could set up a foreign-body reaction, e.g., dirt in the lumen of a needle.

To avoid the above hazards, the health worker must observe the following guidelines:

1. Carefully select the injection sites to avoid major nerves, blood vessels, and organs. An accurate and extensive knowledge of anatomy and physiology of all age groups is therefore required.

2. Utilize only sterile, preferably disposable, needles and syringes.

3. <u>Always pull back on the plunger to determine if you have entered a blood vessel before injecting the medication.</u>

4. Select an injection site that is relatively normal, i.e., free of lesions, inflammation, rashes, moles, freckles, and the like.

5. <u>Avoid hairy sites for injections.</u> Shave the area before inserting the needle if alternative sites are not available. This will minimize possible displacement of a hair follicle into the underlying tissue, which would set up local tissue reaction.

6. Rotate injection sites for patients receiving many injections by establishing a predetermined plan, thereby decreasing the probability of local tissue reaction, pain and fibrosing.

7. Select the appropriate length of needle to assure deposition of the medication within the proper tissue layer.

8. Obtain assistance as needed in giving an injection, e.g., when your patient is a frightened child, or a belligerent, uncooperative adult.

PREPARATION AND ADMINISTRATION OF MEDICATIONS

B. Preparation of Subcutaneous Injection

Important Steps	Key Points
1. Wash your hands.	
2. Gather all the necessary equipment.	Obtain the medication record (card or Kardex chart), appropriate syringe, needle, antiseptic sponges and medication tray. NOTE: Within the last decade there have been studies indicating that preliminary cleansing of the skin before injection may not be required because it may negate the antibacterial action of the skin.
3. Compare the medication record with the order.	This will assure accuracy. Verify the patient's name (room number and identification number, if indicated), drug, dose, time to be given, route of administration, and date to be discontinued if the medication is a timed medicine (one given for a stated number of doses).
4. Identify and remove the patient's medication from storage.	Medication vials or ampules are usually kept in a box or drawer labeled with the patient's name, room number, drug, dose and route. The vial itself is labeled with the drug, dose and route. If the medication is in a unit-dose, it will be individually packaged for your patient.
5. Compare the medication record with the label on the medication.	Hold both items in your hands, so that they are close together for ease in reading and verifying the information.
6. Calculate the correct dosage to be given.	If the unit-dose system is in use, the correct dosage is already prepared, and therefore this step is omitted. Use the mathematical calculation you learned in your math classes. The vial or ampule is labeled 50 mg = 1 cc. The amount of medication prescribed is 25 mg. How much of the solution will you give? (See answer at the end of this item).

PREPARATION AND ADMINISTRATION OF MEDICATIONS

Important Steps	Key Points
7. Open an antiseptic pledget and clean the vial or ampule.	(a) Vial: Remove the pledget from its container and cleanse the rubber top of the vial with a vigorous rotary motion. This cleanses the top of the vial and decreases the possibility of introducing microorganisms when you insert the needle into the vial to withdraw the medicine.

Discard the pledget in a designated container.

(b) Ampule: Dislodge any drops of medicine caught in the top of the ampule by thumping the ampule with your index finger. Then, with the antiseptic pledget, cleanse the neck of the ampule at the marked line.

Break open the ampule by first filing across the marked line (files are always available with ampules).

Then sharply hit the top of the ampule by striking it on the proximal side so that it will *break away from you.*

For large ampules, you may need to break off the top. Obtain a gauze sponge, antiseptic pledget or paper tissue to cover the top end of the ampule when you *break it away from you.* The sponge will collect the tiny piece of glass and keep you from being injured. Put the ampule on your medication tray.

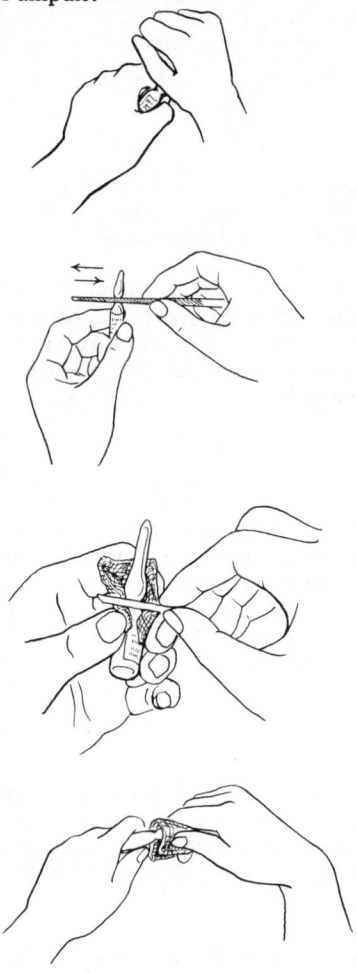

8. Assemble the syringe and needle.

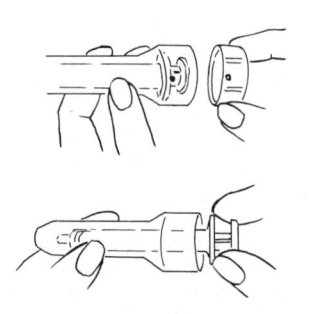

The procedure remains the same for all sizes of syringes. The only difference is the way they are wrapped (except for the single-dose cartridge syringe).

(a) *Rigid plastic package*

    1) Remove the desired syringe from the storage area and twist its cap counterclockwise to break the tamper-proof seal.

    2) Slide the needle sheath and syringe out of the plastic package. (The needle remains protected by the sheath until it is used.)

    3) Place the plastic package upside down on the tray, to serve later as a sterile lodging for the prepared medicine when you take it to your patient.

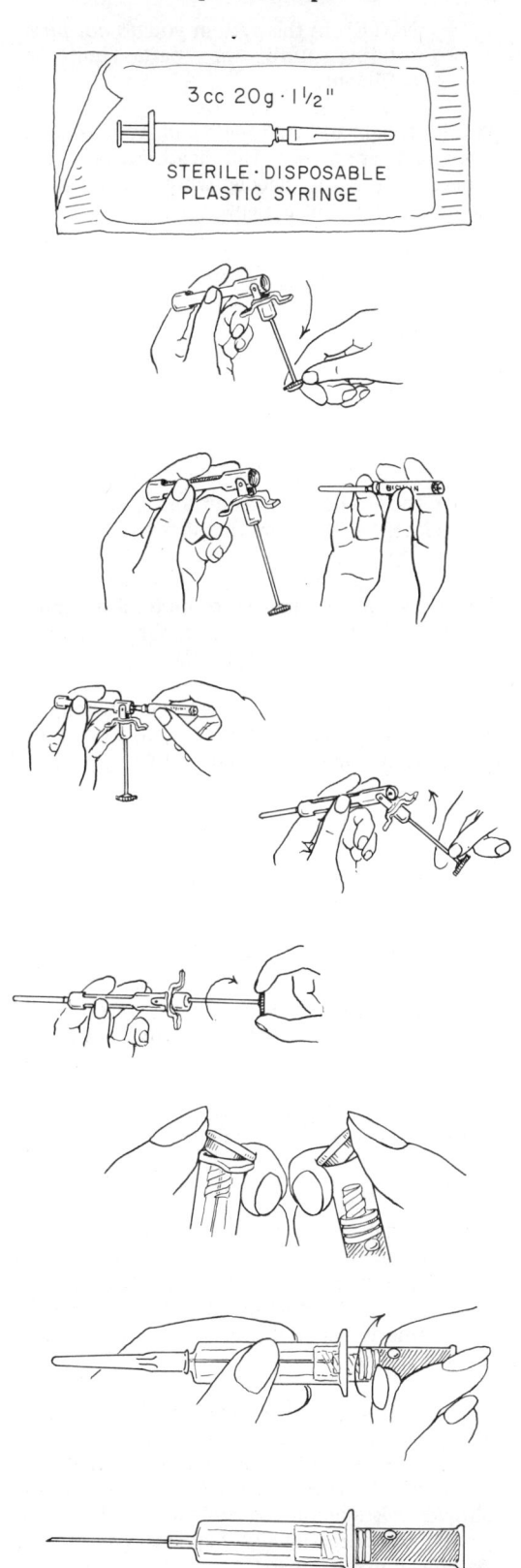

PREPARATION AND ADMINISTRATION OF MEDICATIONS

Important Steps	Key Points

Key Points

(b) *Paper-packaged sterile disposable syringe*

1) Open the package by peeling the outer wrapper off the syringe.

2) Remove the needle with its guard (sheath) by picking it up firmly at the middle of the syringe barrel.

(c) *Tubex metal syringe*

1) Grasp the barrel of the metal syringe in your left hand, and with your right or dominant hand, pull the plunger back firmly. Continue pulling the plunger until it drops downward and locks at a 90° angle.

2) Insert the needle cartridge into the barrel, needle first. (The cartridge can be obtained from the storage area.)

3) Tighten the needle in the front end of the barrel by rotating it clockwise in the threads while holding the barrel and cartridge.

4) Swing the plunger back into place and attach it to the threaded end of the cartridge.

5) To secure the cartridge-needle unit inside the metal barrel, rotate it clockwise until both ends of the cartridge are fully but lightly secured.

Leave the sheath over the needle to maintain sterility until it is used.

This unit is now ready to take to the patient's room.

(d) *Disposable unit-dose system* (select a color-coded syringe and needle to meet your needs).

1) Snap off the protective caps from both the syringe and the medicine vial by placing your thumbs under the lips of the cap and pushing upward.

2) Insert the medicine vial into the syringe and rotate it clockwise to engage the threads on the rubber stopper with the threads on the inside of the syringe barrel.

3) Continue rotating the medicine vial until resistance is felt (about 3 full turns). Then rotate one more full turn to assure that the needle is in contact with the medicine.

PREPARATION AND ADMINISTRATION OF MEDICATIONS

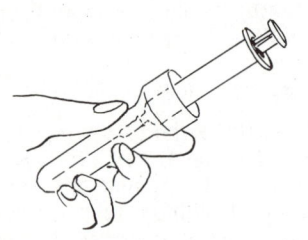

Important Steps	Key Points
	NOTE: In this system you *do not push*; rotating until the parts unite is sufficient.
9. Remove the needle guard (sheath).	Pull it straight off the needle and lay it aside on your medication tray. The sheath can serve as a protector for the needle while carrying the medication to your patient.
10. Test the security of the needle on the syringe.	Grasp the needle at its hub and give it a 1/4 turn clockwise to assure that it is secured to the syringe tip.
11. Pick up the syringe in your left hand.	Pull back on the plunger to obtain a measured amount of air (equal to the amount of medication to be removed from the vial).
	NOTE: This step is unnecessary when obtaining medicine from an ampule, or if the unit-dose or cartridge system is used.
12. Pick up the vial or ampule.	(a) *Ampule*
	Hold the ampule between your left index and middle fingers while grasping the ampule between the left thumb and fourth finger.
	The right hand is used on the syringe plunger to withdraw the medication.
	(b) *Vial*
	The vial is larger than the ampule; hold it between your left thumb and third finger. Your left index finger is used as a counterforce on the bottom of the vial when the needle is inserted through the rubber stopper of the vial.
	NOTE: Since many learners are nervous when first preparing injections, it is absolutely mandatory to discard contaminated syringes or needles, and start with a sterile one if you should mistakenly contaminate it. Don't be upset; this occasionally happens even to experienced practitioners.

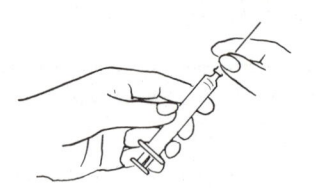

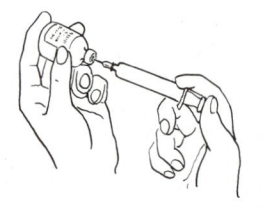

PREPARATION AND ADMINISTRATION OF MEDICATIONS 91

Important Steps

13. Insert the needle into the ampule or vial.

Key Points

(a) *Ampule*

Insert the needle into the distal end of the ampule, being careful to insert the needle of the syringe into the ampule without touching the sides of the ampule.

(b) *Vial*

With the plunger of the syringe pulled back to the exact mark on the barrel indicating the prescribed amount of medicine, insert the needle into the cleansed rubber stopper with the bevel of the needle facing up so that you can see it.

Insert the needle at a slight angle with a forward thrust while simultaneously exerting a slight lateral pressure (less pressure than is needed to bend the needle). Continue pushing the needle until it is through the rubber stopper.

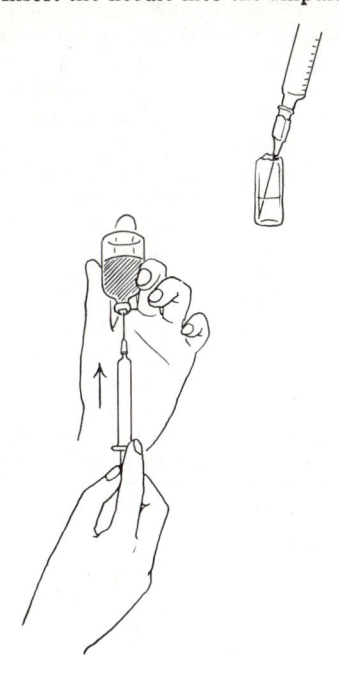

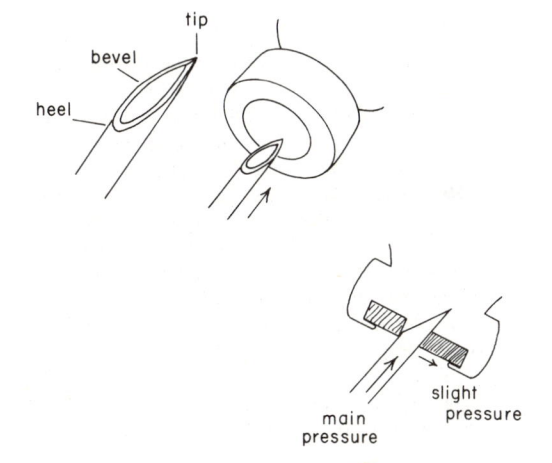

By properly inserting the needle into the rubber stopper as described, you will avoid cutting a core (plug) of rubber out of the stopper, which could then be pushed on into the vial.

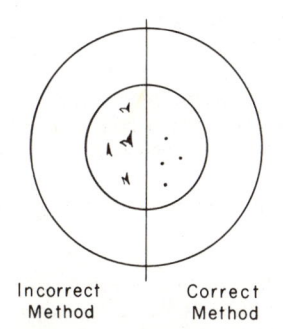

Appearance of stopper using:
(A) incorrect method (B) correct method

Important Steps

14. Withdraw the medicine into the syringe.

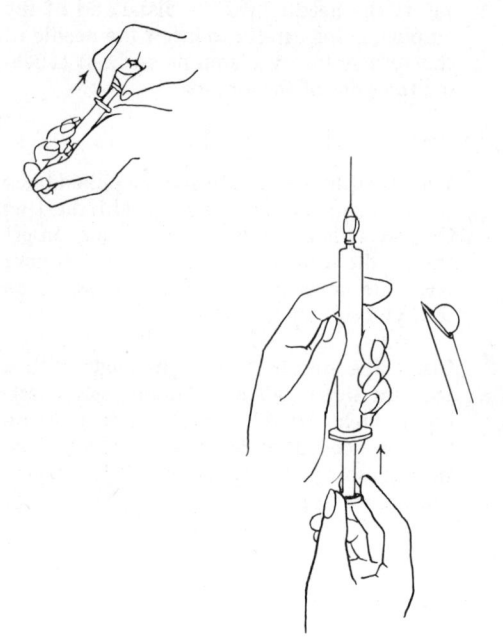

Key Points

(a) *Ampule*

While holding the ampule and barrel of the syringe securely in the left hand, pull the plunger up and back to the desired calibration on the barrel of the syringe. It is wise to withdraw an extra minim or two so that you have enough medicine left after the air bubbles are expelled. Any air that you draw up into the syringe must be expelled before you read the dose. Remove the needle from the ampule and put the ampule on the tray. <u>Turn the needle upward, then slowly and gently push on the plunger to expel air bubbles. Stop when one drop of liquid appears in the bevel of the needle.</u> Verify your calculation and the amount of medicine in the syringe with the medication record. <u>Reinsert the needle in the ampule and put it aside on the medicine tray.</u>

(b) *Vial*

With the needle tip through the stopper and *above the liquid line*, push the plunger into the barrel. This provides for air replacement when the medicine is withdrawn to prevent a vacuum in the bottle. If a vacuum occurs, you cannot withdraw the medicine while holding the vial at eye level. Turn the vial upside down; with the needle *inserted into the medicine*, pull the plunger down the barrel of the syringe until slightly more than the required amount of medicine is in the syringe.

Remove the needle quickly from the vial and put it aside on the medicine tray.

To assure correct dosage, the air bubbles must be expelled from the syringe. While continuing to hold the syringe with the needle pointing upward, gently and slowly push the plunger into the barrel. Stop when a drop of the medicine appears in the bevel.

Verify the amount in the syringe with your medication record.

Replace the needle in the needle guard (do not contaminate the needle by touching the outside of the sheath). Place it on the medicine tray with identification (card, label) and go to the patient's room.

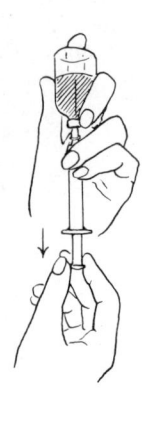

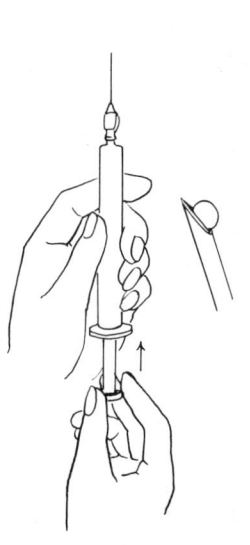

PREPARATION AND ADMINISTRATION OF MEDICATIONS

Important Steps	Key Points
15. Replace the vial in the storage unit.	Read the label again as you replace the vial. Usually vials are multi-dose and therefore can be used for several doses. Everyone who uses the vial to withdraw the medicine must observe scrupulous sterile technique. If the vial is contaminated, the patient could become infected.
	NOTE: Ampules are discarded after use. Because the ampule is opened to air, the contents could partially evaporate and change the strength of the remaining medicine; this could be harmful if injected into the patient.
16. Assemble all items on a clean medicine tray.	This includes the filled syringe with needle protected by covering, medicine identification (card, label), and antiseptic sponges.
	Answer to question in Step 6, page 87. Give 1/2 cc. of solution.

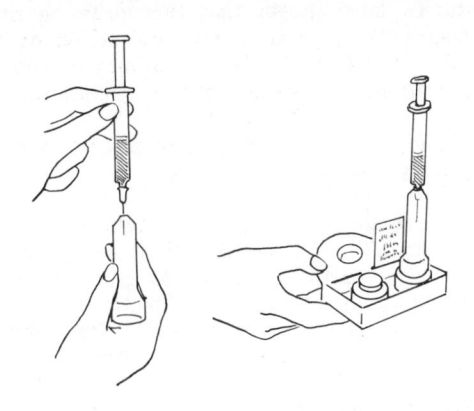

C. Administration of Subcutaneous Injections

Important Steps	Key Points
1. Wash your hands.	Obtain all necessary equipment and supplies.
2. Approach, identify, and explain the procedure to the patient.	Check the patient's identification (Identaband, patient chart, or name if in a home, clinic, or office setting). Tell him that you are going to give him a shot in the arm, and that it will hurt momentarily.
3. Select the site of injection.	Review the sites of injection described on pages 83–85 and select the best one. For this lesson, use the posterior aspects of the upper arm.
	Expose the area so that you have good visibility. Be sure that you have ample lighting so that you easily see the injection site, read the syringe calibrations, and observe your patient.
4. Open the antiseptic sponge package.	Remove the sponge and cleanse the selected site by using a circular motion. Begin at the center point and continue in an ever-widening circular movement until approximately a 2-inch space is cleansed. Hold the sponge between your left index and middle fingers.

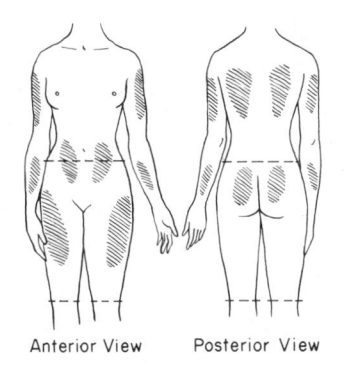

Important Steps	Key Points
	NOTE: In the past decade, some research studies have shown that this cleansing may destroy the normal antibacterial action of the skin. Therefore, follow your agency procedure concerning the cleansing of the injection site.
	Allow the skin to dry (antiseptic evaporates quickly from the skin).
5. Pick up the prepared syringe in your right hand.	Remove the needle guard (or remove it from the ampule). Take care to pull it straight away from the guard or ampule to avoid contaminating it. If you contaminate the needle, it must be removed and replaced with a sterile needle.
6. Expel air bubbles.	Hold the syringe in your left hand with the needle pointing upward. With your right hand, slowly and gently expel the air bubbles. Stop pushing the plunger when a drop of the medicine appears in the needle bevel.
7. Prepare skin site.	(a) You can pinch the skin gently between the thumb and index finger, or
	(b) You can spread the skin lightly by moving the left index finger and thumb in opposite directions, or
	(c) Do nothing to the skin, i.e., do not stretch or pinch, but leave it as you find it. (Follow your agency procedure.)
8. Insert the needle at a 45° angle into the skin.	Hold the barrel in your right hand between the thumb and index finger, letting the syringe rest on the remaining three fingers. Then insert the needle through the skin with a firm, quick, forward thrust.
9. Release the skin.	Hold the barrel securely between your left thumb and index finger.
10. Pull back on plunger with right hand.	This is to determine if your needle has hit a blood vessel. If so, you can injure the inner blood vessel wall by injecting medications that are not prepared for IV use. Also, if you inject the medication directly into the circulatory system, the effect from the drug is almost instantaneous, and this can produce a shock effect.

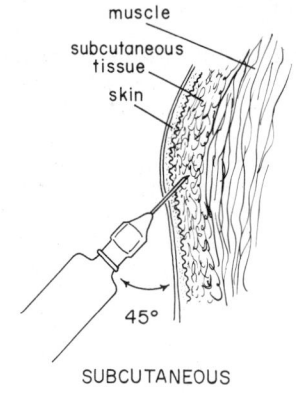

Important Steps	Key Points
	If blood appears in the syringe, withdraw the needle a bit, redirect and reinsert it, and again pull back on the plunger to determine if you have hit a second blood vessel. (If so much blood has come back into the syringe that you cannot recognize the medicine, withdraw the needle and discard both the needle and the syringe, and start again.)
11. Inject the medicine.	With your right thumb, press the plunger into the barrel slowly and steadily until all of the medication is injected.
12. Remove needle.	Do this quickly, and by pulling straight out at the same angle at which it was inserted. Put the used needle back in its guard on the tray (this is for your own protection so that you won't be pricked with the contaminated needle).
13. Massage the site with an antiseptic sponge.	Use a gentle circular motion to help disperse the medication in the subcutaneous tissue so that it will absorb readily. The peak action of a subcutaneous injection is expected within 30 minutes. Discard the sponge in a designated container.
14. Place a BAND-AID over the injection site.	A BAND-AID is rarely needed for a subcutaneous injection, but occasionally a few drops of blood may be spilled from a superficial capillary vessel as the needle is being withdrawn.
15. Leave the patient safe and comfortable.	Position him for comfort: adjust the bed linens and siderails (if indicated); leave the bedside stand and call signal within his reach. Ask if there is anything else you can do, and tell him when you expect to return.
	NOTE: If you administer a hypnotic, the patient may become sleepy or disoriented. Siderails should be raised as a precautionary measure in this instance. (Follow agency procedure.)
16. Return supplies to the medication preparation area.	Reusable syringe: Rinse the glass syringe and needle by drawing tap water into the barrel, and then expelling.
	Repeat the process until the syringe and needle are clean (this is especially important for oily or colored preparations).

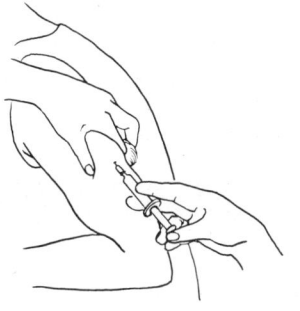

Important Steps	Key Points
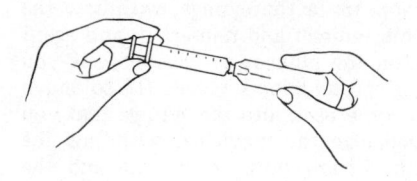	Disposable syringe: Holding the syringe in your left hand and the needle guard in the right hand, bend the needle to and fro at the hub so that the tip breaks off the syringe and remains lodged within the hub of the needle. (In this way, would-be drug users cannot use these syringes again.)
	Discard the broken syringe and needle in a designated container.
	When the needle container is full, it must be sent to the incinerator.
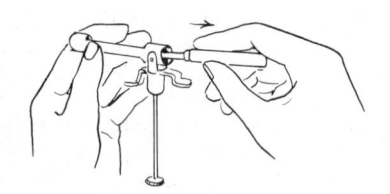	Tubex metal syringe with cartridge: With the needle sheath in place to prevent hooking, disengage the plunger from the piston by turning it in a counterclockwise direction. Then, grasping the barrel in your left hand, pull back on the plunger with the right hand until it leaves the barrel, and swing the handle downward so that it locks in place.
	Rotate the medication cartridge counterclockwise between your left thumb and index finger to disengage it at the front end of the syringe.
	Remove the cartridge from the barrel of the syringe, and discard it in a designated container.
	Replace the metal holder in the designated location. Be sure to wipe it clean with a damp paper towel if medicine was accidentally spilled on it.
	Leave the work area clean and tidy. Doors and drawers should be closed and locked as indicated by agency policy.
	Return the medication card or Kardex to the designated place.

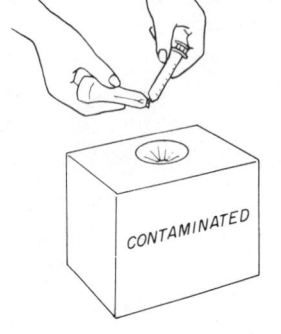

PREPARATION AND ADMINISTRATION OF MEDICATIONS

Important Steps	Key Points
17. Record the procedure on the patient's record.	Depending upon the agency for which you are working, this could be done on the medication Kardex or on the patient's chart or record.

Charting example:

10:00 A.M. — Thiomerin 0.2 cc "H" in posterior aspect, upper arm.

J. Kula, R.N.

ITEM 4: HANDLING STUCK HYPODERMIC NEEDLE OR FROZEN SYRINGE

Removing a stuck hypodermic needle can be done easily by grasping the hub of the needle with a straight hemostat, and giving a firm counterclockwise turn. You may need to wiggle the needle back and forth to break the seal. Since the advent of disposable needles and syringes, stuck needles and syringes are not a problem since the entire unit is discarded after use.

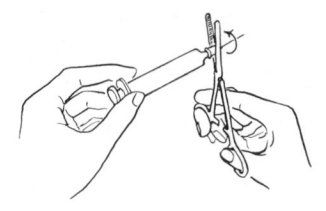

Unsticking a frozen syringe takes more skill. Usually, the processing department has a syringe opener which will assist in the procedure. The instrument looks much like a syringe except that it is placed on the tip end of the frozen syringe. As you insert the plunger in the syringe opener, air is injected into the frozen syringe with the intention of breaking the seal. It is easy to break glass syringes by using this method, and therefore you must take care not to get cut from flying glass fragments.

<u>You can prevent syringes from sticking by rinsing the syringe barrel and plunger with clear cold water immediately after use.</u>

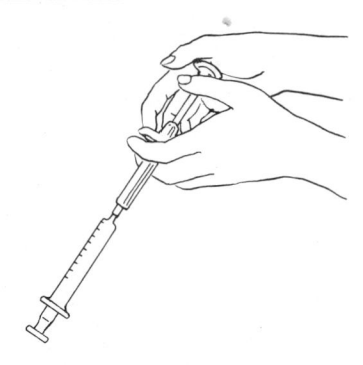

ITEM 5: INTRAMUSCULAR (IM) INJECTIONS

Intramuscular injections are utilized when the patient cannot take the medicine orally, or if the medication is not prepared in an oral form. IM injections provide a quick but sustained action because muscular tissue is highly vascular.

Selection of the injection site is a critical decision for the health practitioner. Improper site selection can result in damaged nerves, (leading to possible paralysis), delayed deformities, or atrophy of a limb, among other sequelae. Therefore, age (child or adult), build, and the individual's physical condition must be considered when giving an injection. From 2 to 5 cc of fluid may be injected into a muscle, depending on the size of the patient. If more than 5 cc of medication must be given at one time, the doses should be divided into two and given in two different sites.

A. Anatomical Injection Sites

The most common sites for IM injection in the adult are the deltoid muscle in the arm, the gluteal muscles, and the ventrogluteal and vastus lateralis muscles of the thigh. Because the gluteal region in infants is poorly developed, the site of choice for infants is the lateral vastus muscle, but the gluteal region can usually be safely used after the child has reached three years of age. By that time, he may have been walking a year or more and the gluteal muscles will be generally developed.

The mid-deltoid muscle is a common site for IM injection; however, the actual area involved is limited because of the major vessels, nerves, and bones. Only small amounts of medication can be injected in this site. The area for the arm injection is a rectangular area bounded on the top by the lower edge of the acromion, on the bottom by the axilla, and by the lateral one-third of the arm.

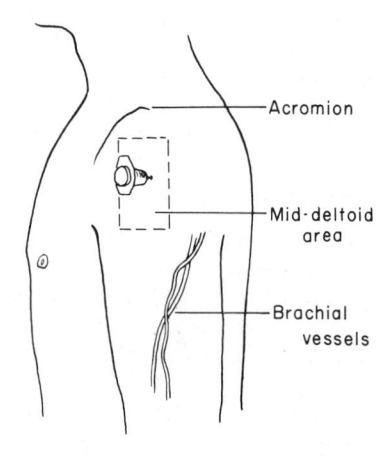

The gluteal muscles are probably the most commonly used for IM injections. The preferred injection site is in the upper outer quadrant in the gluteus medius. Strict location and utilization of this site will prevent injury to the sciatic nerve, or to the superior gluteal artery.

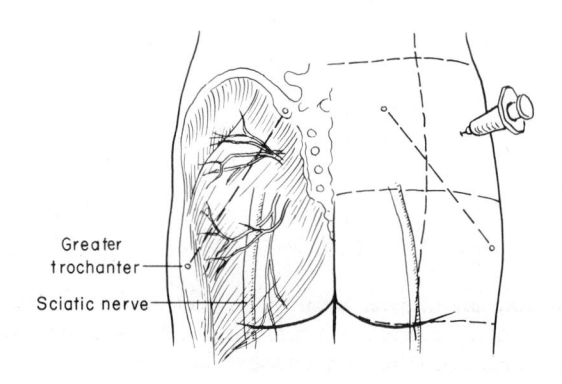

PREPARATION AND ADMINISTRATION OF MEDICATIONS

The ventrogluteal area, commonly known as von Hochstetter's site, is gaining recognition as a safe, proper IM injection site. It usually has a very small fatty layer, and the muscle layer is thick. This site can be used both for adults and children, and is especially helpful if the patient must recline in either the Sims or the prone position.

To locate the injection site, place your left palm to the right of the greater trochanter, put your index finger on the anterior iliac spine, and spread your middle finger posteriorly as far as possible to touch the iliac crest. (Reverse the hand position for a patient who is lying on his right side.) The center of the triangle bounded by your fingers is the precise injection site to be used.

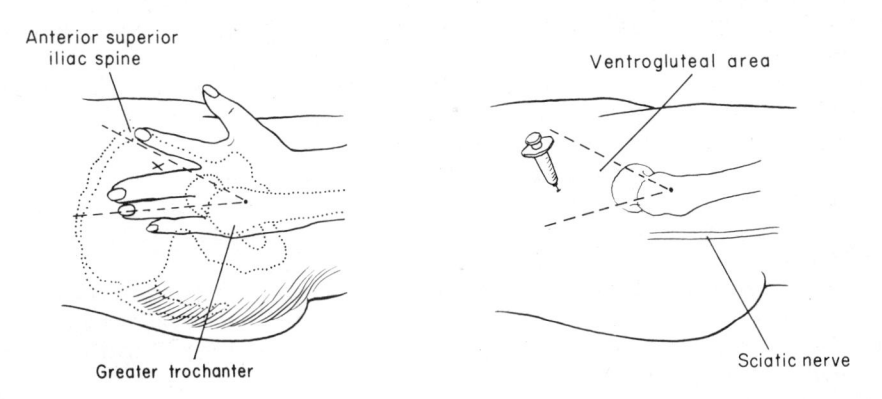

The vastus lateralis muscle is also a common IM injection site for both adults and children. The area extends from the mid-anterior front of the thigh to the mid-lateral thigh, a hand's width below the proximal end of the greater trochanter, and a hand's width above the upper knee.

This muscle can be used when the patient is lying prone, in a Sims position, or sitting upright.

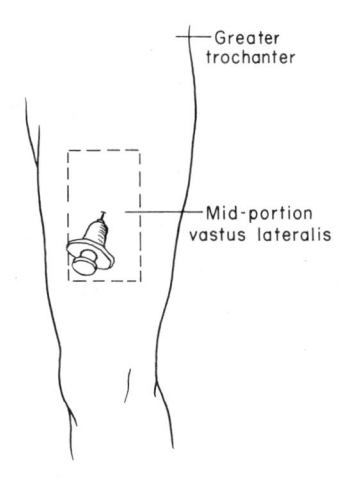

For newborns and infants, there are three sites used for IM injections: mid-anterior (rectus femoris) muscle of the thigh, mid-lateral (vastus lateralis) muscle, and the deltoid muscle in the upper arm. Your margin of error in giving IM injections is considerably increased because of the smallness of the child's anatomical features.

When giving injections to children, you must assess and understand their level of biophysical and psychosocial development. By knowing the various stages of growth and development, you will be able to provide the child with the essential explanation and support before, during, and after the injection.

For example, an infant's physical responses are diffuse; he will probably cry immediately, flex his legs, and exhibit general body movement. In the older infant the cry may be delayed, and there will be considerably less movement. By the time he is six to eight months old, he will begin to cry as soon as he sees the needle and syringe (after the first injection, of course). Safely restraining the child is essential to avoid injury, and therefore you may need someone to assist you in restraining him, gently and with concern. Reassure the child by your manner. If he is old enough to understand, be honest with him. Tell him, "It will hurt for a minute." After the injection, cuddle the infant and talk quietly to him. This will help him to learn to trust—an important aspect of growth and development. (Ask your instructor to give you readings from Eric Erickson and other experts on the subject of growth and development.)

Although the toddler does not have an instinctive fear of an injection, the situation he finds himself in may be unfamiliar, and therefore he is frightened. After the first injection, his perception of the pain may be exaggerated and he may try to avoid successive injections by hiding or running away. After the injection, he needs to be held while he displays aggressive acts, such as hitting the health worker.

The pre-school child is learning and becoming aware of his body and what he can do. Play-acting is helpful for explaining procedures to a child this age. Let him feel the syringe. Demonstrate the entire procedure on a doll, so that the child will know exactly what will be done to him. Explain that the medicine will help him get better, and he can soon play outdoors again.

The school-aged child wants to know how and why things work; a clear, simple explanation of what the health worker is going to do and why it is being done is vital to his understanding of the grown-up world. Tell him that he is good; children thrive on praise, and of course this is true for almost everyone.

The average adolescent, who is trying to be an adult, will avoid expressing his real feelings. Many adolescents are extremely modest, and therefore you must be constantly mindful to provide for this sensitivity.

To locate the correct injection site for children over 2 years of age who have well-formed gluteus muscles, feel the posterior iliac crest and the head of the trochanter; imagine a line connecting the two locations. Injections should be given above this imaginary line in an area that is almost free of major vessels and nerves. This site is *not used for children under two*, or for those who are undernourished.

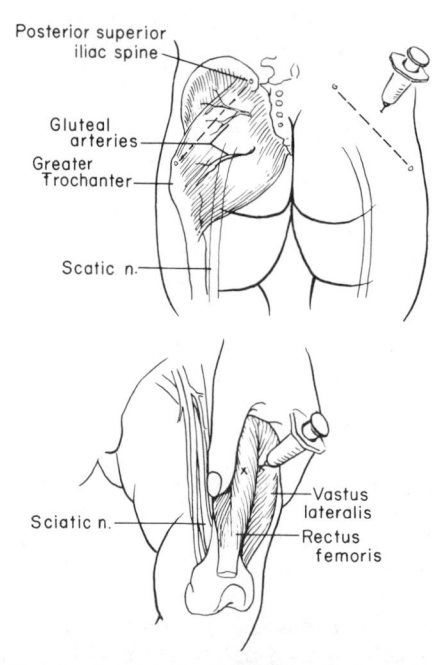

The most common IM injection site in the infant is the vastus lateralis or the anterior muscle, the rectus femoris. The needle size and the angle of injection will depend upon the size of the infant. However, a one-inch needle inserted at a 45° angle is customary.

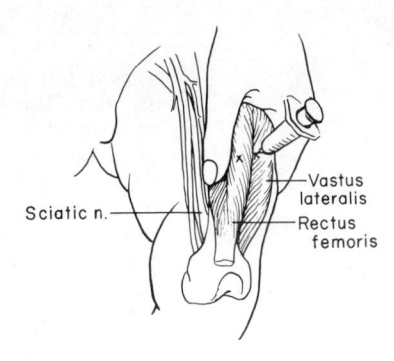

Figure: Injection site on infant thigh showing Sciatic n., Vastus lateralis, Rectus femoris.

With the infant lying on his back, grasp the thigh and gently pinch the muscle to concentrate the tissue for a good injection site. The needle can be inserted in either of the locations indicated in the above picture.

Although the deltoid muscles can be used for infants and children, only very small amounts of liquid can be injected because this muscle is very thin. The injection should be given in the thickest part of the muscle; the needle should point at a slight angle toward the shoulder.

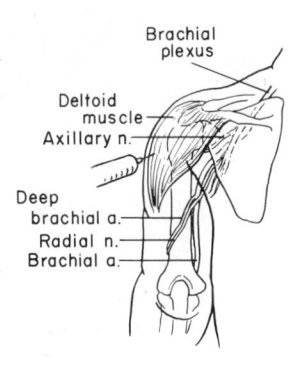

Figure: Deltoid injection site showing Brachial plexus, Deltoid muscle, Axillary n., Deep brachial a., Radial n., Brachial a.

B. Administration of an Intramuscular Injection

Preparation of the needle and syringe follows the same procedure that you learned in Item 3,C on preparing for subcutaneous injection. Remember to read your labels three times so that you can check the accuracy of the medication and desired dose as you remove the medication from storage, as you pour the medication, and as you return the unused medication to the storage area.

Note: If you are using the unit-dose system, you will compare the label of the individual dose with the medication record when you take it from storage, and also just before you give it to the patient. A third check is possible while comparing the label from the package as you record the medication on the patient's chart.

Important Steps	Key Points
1. Wash your hands and obtain necessary equipment and supplies.	Place the prepared medication on a tray and take it to the patient, together with the record.
2. Approach, identify, and explain the procedure to the patient.	Verify the identification of the patient (Identaband, patient's record, depending on where the patient is being treated: ambulance, hospital, clinic, office, or home.

PREPARATION AND ADMINISTRATION OF MEDICATIONS

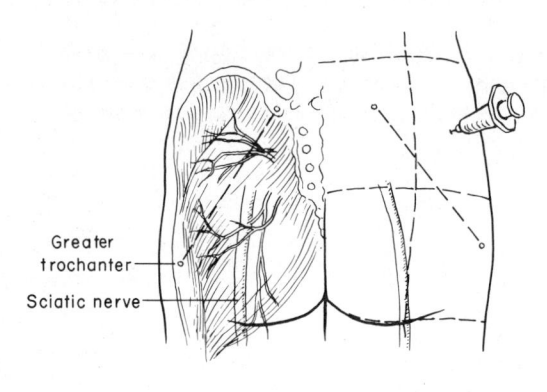

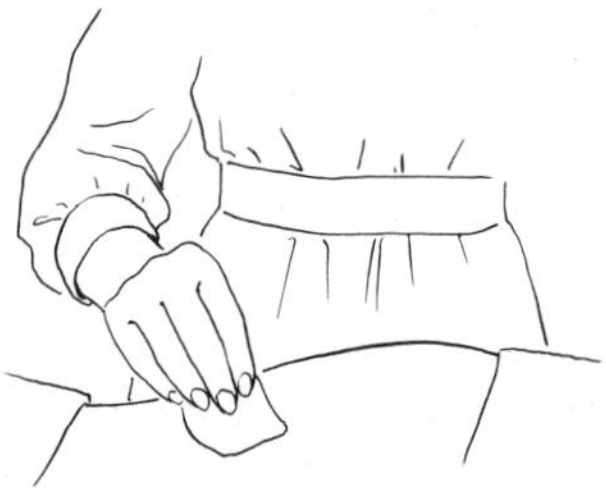

Important Steps	Key Points
	Always tell the patient what you are going to do even though you may think he cannot understand, e.g., infant, small child, confused or unconscious person.
	If you need assistance because of the patient's condition, be sure to have another health worker help you, e.g., your patient may be a small, scared, belligerent child, or a frightened, violent adult.
3. Select the injection site.	Expose the injection site so that you will have an unobstructed view.
Greater trochanter — Sciatic nerve —	If the gluteal region is being used, have the patient lie on his abdomen with his toes turned slightly inward. This position provides for the greatest muscle relaxation.
	Follow the directions in Item 5,A for selecting the site of injection as well as hand placement, which serves as a boundary line to avoid major nerves, vessels, and other structures.
4. Open and remove an antiseptic sponge from the package.	Cleanse the injection site, using a firm but gentle circular motion, moving from a central point in ever-widening circles until about a 2-inch space is cleansed. Hold the sponge between your last two fingers for use later when you remove the needle.
	Allow the area to dry.
5. Pick up the syringe and position your hands.	Expel air bubbles from the syringe and check anatomical landmarks. Place your non-dominant hand on the area. Tell your patient you are going to insert the needle; he will automatically tighten his muscles, (you can feel this taking place). Tell him to relax, and wait until you can feel the muscles loosen.

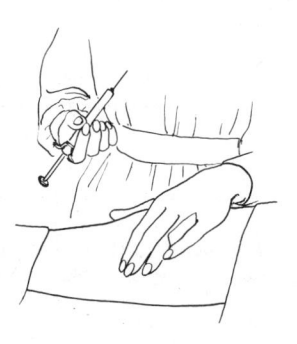

PREPARATION AND ADMINISTRATION OF MEDICATIONS

Important Steps

6. Insert the needle.

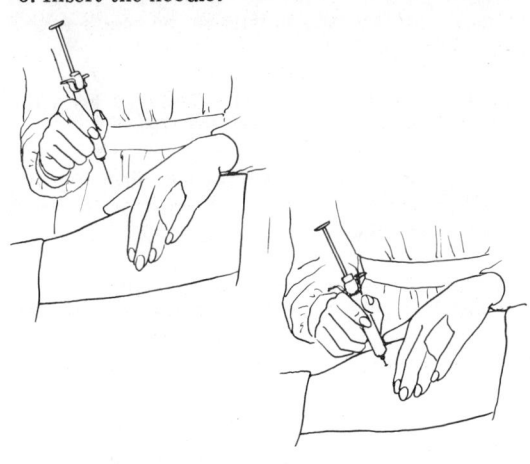

7. Pull back on the plunger.

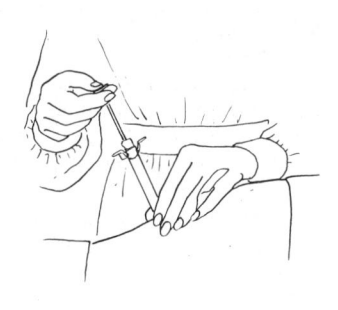

8. Inject the medication.

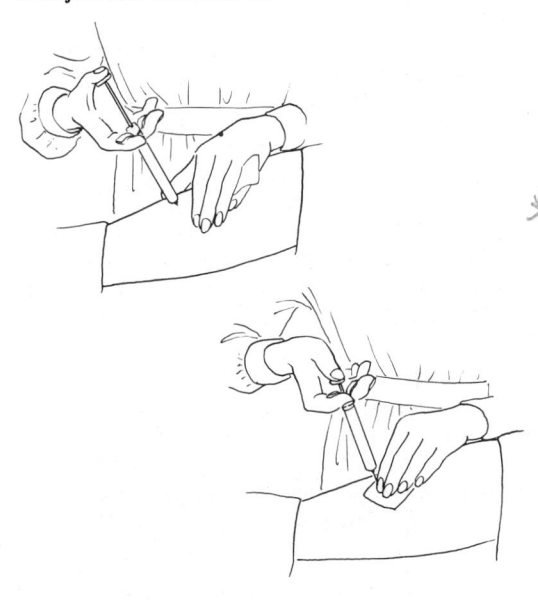

Key Points

Grasp the barrel of the syringe *firmly* between the dominant thumb and index finger and plunge the needle firmly into the muscle at a 90° angle to about one-half the depth of the needle. Complete the insertion with an additional quick, forward thrust of the needle to the desired depth.

You will feel a moderate resistance to the needle as you puncture the skin; however, it moves easily through the subcutaneous and muscle tissue.

You will remember that you do this to see if you have entered a blood vessel. Withdraw the needle slightly, redirect, and reinsert; then aspirate again to check for blood.

You will need to reposition the non-dominant hand to hold the barrel of the syringe and to steady the needle while you draw back on the plunger with your dominant hand.

This step will take some practice; however, since you will use it for *every injection* regardless of type, it soon becomes automatic. Rarely will you hit a blood vessel if you follow the anatomical landmarks described in this Unit, and you will seldom need to reinsert the needle.

Observe the patient for symptoms of shock, unusual pain, etc.

Shift the finger on the dominant hand so that the thumb rests on the plunger and your index and middle fingers rest under the upper tip, or hooks, of the syringe barrel. Using the fingers as a counterforce, push the plunger into the barrel with a slow, continuous downward movement as far as the plunger will go.

NOTE: The last air bubble to disappear is important because it cleans the needle lumen of the medication and keeps the medication from dribbling into the tissue as the needle is removed. Medication prepared for IM absorption may cause local tissue reaction if left in the fatty subcutaneous or intradermal tissues.

Important Steps	Key Points
9. Withdraw the needle.	Apply pressure with the antiseptic sponge at the needle site as you remove the needle with a quick, upward motion.
	This external pressure also helps to keep the medicine from leaking into the tissues.
10. Massage the injection site.	Doing this with a gentle but firm circular motion helps to disperse the medicine so that it can be absorbed more quickly.
	Apply a BAND-AID if there happens to be superficial bleeding. Some people have a very intricate superficial vascular system and they will bleed slightly regardless of how careful you are.
11. Position the patient for comfort and safety.	Replace linens or clothing. Locate the signal and bedside stand within easy reach. Adjust the bed and siderails if indicated.
	While continuing to observe the patient for unusual reactions (such as rash or shock), ask him if there is anything else you can do. Tell the patient when you expect to return.
12. Remove the equipment.	Take the syringes and needles to the work area and dispose of them in the designated needle and syringe container. Replace the cleaned medicine tray.
13. Record the procedure.	For example:
	12:15 A.M. — Demerol 50 mgm IM in RUQ, buttock given for severe pain.
	H. Johnson, R.N.
	12:45 A.M. — Pain has subsided substantially; patient dozing.
	H. Johnson, R.N.
14. Return the medication record to storage.	The patient's chart should be returned to the chart desk; the medication Kardex may remain in the medication room or on the medication cart; the medication card should be returned to the medication card storage in the medication room.

It is the health worker's responsibility to check the patient after 20 or 30 minutes, and periodically during the intervening time until the next dosage is to be given. This is done to see if the desired response to the medication has been obtained; e.g., relief from pain, nausea, bleeding, etc. Record the observation on the patient's record. This step of the medication procedure is frequently omitted. As you begin to give medications, develop the habit of not only observing the patient's response to the medication, but also recording it accurately on his chart.

PREPARATION AND ADMINISTRATION OF MEDICATIONS

C. Z-Track Technique

The alternate IM injection method is called the *Z-track technique*. It may be used for injecting a drug called Imferon. The upper outer quadrant of the *gluteal region* is the preferred site of injection.

Important Steps	Key Points
Follow steps 1 through 7 as above.	
8. Retract the skin laterally.	
9. Insert the needle at a 90° angle. (Use at least a 2-inch needle).	Withdraw the plunger slightly to assure that you are not in a blood vessel. If you are, remove the needle and replace it with a sterile one; then begin again. *Keep the skin pulled laterally during injection.*
skin stretched	
10. Inject the medication.	Wait for 10 seconds.
11. Remove the needle.	Put it aside, out of the patient's way. DO NOT MASSAGE THE SITE; this may force the medication out into the muscle or subcutaneous tissue. Imferon is absorbed rapidly from muscle, but not from subcutaneous tissue.
12. Release the skin.	This seals off the skin opening and stops leakage of the drug, thus preventing tissue stain.
	NOTE: Walking helps absorption. Use alternate buttocks for subsequent injections.
skin relaxed	

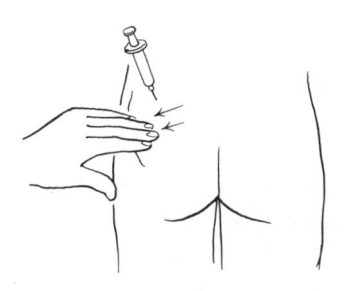

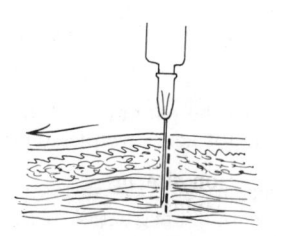

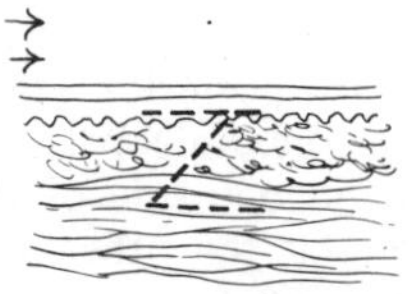

Continue with steps 11 through 14 of the foregoing item.

ITEM 6: INTRADERMAL INJECTIONS

Intradermal injections are customarily given in the dorsal site of the forearm, but the lateral or posterior sides of the arm can also be used. These are selected so that the site can be easily observed for various reactions (such as redness or swelling) as well as for keeping clothing from rubbing the area. Injections of this type are commonly used for various skin tests to determine sensitivity to a disease (for example tuberculosis, coccidioidomycosis, and histoplasmosis) as well as sensitivities (allergies) to drugs or foreign objects such as tetanus antitoxin, tetanus toxoid, dust, grass, food substances.

Since very small quantities of solution are administered (0.1 ml to 0.3 ml), a tuberculin syringe is normally used because of its fine calibrations, providing an easy means for giving minute quantities of medicine.

Frequently, the injection of the solution into the dermis causes a stinging, burning sensation, which is in direct proportion to the amounts of solutions that are administered. You must alert the patient to this possible discomfort.

Preparation of the needle and syringe is the same for the intradermal injection as for the subcutaneous and IM types of injection, except that you should select a needle with a fine lumen (26 or 27 gauge), and one that is short (3/8 to 1/2 inch); also select the tuberculin syringe for accurate measurement of the medication.

Important Steps	Key Points
1. Wash your hands.	Take the prepared needle and syringe on a medicine tray with the medication record to the patient.
2. Approach, identify, and explain the procedure to the patient.	Verify his identification (Identaband, patient chart, etc.)
	Always explain to the patient even though you may think he cannot hear or understand.
3. Select the injection site.	Expose the area, usually the anterior forearm, so that you have an unobstructed view.
4. Open and remove the antiseptic sponge from the package.	Cleanse the injection site using a firm, gentle circular motion, cleaning an area approximately 2 inches in diameter.
	When you are finished with the cleaning, hold the sponge between the last two fingers for later use when you remove the needle.
5. Pick up the syringe.	Expel air bubbles by holding the syringe vertically and gently pushing on the plunger.
6. Grasp the forearm to be injected.	While standing in front of the patient, turn the patient's anterior forearm upward, facing you. Grasp his arm on the posterior side, toward the middle of the forearm. With your non-dominant thumb on one side of the arm and your index finger on the other side, pull the anterior skin taut.
7. Insert the needle.	With the bevel of the needle facing upward, insert the needle through the skin at an angle almost parallel to the skin (10 to 15 degrees). Insert the needle so that only the bevel penetrates the skin. Avoid hair follicles.
8. Inject the solution slowly.	If you have inserted the needle correctly, a small circular bump (wheal) that is blanched (white) will appear in the skin.

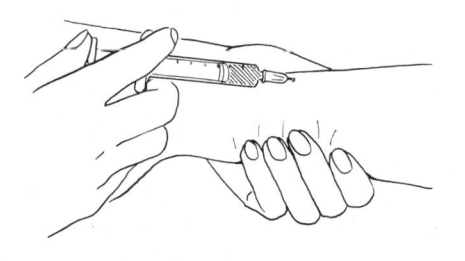

Important Steps	Key Points
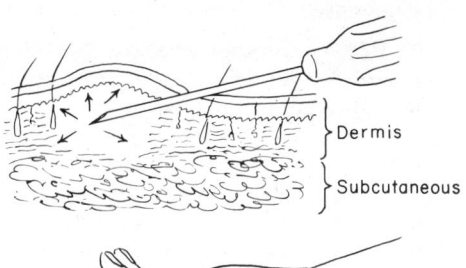	<u>You should be able to feel some resistance at the needle point if you are in the dermal layer. If the tip moves freely, you have inserted the needle too deeply. In this event, withdraw the needle slightly and check again for resistance.</u>
	Continue to reassure your patient as you inject the solution.
	Observe the patient for unusual reactions (e.g., shock).
9. Withdraw the needle.	Wipe the area *very gently* with the antiseptic sponge as you remove the needle. *Do not apply pressure.* You must not disperse the medicine into the underlying tissues.
10. Position the patient for comfort and safety.	Have him lie down if he feels faint. Ask him to sit a few minutes to assure that he feels all right, and that no unusual effects are occurring.
	Put the call light signal and bedside stand near the patient, as necessary. Adjust the bed and siderails if indicated.
	While continuing to observe the patient for unusual reactions, ask if there is anything else you can do, and tell him when you expect to return.
	Observe the skin reaciton (for redness or swelling) to record on the chart. The size of the reaction determines what the treatment will be; e.g., if the reaction to the test dose of tetanus antitoxin is negative (described in the tetanus antitoxin brochure accompanying the drug), the prescribed dose of tetanus antitoxin can be given to the patient. But if the patient has a positive reaction to the test, the antitoxin may have to be given in divided doses over a period of several hours.
	Since there are various interpretations of each of the intradermal solutions, the specifics of these will not be discussed here. You will learn about these responses in your pharmacology course when you learn about various drugs.
11. Remove the equipment.	Return the supplies to the designated storage area and dispose of the used needle and syringe in the designated containers (for reprocessing if reusable syringes were used, or for incineration if disposable syringes were used).

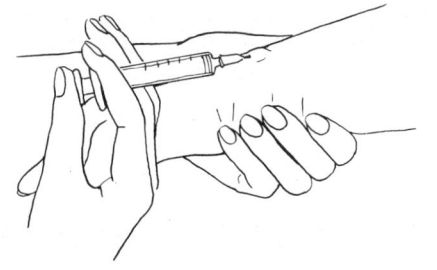

Important Steps	Key Points
12. Record the procedure.	For example:

8:10 P.M. — Tetanus antitoxin 0.1 ml given intradermally on right anterior forearm; 1 cm wheal appeared within 15 minutes.

J. Fish, R.N.

NOTE: The wheal reaction is read at varying times within 48 hours, depending on the particular medication used. Follow the directions accompanying the medicine for the reading and interpreting schedule.

ITEM 7: INTRAVENOUS (IV) INJECTIONS

Medications injected directly into the circulatory system produce almost immediate response to the drug, usually within 30 to 60 seconds.

For many years, nurses were not permitted to give IV medications or volume solutions; this remained the responsibility of physicians. However, in the 1960's many state laws and agency policies authorized designated RN's to administer medicines via the circulatory route in special instances: e.g., upon completion of a physician-supervised training program; within certain boundaries prescribed by agency procedure such as specified volume solutions and specified small-dosage medicines (1 to 10 cc).

In some states, LPN/LVN's are now allowed to insert needles into veins to withdraw blood for test purposes after having completed a physician-supervised training program. This activity will probably be expanded within the next decade so that LPN/LVN's can legally give medicines via the IV route, particularly with the expansion of the unit-dose system of medications. In other words, the IV medicine would be prepared, packaged and labeled by the pharmacist for the individual patient, thereby practically eliminating errors in preparing IV medications for administration. The technique of administering an intravenous injection is not difficult to learn.

Preparation of IV medications for direct injection into the vein follows previously described procedures. The size of syringe selected is based on the amount of IV medicine to be injected, from 1 to 50 cc. The only exception is the preparation of volume IV solutions (250, 500, 1000 cc). Volume fluids are given directly into a vein (infusion) via a needle or catheter for patients unable to take fluids by mouth. The insertion of the intravenous catheter is usually done by the physician and therefore will not be discussed in this unit. Infusions permit the patient to receive complementary nutrients that are essential to carrying on life functions. Hyperalimentation is a comparatively new method for providing total parenteral nutritional needs for patients who cannot take medicines or food orally, or whose disease or condition requires that the bowel rest during the healing processes. In the case of hyperalimentation, the catheter is inserted into (1) the axillary vein, through the subclavian vein, and hence into the superior vena cava; or (2) the external or internal jugular vein and is then threaded into the superior vena cava; or (3) the femoral vein, and is then threaded up to the superior vena cava. Hyperalimentation can be utilized for selected patients during a period of six weeks or more.

Infusions, on the other hand, are more common and are utilized for shorter periods of time, from a few hours to several days. The actual site of the venipuncture is dependent not only upon the condition of the patient's veins, but also upon his safety and comfort. If a patient must have his leg or arm extended and restrained for long periods of time, he can suffer great discomfort. If this happens, he may become restless, dislodging the needle from the vein and injuring the vein and surrounding tissue. This in turn would inject solution that is intended only for intravenous use into the surrounding tissue, possibly causing irritation and, on a long-term basis, necrosis of the tissue. Either of these situations is extremely painful.

ITEM 8: PREPARATION OF IV INFUSION

Important Steps	Key Points
1. Wash your hands.	
2. Obtain the required equipment.	This will include a bottle of the prescribed IV solution, IV or blood transfusion tubing, needles (16-20 gauge), antiseptic sponges, tourniquet, extra needle and syringe (3 cc, 5 cc), tape, and arm board. An IV tray is required to carry the prepared medication to the patient's bedside.
	Inspect the solution or blood package for sediment, abnormal cloudiness, or change in color. *If any of these conditions is present, the blood or solution must not be used.* Follow your agency procedure for returning unusable solutions or blood.
3. Verify the medicine with the patient's medication record.	Be sure that you have the correct solution and equipment. Compare the label on the IV solution (medicine) with the patient's record: i.e., name, dose, route, hours of administration, patient's identification.
4. Remove the metal protector and rubber diaphragm from the solution bottle.	Follow the directions on the cap for removal. Avoid cutting your finger on the edges of the cap. Discard the cover at once in a designated container.
5. Open and remove the antiseptic sponge.	Discard the wrapper in a designated container.
6. Wipe the rubber stopper of the solution bottle.	Holding the antiseptic sponge in your dominant hand, wipe the stopper with several firm, brisk, back-and-forth motions. Discard the sponge in a designated container.
7. Open the sterile tubing package.	These packages are clearly labeled with directions for opening them, and for inserting the tubing.
	<u>A single tube is utilized for most infusions.</u>
	A "Y" tube is used for the blood transfusion. One branch of the "Y" is inserted into the normal saline solution, while the other branch is inserted into the package (bottle) of blood or a second solution. The distal extension is inserted into the needle that is to be inserted into the vein. The "Y" tube also has a filter attached within the tubing, to filter out larger particles in the blood that may have developed during storage.
8. Remove the protective cap from the drip chamber.	The solution bottle is frequently called a Vacoliter because it is a one-liter bottle filled under vacuum. Other size bottles are in use, however (250 cc, 500 cc).

Important Steps	Key Points
9. Insert the drip chamber tip into the rubber stopper.	The rubber stopper is marked with a circle and an "X". Holding the Vacoliter bottle securely in your non-dominant hand, bracing it against your body so that it won't slip, make a fist around the drip chamber, being careful to avoid touching the sterile tip of the chamber and the clean stopper. Grasp the drip chamber tip firmly with your dominant hand, and with a straight down and forward motion, push the tubing tip into the rubber stopper. This pushing action takes considerable strength, which is why you must hold the Vacoliter very securely to keep it from slipping and falling to the floor. Breaking the Vacoliter is dangerous because of the broken glass; it is also very costly to the patient or the agency. (Some agencies charge the unused solution or blood to the patient, while others may have a charge system wherein the unit or floor is charged for losses.)
10. Clamp the tubing.	With the tubing clamp, close off the flow of solution into the tubing. (Since there are several types of clamps, follow the directions on the package for the specific kind being used in your agency.)
11. Attach the distal end of the tubing to the needle.	Remove the protective guard from the needle holder. Hold the tubing between your non-dominant middle and index fingers, taking care not to contaminate the tip of the needle holder. Remove the protective guard from the tip while holding the cap in your dominant hand between thumb and index finger, with the needle casing between the thumb and index finger of the non-dominant hand.

Discard the needle cap from the dominant hand. Tip the needle package slightly downward so that the needle hub is visible, and insert the tubing end into the needle. Keep the needle protected with the needle cover until you are ready for the injection. |
12. Verify the solution with the patient's record.	NOTE: If your agency uses the unit-dose system, your IV Vacoliter will come to you labeled with additives and ready to insert the tubing.
13. Take the solution to the patient's room.	Put it on the bedside stand and prepare the IV stand. It should be placed on the side of the bed nearest the injection site; e.g., if giving the injection in the right area, the IV stand should be placed on the right side of the bed near the patient's head.
14. Invert the bottle and hang it on the IV pole.	Remove the needle protector, release the clamp, and allow some fluid to run through the tubing to remove all the air bubbles. This bit of solution can be directed into the nearby wastebasket. Air injected into the vein can cause an air embolus, which could kill the patient.

Important Steps	Key Points
	Close the clamp, replace the protective cover on the needle, and lay it aside while you prepare the patient.
15. Tear off three or four pieces of tape.	These are for securing the needle when you have finished the procedure. Hang the tap on the bedside stand within your reach.

ITEM 9: ADMINISTRATION OF AN IV INJECTION

Important Steps	Key Points
1. Wash your hands.	
2. Approach, identify, and explain the procedure to the patient.	Tell him that he will be receiving fluids (food) in his vein for the specified period of time (hours, days, or whatever). He will have to refrain from moving too much to keep from dislodging the needle. Assure him that you will find a site in which to put the needle that will give him the greatest possible mobility as well as the least pain.
3. Select the site for the venipuncture.	(a) The basilic or cephalic veins on the inner aspect of the upper forearm are used frequently because of their accessibility. However, since the patient must usually be immobilized to prevent dislodgement of the needle, this area should be selected only for short-term IV's. (This site is usually the easiest for the novice.)
	The lower forearm cephalic and basilic veins may be used for long-term therapy because the patient can move more fully.
	(b) The metacarpal veins on the back of the hand are also used for long-term infusions because this area, too, allows the patient mobility. These veins are usually superficial and easily seen; however, the venipuncture is often painful for patients. Also, there is greater likelihood of inserting the needle completely through the vein.
	If patients must have repeated infusions, it is best to start your IV's first in the most distal veins in the extremity, and progress proximally as you start each successive infusion.
	(c) The saphenous or femoral veins in the thigh can be used. Because of the danger of phlebitis, however, leg veins should be used with discrimination. Your agency may have special regulations regarding the usage of leg veins for infusions. Be sure to follow these rules.

— proposed point of entry

— Femoral vein

— Saphenous vein

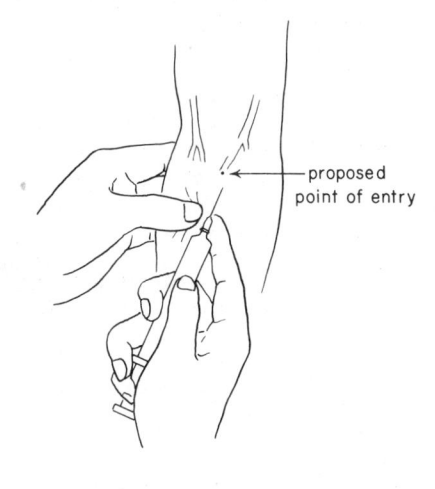

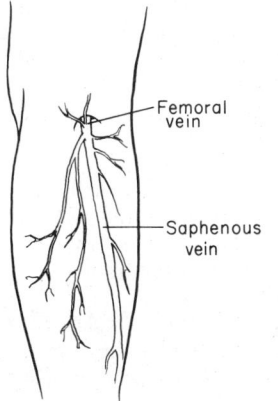

Posterior View

Important Steps	Key Points
	(d) The saphenous and the marginal veins in the lower leg and foot can also be used. Obviously, fluid administration is easier and more rapid when infused in the larger veins. Thus site selection is a very important consideration.
4. Place the extremity on a board for restraining.	This measure is usually required if you select a site near the bend of the elbow or ankle. It immobilizes the extremity to keep from dislodging the needle. Secure the extremity on the padded board with tape or gauze bandage. Whichever is used, do not secure it so tightly that the circulation is restricted.
5. Place tourniquet around extremity.	For purposes of this lesson, we will use the patient's right arm. A tourniquet is applied above the site of injection to provide proper visibility and distention of the vein. NOTE: There is an alternate technique without using a tourniquet which will be given in the next item. A soft, 1-inch Penrose rubber tubing is preferred, or blood pressure cuff can be used. The tourniquet is applied about 2 or 3 inches above the injection site. Of course, you would never apply a tourniquet around a limb that already has an infusion going. Sometimes, because of the patient's condition, two or more limbs may be used to administer infusions simultaneously.
6. Grasp the ends of the tourniquet with your dominant hand.	Cross one end with sufficient tension for your purposes, and for the patient's comfort. Press the crossing point with your thumb and middle finger to retain the tension. With your index finger, tuck a loop of the upper end under the circle of tubing, then remove your fingers. Tension will hold the tucked loop in place and prevent it from slipping loose.

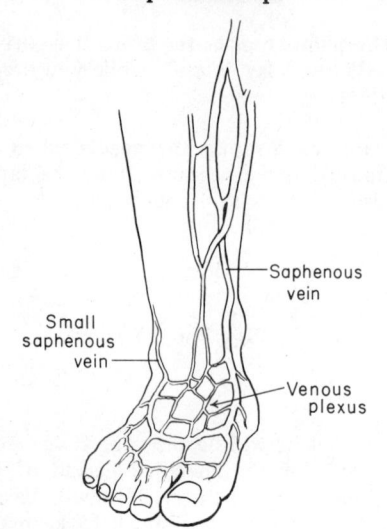

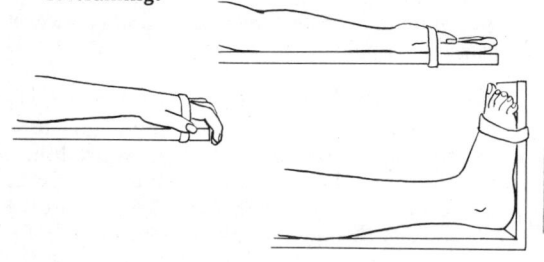

PREPARATION AND ADMINISTRATION OF MEDICATIONS

Important Steps	Key Points
7. After releasing your fingers, check the tension.	If the tension is too tight, the patient will complain; if the tension is too loose, there will be no distention of the vein. In either case, untie the tourniquet and retie it until a reasonable tension is obtained. This will have to be practiced under supervision until you can judge the appropriate constriction of the veins. NOTE: The two ends of the tourniquet can be clamped snugly on the extremity if you have a hemostat available.
8. Locate the vein.	Ask the patient to make a fist, and to open and close it a few times. Next, have him hold the fist. This allows time for the blood to build up in the distal portion of the extremity below the tourniquet, making the veins distend and become more visible either to sight or palpation. The tourniquet cuts off circulation, and the patient may complain of pinpricks or tingling or say that his fingers are "going to sleep." Therefore, you must work rapidly so that you can release the tourniquet quickly after the needle is in place. Allowing the extremity to hang down off the bed for a short time will also speed up the engorgement of the veins in the extremity. Wrapping the extremity in a warm pad is another way to distend the veins.
9. Examine the selected vein.	Tap your dominant index finger lightly against the vein. You should be able to feel the distended vein. It should feel like a spongy, elastic tube under your fingers; you may be able to feel pulsating ridges, but the vein should not roll freely about. Move your finger an inch or two in either direction so that you can be sure of the size and direction of the vein.
10. Cleanse site with an antiseptic sponge.	*Do not touch* your finger to the site again. If you must feel the vein again, the site must be cleansed with another antiseptic sponge. Place the used sponge just above the injection site for use again, if needed.
11. Check for air bubbles in the IV tubing.	Remove the protective covering from the needle and release the tubing clamp once more, allowing a few drops of fluid to run. Reclamp the tubing.

PREPARATION AND ADMINISTRATION OF MEDICATIONS

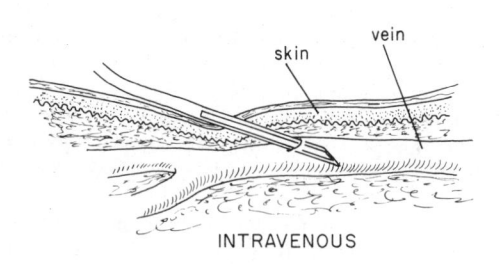

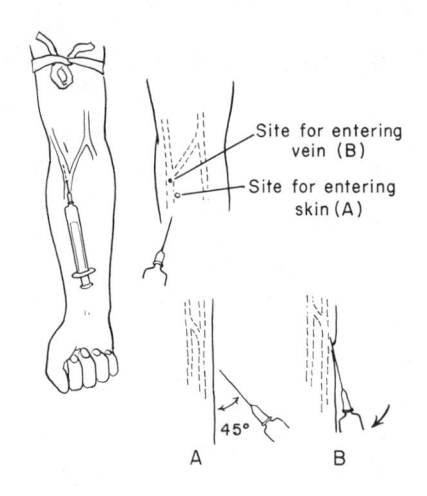

Important Steps	Key Points
12. Pick up the needle.	(a) If you are using a syringe and needle to start the IV, grasp the syringe with your dominant hand, using the index finger to stabilize the needle at the hub, and the palm of your hand and little finger to stabilize the plunger.
	(b) If you are using the IV tubing attached directly to the needle, grasp it between the thumb and index finger of your dominant hand.
13. Stretch the skin near the injection site.	With the non-dominant hand, grasp around the extremity. Place the thumb about 1 inch directly below the injection site; with a firm downward pressure of the thumb directly over the vein, pull the skin taut toward you.
14. Point the needle in the direction of the selected vein.	In the dominant hand, hold the needle at about a 45° angle with the bevel up about 1/2 inch below the injection site.
15. Pierce the skin.	(a) If the vein is large and stable, you can probably enter the skin and vein in one quick, steady, forward thrust with the needle. You will feel a decreased resistance to the needle as you enter the vein.
	(b) If the vein is sclerotic, buried in adipose tissue, or very small, you may prefer a two-step insertion. First, pierce the skin directly parallel and immediately to the side of the vein, then move the tip of the needle toward the vein and gently into the vein.
16. Check the entry into the vein.	If you are in the vein, the pressure of the blood flowing into the vein will cause the plunger to move back in the barrel, or the blood to back-flow to the IV tubing. At any rate, when you are in the vein, you will be able to see the blood return, either into the tubing or the syringe.

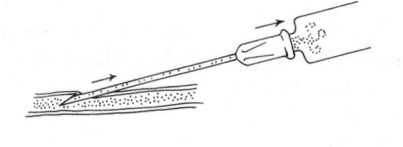

PREPARATION AND ADMINISTRATION OF MEDICATIONS

Important Steps	Key Points
	The amount of blood flowing into the syringe or tubing may be minimal or nearly nonexistent when a patient is in shock. Therefore, you must have substantial practice before initiating an infusion into a patient who is in shock.
17. Settle the needle in place.	After you make sure that you are in the vein, slowly move the needle tip forward so that it is anchored securely in the vein (usually the length of the needle — 1-1/2 to 2 inches). If you gently lift the needle and point the tip very slightly upward you will avoid puncturing the posterior vein wall as you settle the needle into place.
	NOTE: If you go through the vein, withdraw the needle to the dermis and reinsert.
	You should not attempt the venipuncture more than twice without success. Call for assistance; do *not* put your patient through a continuing painful procedure. Even those individuals who are most experienced at starting infusions will occasionally find a patient with whom they have difficulty.
	If you were using a syringe, quickly remove the syringe from the needle. Be sure to hold the hub of the needle securely between the thumb and index finger of your non-dominant hand. Remove the tubing with the needle tip from its protective guard and insert it quickly and tightly into the needle.
18. Release the tourniquet.	Ask the patient to open his fist; unclamp the IV tubing and watch the fluid enter the vein.
19. Regulate the solution flow.	The rate will vary depending on the patient's condition and the concentration of the liquid. The rate must be regulated according to the order and type of IV drip chamber that is being used:
	(a) Regular drip meter releases 15 gtt/cc
	(b) Blood drip releases 10 gtt/cc
	(c) Micro-drip releases 60 gtt/cc
	Most of the companies that distribute intravenous solutions supply full charts that display the various conversion tables.
20. Place a piece of folded gauze under the hub of the needle.	This will stabilize the needle. As you put the gauze under the hub, observe the flow rate; it may speed up or slow down. Adjust the thickness of the gauze to obtain the rate of flow that is ordered.

Important Steps	Key Points
21. Secure the needle in place.	Apply the tape gently in a criss-cross fashion across the hub of the needle. Loop the tubing on the extremity and secure it again with tape. This will prevent direct pull on the needle, which could possibly dislodge it if the patient should move around. Once more, verify the label on the bottle with the medication record.
22. Leave the patient safe and comfortable.	Adjust the bed for comfort, put the call signal and bedside stand within his easy reach. Ask if there is anything else you can do and tell him when you will return. You or your designate should check the infusion every 15 minutes. Ask the patient to call you if his arm begins to sting (possible infiltration) or if the solution stops dripping (clogged needle, tubing, or filter).
23. Leave the IV tray at his bedside.	You will have antiseptic sponges, gauze, tape, etc., available if you need to remove or adjust the infusion. The tray will be removed later, when the infusion is completed.
23. Record the procedure on the patient's record.	Charting example: 10:00 A.M. — 1000 cc 5% Dextrose in water started IV in the right antecubital area. IV regulated at 60 gtt minute. M. Hoyaski, R.N. NOTE: Agencies sometimes initiate the infusion by injecting 20 milliliters of one per cent sodium bicarbonate into the vein to decrease the probability of a phlebitis. Some agencies routinely apply Bacitracin ointment and a sterile gauze daily over the injection site to prevent an infection from developing at the venipuncture site. In any case, follow your agency procedure. If the intravenous injections are to be given over a period of several days, the tubing should be changed every 24 hours to minimize the danger of infection.

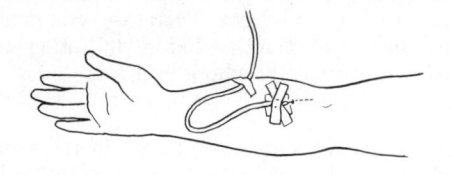

ITEM 10: ALTERNATE VENIPUNCTURE TECHNIQUE

Recent research studies indicate that it may be better not to use a tourniquet nor to have the patient make a fist for the venipuncture. The venous stasis that occurs may alter blood chemistries if the tourniquet is improperly applied; the effect would change the blood chemistry reports. A sustained fist during the venipuncture may increase the ammonia concentration in the blood, and this could alter the various ammonia tests done in the clinical laboratory.

The procedure for selecting and preparing the injection site remains the same as for the previous item, as does the actual injection procedure itself.

It is recommended that the syringe be operated with one hand so that you can stabilize the extremity with your other hand. In addition, if you use both hands on the syringe, the needle may easily slip out of the vein.

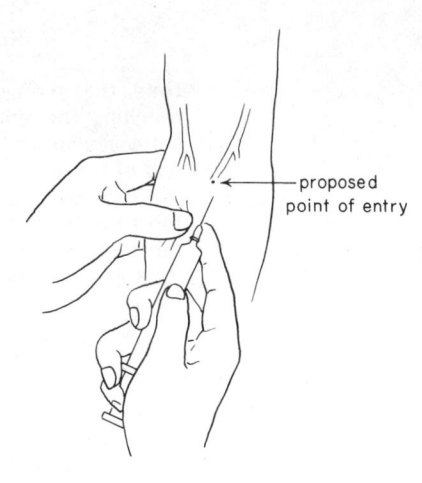

PREPARATION AND ADMINISTRATION OF MEDICATIONS

proposed point of entry

If you are taking a blood sample, pull back slightly on the plunger with your free hand until you have the required amount of blood for the particular laboratory test to be done. Then remove the needle as in the previous item.

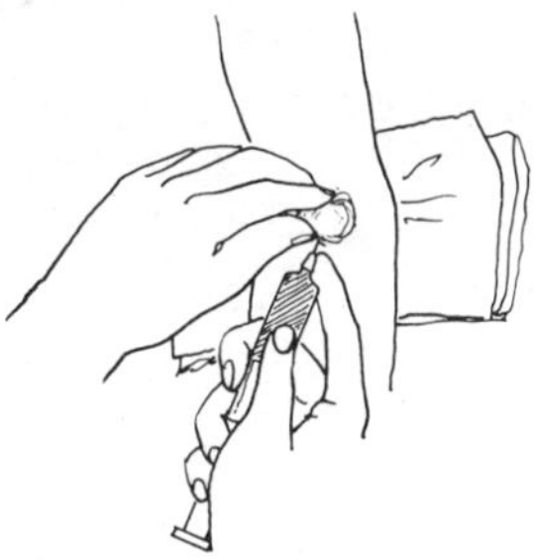

Transfer of Blood to Tube

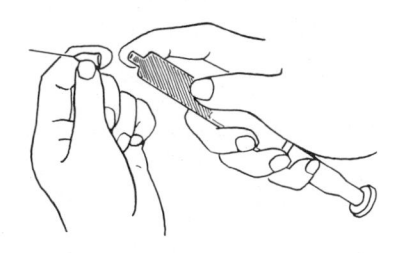

Important Steps	Key Points
1. Remove the needle from the syringe and put it in the needle holder.	Ask the patient to apply pressure to the puncture site.
	If the needle is not removed from the syringe, the blood will move rapidly through the lumen and hemolyze (rupture) the red blood cells thereby causing erroneous results of blood tests done in the laboratory.
2. Divide the blood specimen.	The blood is divided into several tubes as required for the tests to be done. This requirement should be anticipated before the patient's blood is drawn. Your agency's laboratory procedure manual will instruct you concerning the use of one or more extra tubes containing an anticoagulant. Let us assume that a procedure calls for two tubes, one containing an anticoagulant and the other being empty (plain).

PREPARATION AND ADMINISTRATION OF MEDICATIONS

Important Steps	Key Points
3. Inject blood into the tubes. 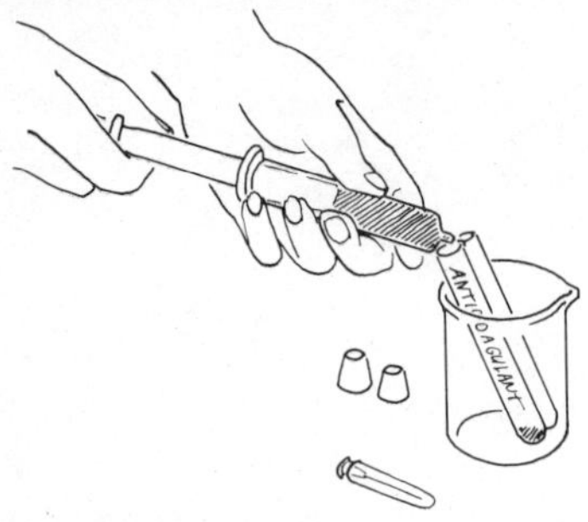	Hold the syringe at an angle with the end touching the side of the tube containing the anticoagulant. Slowly push the plunger until half of the blood (3 ml) runs down the inside of the tube with the anticoagulant. Blood that is too forcefully transferred to the bottom of the tube will tend to hemolyze, a condition that is indicated by the appearance of froth on the blood surface.
4. Expel the remainder of the blood into the plain tube.	Use the same procedure and caution as above.
5. Put the syringe down.	Pull the plunger of the syringe about halfway out of the barrel and place it on a working surface nearby to avoid breaking the tube or injuring the patient.
6. Place the stopper in the tube containing the anticoagulant. 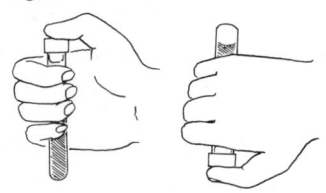	Completely invert the tube ten times to mix the contents thoroughly. Do not shake because hemolysis could occur.
7. Place the stopper or cork in the plain test tube.	*Do not mix.*
8. Label the blood tubes.	The patient's identification includes his name, room number, and other pertinent information.
9. Rinse the syringe in cold water as soon as possible.	Discard it in containers designated for disposal or reprocessing.

ITEM 11: TAKING A BLOOD SAMPLE WITH A VACUTAINER*

The Vacutainer is a type of syringe that has a special vacuum tube, a double-ended needle, and a plastic holder with a guideline.

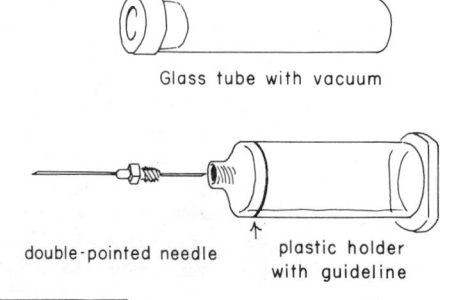

Glass tube with vacuum

double-pointed needle   plastic holder with guideline

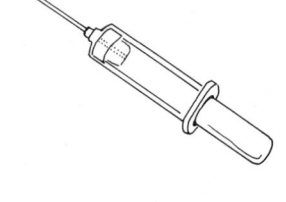

---

*Manufacturer: Becton-Dickinson and Co.

The glass tubes may be empty or they may contain a measured amount of anticoagulant, with sufficient vacuum (empty) space to permit drawing a predetermined volume of blood into the tube.

Since most blood specimens do not need to be sterile, the stopper on the glass tube is not sterile. However, the needle that is inserted into the vein must be sterile. In the event that sterile blood specimens are required for bacteriologic studies or cultures, the Vacutainer system is not used.

Advantages of the Vacutainer system:

1. It is easy to use.

2. It enables filling as many tubes as necessary to obtain as many blood samples as needed with only one needle stick.

Disadvantages of the Vacutainer system:

1. It seems to be more difficult to control the needle entry into the veins because the needle is quite short and therefore not easily palpated within the vein.

2. The vacuum tube makes it impossible to draw back on the plunger to determine if you are in the vein. If you break the vacuum in the tube and you are not in the vein, another tube must be used.

3. The pressure of the vacuum sometimes can collapse the vein.

Important Steps	Key Points
1. Screw the short-ended needle into the plastic holder.	Use a clockwise motion.
2. Insert the Vacutainer tube into the holder.	Introduce the rubber-stoppered end first. Advance it into the barrel to the guideline. The short needle is embedded in the rubber stopper, but does not break the vacuum.
3. Insert the needle into the vein.	Do this as directed in Item 9, step 15. Authorities disagree as to whether the bevel of the needle should face up or down. (Follow your agency procedure.)
4. Advance the Vacutainer tube to the end of the holder.	This breaks the vacuum by pushing the needle completely through the rubber stopper; the blood will start to flow.
5. Remove the needle when the desired amount of blood is obtained.	This occurs when the tube is filled or the blood stops flowing. NOTE: If more blood is needed, leave the needle in the vein, remove the Vacutainer tube from the holder, and lay it aside. Insert another Vacutainer tube as before. Repeat as often as necessary to obtain the required amount of blood. When removing the syringe, place an antiseptic sponge over the injection site and apply pressure as the needle comes out.
6. Discard the needle and holder.	Put it in the designated container.

Important Steps	Key Points
7. Label the blood tubes.	Information must include the patient's name, identification, and successively numbered tubes: #1, #2, #3, and so on.
8. Leave the patient comfortable and safe.	Remove the supplies and discard them in designated containers.
9. Send the specimens to the laboratory at once, along with the appropriate requisition.	
10. Record the procedure.	Charting example: 12 P.M. 10 cc blood specimen obtained from right antecubital area. Sent to laboratory with requisition. M.O.Hare, R.N.

ITEM 12: REMOVAL OF INFUSION

When the desired amount of nutrient has been given, or upon an order to discontinue, proceed to the patient's room to remove the infusion as follows:

Important Steps	Key Points
1. Wash your hands.	
2. Loosen restraints (tape, gauze).	Take care not to dislodge the needle.
3. Open and remove an antiseptic sponge from the package.	Place it over the needle site.
4. Clamp the tubing.	This stops the flow of solution and keeps it from leaking into the tissue as the needle is removed, or from soiling the bed linens after removal.
5. Remove the needle.	Use your non-dominant hand to hold the antiseptic sponge firmly over the injection site; grasp the needle at the hub with your dominant hand and, using a quick, backward motion, withdraw the needle. Hang the tubing on the IV stand momentarily.
6. Inspect the injection site.	Look for rash, redness, swelling, pallor, etc.
7. Place a bandage over the injection site.	A BAND-AID may be used, or you may use the antiseptic sponge secured in place with a piece of tape.
8. Leave the patient comfortable and safe.	Adjust his position and the height of the bed and siderails as indicated. Put the call-light and bedside stand within easy reach of the patient. Ask if there is anything else you can do and tell the patient when you expect to return.

Important Steps	Key Points
9. Remove the equipment.	Dispose of the Vacoliter, tubing and needles in the designated containers. Return the IV tray with additional supplies to storage. Replenish them as necessary.
10. Record the procedure.	Charting example: 5 P.M. IV removed, 1000 cc 5% glucose in water absorbed. No redness, swelling observed. Backrub given. Patient resting comfortably. J. Hayashi, R.N.

ITEM 13: PREPARING LIQUID ADDITIVE TO BE INJECTED INTO IV SOLUTION

Note: This procedure will be done in the pharmacy if your agency has a total unit-dose system.

Important Steps	Key Points
1. Draw additive up into syringe.	Select the syringe size according to the amount of additive to be drawn into the syringe. The additive may be contained in a vial or ampule.
2. Remove the needle from the vial (ampule).	Verify the label with the patient's record, then set the vial (ampule) aside on a nearby working surface.
3. Cleanse the rubber stopper of the Vacoliter.	Use an antiseptic sponge; work with a firm, brisk to-and-fro motion. Discard the sponge in a designated container.
4. Insert the needle into the rubber stopper.	Select site marked "X".
5. Inject the additive directly into the IV solution.	Air bubbles that may have been in your syringe will be inserted into the Vacoliter and then will escape out the airway in the Vacoliter.
6. Withdraw the needle.	Rinse the needle and syringe under clear running water.
7. Discard the needle and syringe.	Dispose of them in a designated container or return to processing.
8. Thoroughly mix the solution and additive.	Pick up the Vacoliter in both hands and gently rotate it to assure thorough mixing.
9. Label the Vacoliter.	Identify the additive names and amount.
10. Verify the label on the Vacoliter and ampule (vial) with the patient's record.	Discard the ampule or vial in a designated container; leave the work area neat and tidy. Continue the IV procedure by inserting the tubing and taking the prepared Vacoliter to the bedside. NOTE: This procedure is unnecessary if your agency uses the unit-dose medication system; then the pharmacist prepares the IV solution per order.

ITEM 14: PREPARING SOLID ADDITIVES FOR INJECTION INTO IV SOLUTION

Vials or ampules of solid additives are accompanied by a vial or ampule of liquid (diluent) in each package for mixing the medication before introducing it into the Vacoliter. The additives are usually sent to you with specific mixing instructions included in the package.

Note: This procedure will be done in the pharmacy if your agency is on a total unit-dose system.

Important Steps	Key Points
1. Open the ampule or remove the cap from the vial.	
2. Prepare the needle and syringe.	Follow the instructions in Item 3.
3. Draw the diluent into the syringe.	Follow the directions provided with the package; usually the entire amount of the diluent is used.
4. Remove the needle from the vial (or ampule).	Set the vial or ampule aside on the working surface nearby.
5. Insert the needle into the solid vial or ampule.	The solid medicine is in a powder or crystal form.
6. Inject the diluent into the solid vial or ampule.	
7. Mix the contents thoroughly.	This can be done by withdrawing the solutions into the syringe and reinjecting solution into the vial or ampule until the solid is dissolved in the solution.
8. Withdraw the needle and syringe.	Do this after you are satisfied with the complete mixing of the additive.
9. Cleanse the rubber stopper of the Vacoliter.	Use an antiseptic sponge with a firm, brisk to-and-fro motion. Discard the sponge in a designated container.
10. Insert the needle into the rubber stopper.	Use the site marked "X".
11. Inject the additive with the solution.	
12. Withdraw the needle and syringe.	Rinse the needle and syringe under clear running water. When dried these additives often cause the needle and syringe to stick together.
13. Discard the needle and syringe.	Put them into a designated container for disposal or reprocessing.
14. Mix the additive in the solution.	Pick up the Vacoliter with both hands and rotate it to assure even distribution of the additive throughout the solution.
15. Label the Vacoliter.	Write the name and dose of the additive on the label.

PREPARATION AND ADMINISTRATION OF MEDICATIONS

Important Steps	Key Points
16. Verify the label on the Vacoliter and the vial or ampule by checking the patient's record.	Discard the vial or ampule in a designated container. Leave the work area neat and tidy.

Continue the IV procedure as before.

NOTE: This procedure is unnecessary if your agency utilizes the unit-dose system; in this case the pharmacist prepares the IV solution per order.

ITEM 15: GIVING DRUGS BY INHALATION

Inhalation drug therapy is utilized for patients with respiratory conditions. Such conditions may originate in any area from the nasal passageways to the deep lung tissues.

Steam humidity or vaporizers are used to relieve upper respiratory congestion, while oxygen attached to mist nebulizers are used for respiratory infections deep within the lung tissues. Respiratory and heart stimulants, e.g., aromatic ammonia capsules or smelling salts, are also available to promote rapid absorption into the blood stream.

Drugs used for inhalation therapy are always water-soluble to insure quick absorption into the respiratory system without creating tissue inflammation (*Warning*: Oil-based medicines may lead to lipid pneumonia).

Various mechanical devices are designed for aerosol treatment; these include: atomizers, sprays, hand nebulizers (all of which are either disposable or reusable). Steam inhalators, cold humidifiers, and various methods of oxygen treatment (catheter, mask, tent nebulizers, and oxygen given under pressure—e.g., IPPB, etc.) are also used, but such equipment will be discussed in detail in the volume on Respiratory Skills.

Nebulizers and nasal sprays normally come in containers labeled with directions for using them. The patient must hold his head upright as the tip of the spray is placed in each nostril. The bottle (or bulb) is squeezed, or depressed into a mechanism that releases a spray of the medication into the nostril. One or two sprays per nostril is the usual treatment. Similar devices are used for oral inhalants.

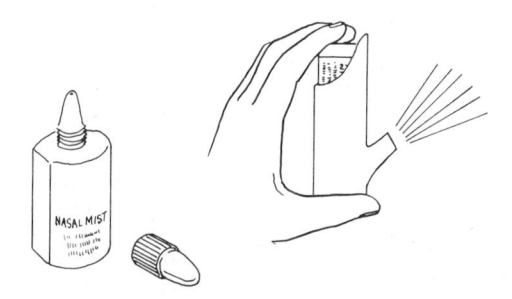

An atomizer can be filled with any one of a variety of solutions: decongestants, antihistamines or antibiotics, depending on the patient's needs.

Nebulizers can be used with antibiotics, antispasmodics, various bronchodilators, mucolytic agents, proteolytic enzymes, and anti-inflammatory drugs. The hand-operated nebulizer is convenient, lightweight, and easy to handle. However, the hand-operated nebulizer is the least effective method because the droplets of medicated solution are quite large and frequently fall out of the mist in the upper respiratory tract before reaching deep into the bronchioles; they may also condense within the nebulizer.

As a treatment for temporary respiratory or heart sluggishness (e.g., fainting), aromatic capsules of ammonia can be crushed within their netted covering and held directly under the patient's nostrils. The ammonia acts as a respiratory stimulant by irritating the mucous membranes, causing the recipient to gasp and take in large breaths of air. Spirits of ammonia are commonly called "smelling salts"; this type of ammonia salt liberates a strong alkali that causes excessive flow of secretions from the nose, bronchi, and tearducts.

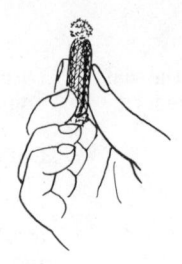

Amyl nitrate capsules are also crushed and inhaled. They are used to dilate the blood vessels surrounding the heart when a patient suffers an attack of angina pectoris.

ITEM 17: TOPICAL DRUGS

Topical drugs come in the form of lotions, ointments, or liniments. Lotions are liquid preparations of drugs which are applied to the skin for the purpose of protecting, soothing (emollients), softening, relief from itching, and for checking the growth of bacteria. Ointments are preparations of medication in lard, petroleum jelly, oils, or other fatty substances; after being applied to the skin or mucous membranes, they are melted by the body heat, and the drug is thus absorbed. They are used as antiseptics and antibiotics. Liniments are liquid preparations of drugs that are applied to the skin by rubbing; they act as vasodilators and warm the affected area. This serves to dilate the superficial blood vessels, which in turn relaxes tight muscles.

ITEM 18: APPLICATION OF A LOTION OR LINIMENT

Important Steps	Key Points
1. Wash your hands.	
2. Assemble the necessary equipment.	You will need a medicine tray, bottle of lotion (liniment), two packages of sterile 2 × 2 gauze or cotton balls, and a sterile glove.
3. Verify the medication with the patient's record.	Take the bottle from storage and compare its label with the order. Read it at eye level and verify the patient's name, identification, drug, dose, and administration time.
4. Take the medicine to the patient's room.	Place the tray on a convenient working surface near the part of his body on which you will be applying the medication.
5. Approach, identify, and explain the procedure to the patient.	Verify his identification (Identaband, patient record, etc.). Tell him that you will be applying calamine lotion to the right lower leg to help relieve the itching.
6. Expose the area to be medicated.	Maintain the patient's warmth and modesty at all times.
7. Open the bottle.	Lay the cap *upside down* on the medicine tray.
8. Open the sterile gauze or cotton balls.	Leave the package open on the medicine tray.
9. Put the sterile glove on your dominant hand.	Only one glove is needed for this procedure.

Important Steps	Key Points
10. Pick up the sterile gauze (or cotton balls).	Use you gloved hand and pick the gauze (cotton balls) straight up and away from the package without contaminating it.
11. Pour some lotion (or liniment) onto gauze (cotton balls).	Pick up the bottle in your non-dominant hand with the label facing upward. This will prevent soiling of the label if some of the medicine drips down the side of the bottle while pouring. (Soiled labels are difficult to read. You must insure absolute clarity of labels so that the proper medication is obtained.)
	The amount to pour will depend on the extent of the area on which the liquid is to be applied.
12. Apply the liquid to the affected area.	Pat the area lightly. DO NOT RUB. Since most lotions are applied to relieve itching, rubbing would only increase the pruritus. Also, if a lotion is applied over a rash, friction would irritate the lesion.
	Repeat steps 11 and 12 until the area is sufficiently covered.
	Observe the skin while applying the liquid for change in color, swelling, rash, etc., to be recorded later on the patient's record.
13. Discard the gauze (cotton balls).	Put them in the designated container and then remove your rubber glove. Replace the cap on the medicine.
14. Leave the patient safe and comfortable.	Replace linens as indicated; adjust the height of the bed and siderails, as indicated. Leave the call-light and bedside stand within easy reach. Ask if there is anything else you can do, and tell him when you expect to return.
15. Return all supplies to storage.	Put them in the medication cart or cupboard.
16. Record the procedure.	Charting example:
	10 A.M. Calamine lotion applied to right lower leg. Itching is considerably less severe today.
	J. O'Hara, R.N.

ITEM 19: APPLICATION OF OINTMENT

Important Steps	Key Points
1. Wash your hands.	
2. Assemble the necessary equipment.	You will need a medicine tray, sterile tongue blade, sterile gauze and tape if the area must be covered with a dressing, and the medication (tube or jar of ointment).

Important Steps	Key Points
3. Verify the medication with the patient's record.	Take the medicine from storage (cart or cupboard). Compare the label with the record, reading at eye level. Verify the patient's name, identification, drug, dose, and administration time.
4. Take the medicine to the patient's room.	Place the tray on a convenient working surface near the part of the patient's body where you will be applying the ointment.
5. Approach, identify, and explain the procedure to the patient.	Verify his identification.
6. Expose the area to be treated.	Maintain the patient's warmth and modesty.
7. Open the tube (jar).	Place the cap *upside down* on the tray.
8. Open and remove the sterile tongue blade from package.	Hold the proximal end of the tongue blade, keeping the distal end sterile.
9. Squeeze or scoop the ointment onto the tongue blade.	The amount will depend on the area to be medicated.
10. Apply the ointment to the designated area.	Use a gentle but firm stroke to spread the ointment. NOTE: You cannot return the used tongue blade to the jar of ointment for additional medicine. If more is needed, discard the used tongue blade and obtain a new sterile tongue blade. Break and discard the used tongue blades in the designated container. Observe the skin for color, swelling, rash, etc., to be charted later.
11. Apply a sterile dressing, as indicated.	Generally, a protective covering will be applied if the area is covered by clothing or linen so that the ointment cannot be entirely wiped off and thereby soil clothing or linens. Secure the dressing lightly in place with gauze or tape (whichever is best for the area to be dressed).
12. Leave the patient safe and comfortable.	Replace linens if necessary. Adjust the bed height and siderails as indicated. Leave the call light and siderails within easy reach; ask if there is anything else you can do and tell the patient when you expect to return.
13. Return all supplies to storage.	
14. Record the procedure.	Charting example: 9:30 A.M. Furacin Ointment appplied to back of right hand. Sterile gauze bandage applied. Area very red, no blisters observed. J. O'Hara, R.N.

VI. ADDITIONAL INFORMATION FOR ENRICHMENT

There is a wealth of information regarding improved medication techniques as well as current pharmacological products. Ask your instructor for additional assignments in your area of particular interest and need.

POST-TEST

1. Name seven routes by which medications can be administered.
   Oral, IM, S.C., Intradermal, IV, Inhalation, inunction

2. Standardization of drugs by various national bodies ensures uniformity of *Preparation* and *Strength*.

3. The initials U.S.P. stand for *United States Pharmacopeia*

4. The official book on drugs and their method of preparation published frequently by the American Pharmaceutical Association is called the *National Formulary*.

5. The Federal Food, Drug and Cosmetic Act of 1938 is implemented by which Federal agency? *Food & Drug Administration*

6. What Federal regulation establishes specific guidelines for narcotic control? *Harrison Narcotic Act*

7. Describe the unit-dose medication system. *Premeasured, prepackaged, prelabeled, ind. portions of med for/pt.*

8. List at least five advantages of the unit-dose medication system.

9. List at least five nursing responsibilities that remain in unit-dose medication administration.

10. Name the five patient rights during medication administration.
    Drug, Dose, Patient, Method, Time.

POST-TEST ANNOTATED ANSWER SHEET

1. Oral, intramuscular, subcutaneous, intradermal, intravenous, inhalation, inunction. Page 66

2. Preparation, strength. Page 66

3. United States Pharmacopeia. Page 66

4. National Formulary (N.F.) Page 66

5. Food and Drug Administration (FDA) a department within N.E.W. Page 66

6. The Harrison Narcotic Act of 1917 and its amendments. Page 67

7. It is a medication system that provides premeasured, prepackaged, prelabeled, individual portions of medicine for a patient. Page 67

8. Time saver because medication order need not be transcribed for the pharmacist; drug refills are handled entirely by the pharmacist; pharmacy delivers the medications to the nursing unit; elimination of proof-of-use forms; elimination of credit processing for unused drugs; medication preparation by pharmacy saves many hours of nursing time, which can be directed to direct patient care; decrease in floor stock and pharmacy inventory. Pages 68, 69

9. To insure safe patient care; to observe medication effects on patient; to report patient's response to drugs to appropriate health team members; to record patient's response to drugs; to utilize pharmacologic knowledges to plan nursing care; to teach patient about his medications on discharge; and to assess the patient's needs for PRN medications based on scientific principles of chemistry, physiology and psychology. Pages 69, 70

10. Right drug, right dose, right patient, right method, right time. Pages 69, 70

PERFORMANCE TEST

Discuss at least five nursing responsibilities that you must be concerned with during preparation or administration of medication. Discuss also the patient's rights during medication administration.

PERFORMANCE CHECKLIST

The student will demonstrate the preparation and/or administration of medications.

PREPARE ORAL MEDICATIONS

1. Check patient medication record and compare with medication order.
2. Wash hands and assemble equipment.
3. Select medication and compare with medication record.
4. Calculate correct dose to be given, if applicable.
5. Remove bottle cap or lid and pour medication.
6. Verify poured medication with medicine order.
7. Place the medicine on tray.
8. Return the stock bottle to shelf or drawer.

ADMINISTER ORAL MEDICINES

1. Wash hands and take medication to patient.
2. Identify patient and explain procedure.
3. Hand medicine and water (if applicable) to patient.
4. Observe patient for reactions.
5. Discard medicine cup in designated container.
6. Record medication on appropriate record.
7. Leave patient safe and comfortable.
8. Replace supplies.

PREPARE SUBCUTANEOUS INJECTION

1. Wash hands and assemble equipment.
2. Compare medication record with order.
3. Select medicine and compare with medication record.
4. Calculate correct dosage.
5. Open antiseptic sponge and cleanse ampule or vial.
6. Assemble needle and syringe.
7. Remove needle guard and test for secure syringe attachment.
8. Pick up ampule or vial and insert needle.
9. Withdraw medicine into syringe.
10. Replace vial in storage or discard ampule.
11. Place on medicine tray.

ADMINISTER SUBCUTANEOUS INJECTION

1. Wash hands and assemble supplies and equipment.
2. Identify patient and explain procedure.
3. Select and prepare injection site.
4. Expel air bubbles from syringe and needle.
5. Insert needle at 45° angle and inject medicine. Observe patient.
6. Remove needle and place needle and syringe on tray.
7. Massage site with antiseptic sponge.
8. Place adhesive bandage over injection site, if applicable.
9. Leave patient safe and comfortable.
10. Return supplies to medication area and discard as indicated by type of equipment in use.
11. Record medication and observations on medication record.

ADMINISTER IM INJECTION

1. Wash hands and assemble equipment.
2. Identify patient and explain procedure.
3. Select and prepare injection site.
4. Pick up syringe, expel air bubbles, and insert needle at 90° angle.
5. Pull back on plunger, inject medicine, observe patient.
6. Withdraw needle and gently massage site.
7. Leave patient safe and comfortable.
8. Discard equipment.
9. Record the medication administration.

Z-TRACK INJECTION TECHNIQUE

1. Wash hands and assemble equipment.
2. Identify patient and explain procedure.
3. Select and prepare injection site.
4. Pick up syringe, expel air bubbles, and retract skin laterally.
5. Insert needle at 90° angle, pull back on plunger, and observe patient.
6. Inject medicine and wait ten seconds.
7. Remove needle, release skin. DO NOT MASSAGE.
8. Leave patient safe and comfortable.
9. Discard equipment.
10. Record medication administration.

ADMINISTER INTRADERMAL INJECTION

1. Wash hands and assemble equipment.
2. Identify patient and explain the procedure.
3. Select and prepare injection site.
4. Pick up syringe and expel air bubbles.
5. Insert needle at 10 to 15° angle. Inject slowly.
6. Observe wheal and patient reaction.
7. Withdraw needle; do not apply pressure over injection site.
8. Position patient for safety and comfort.
9. Discard equipment and record procedure.

PREPARE IV INFUSION

1. Wash hands and assemble equipment.
2. Verify medicine with medication orders.
3. Prepare Vacoliter, open sterile tubing set.
4. Insert sterile tubing into rubber stopper of Vacoliter.
5. Clamp tubing, attach needle to distal end of tubing.
6. Take solution to patient room and hang inverted bottom on IV pole.
7. Tear off tape.

ADMINISTER IV INJECTION

1. Wash hands, identify patient, and explain procedure.
2. Select and prepare injection site.
3. Place extremity on restraint board.
4. Apply tourniquet *above* injection site.
5. Locate and examine selected vein.
6. Cleanse site and check air bubbles and IV tubing.
7. Pick up needle and insert needle at 45° angle.
8. Check entry into vein and settle needle in place.
9. Release tourniquet and regulate solution flow.
10. Secure needle in place and leave patient safe and comfortable.
11. Record procedure.

PREPARATION AND ADMINISTRATION OF MEDICATIONS

ALTERNATE VENIPUNCTURE TECHNIQUE

Transfer blood to tube.

1. Remove needle from syringe and place in needle holder.
2. Divide blood specimen into specimen tubes.
3. Inject designated amount into tube containing anticoagulant and plain tube.
4. Place syringe to one side and place stoppers in tubes.
5. Label blood tubes.
6. Rinse syringe in cold water.

Take blood sample with Vacutainer.

1. Screw needle into plastic holder.
2. Insert Vacutainer tube into holder.
3. Prepare injection site and insert needle into vein.
4. Advance Vacutainer to end of holder.
5. Remove Vacutainer tube and lay it aside. Insert another Vacutainer tube. Remove as much blood as needed.
6. Remove needle and discard.
7. Label blood tubes.
8. Leave patient safe and comfortable.
9. Send specimens to laboratory and record procedure.

REMOVE INFUSION

1. Wash hands and loosen restraints (tape, gauze).
2. Place antiseptic sponge over site, clamp tubing, and remove needle.
3. Inspect injection site and bandage as needed.
4. Leave patient safe and comfortable.
5. Remove equipment and record procedure.

PREPARE LIQUID ADDITIVE FOR IV

1. Draw up additive into syringe.
2. Cleanse rubber stopper of Vacoliter.
3. Insert needle into rubber stopper and inject directly into IV solution.
4. Withdraw needle and discard syringe and needle.
5. Mix solutions thoroughly and label Vacoliter.
6. Verify Vacoliter with patient's record.

PREPARE SOLID ADDITIVES FOR INJECTION INTO IV SOLUTION

1. Open ampule or vial.
2. Prepare needle and syringe and draw diluent into syringe.
3. Insert filler syringe into vial or ampule with dry medicine and inject diluent.
4. Remove needle and syringe and mix thoroughly.

5. Cleanse rubber stopper on Vacoliter and insert needle into rubber stopper.

6. Inject thoroughly mixed additive solution.

7. Withdraw needle and syringe and discard.

8. Mix additive in solution.

9. Label Vacoliter and verify with patient's record.

ADMINISTER TOPICAL DRUG

1. Wash hands and assemble equipment.

2. Verify medication with patient's rocord.

3. Take medicine to patient's room, identify patient, and explain procedure.

4. Select application site.

5. Pour lotion (liniment) on gauze (cotton ball).

6. Apply liquid to affected area and discard gauze.

7. Leave patient safe and comfortable.

8. Return supplies to storage and record procedure.

APPLY OINTMENT

1. Wash hands and assemble equipment.

2. Verify medication with patient's record.

3. Take medicine to patient's room, identify patient, and explain procedure.

4. Expose area to be treated.

5. Open tube or jar and squeeze ointment onto tongue blade.

6. Apply ointment to designated area.

7. Apply sterile dressing as ordered.

8. Leave patient safe and comfortable.

9. Return supplies and record procedure.

Unit 3

PREPARING FOR AND ASSISTING WITH EXAMINATIONS

I. DIRECTIONS TO THE STUDENT

Please read the following paragraphs carefully. They will tell you what you will be expected to know and perform at the end of this unit.

When you have completed your study of the unit and practiced the procedures, you should arrange with your instructor to take the Performance Test. You will be expected to understand the rationale for the examination of the patient, and to demonstrate your skill in carrying out the procedures.

II. GENERAL PERFORMANCE OBJECTIVE

Upon the completion of this unit, you will be able to assemble the equipment to be used for the specified type of physical examination, prepare the patient (which includes correct positioning and draping), and assist both the patient and the physician during the examination.

III. SPECIFIC PERFORMANCE OBJECTIVES

When you have completed this unit, you will be able to:

1. Assemble all the supplies and equipment required by the physician for a general physical examination of a patient, including everything needed for a rectal and vaginal examination when required.

2. Prepare the patient for the examination by providing instructions which he can understand, position him to facilitate the examination, and drape him to avoid unnecessary exposure or embarrassment.

3. Assist the physician in the physical examination by taking certain physiological measurements, supplying items as requested, and carrying out other tasks which may be required.

4. Assemble the supplies and equipment required by the physician for the examination of specific areas of the body, prepare the patient for the examination, and assist the physician and the patient as needed during the actual examination. These specialized examinations utilize clean, nonsterile technique and include proctoscopy, sigmoidoscopy, gastroscopy, neurological examination, and those procedures related to ear, eye, nose, and throat.

IV. VOCABULARY

Read the definitions of the terms listed below. Do not attempt to memorize these definitions before proceeding with the lesson. Each term will be explained or defined again in the text. On completion of the lesson, however, you should know the correct definitions of these terms.

auscultation—a method of examination in which a stethoscope is used to listen to sounds in a cavity (especially the chest and abdomen) to detect an abnormal condition.

bronchoscopy—internal examination of the bronchus by means of an instrument called a bronchoscope.

cystoscopy—internal examination of the bladder by means of an instrument called a cystoscope.

endoscopy—examination of a hollow organ of the body by using a special instrument (e.g., proctoscope, otoscope, etc.).

fiberoptics—a bundle of flexible glass fibers capable of transmitting light, used in certain instruments (endoscopes) to permit inspection of a cavity without the trauma of a surgical operation.

gastroscopy—internal examination of the stomach by means of an instrument called a gastroscope.

insufflator—a bag used to blow air into some opening or part of the body.

integument—the skin covering the body.

laryngeal mirror—an instrument used to visualize the larynx and pharynx.

lithotomy position—lying on the back with thighs flexed upon the abdomen and the legs flexed upon the thighs which are abducted.

otoscope—an instrument used to look into the ear canal.

ophthalmoscope—an instrument used to look within the eye.

palpation—a method of examination by applying the hands to the external surface of the body to detect evidence of disease in an organ.

Papanicolaou smear—a microscopic laboratory examination used to determine the presence of malignant cells from body secretions (respiratory, genitourinary, or digestive tract). This test is performed most commonly to detect malignancy in the female reproductive tract.

patency—the state of being freely open (e.g., a patent airway).

percussion—a method of examination using a light tapping of the body to detect variations in the sounds emitted. Sound variations can be evidence of disease.

proctoscope—an instrument used to look into the rectum.

sigmoidoscope—an instrument used to look into the sigmoid colon.

speculum (plural, specula)—short, funnel-like tube for the examination of canals, such as nasal canal and the vagina.

symmetry—correspondence in shape, size, and relative positions of parts of opposite sides of the body.

V. INTRODUCTION

Probably most people in this country have had a general physical examination at some time in their lives. Physical examinations are required for entry into most schools, for the issuance of insurance policies, and for induction into the military service. They are performed as a general health measure and whenever a person seeks medical attention for an illness.

The general physical examination is one of the most valuable diagnostic tools used by the doctor to gather information about the physiological state of an individual. As a nurse you will frequently be called upon to assist the doctor in his physical examination of the patient. The information gathered from the examination can be used by the doctor for a variety of purposes. These include:

1. Ascertaining the individual's level of health or physiological functioning.

2. Arriving at a tentative diagnosis of a health problem or disease.

3. Confirming a diagnosis of dysfunction or disease.

4. Indicating specific body areas or systems for additional examination or testing.

5. Evaluating the effectiveness of prescribed treatment and therapy.

PREPARING FOR AND ASSISTING WITH EXAMINATIONS

The nurse's part in the physical examination has a dual focus. In patient-centered nursing, the primary focus is the comfort and welfare of the patient. The nurse is concerned with the psychological, social and physiological needs and responses of the patient before, during, and following the physical examination. The other focus is on assisting the physician. This consists of preparing the patient, providing the supplies and equipment needed, and helping the physician during the actual examination.

ITEM 1: THE GENERAL PHYSICAL EXAMINATION

The general physical examination may be referred to as the "physical," the physical exam, or simply as a "P.E." Doctors are taught early in medical school education to perform a physical examination; to gather information in a systematic, organized way; and to record their findings. The method of performing the examination is to look at each body system, examine parts of the system, assess their functioning, and make sure measurements and tests as are appropriate. The physician uses all sources available to gather information about the health status of the patient. These sources include the senses of sight, hearing, smell, and touch; the use of diagnostic instruments; and the services of other specialized technicians, such as those in the laboratory, X-ray, ECG, and so forth.

The general physical examination is performed in a variety of settings where doctors care for the health needs of people: in the doctor's office, in clinics, in the home, in health centers, in hospitals, and in schools. The examination is usually performed by the physician, although some basic measurements may be taken by the nurse. Nurses are also beginning to do physical exams as a part of their new "extended roles," i.e., family nurse practitioner, adolescent nurse practitioner, and so forth.

In performing the physical examination, the physician checks the anatomical and physiological functioning of the individual from head to toe. This may be done by body systems, or by body parts such as head, throat, chest, extremities, and so forth. Regardless of the method used, the physician will observe, test, and measure for evidence of normal or unusual function of the part or system.

As an example, in an examination of body systems, the physician would examine the following for evidence of proper functioning:

Musculoskeletal system—symmetry of parts, mobility, coordination, etc.

Integument—intactness of skin, presence of scars or rashes, color, warmth, unusual texture, etc.

Eye, Ear, Nose, and *Throat*—receptivity of sense organs, equilibrium, patency of passages and cavities, etc.

Cardiovascular system—heart rate and action, adequacy of circulation systemically and peripherally, etc.

Respiratory system—respiratory rate, adequacy of ventilation and gas exchange membranes, adequacy of digestive process, etc.

Neurological system—normal reflexes, adequate motor and sensory innervation, development of intellectual and psychological processes, etc.

Genitourinary tract—adequacy of urinary control and elimination, patency of membranes and passages, appropriate development of reproductive (sexual) organs.

Endocrine glands—adequacy of hormonal activity shown by certain characteristics of body function or development, size of glands, etc.

Various physiological measurements are also part of the examination. Often these measurements are taken and recorded by the nurse. These measurements include:

Temperature, pulse, and respiration.

Blood pressure.

Height and weight.

Visual acuity and hearing (may be optional).

Other tests that the physician may request as part of the general physical examination include a complete blood count, a urinalysis, and a chest X-ray.

ITEM 2: SPECIAL EXAMINATIONS

Certain kinds of physical examination are restricted to special areas or special functions of the body. They are extensive and detailed, in order to obtain definitive information of a complex nature. Special exams are also used to investigate the interior of body cavities and passages.

Some of the special examinations are endoscopic (*endo*—within, or interior; *scopic*—instrument of viewing); these include proctoscopy, sigmoidoscopy, bronchoscopy, cystoscopy, and gastroscopy. Other types of specialized examinations include neurological, ophthalmological, cardiac catheterization, among others. Some procedures require strict aseptic technique and are usually performed in a surgical suite (operating room). Others are performed as clean procedures. The principle determining whether a sterile or a clean technique is required is the need to avoid possible introduction of a source of infection into the body cavity or passage.

ITEM 3: METHODS OF PHYSICAL INVESTIGATION

The physician uses several methods to learn about the patient's condition. The most common is inspection or observation of the various parts of the anatomy. He observes such signs as color, condition, deformities, rashes, scars, general body contour, type of respirations, etc.

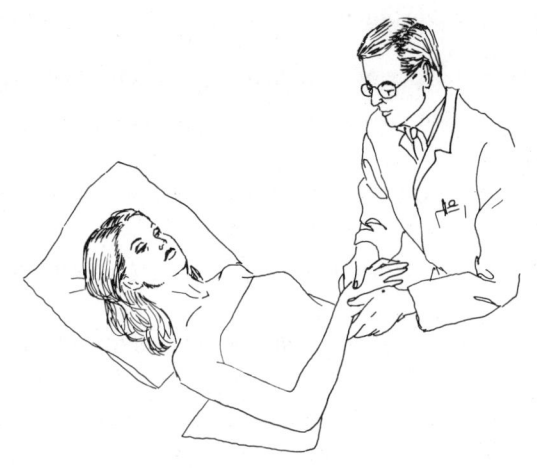

Observation

Palpation, another common method of examination, uses the sense of touch to determine the firmness and size of parts of the body that cannot be seen (e.g., internal organs). By palpation (or feel) the physician can determine if the organ or part is displaced or if pain or tenderness is present. Any deviation from normal with respect to size, tenderness, placement, etc., may indicate illness or disease, and further study would be indicated. The physician never bases a diagnosis on a single factor, but on a combination of clinical observations and test indicators.

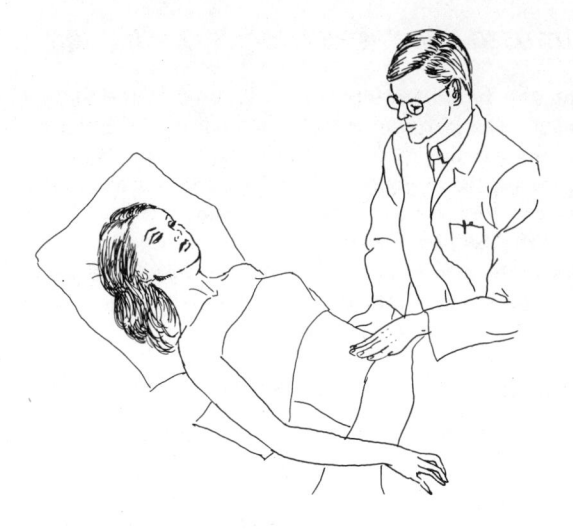

Palpation

Percussion is a method of tapping parts of the body to assist in making a diagnosis from the sound that is emitted. The physician places one hand firmly against the patient's body. With the fingers of the other hand, he taps the fingers that are on the patient's body. As he moves the first hand about, he listens to the differences in sounds that are emitted as he continues tapping with his other hand. You may have had the doctor do this to your chest. Variations from the usual sound may indicate disease. It takes a great deal of practice to be able to distinguish between normal and abnormal sounds and to know what they indicate.

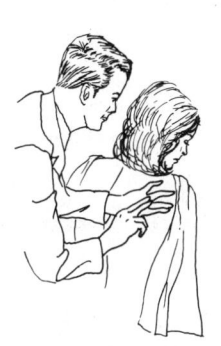

Percussion

Auscultation is the process of listening with the aid of a stethoscope to sounds produced in a body cavity, particularly the chest and abdomen.

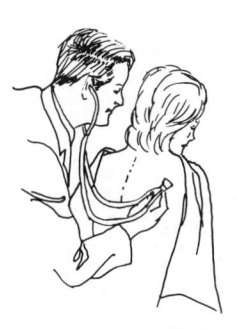

Auscultation

ITEM 4: EQUIPMENT USED FOR THE PHYSICAL EXAMINATION

The exact amount and type of equipment to be used in the physical examination will depend on several factors—the purpose of the examination, its scope and thoroughness, the physician's preference, the location of the facilities, and the condition of the patient.

In some health agencies, the equipment used for a physical examination will be available on a special tray, or kept in a central location. However, it may be necessary for you to assemble the equipment that will be needed.

If you were to use problem-solving to assemble the equipment needed for the physical examination, and given the information in Item 1, you would probably come up with a list of supplies and equipment similar to the following:

Examination gown for patient	Percussion hammer
Draping material—bathblanket, sheet, etc.	Tongue blades
Blood pressure cuff	Laryngeal mirror
Stethoscope	Head mirror
Thermometer	Tissues
Scale with height measure rod	Cotton balls in antiseptic solution (or pre-packaged antiseptic pledgets)
Tape measure	
Tuning fork	Flashlight and spotlight or gooseneck light
Otoscope	Urine specimen bottle
Ophthalmoscope	Laboratory request forms and X-ray request form
Nasal speculum	

Additional equipment may be needed for eye, rectal, or vaginal examination. Depending on the purpose of the physical and the condition of the patient, you may need the following:

Gloves	Papanicolaou smear slides and request form
Lubricant	Eye chart, such as the Snellen chart
Vaginal speculum	Cotton applicators

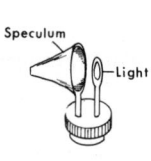

Otoscope head

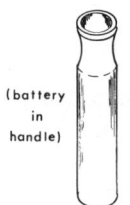

Combination handle with otoscope head and ophthalmoscope head

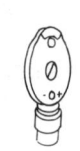

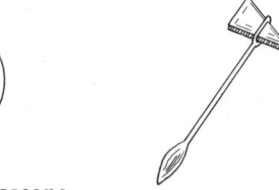

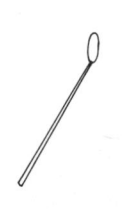

Ophthalmoscope

Percussion hammer

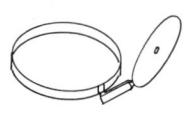

Head mirror

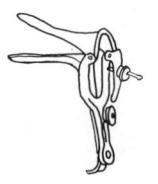

Vaginal speculum

Laryngeal mirror

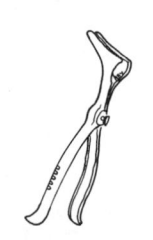

Nasal speculum

Gooseneck lamp   Glove

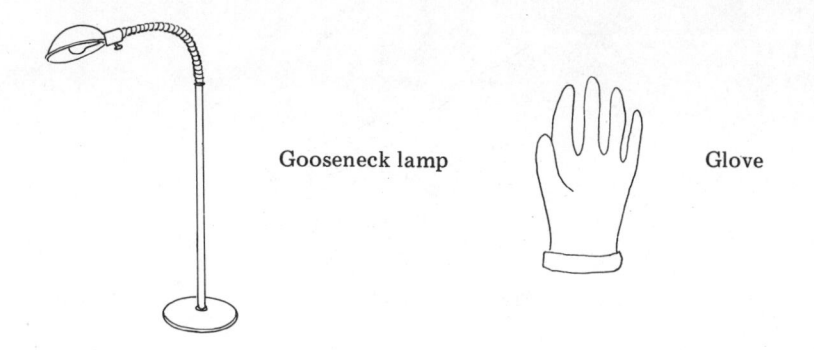

ITEM 5: POSITIONING THE PATIENT

The physical examination of the patient is facilitated by the use of an examining table. A common type of examining table found in clinics, hospital examining rooms, and doctors' offices is shown below. The short table unit is convenient for the patient in a lithotomy position and allows better visibility and accessibility for the physician for his examination of the genitorectal areas. The table is extendable by a pull-out section, which provides support for the patient in other positions.

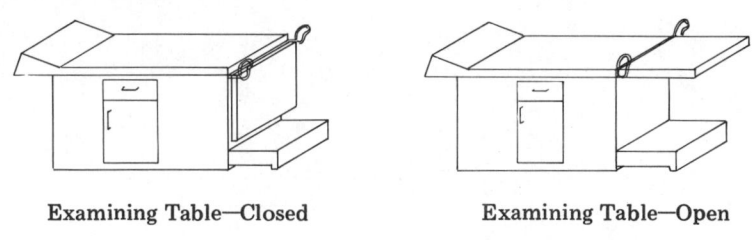

Examining Table—Closed   Examining Table—Open

It is not always possible or advisable to perform the physical examination with the patient on an examining table. The examination can be done with the patient lying on a stretcher, in a bed, on a cot, etc. Adjustments in the positioning of the patient are made according to the circumstances and the condition of the patient.

You will recall that there are three basic positions and variations of these positions. The basic positions are the supine, the lateral, and the prone. The variations are the Fowler's (or sitting) position, the Sims', the semi-Fowler's, and the Trendelenburg. In positioning the patient for physical examination and for other medical procedures, the lithotomy position and the knee-chest position are frequently used. The various positions of the patient most frequently used in the general and special physical examinations are shown below.

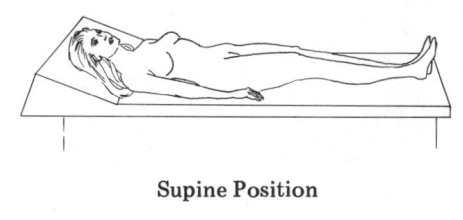

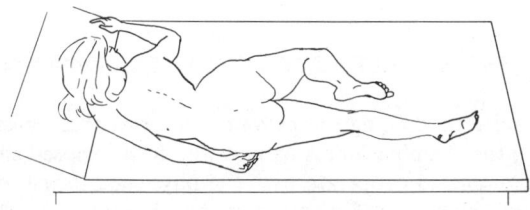

Supine Position

Sims Position

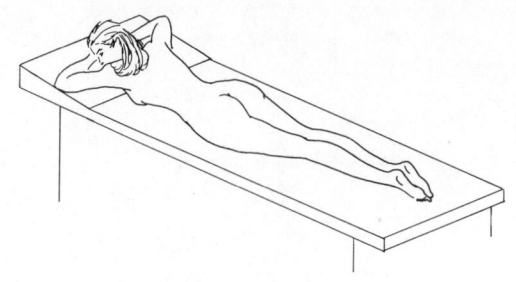

Prone Position

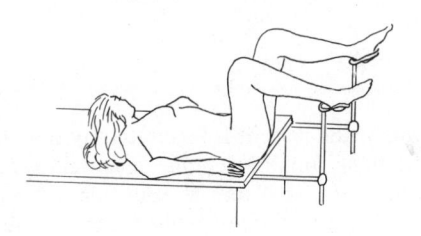

Lithotomy Position

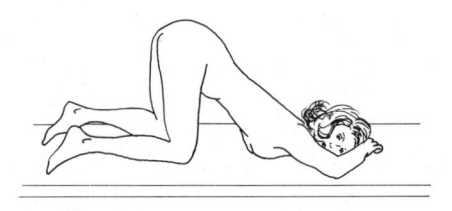

Knee-chest Position

The lithotomy position is generally used for the pelvic examination of female patients. The patient's knees are separated and flexed. The feet are placed in stirrups which are attached to the examining table, or may be placed flat on the bed with the hips and knees abducted to afford good visualization of the area to be examined.

The knee-chest position is used to examine the anal and vaginal areas. In this position, the patient kneels, keeping buttocks elevated and back straight, and supports her chest and her arms. In many proctoscopic and sigmoidoscopic examining units, a special table is used that provides support for the patient's body and can be tilted by the physician to obtain the best exposure during the examination.

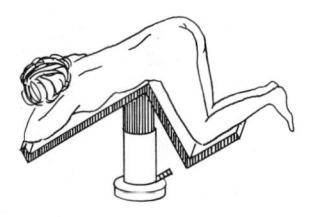

Special table used for proctoscopic or sigmoidoscopic examinations.

ITEM 6: DRAPING THE PATIENT FOR PHYSICAL EXAMINATION

The primary purpose of draping the patient is to prevent unnecessary exposure of the patient's body during the examination. A patient who feels exposed and embarrassed will be tense, restless, and less able to cooperate with the physician. Proper draping contributes to the patient's feeling of being cared for and promotes his relaxation. The drapes also provide some warmth and help avoid chilling the patient.

The drapes may be of cloth or of paper. The usual items are the bathblanket, one or two sheets, or a sheet and a towel. Some agencies provide a loose fabric or paper boot to fit over each leg in the lithotomy position; this "boot" extends over the thigh to the groin area. The cloth or paper examining gown worn by the patient may also be considered part of the drape since it covers part of the body and can be rearranged to expose and cover different parts as needed.

To drape the ambulatory patient, provide a patient gown and a folded sheet over the lower trunk and extremities.

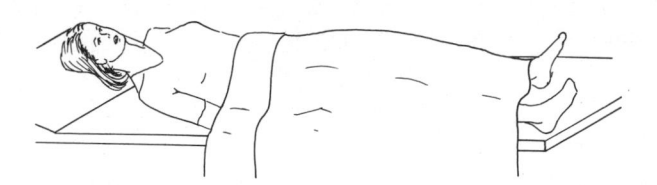

To drape the patient for the supine, prone, or Sims' position, provide a patient gown or towel to cover the upper chest and a bathblanket or sheet to cover the rest of the body. The draping sheet is placed in a rectangular arrangement over the patient's body for the general physical examination (see below).

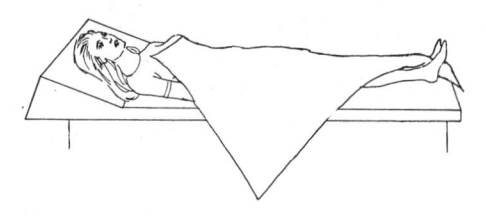

To drape for the lithotomy or knee-chest position, provide a draping sheet or a bed sheet with booties (if used in your agency). The draping sheet is placed in a diamond-shaped arrangement (rectangular) over the patient's body. One point of the sheet faces the patient's chin, while the opposite corner points toward the patient's toes. The lateral corners point laterally toward the sides of the table. With the patient's knees flexed, and the feet placed firmly on the table, the lateral corners of the sheet are wrapped around the feet in a spiral fashion (see diagram).

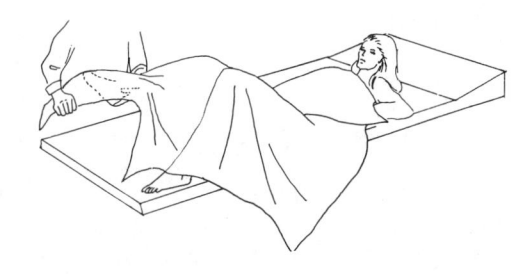

The corner of the sheet toward the head of the table is used to drape the upper chest of the patient. *Do not cover the face.* The corner of the sheet extending toward the foot of the table (or bed) is drawn downward to cover the perineal area until the examiner is ready to proceed with the examination (see diagram).

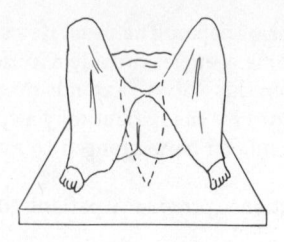

The corner of the sheet extending over the perineum is later pulled back and upward toward the head of the bed to expose the perineum when the examination begins (see (diagram). That corner of the sheet is then fanfolded neatly over the patient's abdomen.

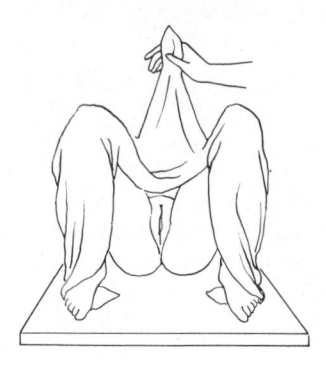

The rectangularly placed sheet can be used to drape the patient in the lithotomy position, except that in this position the legs are suspended in stirrups and the lateral corners of the sheet are wrapped around the foot and legs in the same manner as above and the legs are then gently supported in the padded stirrup (see diagram).

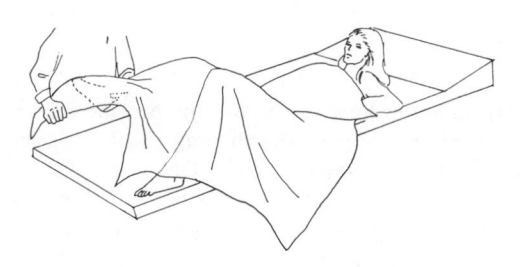

ITEM 7: PREPARING THE PATIENT

The physical examination may be done by the physician without any special preparation of the patient, such as restricting fluids, refraining from breakfast, giving medications, etc. However, the patient is not to be overlooked or ignored. As the nurse, you must evaluate the patient's condition and his need for assistance. Factors that you should consider in assessing this need include age, level of understanding, the ability to move, the state of health, etc. The very young, the very old, the mentally impaired, the handicapped, and those who are acutely ill are most likely to require assistance during the examination.

As a nurse, you must also be concerned with the psychological preparation of the patient for the examination. Every patient, whether healthy or ill, wants to be considered as an individual and important in his own right. He is apt to have feelings about his health, fears of the unknown, and apprehension about what the examination may reveal. The nurse can do much to reassure the patient by listening, and by showing an accepting, understanding manner in both verbal communication and actions

ITEM 8: PROCEDURE FOR THE GENERAL PHYSICAL EXAMINATION

In the classroom or the clinical laboratory, you should practice the steps of the procedure until you are familiar with them and have achieved a beginning level of skill in performing the required tasks.

Important Steps	Key Points
1. Assemble the necessary equipment and supplies.	Required equipment and supplies are listed in Item 4. Some agencies keep P.E. articles on a special tray, or in a special space, for convenience. Be sure to see if electrical appliances are plugged in and working. Test battery-operated equipment to see if it is working.
2. Approach the patient, check his identification band, and secure his cooperation if possible.	It is often helpful to describe what will be done and how the patient can help in the examination. If the examination is to be done in the treatment room, take him to it. Wash your hands.
3. Proceed to take physical measurements and record: a. Temperature. b. Pulse. c. Blood pressure. d. Respiration. e. Height. f. Weight. *g. Visual acuity. *h. Hearing acuity.	If the patient is acutely ill, you may not be able to measure his height or weight. In that case, get the information from the patient, the family, or by estimating, if permitted in your agency. Visual and hearing tests may be done by the physician or a special technician.
4. Prepare the patient for the examination.	a. Ask the patient to void in order to empty the bladder. Save the urine specimen for urinalysis. NOTE: This step may be done before taking the patient to the treatment room in Step 2. b. Have the patient undress and put on an examining gown. NOTE: This is optional if the patient is in a hospital gown. c. Provide a draping sheet. d. Have the patient lie or sit on the examining table or bed. (The acutely ill patient will be examined in the supine and lateral positions, while the ambulatory patient would use the supine and sitting positions.)

---

*Optional. May not be required by your agency.

PREPARING FOR AND ASSISTING WITH EXAMINATIONS

Important Steps	Key Points
5. Stand by to assist the physician in the examination.	You should be available to hand the physician instruments and supplies when needed. He will proceed from head to toe.
	NOTE: When handing the tongue depressor (blade) to the physician, hold it at the center. When accepting it from the physician, again hold it in the center. After use, break the tongue depressor (without touching its ends) and discard it in the emesis basin or waste container.
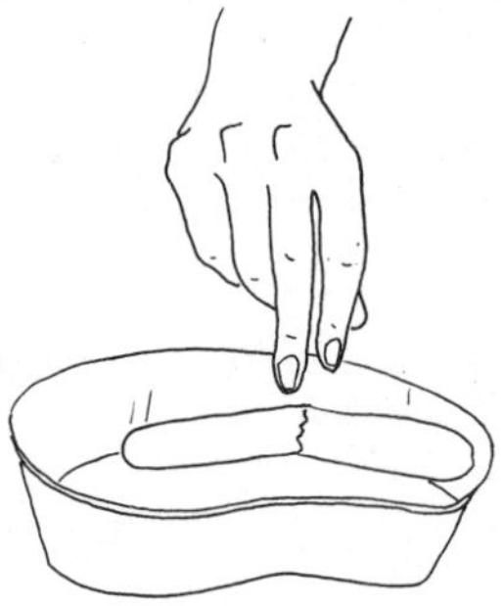	NOTE: If the laryngeal mirror is used, it must be warmed to prevent fogging. This is done by placing the mirrored end in a glass of warm water (or holding it in the palm of your hand). Be sure to dry the mirror after removing it from the water.
6. Assist the patient during the examination.	Be available for changes in position and give reassurance and comfort to the patient. You should be available to assist all patients—male, female, young, old, ill, or healthy. Some parts of the examination may be uncomfortable or painful for the patient; the nurse's touch can be very comforting.

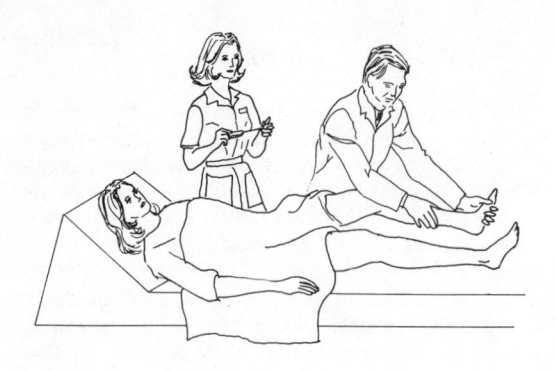

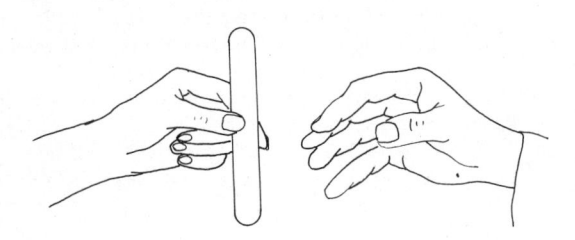

Important Steps	Key Points
*7. Assist during vaginal or rectal examination.	a. Position patient in the lithotomy position.
	b. Drape securely.
	c. Provide equipment and supplies as needed.

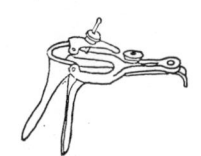

Vaginal speculum

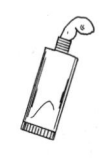

Lubricant

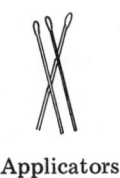

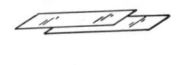

Applicators

Glass slides

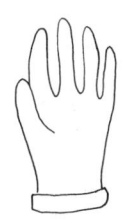

Rubber glove

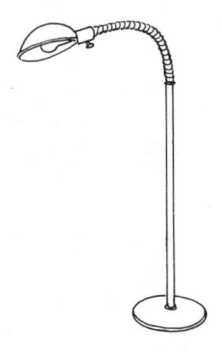

Gooseneck lamp

This part of the examination is the most distressing and painful for most patients:

a. The vaginal speculum is freely immersed in lubricant for easy insertion into vagina.

b. The speculum is inserted into the vagina.

c. The speculum is then opened so that the examiner can see the cervix clearly.

d. A cotton applicator or a narrow tongue blade may be inserted and drawn across the cervix to obtain a specimen which is then rubbed across a sterile slide and immersed in a special fixative. This will be sent to the laboratory for a Papanicolaou smear (this is a routine part of a vaginal examination in many agencies). The applicator or tongue blade is discarded in an appropriate container.

e. The speculum is removed and discarded in a designated container.

f. The examiner then inserts the gloved finger of the dominant hand into the vagina to palpate internally for displacement or growths on the cervix or uterus. The other hand is placed on the patient's abdomen to apply counterpressure during the examination so that the movable abdominal organs can be felt more easily.

g. The finger is removed from the vagina and then inserted into the rectum (Additional lubricant may be needed before inserting the finger into the rectum.)

h. The rectum is palpated internally to determine if there are growths or obstructions in the lower rectum. This is often painful for the patient and must be done gently and slowly.

The physician usually wants a good light (gooseneck light) for the vaginal examination.

---

*Optional. May not be done as part of the routine examination.

Important Steps	Key Points
8. Provide for the patient's comfort and welfare at the conclusion of the examination.	Remove drapes and assist patient to dress, if needed. Assist the patient back to her hospital room, if appropriate.
9. Carry out the physician's requests for further tests or examinations.	The examining physician may request further laboratory and X-ray tests, or special tests of the patient. Make out the required request forms and give the instructions to the patient.
10. Collect all used equipment and supplies; return, dispose of, and replace as needed.	
11. Record the examination on the chart.	Charting example: 10:10 A.M. Vaginal exam done in treatment room by Dr. Meek. Vaginal smear sent to laboratory. Returned to bed. M. King, S.N.

ITEM 9: PREPARING PATIENT FOR PROCTOSCOPY AND SIGMOIDOSCOPY

When preparing the patient, refer to the specific instructions of your physician or your agency. The usual preparation includes:

1. Laxative the evening before the examination (type and amount are prescribed by each agency).

2. Only liquids allowed for breakfast.

3. Enemas until the return flow is clear of fecal material (at least one hour before examination).

Equipment used for the proctoscopy or sigmoidoscopy are:

a. Specimen bottles.

b. Proctoscopes and sigmoidoscopes.

c. Biopsy forceps.

d. Suction tip for the suction machine.

e. Gloves.

f. Lubricant.

g. Insufflator.

h. Suction machine.

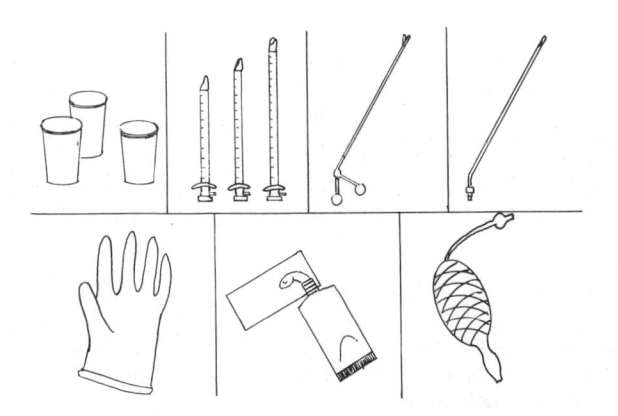

ITEM 10: PROCEDURE FOR PROCTOSCOPY AND SIGMOIDOSCOPY EXAMINATIONS

The procedure used to examine the rectum or the sigmoid colon is outlined below. The steps are similar to the general physical examination.

Important Steps	Key Points
1. Assemble the necessary equipment and supplies.	Be sure to test the lights on the scopes and the suction apparatus to see that these are in working order. NOTE: Some agencies may provide disposable scopes.
2. Approach the patient, check his identification band, and secure his cooperation if possible.	This procedure produces a good deal of discomfort for many patients; therefore full explanation is vitally important. Explain that you will stay throughout the procedure. Continue to reassure the patient throughout the procedure. Wash your hands.
3. Prepare the patient for examination by the examiner.	a. Have patient empty bladder. b. Have patient put on examining gown (patient gown is acceptable). c. Position in knee-chest position; this is preferred since it permits the abdominal contents to fall away from the pelvis, making it easier and less painful to scope the patient. (A pillow may be needed under the head to provide additional comfort.) A left Sims' position can be used if the patient cannot tolerate the knee-chest position. d. Drape patient completely. (Some agencies have a special large sheet with a cut-out circular opening in the center which is placed directly over the anus. If the special sheet is not available, use a regular bed sheet. Place the sheet diagonally across the patient's back. Tuck the lateral corners around each leg. Fan-fold the top corner of the sheet back upon the patient's shoulders so that his head will not be covered. the proximal corner of the sheet can be lifted up and back and fan-folded on the patient's lower back so that the anus can be exposed when the examiner is ready to proceed. Many "procto" examining rooms have a special tilted table to support the patient in the knee-chest position (see diagram). Draping remains the same. NOTE: This is a particularly uncomfortable position for the patient and one that cannot be tolerated for long periods of time.

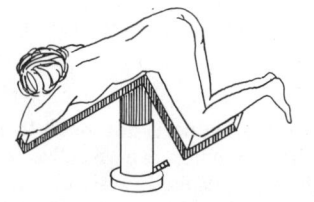

Important Steps	Key Points
4. Do manual rectal exam.	The examiner may use a finger cot or a rubber glove; be sure that a liberal amount of lubricant is applied to the index finger (of the dominant hand) for ease of insertion into the rectum.
5. Stand by to assist the examiner.	a. Warm the metal scopes by placing in warm water or by holding in your hand. Plastic scopes (disposable) do not need warming.
	b. Lubricate the distal end of the scope and obturator generously with lubricant before handing it to the examiner. Attach the inflation bag to the scope.
	c. Tell the patient to bear down slightly as though he were having a bowel movement when the scope is inserted. This will relax the anal sphincter and make it easier to insert the scope.
	d. The examiner will separate the buttocks with the thumb and finger of the left hand, and will insert the scope gently and slowly with the right hand (reverse positions if left-handed). Scope is initially inserted about 3 to 4 cm. Remove the obturator and place in a designated container.
	e. The light source is then attached to the scope.
	f. As the scope is advanced to its full length, the examiner can visualize the walls of the bowel. Inspection should be leisurely and complete. The best observation occurs during the withdrawal of the scope when the patient is having the least pain.

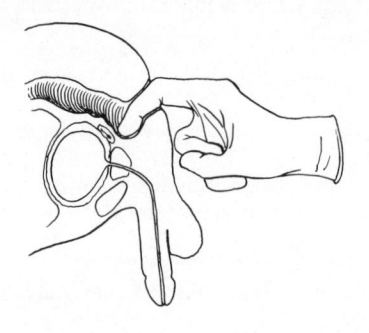

Important Steps	Key Points
	g. Inflation of the bowel with the inflator bag attachment is used sparingly since this causes considerable pain for the patient, but it is necessary to get good visualization of the bowel. The inflator bag is pumped just like the inflator bulb on the blood pressure cuff to inject a small amount of air into the bowel. (Air insufflation is avoided in cases of extreme bowel fragility, e.g., ulcerative colitis, diverticulitis, etc.) *Force is never used* to insert the scope. Tearing of the bowel commonly occurs when force is used.
	h. If a biopsy is to be taken, hand the biopsy forceps to the examiner.
	i. When the specimen is obtained collect it immediately and put it into a labeled specimen jar.
	j. If bleeding occurs, the examiner may need the suction tip. Stay alert at this time to assist the examiner and to reassure the patient.
	NOTE: Your speedy actions to assist the examiner, as well as your touch and words of assurance to the patient during the examination, will make the procedure flow quickly and smoothly and with minimal discomfort for the patient.
6. Assist the patient during the examination by reassuring and giving comfort.	You can encourage the patient to take deep breaths through his mouth to relax the anus and rectum when the scope is being inserted.
7. Provide for the patient's comfort and welfare at the conclusion of the examination.	Some patients continue to have an urge to defecate following withdrawal of the scope. Use of the hand to provide pressure against the anus will often relieve this. Others may feel faint when standing up at the end of the exam, and should be encouraged to rest in a supine position for a few minutes. Return patient to his room via stretcher or wheelchair as indicated.
8. Carry out the examiner's requests for further tests or examinations.	If specimens were taken, prepare the proper forms and be sure they are sent with the specimens to the lab. Be sure specimens are correctly labeled.
9. Collect all used equipment and supplies; rinse, return, dispose of, and replace as needed.	Follow your agency's instructions for the cleaning and disinfection of the proctoscopes and sigmoidoscopes.
10. Record examination on chart.	Charting example:
	2:45 P.M. Proctoscopy done in treatment room by Dr. Meek. Tissue specimen sent with requisition to laboratory. Returned to bed via stretcher. Complained of weakness.
	J. King, S.N.

152 PREPARING FOR AND ASSISTING WITH EXAMINATIONS

ITEM 11: SPECIAL EXAMINATION: GASTROSCOPY

For preparing the patient, refer to the specific instructions of your physician or your agency. This examination is usually done in a special examining room. The usual preparation includes:

1. Nothing by mouth for 8 hours prior to the examination.
2. Injection of an atropine-type drug and sedative about 1/2 hour before the examination.
3. Local anesthesia sprayed on pharynx before gastroscope is inserted.
4. Nothing by mouth for several hours after the examination until the anesthesia has worn off and the patient can swallow without difficulty.

Equipment used:

Topical (surface) spray anesthesia.

Gastric lavage set.

Lubricant.

Gloves.

Specimen bottles.

Gastroscope (fiberoptic endoscope).

Suction equipment.

ITEM 12: PROCEDURE FOR GASTROSCOPY

Important Steps	Key Points
Steps 1 and 2 are the same as in Item 8.	
3. Prepare the patient for the examination by the physician.	a. Have him undress and put on examining gown (patient gown is acceptable).
	b. Position him in a left lateral position.
	c. Drape him completely using the large examining sheet, covering him as though he were lying on his side in bed.
4. Stand by to assist the physician during the examination.	A gastric lavage is usually done to drain secretions from the stomach so the walls can be visualized. The nurse may be the one to insert the gastric tube and lavage the stomach.
Steps 5, 6, 7, and 8 are the same as in Item 8.	

ITEM 13: OTHER SPECIAL EXAMINATIONS

There are numerous other special types of examinations that are performed to gain additional information about a body organ or system. Some of these examinations will be described briefly.

Neurologic examination. The neurologic examination tests the cranial nerves and the motor and sensory responses of peripheral nerves. There is no special preparation needed for the patient. The required equipment and supplies include pins, tuning fork, tongue depressor, ophthalmoscope, flashlight, hot and cold water, several bottles of volatile oils to test sense of smell, and bottles of sweet, sour, salty, and bitter solutions for the sense of taste.

The neurologic examination by nurses consists of observations made of cerebral function in patients. Change in the reaction and equality of the pupils, the level of consciousness, the presence or absence of the corneal and gag reflexes, and changes in motor and sensory function can be tested and observed by the nurse.

Hearing examinations. Patients with impaired hearing may be examined with an instrument as simple as the tuning fork, or with audiometry which utilizes a soundproof room, earphones, sound wave generators, timing circuits, and other complex equipment. Usually there is no special preparation of the patient. However, very young infants suspected of having a hearing impairment may be sedated prior to undergoing complex audiometric examinations. This examination is usually done by a physician or an audiometric technician.

Pulmonary function examinations. Tests of the respiratory functioning of patients are becoming more common. Most pulmonary function examinations are performed in a special examining area or center. Some of the instruments used include the bellows or spirometer for measurement of vital capacity, a flow-meter for ventilation studies, the plethysmograph for volume of gases, and radiation counters to detect radioactivity in tissues. In most instances, no special preparation is required for the patient. These tests will be explained in detail in the companion text *Inhalation Therapy Skills for Allied Health Services.*

Urological examinations. The urological examination of the patient involves extensive examination of urine specimens and tests of kidney function, such as intravenous pyelography, cystoscopy and cystography, and retrograde pyelography. There are specific requirements for the preparation of the patient for these examinations, but these vary. You will need to refer to your agency's instructions. Many of the urological examinations are conducted under sterile conditions to reduce the possibility of introducing infections into the urinary system. You will learn more fully about these examinations when you have your clinical experience in the operating room.

ITEM 14: CONCLUSION OF THE UNIT

You have now completed the unit "Preparing for and Assisting with Examinations." When you have practiced the procedures and feel that you know the equipment and the steps of the procedures, you should arrange with your instructor to take the Performance Test. You will be expected to demonstrate accurately your ability to prepare for and to assist with a general physical examination and with a special examination.

PERFORMANCE TEST

In the skills laboratory, your instructor will ask you to demonstrate your skill in carrying out the following procedures without referring to source materials. For these activities it would be helpful to have another person play the part of the patient.

1. Given a patient with a health problem who is ambulatory and able to go to an examining room, you are to prepare for and assist in the general examination of the patient. For purposes of this test, the examination will not include testing of visual and hearing acuity, but will include a rectal examination.

2. Given a patient who is to have a sigmoidoscopic examination, you are:

    a. to describe the preparation of the patient for the examination.

    b. to list the equipment used in the examination.

    c. to assist with the examination.

PERFORMANCE CHECKLIST

PREPARING FOR AND ASSISTING WITH GENERAL PHYSICAL EXAMINATION

1. Assemble the equipment and supplies needed for the examination.

2. Approach the patient, check his identification band, and obtain his cooperation.

3. Take the following physical measurements of the patient and record results on chart:

    a. temperature, pulse, and respiration.

    b. blood pressure.

    c. height and weight

4. Prepare the patient for the examination:

    a. have patient void, and save the specimen.

    b. have patient undress and put on examining gown.

    c. position patient on examining table in supine or sitting position.

    d. drape the patient.

5. Assist the physician during the examination (hand him appropriate supplies and equipment as needed).

6. Assist the patient during the examination, giving reassurance and comfort.

7. Change patient's position to lithotomy for rectal examination, drape the patient, and have needed equipment ready for the patient.

8. Provide for patient's comfort at conclusion of the exam by removing drapes, assisting to dress, etc.

9. Carry out physician's orders for additional tests or examinations.

10. Collect, clean, return, dispose of, and replace all used equipment as needed.

11. Record on chart.

PREPARING PATIENT FOR SIGMOIDOSCOPIC EXAMINATION

1. Describe the preparation to the patient for the sigmoidoscopic examination:
   a. laxative the evening before.
   b. liquids only for breakfast.
   c. enemas until clean one hour before examination.
2. List the equipment needed for the examination (in any order):
   a. gloves.
   b. lubricant.
   c. sigmoidoscopes.
   d. biopsy forceps.
   e. insufflator.
   f. suction.
   g. specimen bottles.
3. Assist with the procedure by doing the following:
   a. Approach the patient, identify him, and secure his cooperation.
   b. Prepare the patient for the examination:
      1) have patient void.
      2) have patient undress and put on examining gown.
      3) position patient in the knee-chest position.
      4) drape patient securely.
   c. Stand by to assist the physician (hand appropriate supplies and equipment).
   d. Assist the patient during the examination.
   e. Provide for the patient's comfort at the conclusion of the examination.
   f. Carry out the physician's requests for other tests or examinations.
   g. Collect, clean, dispose of, and replace all used equipment and supplies.

Unit 4

IRRIGATIONS AND INSTILLATIONS

I. DIRECTIONS TO THE STUDENT

Study this unit on irrigations and instillations. Be prepared to demonstrate your proficiency in manual skills and written knowledge of this unit.

II. GENERAL PERFORMANCE OBJECTIVE

Upon completion of this unit, you will be able correctly to irrigate and instill medications into a body part or cavity.

III. SPECIFIC PERFORMANCE OBJECTIVES

Upon completion of this lesson, you will be able to:

1. Approach your patient with a general understanding of the body part to be irrigated or into which a medication is to be instilled.

2. Carry out the procedure of irrigation or instillation of the body part with proper technique (bladder, kidney, ear, eye, nose, throat, vagina, wound).

3. Discuss the ramifications of microbiology, chemistry, pharmacology, physics and psychosocial aspects associated with the procedure and with the body part.

IV. VOCABULARY

Read the definitions of the terms listed below. Do not attempt to memorize them before proceeding with the lesson. Each term will be explained or defined again in the text. Upon completion of the lesson, however, you should know the correct definition of each term.

acoustic nerve—the eighth of twelve cranial nerves, concerned with hearing.
anodyne—(antalgesic or antalgic) a drug with pain-relieving properties (e.g., morphine, codeine, acetylsalicylic acid).
anxiety—a state of tension or distress akin to fear, but produced by a threatened awareness of an unacceptable feeling rather than by an external threat.
astringent—a drug that checks secretions from wounds or mucous membranes, and hardens tissue.
cavity—a hollow space, such as a body organ (e.g., abdominal cavity).
clitoris—organ of female genitalia homologous with the penis in the male.
cochlea—a coiled, tubular structure located in the inner ear.
colostomy—an incision into the colon to form an artificial anus (stoma).
cystitis—inflammation of the bladder.
esophagus—a tube connecting the pharynx and stomach.
genitalia—organs of reproduction.
guilt feelings—self-recriminating blame.
labia majora—outer, lip-like structure forming the sides of the vulva.
labia minora—inner and delicate fold beneath the labia majora and enclosing the vestibule.

lavage—a washing-out of a part, e.g., washing out the stomach in gastric lavage.

miotic—a drug that causes the pupil of the eye to contract.

mydriatic—a drug that causes the pupil to dilate.

nasopharynx—part of the pharynx situated above the soft palate.

ophthalmologist—a physician who specializes in the treatment of eye disorders.

optometrist—a person who measures the eye's refractive powers and fits glasses to correct ocular defects.

otologist—a physician who specializes in the treatment of ear diseases.

otosclerosis—a disease of the ear characterized by a fixation (hardening) of the stapes (a part of the middle ear).

perineum—surface between external genitalia and anus.

pH—chemical symbol indicating the degree or concentration of acidity or alkalinity in a solution.

pharynx—a five-inch tube extending from the oral cavity to the esophagus; also called the throat.

precipitate of phosphates—ingredient needed to help maintain the acid-base balance in the body.

urinate (micturate, void)—the act by which urine is expelled.

vaginal orifice—the mouth-like opening of a passageway between the uterus and the outside of the body.

ventral—front side of the body.

vestibule—a small space at the entrance of a canal.

V. INTRODUCTION

Irrigation is a process of instilling or flushing a wound or body part with a solution. It is used as a cleansing action to remove bits of tissue or to loosen clots. Irrigations may be used to bathe tissue cells with drugs or with drugs in solution. An irrigation may be intermittent or continuous.

Ramifications of principles of microbiology, chemistry, pharmacology, and physics, and psychosocial aspects pertaining to each body part discussed in the following procedures, will be found in the enrichment section at the end of this unit.

Instillation differs from irrigation only slightly. *Instillation* is the pouring in of a liquid drop by drop, while irrigation is the cleansing of a canal by using varying amounts of water or other solutions. Each of the following cavities or organs may be irrigated or have fluids instilled:

1. rectum or colon (enema or colonic irrigation);
2. bladder (via catheters);
3. kidney;
4. kidney pelvis;
5. ureters;
6. wounds;
7. colostomy, ileostomy, or gastrostomy;
8. gastrointestinal tract;
9. mouth and throat;
10. perineum;
11. vagina;
12. special sense organs, such as the ear, eye, or nose.

Usually the irrigations and instillations of body cavities or openings are carried out using aseptic technique. An exception may be the external irrigation of an ear to remove accumulated wax.

TYPES OF IRRIGATORS

The Asepto syringe is a plain glass or plastic syringe that comes in varying sizes: 1 oz., 2 oz., 4 oz. Each has a rubber bulb on the distal end that works either as a suction to pull solution from a cavity, or as an instiller to push liquid into a cavity.

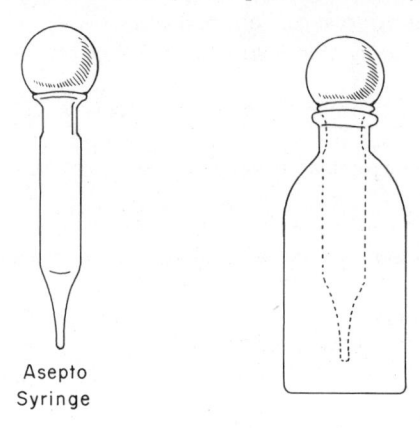

Asepto Syringe

The rubber bulb syringe is made from a resilient rubber. It is commonly called an ear or ulcer syringe and is often used to aspirate mucus from the nasal passageways or mouth of the newborn infant. It may be used to irrigate an eye or a small wound. It comes in 1-, 2-, or 3-ounce sizes.

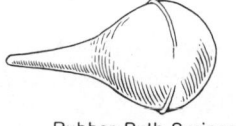

Rubber Bulb Syringe

Glass or plastic irrigating syringes are of several types, about 50 to 60 cc in size. Typical is the catheter syringe, which has a 2-ounce glass barrel and plunger. The irrigating tip is reinforced with a permanently attached, unbreakable, tapered metal tip. This syringe is commonly used to irrigate the stomach or bladder, and to gavage adults.

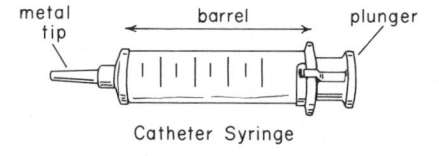

Catheter Syringe

Another common type of irrigating syringe is made of a special heat-resistant glass that can withstand repeated sterilizations. Since this large syringe is costly, the reusable glass syringe is frequently preferable to its counterpart, the disposable plastic syringe. However, both syringes are used successfully by practitioners. The plunger and barrel are accurately ground to insure a tight leak-proof fit. The long tapered tip fits any size catheter and is used to irrigate urethral and duodenal catheters. The 2-ounce irrigating syringe is calibrated in 1/4-ounce markings.

Irrigating Syringe

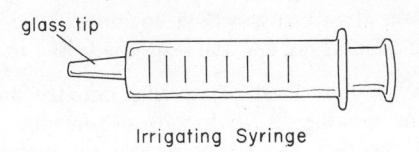

There are two bladder evacuators in common use. The Toomey bladder evacuator is a glass syringe with a removable metal tip. Its capacity is approximately 50 cc, and it is used by the physician to evacuate clots from the bladder following bladder surgery, or to evacuate tissue or stone fragments following tissue resections or removal of stones (litholapaxy). The Toomey evacuator costs at least twice as much as the two syringes described above, and therefore special care must be taken to avoid breakage.

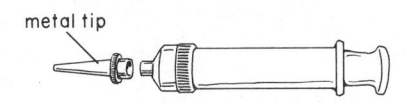

Toomey Bladder Evacuator

The Ellick bladder evacuator has an unusual shape that creates a whirling action of the water and permits resected tissue (e.g., prostatic) to fall into the trap as it is evacuated. The pieces of tissue remain in the lower portion, while the water moves to and fro from the pressure of the rubber bulb pushing a stream of water into the bladder. The Ellick evacuator is usually employed by the physician during an operative procedure in which tissue is removed from the bladder.

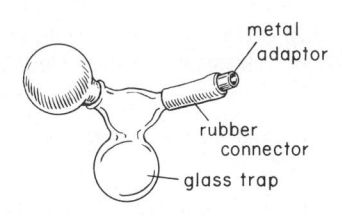

Ellick Evacuator

In caring for patients who are receiving irrigations or instillations, you should be knowledgeable about and practice the following guides:

1. Understanding the body part or area to be irrigated, which ensures:

   a. observation of deviations from normal structure;

   b. knowledge of areas of extreme sensitivity;

   c. awareness of possible dangers in use of equipment, pressure, adverse medications, and so forth;

   d. proper health instruction as needed by the patient.

2. Explaining the procedure benefits the patient by helping him understand what is being done and also encourages his cooperation.

3. Providing privacy during the procedure which reduces some of the psychosocial trauma.

4. Correct positioning of the patient, which improves results of the procedure.

5. Adhering to strict safety measures, which includes: ensuring correct temperature of solution, maintenance of correct height of irrigator, avoidance of conversation to prevent spreading germs.

6. Proper charting of the treatment, which includes: time, amount of irrigation solution, temperature of solution, and the response to the treatment.

7. Knowing limitations of your level of nursing practice and staying within these bounds, which means seeking assistance from someone who has the necessary knowledge and skill if the procedure is not within your realm of practice.

8. Verifying the identification of the patient before beginning the procedure.

9. Reviewing the physician's orders for correct irrigation solution, body part to be irrigated, and evaluating the order for correct medication dosage, and time. If you suspect there is an error in the order, confirm the order with the physician *before* carrying out the procedure.

10. Evaluating and charting the patient's mental condition, in addition to recording the procedure as indicated. Chart all allergic reactions.

11. Using only clearly labeled medications to prepare solutions for irrigations.

12. Using a thermometer to check the temperature of a solution. *Don't guess.*

13. Washing your hands before each procedure. If a lavatory is provided in the patient's room, wash them there to insure the highest degree of cleanliness. (Patients observe actions of this sort and thus will have more confidence in the care you give them.)

14. Disposing of soiled dressings in paper container (or plastic) to be burned later in an incinerator.

15. Working in an organized fashion to economize on your time and effort. Foresee the need for additional equipment and bring it into the room with you.

16. Washing hands between each irrigation if more than one body area or part is to be irrigated, in order to prevent transfer of microorganisms from one body part to another.

17. Using sterile equipment and solutions as the procedure requires. (If in doubt, use sterile solution and equipment.)

18. Working cooperatively with other members of the health team to ensure smooth, efficient functioning.

19. Avoiding discussion regarding the work of the physician and other health workers.

ITEM 1: BLADDER IRRIGATION WITH CATHETER IN PLACE

Check the treatment order to ascertain the type of solution to be used and the exact treatment that is ordered.

Important Steps	Key Points
1. Obtain the equipment from storage.	The equipment may be a sterile disposable set or it may be a set which must be reprocessed between use. Use whichever is available at your agency.
	The complete set-up will include:
	a. Container of irrigation solution (e.g., sterile water, normal saline, potassium permanganate 1:5,000, bichloride of mercury 1:10,000);
	b. Sterile tubing, clamp, and connector tip, if necessary;

Important Steps	Key Points
	c. Sterile syringe;
	d. Container for solution;
	e. Drainage basin;
	f. Drapes (towels) to protect bed;
	g. Antiseptic sponge (usually individually pre-packed);
	h. Sterile catheter plug or sterile gauge to cover the end of the catheter after the irrigation.
	Be sure to include medication, if one is to be instilled in the bladder following treatment.
2. Wash your hands.	
3. Approach and identify the patient; explain the procedure to him.	Read his Identaband. Avoid technical terms when you describe the procedure, e.g., "I am going to use this syringe (show it to the patient) to put an irrigating solution through your urinary catheter in order to wash out your bladder. It should not be painful. If you have any discomfort, please tell me at once and I shall stop the irrigation until you are more comfortable."
4. Prepare the patient.	Pull the curtains, or screen the patient to provide for privacy. Adjust the bed (table) to a working height, lower the siderail on the side where you are working. Place the patient in a dorsal recumbent position on the proximal side of the bed (this prevents undue stretching for you).
	Drape the patient so that the perineal area is easily observed and reached. You may use a bath blanket or sterile towels (whichever is indicated in your agency).
5. Prepare the equipment.	Open the irrigation tray. Remove the cap (cover) from the irrigating solution and fill the irrigating container with the desired amount of solution. Replace the cover on the sterile solution and set it to one side. Place the irrigation tray between the patient's legs. Prepare the medication for introduction at the end of the procedure. (Pour the prescribed amount into the container.)
	Mentally review the purpose of the irrigation: (1) to rid the bladder of decomposing urine and bacteria and their products; (2) to reduce inflammation; (3) to soothe the infected lining and promote healing; (4) to cleanse the lining in order to promote absorption of medication if it is to be instilled; (5) to provide relief of such conditions of the bladder as cystitis or tumor; (6) to clean out the lumen of an indwelling catheter.

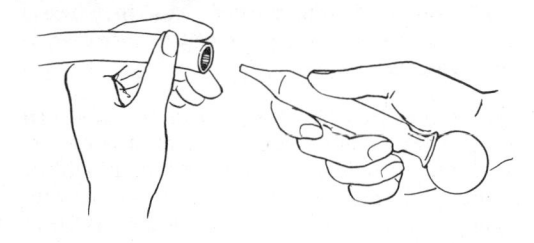

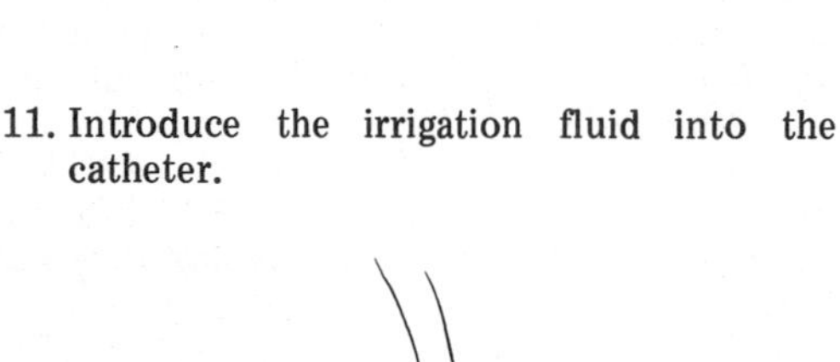

Important Steps	Key Points
	The purpose of the irrigation for your patient will influence the amount of irrigation solution to be used. Normally 60 cc of irrigation solution is used to cleanse an indwelling catheter. If more solution is required, the order sheet will state the amount.
6. Disconnect the drainage tube from the catheter.	Hold the drainage tube in your dominant hand between the middle and index fingers to prevent contaminating the tip. Cleanse the end of the catheter with an antiseptic sponge before attaching it to the irrigating syringe.
7. Insert an irrigating syringe into the catheter.	Gently place the syringe on a sterile towel or tray between the patient's legs.
8. Cover the drainage tube end.	Use a sterile gauze pad from tray or place a sterile plastic cover over the tube end. Use whichever item is available in your agency. Secure the tube to the side of the bed with a catheter clamp or safety pins until the irrigation is completed.
	NOTE: Steps 6 and 7, 8 are optional if a drainage tube is not attached to the catheter.
9. Fill a syringe with the required amount of irrigation solution.	Disconnect the syringe from the catheter, while holding the syringe in your dominant hand. Maintain sterility of the system. *Do not* touch the tip of the syringe or catheter with your unsterile hands.
10. Re-insert the tip of the syringe into the catheter.	Hold the catheter securely in your left hand so that it will not dislodge when the irrigation is in process. However, do not hold the catheter so tightly that you compress the lumen of the catheter and thus prevent the solution from passing through the catheter.
11. Introduce the irrigation fluid into the catheter.	If an Asepto syringe is used, compress the bulb of the syringe until the fluid enters the catheter.
	On releasing the bulb, the fluid will flow back freely if there is no obstructing part.
	Another method to allow return flow is to disconnect the syringe and allow the fluid to flow into the drainage pan. If you use this method be sure that the free end of the catheter is in the irrigating pan.

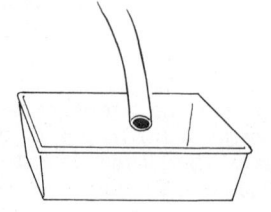

IRRIGATIONS AND INSTILLATIONS

Important Steps	Key Points
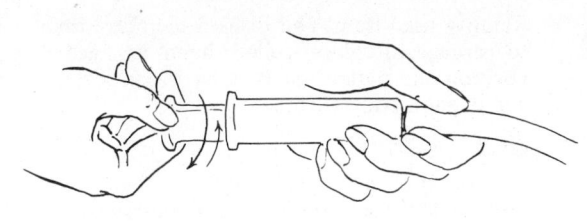	If the plastic "piston" syringe is used, care must be exercised when introducing fluid. Use a "twisting" motion of the plunger to allow control of pressure exerted by pushing the fluid into the bladder.
12. Continue the introduction and withdrawal of the solution.	This should be done until the desired effect is attained, i.e., until the sanguineous solution becomes clear. Do not use force when introducing or withdrawing solution. Stop the procedure immediately and call the physician or genitourinary technician.
13. Remove the syringe.	With the left thumb and forefinger, pinch the catheter tip as your remove the syringe to stop any remaining solution from soiling the bed.
14. Instill the medication. (This step is optional.)	Withdraw the prescribed amount of medication into a calibrated syringe. Unpinch the catheter tip and insert the syringe tip. Push the plunger in to expel the entire amount of medication to be instilled into the bladder.
15. Remove the syringe.	While pinching the catheter closed to prevent medicine from draining out, attach the catheter clamp so that medication can remain in the bladder for the prescribed length of time.
	NOTE: If medication is inserted, the catheter will be clamped off for a stated period of time. The catheter will not be attached to the drainage tube during this time.
16. Reattach the drainage tube to the catheter (if medication was not instilled).	First remove the drainage tip protection with your left hand, then insert the drainage tubing into the catheter. (You may need to release the drainage tube from its location so that you have enough tubing to reach easily the distal end of the catheter.) Secure the tubing to the patient's leg to keep him from pulling on the catheter as he moves about in bed.

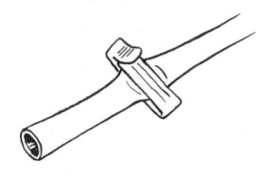

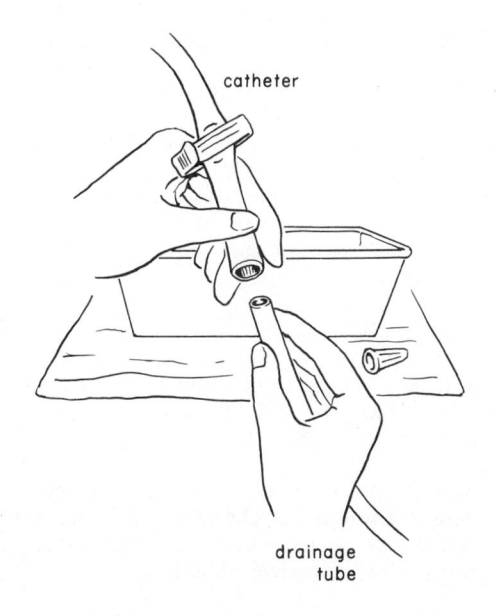

Important Steps	Key Points
17. Provide for patient safety and comfort.	Remove used items and discard or return them to storage. Replace soiled linen as needed. Position the patient so that he is comfortable and in good body alignment.
	Place the call light and bedside stand within easy reach of the patient. Adjust the bed to low position and raise the siderails, if indicated.
	Ask if there is anything else you can do, and tell the patient approximately when you will return. Wash hands.
18. Report and record.	Promptly report any unusual occurrence you may have encountered during the irrigation. Make a note of the irrigation promptly.
	Charting example:
	10:00 A.M. Bladder irrigated with 100 cc potassium permanganate 1:10,000. Many small blood clots removed. Solution was returning clear at the end of the treatment. Complained of severe lower abdominal pain over the pubes during the irrigation.
	M. Hernandez, R.N.

ITEM 2: BLADDER INSTILLATION OF MEDICATION IN THE ABSENCE OF AN INDWELLING CATHETER

Important Steps	Key Points
1. Collect the equipment.	Select the catheter tray and equipment for catheterization.
	Check the patient's orders for type of medication, solution, amount, time for instillation, temperature of solution, and other directions.
	The equipment will include:
	a. sterile container for solution;
	b. ordered medication and solution;
	c. funnel or Asepto syringe with bulb removed.
2. Approach the patient, identify and prepare him physically and mentally.	Read his Identaband and explain the procedure, e.g., "We're going to instill medication through a rubber catheter into your bladder to help reduce the inflammation and give you comfort."
	NOTE: In a clinic setting the patient may not have an Identaband. The patient must be identified by asking his or her name, which you will verify with the patient's chart.

IRRIGATIONS AND INSTILLATIONS

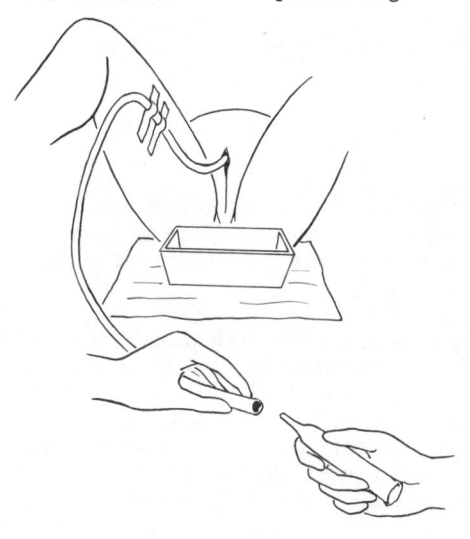

Important Steps	Key Points
	Wash your hands.
	Adjust bed or table to working height. Lower the siderail as indicated. Drape the patient to expose the perineal area, while at the same time providing warmth and privacy.
3. Insert the catheter into the bladder.	Maintain asepsis by using the standard catheterization procedure.
4. Tape the catheter to the patient's leg.	This is done to stabilize the catheter in the bladder during the medication instillation; or, you may hold the catheter securely in your left hand during the medication insertion.
5. Insert the tip of the funnel or glass portion of the Asepto syringe into the catheter.	Reverse hand positions if you are left-handed. Use the syringe or funnel, whichever is provided by your agency.
6. Pour medication into the funnel (Asepto syringe).	Hold the funnel (Asepto syringe) in your left hand at about a 12-inch height from the bed; with the right hand, pour the medication into the funnel (Asepto).
7. Reassure the patient.	Tell the patient what you are doing. Ask her to take a deep breath; this will relax the opening to the bladder and will permit the medication to run into the bladder more easily.
	Ask the patient to tell you if there is any discomfort and assure him that you will stop at once. If pain occurs, stop pouring the medication for a minute or two. Then start pouring slowly again. It may help to lower the Asepto syringe a few inches, too, thereby decreasing the pressure of the solution flowing into the bladder.

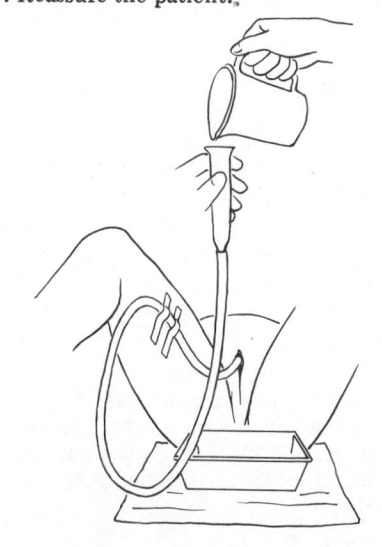

UNIT 4

Important Steps	Key Points
8. Set the pouring container aside after all medication has been introduced.	Continue to observe the patient while you are giving the treatment.
9. Introduce the solution.	NOTE: If the solution does not run into the bladder by gravity, you may need to put the rubber bulb on the Asepto so that you can gently exert pressure to insert the medication.
	In that case: firmly grasp the catheter end that fits over the irrigator tip to prevent it from separating when you insert the solution. If the catheter and Asepto separate, the solution will be sprayed over the patient and the expensive medication will be wasted.
	Continue to observe the patient for discomfort or pain.
	Compress the catheter before the inflow or outflow stops, thus preventing air from entering the bladder. Keep a careful record of the input and output.
	Never use force in introducing fluid or getting fluid to drain out. Gravity drainage is safest.
10. Remove the catheter.	After all the solution is administered, untape the catheter (if this method was used). Dry the perineal area with a towel. Set the catheter tray on the chair or table near the bed.
11. Provide for the patient's safety and comfort.	Replenish linens as needed. Neatly replace the covers. Adjust the bed to low position; adjust the siderails as needed. Place the call signal and bedside stand within easy reach.
	Ask the patient if there is anything else you can do, and tell him approximately when you will return.
12. Remove equipment.	Discard disposable items; return unusable items to processing. Leave the room clean and tidy. Wash hands.
13. Report and record.	Charting example:
	10:00 A.M. 100cc 0.2 per cent nupercaine solution instilled into the bladder for one hour. States bladder pain has decreased markedly since last instillation.
	R. Hernandez, R.N.

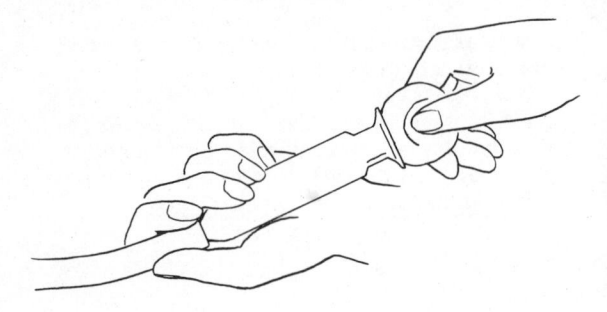

ITEM 3: THROUGH AND THROUGH BLADDER IRRIGATION

When a bladder irrigation is done frequently throughout the day, a calibrated glass or plastic irrigating flask may be suspended on an IV pole and attached with a tubing to the 3-way connector fastened to the catheter and drainage tube. This system is used for irrigating postoperative bladder surgicals or patients with bladder infections or malignancies. Obtain the equipment through your central processing service.

IRRIGATIONS AND INSTILLATIONS

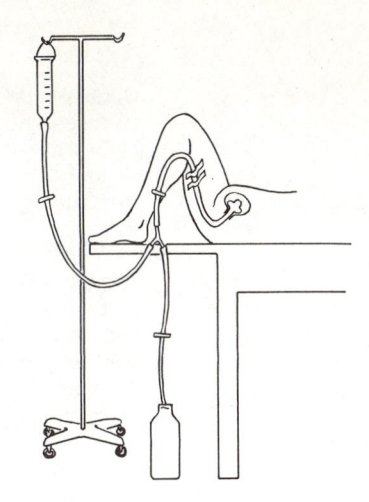

Typical through and through bladder irrigation set up.

Important Steps	Key Points
1. Obtain the equipment from storage.	You will need an IV standard, sterile irrigating solution (this will usually be ordered daily in bulk amounts from the pharmacy), a large calibrated flask, tubing, "Y" connector and tubing clamps (2) and urine drainage bottle (bag). NOTE: Many agencies have this unit set up as a "G.U. Irrigating" set. Some of these units are disposable, some are reusable.
2. Wash your hands.	
3. Approach the patient, identify him, and explain the procedure.	Read his Identaband. Tell him that since you will be irrigating the bladder frequently, this system will enable you to do the procedure with minimal disturbance for him.
4. Prepare the patient.	Pull the curtains or screen him to provide for privacy. Adjust the bed to working height and lower the proximal siderails, if indicated. Have the patient in the dorsal recumbent position and moved to the proximal side of the bed so that you will not have to stretch across the bed to reach him. Drape the patient so that the perineal area is easily observable. Use a bath blanket or sterile towels to drape for privacy and warmth.
5. Prepare the equipment.	Unwrap sterile equipment and hang flask on an IV standard placed at one side of the bed, near the foot. Connect one end of the tubing to the flask, and the other end to the "Y" connector. Attach one clamp about midway on the tubing. Close it securely by turning it counterclockwise.

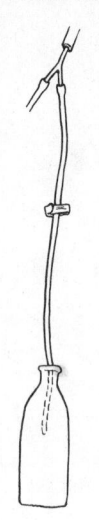

Important Steps	Key Points
	Connect the right-hand branch of the "Y" connector to the exposed end of the indwelling catheter. Be sure that the catheter is attached securely to the leg so that it will not be dislodged from the bladder during the irrigation.
	Attach the remaining tubing to the lower branch of the "Y" connector. Place the distal end of the tubing in the drainage bottle. (Disposable units are usually connected to the drainage bag in the manufacturing process. This of course is preferable to prevent possible bladder infections.)
6. Pour solution into the flask.	Check the label on the solution to be sure that your are using the correct solution as ordered by the physician. Remove cover of solution bottle. Pour carefully so that you do not splatter the solution.
7. Loosen the clamp on the solution tubing.	Turn the clamp clockwise and release it slowly to permit the irrigating solution to flow into the bladder (approximately 75 to 100 cc). Observe the amount introduced on the calibrated flask. Ask the patient to tell you if he feels discomfort at any time. Where discomfort occurs, clamp the tubing off between your left thumb and index finger. Tell the patient to breathe deeply through his mouth; this will help him relax. Wait 30 to 60 seconds, then slowly release the tubing so that the designated amount of solution can run into the bladder.
8. Tighten the clamp on the solution tubing.	Close the clamp securely using a clockwise motion. Allow the solution to remain in the bladder for the stated time (5 to 15 minutes).
9. Loosen the clamp on the drainage tubing.	Open the clamp using a counterclockwise motion. The solution will flow from the bladder into the drainage bottle (or bag) by gravity.
10. Repeat steps 5 to 7.	Do this until the desired goal is achieved (i.e., solution returns clear with no clots or tissue present). Gently palpate the abdomen over the bladder in order to determine if the fluid is draining well and is not being retained in the bladder, and observe the fluid level in the drainage bottle. Leave the lower drainage tubing UNCLAMPED until the next irrigation.

IRRIGATIONS AND INSTILLATIONS

Important Steps	Key Points
11. Provide for the patient's safety and comfort.	Replace soiled linen as needed. Adjust the bed to low position; adjust the siderails as needed. Place the call signal and bedside table within easy reach of the patient. Ask him if there is anything else you can do, and tell him approximately when you will return. Wash hands.
12. Report and record.	Charting example: 10:00 A.M. Bladder irrigated with 100 cc normal saline solution until solution returned clear. Two blood clots the size of pencil eraser tip were expelled. No complaints of pain or discomfort at this time. J. Mikimoto, R.N.

ITEM 4: IRRIGATION OF THE KIDNEY PELVIS

Irrigation of the kidney pelvis via fine ureteral catheters is frequently used in patients who have a pyelostomy or ureterostomy. Since these catheters are extremely small in diameter (much smaller than a small 8 French rubber catheter), the irrigation is done with a 2 or 5 cc syringe connected to the ureteral catheters by a special connector or adapter and/or an 18 or 19 gauge needle. Because the kidney pelvis does not hold much solution, a very small amount of irrigation solution must be used; therefore, by using a 2 or 5 cc syringe, the amount of solution injected can be precisely controlled. The main purpose of this irrigation is to unclog the fine ureteral catheter. Although these irrigations are becoming the responsibility of nurses, the physician or G.U. technician may be the one to carry out this procedure. Nephrostomy tubes may also be used to drain or irrigate the kidney pelvis. However, the catheters used for this procedure are usually large-size Malecot or Pezzar catheters.

Important Steps	Key Points
1. Obtain sterile equipment from storage.	Your agency may have a special ureteral irrigation set-up; however, you may have to collect the items separately. You will utilize strict aseptic technique in carrying out this procedure. Obtain a 2 or 5 cc syringe with adapter to fit the ureteral catheter, or use a #18 or #19 gauge needle, a basin for the drainage, and a basin or medicine cup for the irrigation solution, antiseptic sponge, 4 × 4 gauze, and the prescribed irrigation solution.
2. Wash your hands.	
3. Approach, identify the patient, and explain the procedure.	Read the Identaband. Tell him that you will be inserting a small amount of solution into the catheter to be sure that it is open and draining freely. Tell him he may feel some discomfort during the procedure, but that you will proceed slowly. If he has discomfort, he should tell you at once so that you can stop the procedure and seek assistance, if needed.

IRRIGATIONS AND INSTILLATIONS

Important Steps	Key Points
4. Prepare the patient.	Provide privacy, adjust the bed or table to working height, lower the proximal siderail and position the patient on his back near the proximal edge of the bed for ease in working.
	Drape him to expose the perineal or abdominal area, wherever the catheter is located (usually perineal).
5. Prepare the equipment.	Open the sterile items, and pour irrigation solution into the container. Put on sterile gloves, arrange the sterile items from the tray on the sterile drape. Fill the syringe with irrigation solution; attach the adapter or needle to the syringe and lay it aside while you cleanse the distal tip of the ureteral catheter with the antiseptic sponge.
	NOTE: If the urethral catheter is attached to a drainage tube, disconnect the drainage tube and place it to one side so that the proximal end will not become contaminated (use the catheter guard or cover).
6. Attach the filled syringe to the catheter.	Hold the catheter securely between your thumb and index fingers while you insert the syringe adapter or needle into the catheter.
7. Introduce solution into the catheter.	Push the plunger into the barrel or the syringe very *slowly* and *gently*. *Never* use force; you could rupture the kidney pelvis!
	NOTE: If you encounter any obstacle (obstruction), withdraw the solution, remove the syringe and call the physician at once. Reconnect the catheter to the drainage tube, if indicated.
8. Observe the patient.	Continue to reassure him.
9. Withdraw solution.	Slowly and gently pull back on the plunger. Less solution will return to the syringe than you injected, because some of it will remain in the ureteral catheter.
	NOTE: The solution is not withdrawn if the ureteral catheter is to be reattached to the drainage tube. After the solution is introduced the syringe is disconnected from the catheter and placed at one side of the sterile field. Then the catheter and drainage tubes are reconnected.

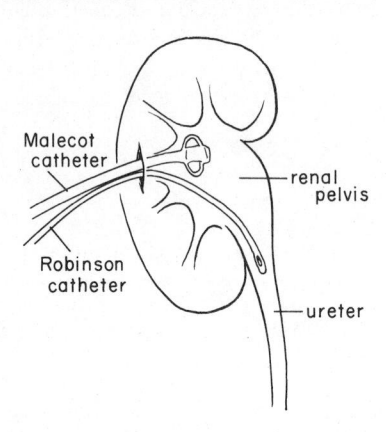

IRRIGATIONS AND INSTILLATIONS

Important Steps	Key Points
10. Remove supplies.	Discard disposable items. Return reusable items to the processing department.
11. Leave the patient safe and comfortable.	Replenish soiled linens as needed. Replace the top covers and adjust the bed and siderails. Put the call light and bedside stand within easy reach. Position the patient in good alignment and ask if there is anything else you can do for him. Tell him when you expect to return. Wash hands.
12. Report and record.	Charting example: 4:00 P.M. 2 cc of NaCl used to irrigate the right ureteral catheter. Solution returned clear. Moderate discomfort exhibited during the procedure. J. Jones, S.N.

ITEM 5: THE EAR

The ear is the organ of hearing and equilibrium. It is composed of three divisions: the external ear, the middle ear, and the inner ear.

For the purposes of this Unit, we are concerned mainly with the external ear (composed of the auricle, or pinna, which is the cartilaginous projection on either side of the head). It also contains some adipose (fat) tissue, muscles, and soft connective tissue. The auricle is covered by skin and joined to the scalp by ligaments and muscles. Sound waves are caught by the auricle and directed toward the external auditory canal.

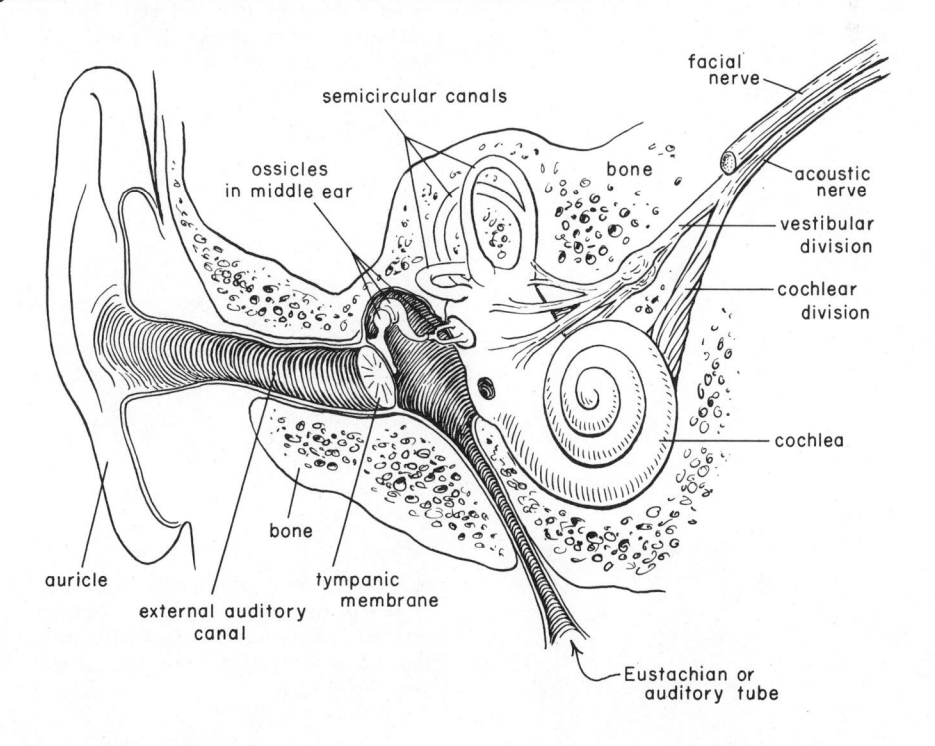

The external auditory canal (external acoustic meatus) is a 1-inch tubular passageway that extends from the outer ear to the typanic membrane, (eardrum) which separates the auditory canal from the typanic cavity (middle ear).

The external auditory canal is an S-shaped curve that goes inward, forward, and upward, then inward and backward. When you lift the auricle upward and backward for irrigating or inspection, you straighten the canal.

The external auditory canal is lined with wax glands (ceruminous glands), which secrete a yellow, waxy substance called cerumen or earwax. It protects the tympanic membrane from injury and foreign objects. There are also fine hairs near the external opening that also filter out foreign objects.

ITEM 6: EAR IRRIGATION

An ear irrigation is usually done to remove foreign objects from the external auditory canal or to cleanse it from purulent drainage or ear wax (cerumen). The irrigation is preceded by a visual examination of the ear through use of an otoscope.

It is better to avoid performing an irrigation if the patient has an acute condition such as a cold, earache, fever etc. The irrigation will just make the patient more uncomfortable.

Ear instillations, on the other hand, can be administered, if ordered, when the patient is suffering from an acute condition such as mentioned above.

Important Steps	Key Points
1. Obtain equipment from storage.	You will need a basin for drainage, drapes (towels), heated irrigation solution, and a syringe. Several types may be used:

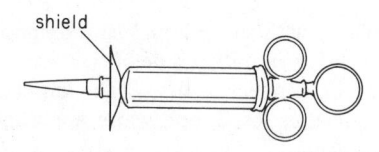

shield

Pomeroy Syringe

The Pomeroy syringe is an all-metal syringe with interchangeable tips. It is available in 2-oz or 4-oz sizes. The metal shield at the tip end protects the health worker from being splattered with solution during the procedure. Although this syringe is preferred by most workers, caution must be exercised to avoid forceful introduction of the solution. Excessive pressure against the ear drum can cause rupture of the typanic membrane.

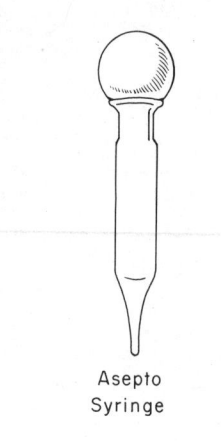

Asepto Syringe

The Asepto syringe, on the other hand, does not permit much force to be exerted. The amount of solution being injected is clearly visible to the worker.

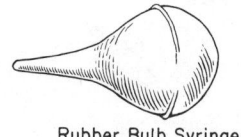

Rubber Bulb Syringe

The rubber bulb syringe is frequently used to irrigate a small child's ear. The force that can be exerted is very limited and thus injury to the delicate internal structures is unlikely to occur.

IRRIGATIONS AND INSTILLATIONS

Important Steps	Key Points

2. Wash your hands.

3. Approach, identify the patient and explain the procedure.

Read the Identaband. Explain why you will wash his ear out e.g., to clean the ear; to remove the wax; to remove purulent drainage.

NOTE: <u>*Do not* irrigate the ear to remove beans or corn. The fluid used to irrigate the ear will make the object swell and thus become more permanently lodged in the ear. Usually this kind of object is removed with tweezers, a hook, or a knife.</u> Extreme caution must be taken to avoid pushing the object further into the ear.

NOTE: If the irrigation is to be done in the treatment room, take the patient and supplies there.

4. Prepare the patient.

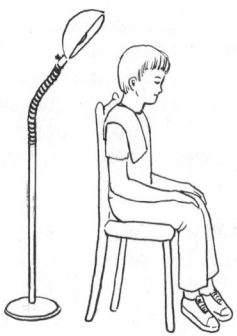

<u>A sitting position is usually preferred.</u> Drape the shoulder on the side you will be working to protect the patient's clothing from being soiled. Be sure that the external ear is well-illuminated (use either a type of flexible light or position the patient so that the ear to be irrigated is near a window light).

5. Prepare the equipment.

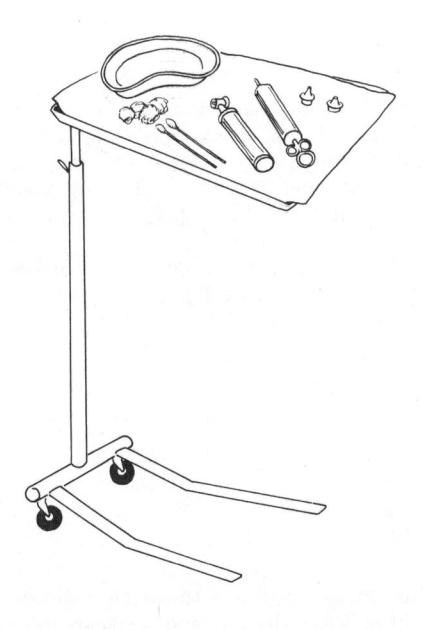

Place items on a stand (bedside, overbed table or Mayo stand) within easy reach. The table should have a comfortable working height.

<u>Fill the syringe with the prescribed warm solution (105°F or 40.6°C). Cool solutions are very uncomfortable for the patient.</u> They make the patient dizzy or nauseated because the equilibrium sensors in the semicircular canals are stimulated. <u>Common solutions used for ear irrigation are: plain warm tap water; 2 to 4 per cent boric acid solution; 0.8 per cent bicarbonate of soda; warm normal saline; hydrogen peroxide; or glycerine and water.</u>

To soften cerumen, you may need to instill a few drops of warm mineral oil or hydrogen peroxide 10 to 15 minutes before the irrigation. In some instances the mineral oil may need to be instilled daily for a few days before the irrigation.

Sometimes an irrigation may be unnecessary because the oil may soften the wax so that it comes out of the ear by itself. Therefore, it is always wise to look into the ear before beginning the irrigation.

<u>Bugs can be killed by putting oil in the ear before beginning the irrigation.</u>

IRRIGATIONS AND INSTILLATIONS

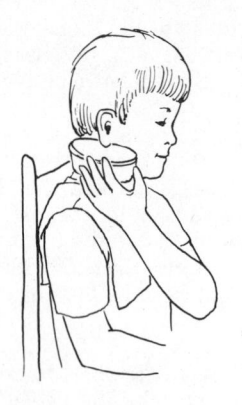

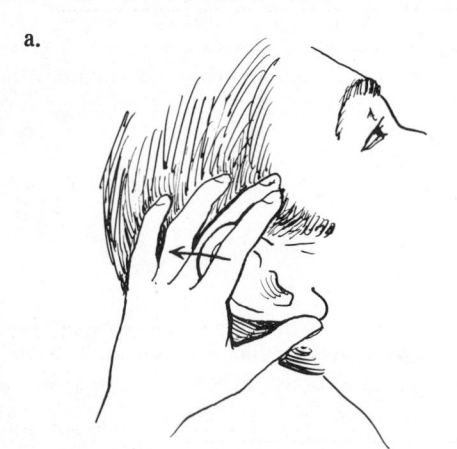

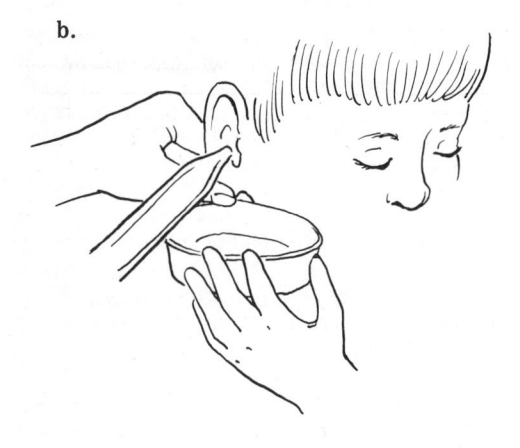

Important Steps	Key Points
6. Have patient hold the drainage pan under his ear.	It should be held firmly against the neck just under the ear to keep the solution from running out of the ear and down the neck.
7. Straighten the auditory canal. a.	With your left hand (or your right hand if you are left-handed), place your thumb on the ear lobe to stabilize your hand. Then grasp the upper portion of the auricle between the middle and index finger. With an *upward* and *backward* motion, straighten the auditory canal. NOTE: Some individuals may prefer to gently hold the auricle of the ear between the thumb and index finger while pulling gently upward and backward.
b.	With your left hand (or your right if you are left-handed), grasp the ear lobe between the thumb and index finger and pull the lobe *downward* and *backward.* This will straighten a child's auditory canal. NOTE: *Always look into the ear* before irrigations so that you do not irrigate if a foreign object is not present!
8. Tilt the head toward the drainage basin.	This must be done to catch solution as it returns from the ear and to keep the patient from getting wet.

Important Steps	Key Points
9. Insert the syringe tip.	Do this carefully to avoid injuring the delicate ear tissue.
	The syringe should enter the external meatus just slightly; then point the tip upward and toward the posterior auditory canal. The flow of solution will then arch forward to carry the debris outside.
10. Inject solution into the external auditory canal.	Push the plunger in *slowly* and *carefully*. If solution is injected into the canal forcefully, it could injure or rupture the ear drum.
	If you are using the Pomeroy syringe, you may wish to rest it against your left thumb as a support. Since it is an all-metal syringe, it is quite heavy.
	Inject all the solution carefully and slowly; observe the returning solution to see what is removed, e.g., wax, foreign object, etc.
11. Remove the syringe, refill and reinsert it in the ear.	Repeat these steps until the returning solution runs clear. You may use no more than one pint of solution to complete the irrigations.
12. Remove the syringe and inspect the ear canal.	When you are satisfied that the ear canal is clear, inspect the ear canal visually to be sure that it is clean.
13. Leave the patient safe and comfortable.	Dry his ear and neck. Remove the drapes and change soiled linen as needed.
	Encourage the patient to keep the ear dry for at least 24 hours. Sometimes the cerumen or foreign body is so tightly lodged in the ear canal that it traumatizes the surface of the ear canal. The warm, enclosed abraded ear canal can become an excellent breeding ground for microorganisms.
	Instruct the patient to refrain from cleaning or drying his ear with a cotton applicator, bobby pin, or any sharp object because he cannot see his own ear and he may seriously damage some of the delicate structures. Scratching the ear with the fingernails is also forbidden because the skin can easily be abraded and become a focal point for an infection.
	Position the patient for his comfort. Return him to bed if the irrigation was done in the treatment room. Adjust the height of the bed and siderails as indicated. Ask if there is anything you can do for him, and put the call light and bedside stand within easy reach.

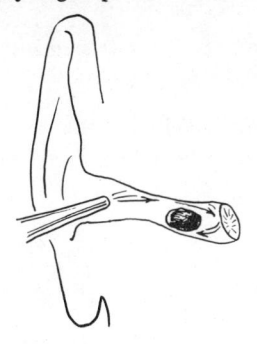

Important Steps	Key Points
14. Remove the supplies.	Take the drainage basin from the patient.
	NOTE: Observe the returned solution for later recording before you empty the basin.
	Remove other equipment and return for processing; leave the room tidy. Wash hands.
15. Report and record.	Charting example:
	3:15 P.M. Right ear irrigated with 500 cc NaCl. Moderate amount of cerumen returned.
	J. deMuir, R.N.

ITEM 6: EAR INSTILLATION

This procedure is generally used to insert a softening agent so that earwax can be removed easily at a later time. It may also be used to introduce an antibiotic suspension of ear drops in cases of ear canal or ear drum infection. Follow the procedure given in Item 5 above, except that you will be using a medicine dropper filled with the prescribed medication instead of an irrigating syringe. Position that patient and explain your intention as before; expose and straighten the ear canal as before.

Important Steps	Key Points
1. Wash your hands.	
2. Withdraw medicine into the medicine dropper.	Check to be sure that you have the right medication and the right dosage.
3. Insert the tip of the medicine dropper into the external ear canal.	Placement should be the same as in Item 5.
4. Inject the medicine.	Compress the rubber bulb on the dropper.
5. Withdraw the dropper.	Place to one side.
6. Plug the external meatus.	Use a cotton ball to keep the medicine from escaping.
	NOTE: Cotton balls should not be used to keep ears from draining; you want them to drain!
7. Leave the patient safe and comfortable.	Remove the supplies. Wash hands.
8. Record procedure.	Charting example:
	4:00 A.M. 5 gtt. mineral oil inserted into left ear. Cotton ball placed in external auditory meatus.
	A. Hopkins, R.N.

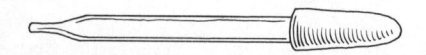

ITEM 7: THE EYE

The eye is the organ of vision. The eyeball, the optic nerve and the visual center in the brain combine to make up the *visual system*.

The eyeball is spherical in shape and is situated in a bony cavity called the *orbit*. Each of the two orbits is funnel-shaped; the large end of the funnel is directed outward and forward, while the small end is directed inward and backward. At the posterior end of the funnel is a large opening through which both the optic nerve and the ophthalmic artery pass, from the cranium to the eye. The orbits contain the eyeballs, nerves, blood vessels, muscles, lacrimal (tear) glands, fat and fascia.

During severe illness, the fat is metabolized at an accelerated rate and the eyeballs appear to be sunken into the orbits. You probably have observed this in members of your family or in friends who have been ill for a period of time.

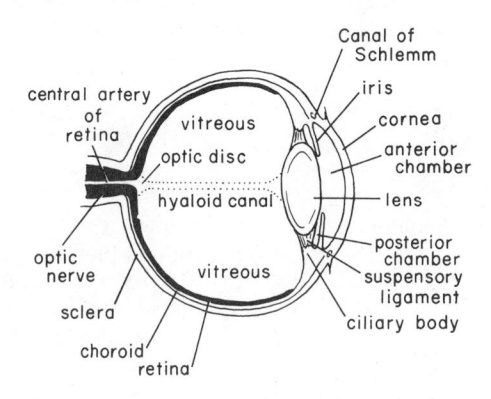

There are three coats (layers or tunics) to the eyeball. The *sclera*, or the white of the eye, is composed of an opaque dense fibrous tissue. It maintains the shape of the eyeball and also acts as a protective covering for the internal structures. Anteriorly this layer is very thin and becomes the transparent layer called the *cornea*. Although it is a fibrous tissue, it is transparent. Sometimes the cornea is called the window of the eye because it is via the cornea that the light is transmitted through the inner structures to the retina. Although the scleral layer has a limited blood supply, there are no blood vessels in the cornea, and surgery on the cornea is therefore bloodless. The cornea does have a good nerve supply and therefore is normally quite sensitive to foreign objects. This, of course, is an important safety factor. The cornea gets its nutritional supply from the lymphatic system, which abounds in the eye. Because the cornea is so delicate, it can be easily injured or scratched. Corneal scarring can result, with possible blindness if the scarring is severe. Corneal transplants, a surgical operation, can restore sight in some of these cases. You may have heard about this procedure, or you may know someone who has had a corneal transplant.

The middle layer of the eye is called the *choroid*. This layer is a thin, dark-brown membrane that lines the inner surface of the sclera. It contains an intricate blood supply system and the pigment cells, which absorb light.

Arising from the choroid layer is the *ciliary body*, a ruffle-like folding of the choroid that encircles the lens. It contains nerves and blood vessels, and supports the ciliary muscles, which are the chief means of accommodation and control of the shape of the lens.

The *iris* (colored part of the eye) is suspended in the aqueous humor in front of the lens (behind the cornea) and it is attached on the distal edges to the ciliary process.

In the middle of the iris is the *pupil*, through which light is admitted to the inner eye. By its contraction-relaxation motion, the iris regulates the amount of light entering the eye, thereby achieving a clear visual image.

A cataract is an opaque lens. Light waves cannot pass through the lens and an individual who has cataract is therefore unable to see. The lens can be surgically removed when it has ripened or matured to a certain degree of opacity. After removal of the cataract, the patient can see again when fitted with corrective lenses (i.e., eye glasses or contact lenses).

IRRIGATIONS AND INSTILLATIONS

The internal layer of the eye is called the *retina*. It is a very delicate tissue that receives the image of objects and transmits the impression via the optic nerve to the sight center in the cerebrum. There are seven layers in the retina, one of which consists of *rods* and *cones*, which are visual receptors. They differ not only structurally but functionally. The cones are important for color vision in bright lights, while the rods are important for light and dark perception (not color). The cones are important in perceiving form and movement in poorly lighted circumstances (e.g., at night). Visual acuity of the rods is less than that of the cones.

The *blind spot* (which contains no receptor cells) is on the inner aspect of the eyeball where the optic nerve enters the eyeball.

An important point on the retina (at exact center) is the *macula lutea* (yellow spot). It is the center of direct vision. When the retina is detached from its moorings, the patient cannot see. Usually the retina can be reattached by a coagulation process using a laser beam, or by surgical procedure. However, some detached retinas cannot be repaired.

Before beginning the eye irrigation or instillation, be sure to check the orders so that you use the right medicine (solution) in the correct dosage in the correct eye!

ITEM 8: EYE IRRIGATION

Important Steps	Key Points
1. Obtain sterile supplies and equipment.	An eye tray may be available in your agency. It should include: container for the solution, cotton balls, eye pads, rubber bulb syringe, designated sterile solution, basin to collect drainage, sterile gloves, and drapes (towels).
2. Wash your hands.	
3. Approach and identify the patient, and explain the procedure.	Read the Identaband. Explain that you will be gently washing the eye to remove the drainage, or to soothe an irritation.
4. Prepare the patient.	Usually the Sims position is preferred (the eye to be treated is closest to the bed).
	The supine position can also be used. In this case, have the patient turn his head in the direction of the affected eye. Be sure that good lighting is available to you for optimal visibility so that you will not injure the eye during the procedure.
	Provide for the patient's privacy. Adjust the bed or table to working height and lower the proximal siderail if one is present. Have the patient move toward the proximal edge of the bed or table for ease in working.

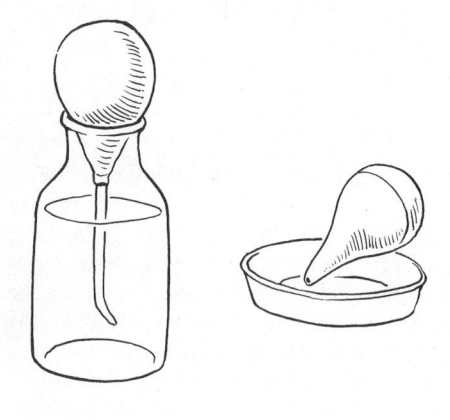

IRRIGATIONS AND INSTILLATIONS

Important Steps	Key Points
5. Prepare the equipment.	Place items on a stand (bedside, or near you) so that it is convenient for you to work. Slip a towel on the bed underneath the patient's head to avoid soiling the sheets. Place an emesis basin close to his face to catch irrigation solution.
6. Cleanse the eyelid with a moistened cotton ball.	The cotton is thoroughly moistened with cleansing solution (e.g., normal saline, boric acid solution). This is done only if there is a crusty discharge on the eyelid. Use one cleansing motion from the inner canthus to the outer edge of the eye. Discard the cotton ball in a designated container.
7. Fill an irrigating syringe with solution.	Depress the bulb and release, drawing the prescribed amount of solution into the syringe. Be sure to read the label on the solution container to be sure you have the right solution for your patient. Warm solution (approximately body temperature) is most comfortable for the patient.
8. Hold the eyelid.	Gently, but firmly, pull the upper eyelid toward the eyebrow with your thumb, and rest your thumb on the bony prominence above the eye. Ask the patient to look downward. This will keep the patient from being blind during the procedure.
9. Inject the solution into the eye.	Hold the syringe about 1/2 to 1 inch above the eye. Direct the flow from the nasal edge of the eye so that the solution drains across the eye to the outer edge.
10. Continue the irrigation.	This should be done until the desired results occur or you have used the prescribed amount of solution.
11. Remove the syringe.	When the irrigation is complete, lay syringe aside on the tray. Dry the eyelid with a cotton ball, and then discard it in a designated container.

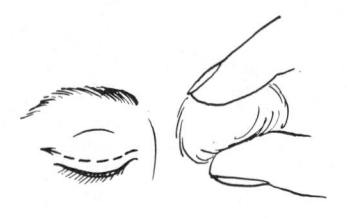

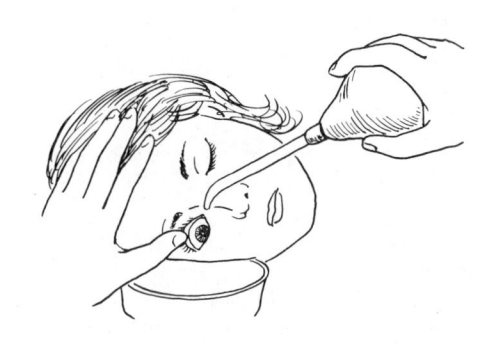

Important Steps	Key Points
12. Leave the patient comfortable.	Remove the emesis basin and place it on the stand. Dry his face with a towel, and change soiled linen as needed. Position him for comfort. Adjust the height of the bed and siderails as indicated. Place the call light and bedside stand within easy reach. Ask if there is anything else you can do, and tell him when you expect to return.

If the treatment is being carried out in the clinic setting, permit the patient to rest on the table a few minutes before he leaves. |
| 13. Remove the supplies. | Discard soiled items, and empty the emesis basin after observing drainage for later recording on the chart. Return reusable items to the processing department. Leave the room clean and tidy. Wash hands. |
| 14. Report and record. | Charting example:

3:00 P.M. Right eye irrigated with 5% boric acid solution. Patient states this is very soothing to his eye. Redness in cornea has decreased markedly since last irrigation.

B. O'Neil, R.N. |

If both eyes are infected, an individual irrigation set should be used for each eye.

ITEM 9: INSTILLATION OF EYE DROPS

Important Steps	Key Points
1. Assemble the required supplies.	Usually medication for instilling comes in a bottle with an eyedropper. Eye medications are ordered for the individual patient and *may not* be used from patient to patient. Cotton balls or paper tissues may be used to catch the excess solution.
2. Wash your hands.	
3. Approach and identify the patient and explain the procedure.	Read the Identaband and explain that you will be putting some eye drops into his eye to control the infection.

In the case of this treatment being done in an office or clinic setting, ask the patient to tell you his name and compare this information with his patient chart (record). |
| 4. Prepare the patient. | The patient may sit or recline in a dorsal recumbent position. Ask him to look upward. This will keep your from touching the cornea with the tip of the medicine dropper in case the patient blinks. It also gives him something to do to keep his eye from moving. |

Important Steps	Key Points
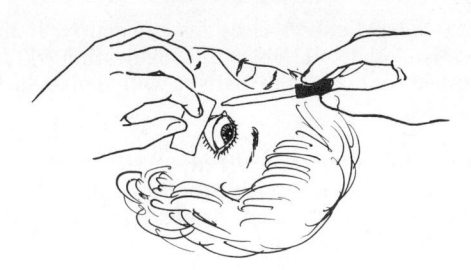	If the patient is supine and if you are right-handed, **pull the lower lid down** with your left index finger and thumb so that the lower fornix is exposed.
	If the patient is sitting in a chair, stand behind the chair and support his head with your body. Expose the lower fornix of the affected eye by pulling the lower eyelid toward the cheek. Again have him look upward to keep the dropper from touching his eye or eyelid.
5. Introduce the medication into the lower fornix. 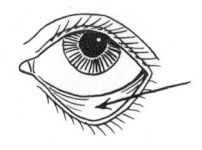	Drop the designated amount of medication directly on the spot indicated in the diagram. Replace the dropper in the medicine container. Be sure to insert the dropper directly into the bottle without touching the sides of the bottle. If you contaminate the eyedropper, you will have to order a fresh medicine supply for the patient.
	NOTE: If a tube of eye ointment is used instead of eye drops, remove the cap from the tube and, standing in the same position as for applying eye drops, apply a thin ribbon of ointment along the entire length of the lower fornix. Eye ointment that is at room temperature applies more easily. To end the ribbon, simply twist the tube with a lateral movement of the wrist. Recap the ointment tube and lay it aside.

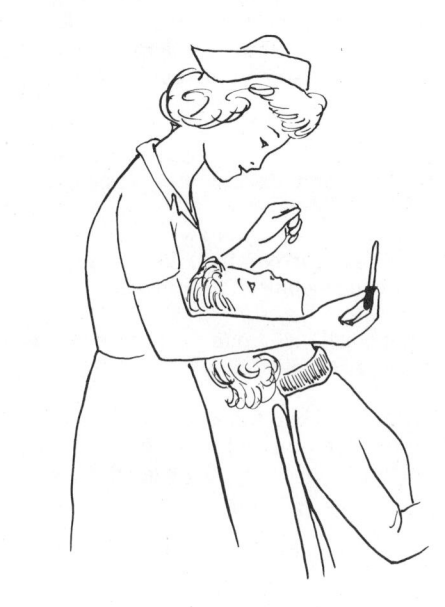

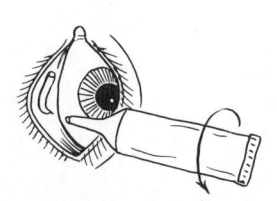

Important Steps	Key Points
6. Close the patient's eyelid.	Ask the patient to close his eye gently. If the eye is closed too tightly, the medication will be pushed out and the patient will derive little benefit.
	If an ointment was instilled, ask the patient to close his eyelid gently and roll the eyeball around to ensure that medication covers the entire exterior eyeball.
	In the case of some poisonous medication (atropine), care must be taken that the medicine does not get into the lacrimal (tear) duct. To avoid this, place your thumb over the inner canthus.
7. Gently dry the eyelid.	With a cotton ball or tissue remove the excess medication, and discard in a designated container.
8. Leave the patient safe and comfortable.	Position him for comfort; adjust the height of the bed and siderails, if indicated.
	Place the call light and bedside stand within easy reach, as indicated.
	Ask if there is anything else you can do, and tell him when you will come back. Return the eye medication to the designated place. Wash hands.
9. Report and record.	Charting example:
	4:00 P.M. 2 gtt. Scopolamine 0.25% given in O.D.
	M. Hayashi, R.N.

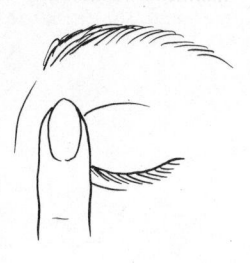

ITEM 10: THE NOSE

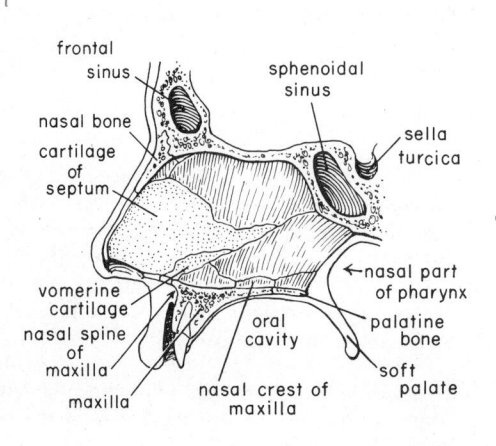

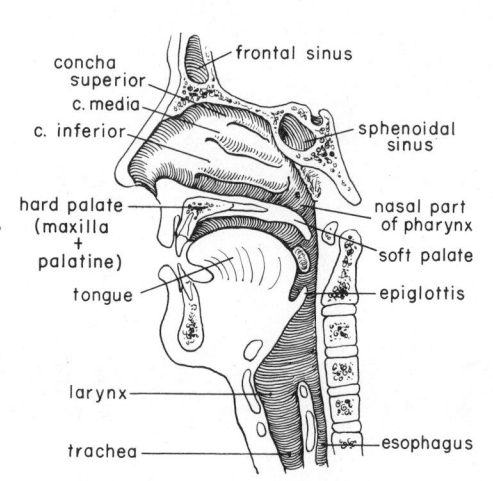

The nose is the organ that provides the sense of smell and acts as the passageway for air going to and from the lungs. It is composed of two parts: the external nose and the internal cavities called the nasal fossae. The nose has a number of important functions, including filtering, warming and moistening incoming air, and assisting in making vocal sounds (phonation).

The external nose is composed of eleven bones and a cartilaginous framework which is covered by skin and lined with a mucous membrane. The two oval external openings are called the nostrils or anterior nares.

The two wedge-shaped cavities are separated by a partition called the septum, which is normally curved more on one side than on the other. This is an extremely important consideration when various tubes must be inserted into the nose or when nasal treatments are given.

The palate, the roof of the mouth, and the maxilla (jawbone) separate the nasal cavities from the mouth. The ethmoid bone separates the nasal cavities from the cranial cavities. The mucous membrane that lines the nasal cavities extends inward to line the sinuses. This is why infections of the nasal mucosa frequently extend to the sinuses. The mucous membranes are well supplied with blood vessels. The olfactory nerve, which is found in the upper third of the septum, assists in smelling.

ITEM 11: NASAL IRRIGATION

This procedure is done for the patient who has chronic rhinitis (inflammation of the nasal mucosa). Nasal irrigations are usually administered at least daily to keep the nasal cavity free of crusts and drainage. This procedure is frequently done in the clinic, the physician's office, or the patient may be taught to do his own nasal irrigation at home.

Important Steps	Key Points
1. Assemble the equipment.	Have the prescribed solution available, at room temperature or no warmer than 105°F.
	You will need an irrigator with a nozzle or catheter (since there are various kinds of appropriate equipment, use what is available in your agency), basin to collect solution, towels, and tissues.
	Connect the irrigator (or syringe) to the irrigating tubing and/or nozzle. Clamp off the tubing. Have irrigating can on the I.V. stand beside the patient at an elevation of about 12 inches above his head. Open the tubing clamp and allow a small amount of solution to run through the tubing into the basin to clear the tubing of air. Reclamp the tubing, and place the tubing nozzle in a tray at the patient's side until you are ready to start the treatment.
2. Wash your hands.	
3. Approach and identify the patient, and explain the procedure.	Read the Identaband, or ask him to give you his name. Check for agreement on his record or chart. Explain that you will have him sit on a stool near the lavatory (sink) so that the solution you inject into his nose can drain into the lavatory.
	If the patient is unable to sit on a chair, he can remain in bed in a sitting position. The emesis basin can be held under his nose to catch the drainage.

Important Steps	Key Points
	Tell him that you will <u>stop the irrigation immediately if he gags, becomes nauseated or uncomfortable</u>. Tell him to signal you to stop by gently touching your arm, or whatever signal you prefer.
	Instruct him to breathe slowly through his mouth without speaking or swallowing during the introduction of the solution.
4. Prepare the patient.	Drape his shoulders and chest with a large bath towel, plastic sheet or cape to protect his clothing.
	Position him on a stool or chair directly in front of the lavatory. Ask him to lean slightly forward so that the return flow is assured and the solution will not flow into other cavities (e.g., sinuses or throat).
	Give him some disposable tissues to use to catch the excess drainage.
5. Insert the catheter or nozzle into the nostril.	With the patient leaning slightly forward over the drainage basin, insert the nozzle gently into one nostril. Remind the patient not to talk and to breathe through his mouth.
	Unclamp the tubing and allow the solution to run gently into one nostril and out the other. Allow approximately 1,000 cc of solution to run in and out. The solution should be at room temperature for patient comfort.
6. Remove the nozzle and insert it in the other nostril.	Clamp off the tubing while transferring the catheter (nozzle) from one nostril to the other, to keep from drenching the patient.
	Unclamp the tubing and allow solution to run into one nostril and drain out the other. Continue the procedure until all the solution is used.
	Stop the treatment as necessary to allow the patient to rest.
7. Clamp the tubing and then remove the nozzle.	Put it back on the tray at the patient's side.
	The patient should continue to maintain his position until all of the solution has drained.
	Tell him *not to blow his nose* because doing so could cause the infection to spread into the connecting eustachian tubes.

IRRIGATIONS AND INSTILLATIONS

Important Steps	Key Points
8. Leave the patient safe and comfortable.	Remove the drapes and dry his face with a towel or disposable tissue. Tell him when the irrigation will be repeated.
	Return the used supplies for reprocessing and discard the disposable equipment in a designated container. Wash hands.
9. Report and record.	Charting example:
	3:10 P.M. 2,000 cc NaCl given as a nasal irrigation.
	K. Sato, R.N.

ITEM 12: NASAL INSTILLATION

The nasal instillation of medications can be done with a medicine dropper, an inhaler, or an atomizer.

Important Steps	Key Points
1. Obtain the required equipment.	Your agency may have a nasal treatment tray. If not, you will need the medication which usually comes in a bottle with a medicine dropper, and disposable tissues, or a towel. Place them on a stand, at bedside or close to the bed, for convenience in carrying out the treatment.
2. Wash your hands.	
3. Approach, identify the patient, and explain the procedure.	Read the Identaband or ask him to tell you his name, and confirm with the record.
	Explain that you will be <u>putting drops in his nose to assist in healing the infection or to shrink swollen membranes.</u>
	NOTE: There are various beliefs as to the effectiveness of nose drops to decrease nasal congestion. Some physicians believe that constricting the blood vessels in the mucous membranes reduces the possibility of infection, while others do not believe this theory.
4. Prepare the patient.	<u>The dorsal recumbent position is the position of choice.</u>
	Place a pillow under his shoulders so that his head can drop back, thus allowing medication to flow deep into the nasal cavity. Or you can move him to the edge of the bed or table so that his head drops backward. Support the head with one hand to avoid undue strain on his neck muscles.
	This treatment can be done in the hospital room, treatment room, clinic, physician's office, or in the home.

Important Steps	Key Points
	There are two head positions commonly used for instilling nose drops.
	The Proetz position is used primarily for treating the ethmoid and sphenoid sinuses.

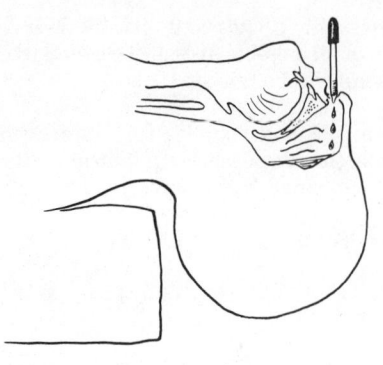

Proetz position

Parkinson position

The Parkinson position is used to treat the nasal passageways and the frontal and maxillary sinuses.

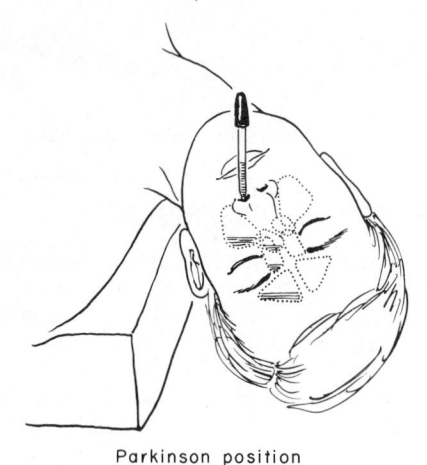

5. Prepare the medication

Unscrew the cap from the medicine bottle. Depress the rubber stopper between your dominant thumb and index finger, and release, drawing the medicine up into the dropper.

NOTE: Oily nose drops should be avoided because of the possibility of inhaling the oily solution into the lungs, which could lead to a lipid pneumonia.

6. Inject the nose drops.

correct   incorrect

Holding the medicine dropper slightly above the nostril, direct the tip of the medicine dropper toward the midline of the superior concha of the ethmoid. This will deflect the medicine toward the back of the nasal cavity. Be careful *not to touch* the nasal surfaces with the medicine dropper, thereby contaminating it. Inject the precise amount of medication that is ordered.

NOTE: If you insert the medicine dropper toward the base of the nasal cavity, the medication will run down the throat and be swallowed without being effective.

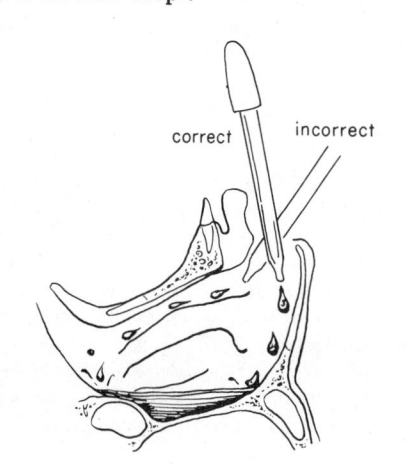

Important Steps	Key Points
7. Withdraw the medicine dropper.	Discard the unused medicine remaining in the dropper in a designated container; replace the dropper in the medicine bottle and set aside. Observe the patient carefully throughout the procedure so that you can chart his reactions.
8. Leave the patient safe and comfortable.	Dry his nostrils with disposable wipes and reposition him comfortably in bed, or on the treatment table. Let him remain in the recumbent position 5 to 10 minutes to allow for absorption of the medication. Wash hands.
9. Record the treatment.	Charting example: 10:30 A.M. 3 gtt ephedrine 0.5% nose drops inserted into both nostrils. Mucous membranes are shrinking and breathing is easier. K. Sato, R.N.

Sometimes medicated nasal inhalers or atomizers containing nasal medications are prescribed for patients because they are more convenient to use. The same principles of administration apply, however, as those described in the above procedure. Insert the inhaler or atomizer into one nostril, and gently close the other nares by depressing the nose toward the septum. Ask the patient to breathe through his nose while keeping his mouth open.

ITEM 13: THE THROAT

The throat (pharynx) is the portion of the respiratory tract that extends from the arch of the palate (roof of the mouth) to the glottis and superior opening of the esophagus. The front of the neck is also called the throat.

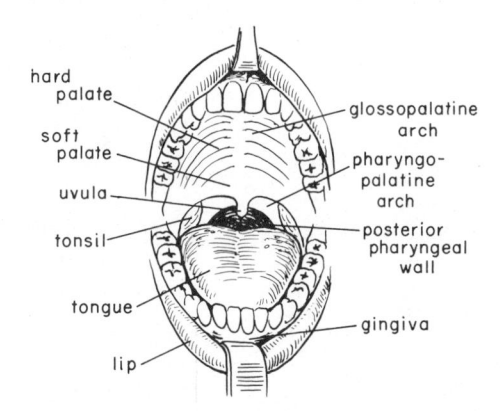

The throat can be examined visually by holding the tongue with a gauze and pulling it forward while depressing the posterior tongue area with a tongue blade or depressor. To enable the examiner to see into the back of the oral cavity, a flashlight beam or head mirror light is employed for illumination by directing it toward the posterior oral cavity (see illustrations on next page). Depressing the back of the tongue often stimulates the gag reflex, and therefore the patient is asked to breathe through his mouth in short breaths (pants). This keeps him occupied and takes his mind off the procedure.

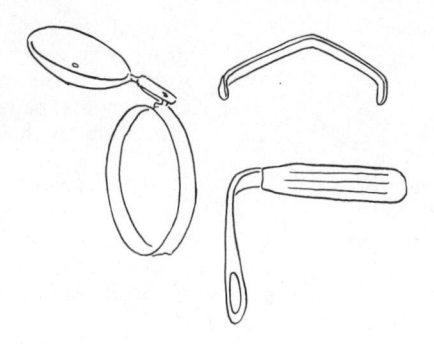

Common infections of the throat are: pharyngitis, tonsillitis, peritonsillar abscess, enlarged tonsils and adenoids. Common solutions used for the throat, mouth irrigations, and gargles are: NaCl, hydrogen peroxide, aspirin solution, and Dakin's solution, among others.

ITEM 14: THROAT IRRIGATION OR GARGLE

Although the throat irrigation is more effective than the gargle because the throat is more relaxed, the gargle is the treatment most individuals prefer. Also, with the advent of antibiotics, the need to use throat irrigations or gargles as a treatment is practically eliminated. However, the saline gargle is still an effective home treatment for a sore throat. If relief of the sore throat (after two or three gargles) is not accomplished, a nurse or physician should be contacted. Throat irrigations or gargles can be carried out in the home, clinic, physician's office or industrial plant.

Important Steps	Key Points
1. Assemble the equipment.	The same equipment is used as for the nasal irrigation (Item 11): the irrigator, catheter, nozzle or syringe, I.V. stand, and solution. The solution should be at room temperature up to 105°F. Attach pieces of equipment together and lay to one side on the treatment tray at patient's side. The tray should be located at working height on a flat, steady surface, easily accessible for use. Follow step 1 in Item 11.
2. Wash your hands.	
3. Approach, identify the patient and explain the procedure.	Read the Identaband or, if the patient is in a clinic or home setting, call him by name and verify with patient's record.
	Explain that you will introduce the solution into the mouth to bathe the throat with the medication to assist in combating the infection and to help decrease the swelling, or whatever is the purpose of the irrigation.
4. Prepare the patient.	He should be seated facing the sink or drainage basin just as he would be for a nasal irrigation.
	Put a plastic cape or bath towel around his shoulders to keep him warm and to avoid soiling him with the drainage solution.

Important Steps	Key Points
	Hand him disposable wipes for use as needed.
	Tell him you will stop the irrigation upon a predetermined signal from him (touch on the arm, raised eyebrows, etc.).
5. Insert the nozzle tip or catheter tip into his mouth.	Stand to one side of the patient, facing him, so that you can see what you are doing.
	Unclamp the tubing. Direct the irrigating tip toward the throat, move the tip slowly back and forth in a fan-shaped motion so that all parts of the throat are reached.
	NOTE: This same procedure can be used for the mouth irrigation, except that the catheter tip is not inserted so far back into the mouth. Direct the tip so that the entire oral cavity can be bathed in the irrigating solution by moving the catheter to and fro in a fan-shaped direction, as above.
6. Interrupt the irrigation.	This must be done to allow the patient to breathe. Clamp the tubing between your thumb and index finger.
7. Continue the irrigation or gargle.	Do this until the prescribed amount of solution is used. Continue to observe the patient throughout the procedure so that you can record any unusual occurence. Talk with the patient in a soothing voice throughout the procedure to keep him calm.
8. Clamp off the tubing.	Remove the irrigator tip and place it to one side while you dry the patient and make him comfortable. Remove the drapes.
9. Leave the patient safe and comfortable.	Position him comfortably and let him rest briefly before moving.
	Examine the contents of the irrigation basin before discarding, for later recording on the chart.
	Return supplies to central processing or discard disposable items in a designated container. Wash hands.
10. Record the procedure.	Charting example:
	6:00 P.M. 2,000 cc Dakin's solution used to irrigate throat. Solution returned clear. Patient states throat is not as sore as it was yesterday.
	K. Sato R.N.

To gargle, the patient takes a deep breath and then takes a moderate amount of the solution into his mouth, tips his head backward and lets the solution run as far back as possible in the throat and holds it there while gently exhaling air to cause the solution to bubble in the throat. When all the air is exhaled, he spits out the solution, takes a deep breath and another mouthful of solution, following the same procedure as above. Prepare at least 8 ounces of solution, generally as hot as the patient can tolerate. Have him repeat the gargle procedure as directed (e.g., hour, q.i.d., etc.).

There are packaged medicated oral sprays that are sometimes prescribed, and in that case, the physician specifies how often, and how much medication is to be used. The exact directions for use of the spray are printed on the label of the spray bottle.

ITEM 15: WOUNDS

Infected or gaping wounds must be kept very clean for proper healing to take place. Wounds must heal from the inside out to avoid formation of pus in the space between the bottom of the wound and the closure of the skin and/or superficial tissue layers. Thus, to keep the wounds healing from the inside out, they may be irrigated frequently with various solutions (e.g., an antiseptic solution such as Betadine 0.5 per cent, antibiotic solutions, proteolytic enzyme solutions such as streptokinase or trypsin, hydrogen peroxide, or Dakin's solution, a germicide and deodorant solution). Review the enrichment section in Unit 1, Aseptic Technique, for additional information about types of wounds and wound healing.

ITEM 16: WOUND IRRIGATION

Important Steps	Key Points
1. Assemble the equipment.	A sterile disposable set may be available. It will include drapes, an irrigating syringe and soft catheter, a basin to collect the drainage, and a calibrated graduate, or other calibrated container, cotton balls and dressings. Open a sterile glove package. Open the irrigating set in a convenient location on a flat surface near the part of the patient's body being irrigated (e.g., abdomen, or extremity). Pour the designated amount of irrigating solution into the calibrated graduate. Tear off the tape for securing the dressing after the irrigation is completed, and place it in a convenient location so that you can easily reach it when you are ready for it.
2. Wash your hands.	
3. Approach, identify the patient, and explain the procedure.	
4. Prepare the patient.	Expose the area to be irrigated. With lifting forceps from the tray, remove the soiled dressing and discard it in the designated container. Set the soiled forceps aside.
5. Put on sterile gloves.	Place drapes around the wound area. Place the irrigating basin against the area of the body to be irrigated.
6. Fill the syringe with irrigating solution.	Often the irrigation order will designate a precise amount of solution to be used.
7. Connect the parts of the irrigating solution.	Attach the catheter to the syringe.

Important Steps	Key Points
8. Insert the catheter into the wound.	The depth of insertion will vary, depending on the wound. Therefore, extreme gentleness and care must be taken during insertion. Insert to a depth where you can feel resistance to the catheter. *Do not force* the catheter deeper.
9. Inject solution into the wound.	Do not use too much force because it may cause the patient to have pains. Inject a slow steady stream into the wound.
10. Pinch the catheter closed and remove the syringe.	This will keep solution from draining out of the wound while you are refilling the syringe.
11. Refill the syringe with irrigating solution.	Repeat steps 10 and 11 until the irrigation solution returns clear or the designated amount of solution has been injected.
12. Withdraw the catheter.	Place the catheter and syringe on the tray.
	Turn the patient to a Sims position and allow 3 to 5 minutes for all of the solution to drain out of the wound.
	NOTE: If the solution is left in the wound, it can become a culture media for pathogenic organisms.
13. Dry the patient's skin with cotton balls or gauze.	Set the irrigating basin on the tray for later disposal. (Refer to Unit 1, Aseptic Technique, as necessary.)
14. Apply a sterile dressing.	Remove your gloves. Secure the dressing with tape or bandage as indicated by the location and condition of the patient's skin.
15. Leave the patient safe and comfortable.	Remove the drapes, change soiled linens as necessary, and position the patient for comfort.
	Tell him when the irrigation will be repeated. Empty the drainage basin, measure the amount, if necessary, and observe the contents for recording purposes.
	Return the reusable supplies for reprocessing. Discard disposable equipment and supplies in a designated container. Wash hands.
16. Record procedure.	Charting example:
	8:00 P.M. Wound on inner aspect of left thigh irrigated with 1000 cc hydrogen peroxide. Solution returned clear. Wound edges are a deep pink. Wound is approximately 1/2" deep. Sterile dressing applied.
	M. Hester, R.N.

ITEM 17: WOUND INSTILLATION

Follow the same procedure as above except for Step 9: a small amount (5 to 10 cc) of the prescribed medicated solution is injected into the cavity and allowed to remain so that it can be absorbed. Usually the medication is an antibiotic and it is applied to stop the growth of pathogenic organisms. Steps 10 and 11 are omitted in this procedure.

Instillation of medications into an open wound is used sparingly. However, when it is done, strict aseptic technique must be carried out.

VI. ADDITIONAL INFORMATION FOR ENRICHMENT

SCIENTIFIC PRINCIPLES RELATING TO THE BLADDER

In a state of health, the bladder is resistant to infection. When the body defense is low, as in a state of illness, microorganisms find a favorable location for multiplication in the bladder. The dark, moist, warm climate of the bladder is conducive to growth of certain bacteria. One of the most common organisms affecting the bladder is the colon bacillus known as *Escherichia*. This organism causes cystitis. Irrigations or instillations may be ordered for treatment of certain diseases of the bladder, or following bladder surgery.

Bacteria may be introduced into the bladder by an unsterile catheter or by using unsterile technique. Thus, adherence to strict aseptic technique during bladder irrigation and instillation is *mandatory*.

SCIENTIFIC PRINCIPLES RELATING TO THE EAR

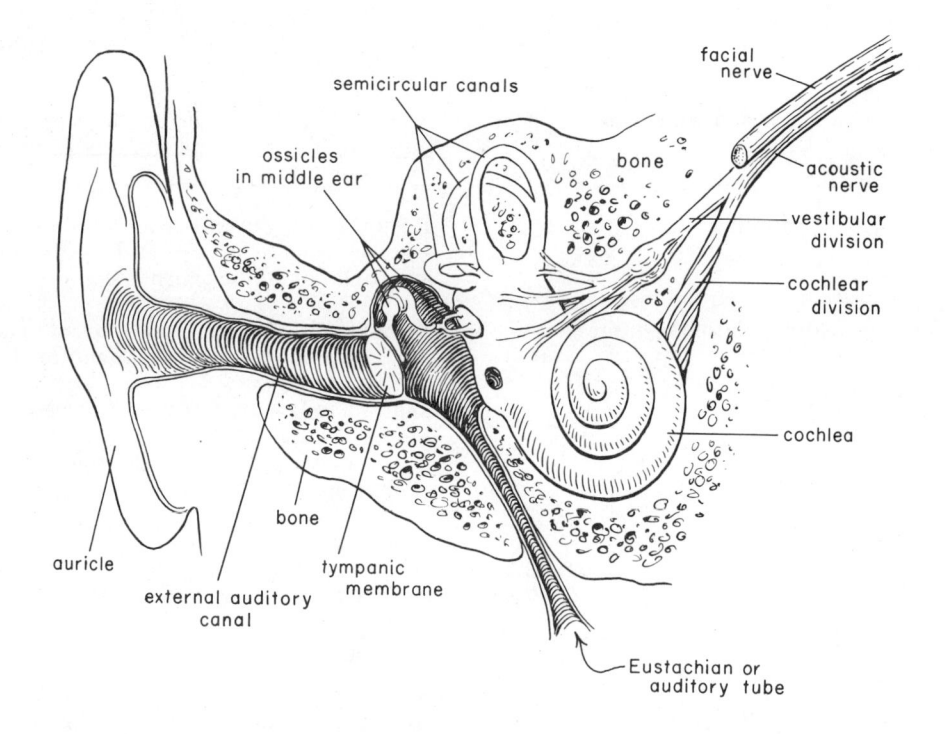

The middle ear is composed of the tympanic membrane (ear drum), the ossicles, and the Eustachian tube. It is located in a hollowed-out portion of the temporal bone of the skull, and is a tiny irregular bony cavity (of a size to hold only 4 to 6 drops of water). It is separated from the external meatus by the membrane and from the inner ear by a very thin bony wall (1/24 inch) in which there are two openings.

In the mastoid wall (posterior portion) there is an opening to the mastoid cells. Because the inner ear is so close to the mastoid, a severe infection in the middle ear can cause a mastoiditis (infection of the mastoid). This condition is especially critical because the infection can easily travel into the brain.

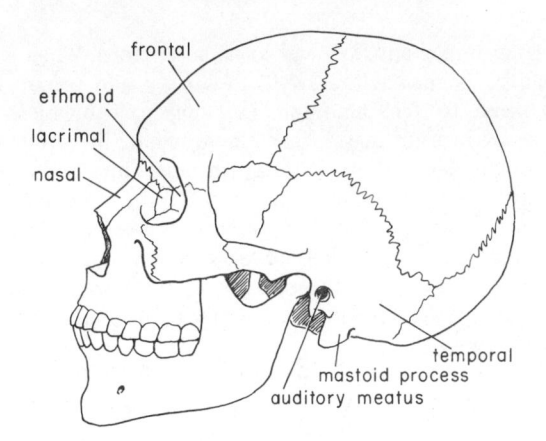

The audiometer is an apparatus that measures hearing acuity for different sound levels and frequencies. The standard unit of measurement of sound is the *decibel*; the frequency of vibrations is called the *pitch*.

The hearing tests are done to measure "threshold of hearing," the lowest intensity of decibels and frequency at which a tone can be heard. An audiometric technician or a physician who is an ear specialist (otologist) performs the test in a quiet room that is specially equipped with devices to measure hearing.

Loss of hearing may be due to auditory nerve impairment, infection of the inner ear, or otosclerosis. Such deafness is remedied by using hearing aids or by performing surgery, depending on the type of hearing deficit.

Infection of the ear can produce disturbing symptoms. Protection from infection and from trauma to the ear are equally important. Nature's protective device is cerumen or ear wax, which serves to shield the ear drum or tympanic membrane from infection.

Normally the cerumen constantly flakes off in small amounts. Sometimes, however, it becomes hardened and requires irrigation to remove it. Boils may form in the external canal and certain molds or fungi find conditions in the middle ear suitable for growth.

The middle ear may become infected (by way of the Eustachian tube) from the nose and throat. Infection may spread to the mastoid area along the continuous mucous membrane extending from the ear. Microorganisms that affect the ear are Treponemata that cause syphilis, the pneumococci that cause pneumonia, and the streptococci from the throat. Complication from the toxins of scarlet fever and other infectious diseases may also affect the ear.

Otitis media, either acute or chronic, is the most common disease of the middle ear. It may be an extension of infection from diseased teeth, tonsils or adenoids. Incorrect nose-blowing could cause viruses of a cold to be forced up the Eustachian tube, possibly resulting in otitis media.

Some ear drops contain an anodyne, a drug that stops pain. Antibiotic powders and various ointments may be instilled in the outer ear to check the growth of fungus infections. Vitamins A and B are used to improve nutritional status in treating conditions of the ear. Streptomycin given in large amounts may cause ringing in the ears.

Alternate condensation and rarefaction of the air produces sound waves. The auricle of the outer ear collects the sound waves and channels them into the auditory canal. This causes the tympanic membrane to vibrate and transfer air to the stapes of the middle ear, and through the inner ear to the auditory nerve. It is thus that hearing takes place, although sounds are also conducted through the bones of the skull.

Temperature changes affect the fluids in the inner ear. Therefore, the temperature of irrigation solutions should be near body temperature. Disturbance of the inner ear fluids in the semicircular canal caused by irrigating fluids that are too hot or too cold can produce dizziness. Pressure of irrigating fluids is controlled by the height of the irrigating container. Pressure should be low so that the tympanic membrane is not injured and therefore *the irrigating can should not be held high.*

Accurate hearing is an important factor in social acceptance. When a person cannot hear unless people talk loudly, he may withdraw from society and refrain from participating. Every person has a need to feel accepted as being part of his social environment. Furthermore, since loss of hearing may affect employment, in certain situations the deaf person may suffer economic deprivation. This in turn causes him to feel even more sensitive, and he may become angry and irritated, and emotional depression could result.

The nurse must make certain that the patient understands what is said to him; "half-truths" may be dangerous. It may be necessary to write messages on a slate to ensure proper understanding. However, some nonverbal communication is possible: a genuine smile communicates acceptance to the patient and buoys up his feelings. Be sensitive to the hearing needs of those around you.

It is essential for the nurse to teach the patient the necessity for immediate treatment of nose and throat infections in order to avoid possible spread of infection to the ear. Earaches should not go unreported; all forms of earache should be studied, to prevent chronic or permanent hearing difficulty.

Sharp or pointed instruments should never be put into the ear by a patient in an attempt "to clean out the ear." Also, there should never be any indiscriminate use of drugs in the ear without a physician's order.

The patient in the home may contact the Visiting Nurse Association or the public health nurse for help with irrigations and instillations that may be ordered. It is impossible, of course, to irrigate one's own ear properly because of the anatomical features of the ear.

Further, it is the duty of the nurse to assist the patient who has a hearing impairment to find his place in the community where he can best realize his social and occupational potential. Referral by the nurse to community agencies helps to direct the patient toward this goal.

SCIENTIFIC PRINCIPLES RELATING TO THE EYE

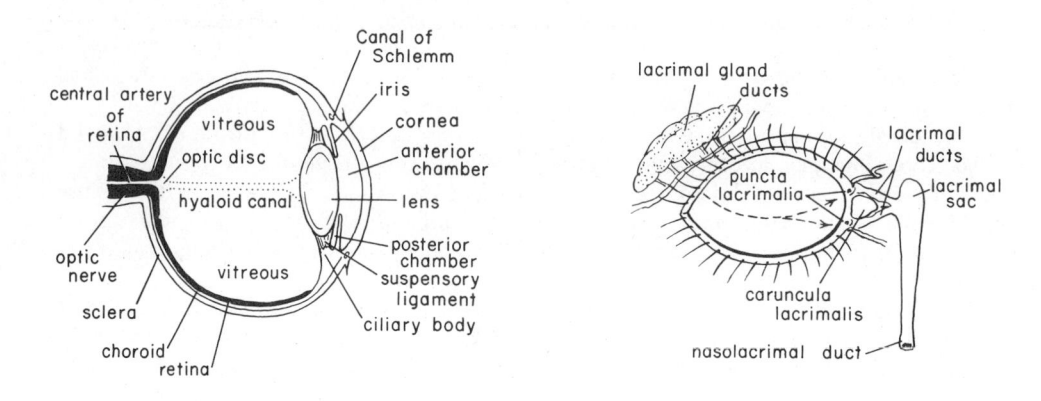

The eye provides sight. Over half of our impressions are gained through the eye; it is referred to as a *special sense organ*. It is well-protected in its orbit by a bony socket with only about one-fifth of it visible. The eye is almost spherical in shape and is approximately one inch in diameter.

It is moved around by six muscles. Loose folds of tissue, called the eyelids, protect it from external injury, drying, and admission of foreign bodies. Eyelashes grow at the edges of the eyelid and further protect the eye from the possible intrusion of foreign objects. A lubricating fluid is secreted from the lacrimal apparatus located at the outer, upper part of the orbit of the eye, and serves to wash out the eye by the process of tearing.

The three coats of the eyeball are covered by a mucous membrane which is continuous with the lacrimal sac, nasolacrimal duct, and the nose. This mucous membrane is called the conjunctiva. A mucous membrane also lines the eyelid.

The eyelids and eyelashes protect the eye from entrance of foreign objects that may carry pathogens such as dust. Tears contain a bactericidal material, called lysozyme, which is protective in nature. Common organisms affecting the eye are the staphylococci (as found in styes), the gonococci (transferred from sex organs), and the Koch-Weeks bacillus (which causes pink eye), among others. Any of these infections is serious inasmuch as the cornea may ulcerate and impair sight. Another danger is the fact that, since the eye is closer to the brain than any other external organ, it is a direct bridge to transfer an eye infection to the brain.

Prevention of transfer of pathogens to the eye includes such measures as:

1. Washing the hands before irrigating the eye.

2. Turning the patient's head to the affected side so that the flow of solution runs toward the outer canthus of the eye, thus avoiding contamination to the other eye.

3. Placing a shield over the eye to protect it from lint or dust.

4. Utilizing only sterile equipment for irrigation.

5. Using clean handkerchiefs or paper tissue, and only clean towels and wash-cloths near the eye.

6. Keeping the fingers away from the eye area.

7. Taking a fresh tissue to wipe each eye.

There are two cavities of the eye. The anterior chamber, which is between the cornea and the lens, is filled with aqueous humor, a clear watery solution. The posterior chamber, located between the iris and the lens, is also filled with aqueous humor.

Behind the lens is the vitreous body, which consists of semiliquid albuminous tissue enclosed in a posterior eye. It helps maintain the shape of the eyeball.

In a condition called *glaucoma* there are intraocular pressure increases that can lead to rigidity of the eyeball, pain, and eventual damage to the visual cells. Glaucoma can usually be kept under control with eye drops, e.g., physostigmine and pilocarpine.

The eyeball is held in place by six external eye muscles. Weakness of one or more of these muscles may lead to a condition called *strabismus* (squinting, cross-eye). It can sometimes be corrected by various muscle-strengthening exercises. As a last resort, a surgical operation can be performed to adjust the pull of each muscle (shortening one or more) so that the eyeball can be recentered.

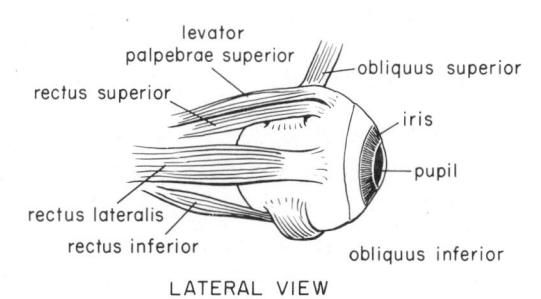

LATERAL VIEW

Normal refraction occurs when the light rays focus clearly on the retina. In order to correct visual problems, the function of the lens of the eye must be corrected (i.e., by eye glasses or contact lenses).

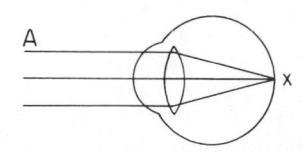

Common refractive conditions are:

- **myopia (nearsightedness)**—the rays of light converge in front of the retina, objects are seen distinctly at very close range, but are indistinctly perceived at a distance. Myopic vision is corrected by the use of a convex lens.

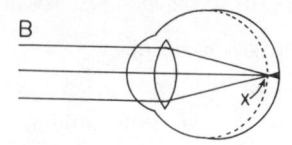

- **hyperopia (hypermetropia, farsightedness)**—the rays of light converge behind the retina. This visual problem can be corrected by using a concave lens.

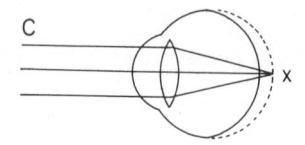

- **presbyopia (old sightedness)**—condition in which the lens begins to lose its elasticity due to aging. This is a physiological process which affects every eye at some point in later life. In this condition, far objects are seen distinctly, while near objects are fuzzy.
- **astigmatism**—the result of an unequal curvature of the refracting surface (cornea or lens). Astigmatism is a common problem, in which images do not properly focus on the retina. It can be congenital or acquired (i.e., due to an injury).
- **accommodation**—the adjustment the eye makes to focus on objects at varying distances.
- **color blindness (daltonism)**—the inability to discriminate colors (chiefly red and green) properly because of the lack of certain pigments in the cone. Nine percent of normal males have some degree of color blindness.
- **binocular vision**—the use of two eyes instead of one. This gives a slight stereo perception and the impression of distance and depth. In order to have binocular vision, normal accommodation and refraction must occur, or at least they can be made normal by use of corrective lenses when there is abnormal accommodation or refraction.
- **floating specks**—small specks of embryonic tissue floating in the vitreous humor. Almost everyone sees floating specks in their eyes: it is usually not an abnormal condition.

Various eye tests may be carried out to check visual acuity:

1. The Snellen test is a chart with letters that vary in size from large to small. It can be administered by a physician or nurse.

2. The lensometer is an instrument used to check the particular lens correction which is prescribed by the ophthalmologist or optometrist. This test may be done by the physician or his assistant.

The pH of normal eyes ranges from 7 to 7.4. This suggests using a neutral irrigation solution. A pH of 9 causes irritation, and a pH of 6.6 to 6.3 causes a feeling of dryness. Boric acid solution is 5 per cent solution, with a pH of approximately 4.2. It produces a slight irritation since it is a weak acid, but it is therapeutic in effect. Boric acid ophthalmic ointment 5 per cent and 10 per cent are used for the eye as well as 5 per cent boric acid solution. Since boric acid preparations have produced some unfavorable effects, they are used less frequently now.

Drugs for the eye are classed as antiseptic, astringent, mydriatic, miotic, and anesthetic. Antibiotic ointments are generally used today, and penicillin ointment is a common antibiotic used to treat eye infections. Common eye antiseptics are Argyrol and silver nitrate solutions. Silver nitrate is put into the eyes of the newborn to prevent gonorrheal ophthalmia, which may lead to blindness.

IRRIGATIONS AND INSTILLATIONS

An example of an eye astringent is zinc sulfate drops used to reduce inflammation. Cortisone is also used to reduce inflammatory conditions of the eye.

Mydriatic drugs e.g., homatropine, are administered to dilate the pupil of the eye for purposes of examination.

Miotic drugs e.g., eserine or physostigmine, reduce the size of the pupil.

An anesthetizing drug may include a derivative of cocaine.

Fluorescein is a stain used as a diagnostic tool to locate lesions and foreign bodies on the cornea.

Vitamins A, B, C, and D all influence eye health. Vitamin A prevents night blindness, Vitamin B affects the condition of the retina (inside coat of the eye) as well as the optic nerve, and Vitamin C affects the metabolism of the normal lens of the eye. Vitamin D is used to increase resistance to infection.

The surface of the eyelid is lubricted by tears, which allow movement of the eyeball without friction. Trachoma, a disease process, causes the conjunctiva to become roughened and the cornea to ulcerate. Friction is increased in trachoma. If the nurse's fingers become moist when she is irrigating the eye, friction that is needed to hold the eyelids open is reduced and the tissue may slip away from her fingers.

Intraocular (within the eyeball) pressure directly affects the eye. It averages between 15 and 25 mm Hg, and it is highest in the morning and lowest in the afternoon. Fluctuation in normal persons is less than 5 mm Hg. However, persons with glaucoma suffer from increased intraocular pressure, and the range is greater. It may vary 25 mm Hg or more. External pressure on the eyeball transmits the same amount of pressure undiminished to the retina or inner coat of the eye. For this reason, the irrigation pressure should be as low as possible and in a steady flow to prevent pain and injury to the eye.

Light glare is tiring to the eyes. Light is measured in foot-candles; one foot-candle is the amount of light cast by 100 candles at 10 feet. This is the minimum recommended for reading. Close, delicate work requires from 10 to 20 foot-candles of light, but more than 20 foot-candles produces fatigue because the pupil constricts to reduce the amount of light entering the eye. (The pupil becomes smaller as more light is admitted.) For general eye work 2 to 5 foot-candles is recommended so that the eye will not have to make continual light adjustments. Other factors contributing to eye fatigue include the size of the print, object, or its color; and the position of the eyes while working.

Visual defects affect the emotional, occupational, and social life of a person. Vision is required for assessment and awareness of the environment. It is an asset in interaction with the environment. Alteration of the person's perception and interaction in the environment may cause serious problems in:

Role change—disengagement or retirement from a given work.

Social isolation—separation from normal social functions. This, together with loss of flexibility, is a prelude to depression.

Sensory deprivation—caused by a restriction of visual sensory input or stimulus and often producing anxiety.

The patient's reaction to anxiety and worry about his eye condition may cause him to be impatient, demanding, depressed, or withdrawn. He may feel helpless and insecure. (Man's desire to be normal and unhandicapped is intense and deep-rooted.) The situation requires great understanding on the part of the nurse and making adjustments in the treatment approach (to allay the patient's fears). The nurse should know about appropriate community agencies if a person does lose his eyesight so that she can refer him to the proper agency, e.g., the Office of Vocational Rehabilitation, American Foundation for the Blind, or Braille Institute of America. A local chapter of the National Society for the Prevention of Blindness may also provide guidance for the patient.

Teaching eye health includes the rules for good lighting, raising the backrest when reading in bed, and proper sitting posture when doing any close work. Protection from infection includes keeping dirty fingers, soiled linens and equipment away from the eyes. Thus, washing the hands and using clean linen or tissues near the eyes by both the patient and the nurse serve to prevent eye infections. The patient should be warned to avoid using home remedies to treat his eyes and encouraged to consult an ophthalmologist when an eye problem exists. Periodic examinations for sight and intraocular tension are a "must" to keep the eyes healthy and to properly treat any eye diseases or conditions.

SCIENTIFIC PRINCIPLES RELATING TO THE THROAT

The throat, or pharynx, is a tube about five inches long extending from the base of the skull to the esophagus. It lies in front of the cervical (neck) vertebrae. The throat has three parts: (1) nasopharynx, located behind the nose, (2) oropharynx, behind the mouth, and (3) larynogopharynx, behind the larynx or voice box.

The throat serves as a hallway for both the respiratory and digestive tracts. It communicates with both the nose and mouth. The adenoids are located in the pharynx, and the tonsils are located in the oral cavity.

Common throat infections include: staphylococcus, streptococcus, meningococcus, and the influenza virus. An intact mucous membrane provides protection against them. A flushing action by the saliva in the mouth and the swallowing action carries bacteria into the stomach where they are rendered harmless by the hydrochloric acid. Frequent oral hygiene also provides protection against the growth of microorganisms.

Certain communicable diseases (such as scarlet fever, diphtheria, pneumonia, tuberculosis, meningitis, septic sore throat and the common cold) begin in the nose and throat. Continuity of mucous membranes throughout the respiratory tract allows for extension of the infection from the throat to the ears and eyes and vice versa. Extension of infection via the olfactory or optic nerves to the brain presents a critical care problem. Thus, careful handling of throat and nose discharges is extremely important in preventing the spread of germs.

Sodium chloride, sodium bicarbonate and boric acid solutions are frequently used for throat irrigations or gargles. Painting or swabbing the throat may be done with iodine, silver nitrate, Mercurochrome, or tincture of benzoin. Ephedrine may be included in medications to constrict the congested mucosa and thus aid in breathing.

Various types of antibiotics are ordered for generalized infections that begin in the nose and throat. Analgesics may be given for pain and antipyretics are given to reduce fever.

Irrigation of the throat can be given at a higher pressure than for other special sense organs. (The height of the irrigation container controls the pressure.) A height as high as 24 inches is acceptable for the throat irrigation. The temperature may be 100°F (37°C).

A patient suffering from a nose and throat infection is very uncomfortable and may not remember how communicable his infection is; therefore remind him to cover his nose and mouth while coughing or sneezing.

For additional information, ask your instructor for further resources.

IRRIGATIONS AND INSTILLATIONS

POST-TEST

Some of the statements are true and some are false. If the statement is true, circle the T preceding the item and do no more. If the statement is false, circle the F and do two things:
1. Underline the word or words that make it false.
2. Write in the blank the word or words that would make it true.

URINARY

T F   1. Two types of syringes most often used in irrigations are the Asepto syringe and the Toomey syringe. _____

T F   2. The Toomey syringe is generally used by the nurse to remove blood clots from the bladder. _____

T F   3. The usual amount of irrigating fluid used to irrigate a catheter in the bladder is 50 to 60 cc. _____

T F   4. The usual amount of fluid to irrigate a ureterostomy or nephrostomy tube is 50 to 60 cc. _____

T F   5. The purpose of the irrigation of the urinary tract will influence the amount of irrigation solution used. _____

T F   6. If a piston-type syringe is used to irrigate the bladder, the best way to introduce fluid to prevent undue pressure of water flow is by rotating the plunger slightly. _____

T F   7. When irrigating the bladder, no more than 60 cc should be put in at one time. _____

T F   8. When instilling fluid into the bladder of a patient who has no indwelling catheter, one way to prevent it from slipping out is to tape it to the patient's leg. _____

T F   9. To prevent separation of the catheter end from the tip of the irrigating syringe, they should be taped together. _____

EAR

T F 10. To irrigate the ear canal, the adult auricle is pulled down and back. _Upward & Backward_

T F 11. To irrigate the ear canal of a child, pull the auricle up and back to provide a straight external ear canal. _Down & Back_

T F 12. The safest irrigator for the ear is the bulb-type syringe. _T_

IRRIGATIONS AND INSTILLATIONS

T F 13. The safest irrigator for the ear is the Pomeroy syringe. _Rubber Bulb_

EYE

T F 14. To open the eyelids, the pressure should be on the lids themselves. _False_

T F 15. Cleansing strokes around the eye should be from the inner canthus out. _True_

T F 16. If infection is present, use separate equipment for each eye. _True_

T F 17. Solutions or medications for the eye should be directed toward the upper conjunctiva and not on the corneal surface. _False - Lower fornix_

T F 18. Ointment from a tube is placed in a line along the lower lid and broken off by a twisting motion of the hand with the tube when the proper amount is administered. _True_

POST-TEST ANNOTATED ANSWER SHEET

URINARY

1. F (p. 159), Ellick
2. F (p. 159), Physician
3. T (p. 162)
4. F (p. 169 (2-5 cc.)
5. T (p. 161)
6. T (p. 163)
7. F (p. 168) (75-100 cc.)
8. T (p. 165)
9. F (p. 165)

EAR

10. F (p. 172) upward & backward
11. F (p. 174) down and back
12. T (p. 172)
13. F (p. 172) Rubber bulb

EYE

14. F (p. 179)
15. T (p. 179)
16. T (p. 180)
17. F (p. 180) lower fornix
18. T (p. 181)

IRRIGATIONS AND INSTILLATIONS

PERFORMANCE TEST

In the practice laboratory, with a partner, you will demonstrate the correct procedure for five of the following procedures:

Bladder irrigation.

Bladder instillation.

Through and through bladder irrigation.

Pyelostomy or nephrostomy irrigation.

Eye irrigation.

Eye instillation.

Ear irrigation.

Ear instillation.

Nasal irrigation.

Nasal instillation.

Throat irrigation.

Wound irrigation.

PERFORMANCE CHECKLIST

BLADDER IRRIGATION WITH CATHETER IN PLACE

1. Obtain equipment.
2. Wash hands.
3. Approach and identify the patient and explain procedure.
4. Prepare the patient (privacy, table at working height, position, and drape).
5. Prepare irrigation equipment.
6. Disconnect drainage tube from catheter.
7. Insert irrigating syringe into catheter.
8. Cover the end of the drainage tube to prevent contamination.
9. Fill syringe with correct amount of irrigating solution.
10. Reinsert syringe into catheter.
11. Introduce irrigation fluid.
12. Remove syringe.
13. Instill prescribed amount of medication (optional).
14. Remove syringe.
15. Reattach drainage tube (*Done only if medication was not instilled*).
16. Provide for patient's safety and comfort.
17. Record procedure.

BLADDER INSTILLATION OF MEDICATION IN THE ABSENCE OF AN INDWELLING CATHETER

1. Collect equipment.
2. Wash hands.
3. Approach and identify patient and prepare patient physically and emotionally.
4. Insert catheter into bladder.
5. Secure catheter.
6. Insert syringe or funnel into distal end of catheter.
7. Pour medication into syringe or funnel. Reassure patient during procedure.
8. Set pouring container aside.
9. Introduce all of solution into bladder.
10. Remove catheter.
11. Provide for safety and comfort of patient.
12. Remove equipment and return supplies.
13. Report and record action.

THROUGH AND THROUGH BLADDER IRRIGATION

1. Obtain equipment.
2. Wash hands.
3. Approach and identify the patient, and explain the procedure.
4. Prepare the patient.
5. Prepare the equipment.
6. Pour the solution.
7. Loosen clamp on solution tubing.
8. Tighten clamp on solution tubing.
9. Loosen clamp on drainage tubing.
10. Repeat steps 6 to 8 until solution returns clear.
11. Provide for patient safety and comfort.
12. Report and record procedure.

IRRIGATION OF THE KIDNEY PELVIS

1. Obtain sterile equipment.
2. Wash hands.
3. Approach and identify the patient, and explain the procedure.
4. Prepare the patient.
5. Prepare the equipment.
6. Attach filled syringe.

7. Introduce solution. Continue to observe the patient throughout the treatment.

8. Withdraw solution.

9. Remove syringe and supplies.

10. Leave the patient comfortable and safe.

11. Report and record procedure.

EAR IRRIGATION

1. Obtain equipment.
2. Wash hands.
3. Approach and identify the patient, and explain the procedure.
4. Prepare the patient.
5. Prepare the equipment.
6. Have patient hold drainage basin under his ear.
7. Straighten the auditory canal (adult, child).
8. Tilt patient's head forward.
9. Insert syringe tip. Tip directed upward and posteriorly.
10. Inject solution into ear canal without injury or pain.
11. Remove syringe, refill, and inject until solution returns clear.
12. Remove syringe and set aside. Inspect ear.
13. Leave patient safe and comfortable.
14. Remove supplies and equipment.
15. Report and record procedure.

EAR INSTILLATION

1. Wash hands.
2. Withdraw medication into medicine dropper.
3. Insert tip of medicine dropper into ear canal.
4. Inject medication.
5. Withdraw medicine dropper.
6. Plug external meatus with cotton.
7. Leave patient comfortable and safe. Return medicine dropper to medicine bottle.
8. Record the treatment.

EYE IRRIGATION

1. Obtain sterile equipment.
2. Wash hands.
3. Approach and identify the patient, and explain procedure.
4. Prepare the patient.

5. Prepare the equipment.
6. Cleanse eyelid.
7. Fill syringe with solution.
8. Secure eyelid.
9. Inject solution.
10. Remove syringe.
11. Leave patient safe and comfortable.
12. Remove supplies and equipment.
13. Record the treatment.

INSTILLATION OF EYE DROPS

1. Assemble supplies.
2. Wash hands.
3. Approach and identify the patient, and explain the procedure.
4. Prepare the patient.
5. Introduce medication into lower fornix.
6. Gently close eyelid.
7. Gently dry eyelid.
8. Leave patient safe and comfortable.
9. Report and record procedure.

NASAL IRRIGATION

1. Assemble equipment.
2. Wash hands.
3. Approach and identify the patient, and explain the procedure.
4. Prepare the patient.
5. Insert nozzle into nostril.
6. Remove nozzle and reinsert it into other nostril.
7. Clamp tubing and remove nozzle.
8. Leave patient safe and comfortable.
9. Record the treatment.

NASAL INSTILLATION

1. Obtain equipment.
2. Wash hands.
3. Approach and identify the patient, and explain the procedure.
4. Prepare the patient.

5. Prepare the medication.
6. Inject the nose drops, directing the medicine dropper toward the middle of superior concha.
7. Withdraw medicine dropper.
8. Leave patient safe and comfortable.
9. Record the treatment.

THROAT IRRIGATION

1. Assemble the equipment.
2. Wash hands.
3. Approach and identify the patient, and explain the procedure.
4. Prepare the patient.
5. Insert nozzle or catheter into patient's mouth.
6. Interrupt irrigation p.r.n. to let the patient breathe.
7. Remove irrigator tip.
8. Leave patient safe and comfortable.
9. Record treatment.

WOUND IRRIGATION

1. Assemble equipment.
2. Wash hands.
3. Approach and identify the patient, and explain the procedure.
4. Prepare the patient.
5. Put on sterile gloves.
6. Connect irrigating equipment.
7. Fill irrigating syringe with solution.
8. Insert catheter into wound without injury.
9. Inject solution into wound without injury.
10. Pinch catheter closed as syringe is removed.
11. Refill syringe and repeat irrigation until desired results occur.
12. Withdraw catheter and turn patient so that the wound can drain freely.
13. Dry skin and apply sterile dressing.
14. Leave patient safe and comfortable.
15. Record the treatment.

Unit 5

URINARY CATHETERIZATION

I. DIRECTIONS TO THE STUDENT

Proceed through this lesson. When you have finished, take the Post-test. After practice in the skills laboratory, make an appointment with your instructor to demonstrate the procedures as soon as you are comfortable with them and feel that you can pass the Performance Test. The Performance Checklist is included for use as a study guide while preparing for your Performance Test.

II. GENERAL PERFORMANCE OBJECTIVE

When you have completed this unit, you will be able to catheterize a patient correctly, obtain a sterile urine specimen, and insert a retention catheter.

III. SPECIFIC PERFORMANCE OBJECTIVES

Following this lesson you will be able to:

1. Describe the indications for the insertion of a retention catheter.
2. Safely and correctly, using aseptic technique, catheterize a patient or a simulated model.
3. Distinguish between retention and suppression of urine and explain the difference.
4. Correctly identify common urinary catheters (e.g., French, Foley), and describe their use.

IV. VOCABULARY

Read the definitions of the terms listed below. Do not attempt to memorize these definitions before proceeding with the lesson. Each term will be explained or defined again in the text. On completion of the lesson, however, you should know the correct definitions of these terms.

abdominal-perineal resection—a surgical procedure to remove a malignancy of the lower bowel; the rectum is excised (removed), the anus is closed, and a colostomy is performed. (Since there are two parts to the procedure, abdominal and perineal, the procedure is called an abdominal-perineal resection.)
aqueous—watery, made with water.
catheter—a tube (plastic, rubber, or metal, glass) used to remove fluid from a cavity, e.g., urinary catheter, cardiac catheter.
catheter guide (stylet)—a slender plug of metal inserted into the lumen of the catheter for stiffening or clearing.
chemotherapy—treatment with a chemical agent, e.g., drugs.
cystoscopy—insertion of a surgical instrument (cystoscope) into the urinary bladder to inspect the wall, irrigate the bladder, or instill a medication.
diuresis—condition characterized by an increased production of urine, as from the use of certain drugs (diuretics) or in certain diseases, e.g., diabetes insipidus.

drape (surgical)—the sterile protective covering used to maintain aseptic technique during a surgical operation or sterile procedure, e.g., catheterization.
dysuria—painful urination.
enuresis—involuntary evacuation of the bladder after the age of 3; enuresis may indicate faulty toilet training or some pathology of the bladder.
fenestrated drape—window-like opening in the center of a sterile drape through which a surgical or sterile procedure can be performed.
Foley catheter—a special catheter frequently used for retention. It has a double lumen; one permits the free flow of urine from the bladder to the drainage tubing. The other lumen is a closed-tube system. When water or air is inserted into the balloon portion surrounding the distal end of the catheter, the lumen serves as an anchor to prevent withdrawal of the catheter from the bladder.
foreskin (prepuce)—loose skin covering the tip end of the penis.
French catheter—a common straight tube used for evacuation or injection of fluid, when the catheter is not retained in the bladder.
frequency—the need to urinate often.
micturition (voiding, urination)—the voluntary act of expelling urine.
nephritis (*nephr* = kidney, *—itis* = inflammation)—inflammation of the kidney caused by bacteria or their toxins, malnutrition, streptococcal infections, etc.
obstetrics—scientific management of a woman during pregnancy, delivery and puerperium.
puerperium—period immediately following childbirth until the uterus (womb) returns to normal size (about 3 to 6 weeks).
pyelonephritis—inflammation of the portion of the kidney tissue called the pelvis, caused by bacteria, malignancy, penetrating wound of the kidney, etc.
sphincter—circular muscle constricting an opening or orifice; e.g., the bladder sphincter is the muscle at the urethral opening of the bladder.
suppression—failure of the kidneys to excrete urine in certain diseases or conditions, e.g., glomerulonephritis, traumatic loss of kidney, kidney stones.
retention—failure to expel urine from the bladder, i.e., from a urethral stricture, or swelling of the urethra following difficult childbirth, or genitourinary surgery.
urgency—the immediate need to urinate.
vaginal repair—surgical procedure to repair or reconstruct the vaginal canal.

V. KNOWLEDGE BASIC TO THIS LESSON

The urinary bladder is a sterile cavity; aseptic technique must therefore be used to avoid introducing pathogenic organisms into the bladder. Pathogenic organisms which are introduced into the bladder can ascend the ureters to the kidney and cause serious kidney disease (e.g., pyelonephritis). Organisms commonly found in bladder infections are: members of the genera *Serratia, Klebsiella, Aerobacter, Proteus,* and *Pseudomonas; Staphylococcus aureus;* and *Escherichia coli.*

Catheterization of the urinary bladder is a sterile procedure done at the specific request or order of the physician after general nursing measures to assist in urination have failed, (e.g., warm external douche, hot sitz bath, hearing running water).

Catheterization may be done for any of the following reasons:

1. to obtain a sterile urine specimen.

2. to relieve a distended bladder in the patient who is unable to void.

3. to measure the amount of residual urine in the bladder.

4. to provide for drainage, irrigation, or instillation of a chemotherapeutic solution by insertion of a retention catheter into the bladder.

5. to prepare a patient for a surgical procedure or obstetrical delivery (childbirth).

6. to assist the incontinent patient in a bladder training program.

7. to maintain cleanliness and dryness of the genitalia following obstetrical or surgical procedures, e.g., difficult delivery of an infant, vaginal repair, abdominal-perineal resection, etc.

8. to dilate urethral strictures.

9. to splint the urethra following surgery on the urethra.

Review the section "Additional Information for Enrichment" in Volume 2, Unit 21, "Urine Elimination" for additional background information.

ITEM 1: FEMALE CATHETERIZATION

Sizes of catheters generally used for females vary from 10 French to 14 French, although catheter sizes may range from 8 French to 18 French, depending on the size of the urethra. The sizes come in increments of 2, e.g., 8, 10, 12, 14, etc. Recommended catheters for routine female catheterization are: 14–16 French, olive-tip coudé (Tieman) or a Tieman-Foley.

Important Steps	Key Points
1. Wash your hands.	
2. Obtain and assemble equipment.	Sterile disposable catheter sets are in general use. The tray will include: a French catheter, antiseptic solution, cotton balls or pledgets for cleansing, lubricant, specimen bottle with cap and label, receptacle for waste urine, drapes, forceps, and sterile gloves.
3. Approach and identify the patient and explain the procedure.	This procedure may cause some embarrassment or anxiety for the patient; therefore, carefully explain the procedure, e.g., "The doctor has requested a special urine test. The urine specimen will be obtained by inserting a small tube into the bladder to remove the urine." Assure the patient that she will not feel pain, but she will feel pressure as the catheter is inserted. Provide for the patient's privacy by drawing the curtains around the bed and closing the hall door.

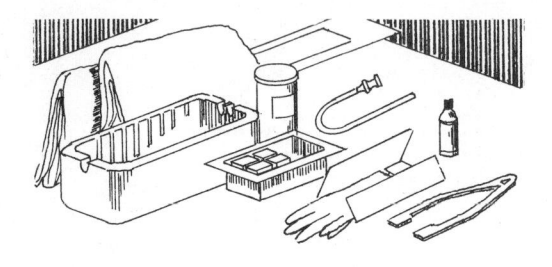

URINARY CATHETERIZATION

Important Steps	Key Points
4. Position and drape the patient.	Raise the bed to working height to avoid back strain while you are working. Lower the siderail on the side where you are working. Move the patient to the proximal side of the bed. Put the bath blanket on the patient and fanfold the top bedding to the foot of the bed. The bath blanket will provide warmth and protect the patient's modesty. Call for assistance if needed, e.g., if the patient is unconscious and cannot hold her legs in position during the procedure. With the patient in the dorsal recumbent position, knees flexed, feet flat on the bed, drape as for a vaginal exam. Position the treatment light (wall-mounted or portable) for best focus on the genital area. Place the light so that there is space for you to work comfortably.
5. Prepare the catheter tray.	Open the catheter tray and place it on the bed between the patient's legs, near (8 to 12 inches) the perineum. Remember the sterile technique; with your *clean* hands open the tray as you grasp the outside of the wrapper. Open the package of sterile gloves.
6. Put on sterile gloves.	Refer to Unit 1, Aseptic Technique.
7. Prepare the work area.	Slip the sterile drape under the patient's buttocks. Cuff the drape to cover your gloved hands to avoid contaminating the gloves while you are placing the drape under the buttocks. Apply another sterile drape over the pubis, with the proximal edge at the top of the labia. (Some sets may have a fenestrated vaginal drape; in this case the opening should be placed over the genital area, exposing the labia.) NOTE: These drapes are made of a waterproof material. The shiny part of the drape should be away from you; the dull, absorbent layer should be next to the patient. Continue to reassure your patient. Explain each step, moving slowly, gently, and firmly. Pour antiseptic solution over cotton balls. Open the package of lubricant and put some on a cotton ball. Place the sterile specimen bottle on the side of the tray, making sure that the cap is removed.

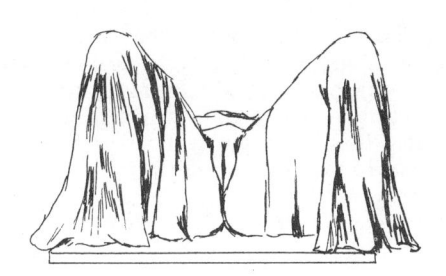

UNIT 5

Important Steps	Key Points
8. Separate the labia, exposing the meatus.	With your left forefinger and thumb, separate the labia minora (reverse hand positions if you are left-handed). A clear view of the meatus is important for ease of insertion of the catheter.

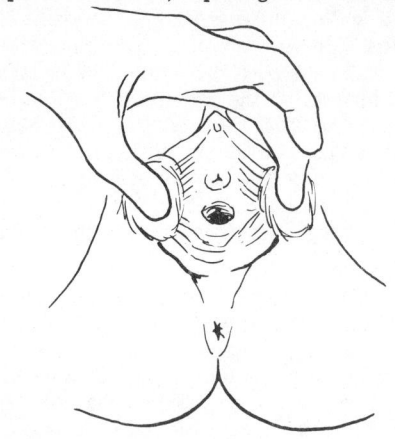

REMEMBER: The left hand is now contaminated and will not be used again to handle sterile objects. You will be using only your right hand or the forceps to handle the sterile objects. The left hand will be used only to continue to expose the meatus. |
| 9. Cleanse the genital area. | With your right forefinger and thumb, pick up an antiseptic cotton ball (or pledget) and with a firm single downward stroke, cleanse the far side of the labia from the pubis to the anus. Discard the ball in the waste container. With the second ball, cleanse the near side of the labia with a single downward stroke. Discard the cotton ball. With the third cotton ball, make a firm single downward stroke in the center of the labia directly over the urinary meatus. Discard the cotton ball. |
| 10. Pick up the catheter with forceps about 3 inches from the distal tip. | Place the distal end of the catheter (the wide end without the eye) in the urine receptacle. By using the forceps, you avoid touching the tip of the catheter, which will be inserted into the bladder. This is an additional precaution to prevent possible introduction of organisms into the bladder.

Apply antiseptic lubricant freely to the proximal tip of the catheter. A water-soluble (aqueous) lubricant is used, which is easily washed away with the urine. |
| 11. Identify the urinary meatus and *gently* insert the catheter. | Insert the catheter about 2 inches, or until the urine flows. The female urethra is about 2 inches long; it lies posteriorly and then moves upward in a slight anterior direction toward the bladder. Therefore, insert the catheter carefully, following the direction of the urethra. You may feel a slight resistance as the catheter passes the internal urethral sphincter. The sphincter will relax if you have the patient exhale. If the urine does not flow, the eye of the catheter may be lodged against the wall of the bladder; gently rotate the catheter between your thumb and forefinger, and carefully insert it another inch further.

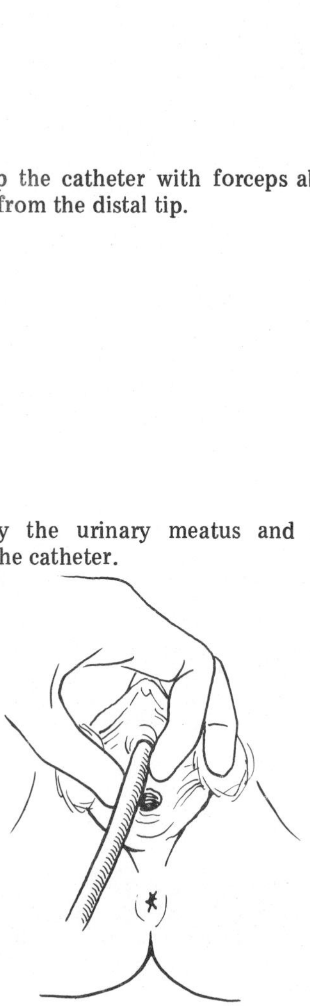

Do not contaminate the catheter during the insertion; if the catheter is contaminated, discard it and rescrub. Begin the procedure again. |

URINARY CATHETERIZATION

Important Steps	Key Points
	CAUTION: Although the patient may be charged for all equipment, you should not risk a bladder infection by using contaminated supplies. You will be the only one to know that you are using contaminated equipment—so follow your conscience. Use only sterile supplies!
	Hold the catheter in place with your left hand while the urine is flowing. You may gently rest your hand on the pubis for support.
	If force is needed to insert the catheter, remove the catheter and call for assistance.
12. Obtain a specimen. (Omit this step if a specimen is not needed.)	After the urine has flowed for a few seconds, pinch the tubing between your forefinger and thumb to stop the urine flow and prevent soiling of the drapes as you transfer the distal end of the catheter from the waste receptacle to the specimen bottle. Lift up the distal end of the catheter with your right hand and transfer it to the specimen bottle.
	Release the catheter and allow at least 30 cc (1 ounce) to flow into the specimen bottle. Again pinch the catheter off to stop flow, and transfer the distal end of the catheter back into the waste receptacle.
13. Complete urine removal.	No more than 1000 cc should be removed at one time. Obtaining more may collapse the bladder wall and cause the patient to go into shock. (Follow your agency procedure on the amount of urine that can be removed at one time.)
14. Remove the catheter.	While slightly rotating the catheter, take it out slowly and gently, removing any residual urine in the neck of the bladder. Place the used catheter on the tray. Dry the genital area and buttocks with a towel or cotton balls. Remove your gloves.
15. Remove the tray and make the patient comfortable.	Place the tray on the chair beside the bed. Replace the bed covers and remove the bath blanket. Return the bath blanket to storage (in the bedside stand, patient's closet, or in a soiled-linen hamper). If the linens were soiled during the procedure, be sure that you change the linen so that the patient is now clean and dry. Position the bed for the patient's comfort. Adjust the siderails, call light, and bedside stand for her convenience. Ask if she needs anything else. Tell her when you will return.

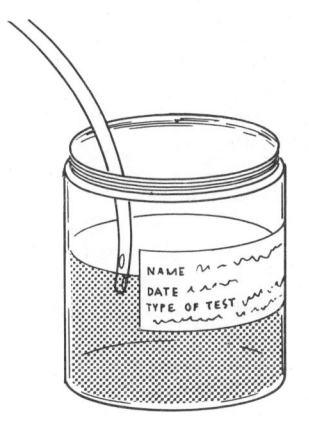

Important Steps	Key Points
16. Remove supplies from the room.	Empty the urine receptacle, noting the amount, color, and odor for later recording. The disposable receptacle is usually calibrated for ease in measuring. If it is not calibrated, use a graduate pitcher (usually kept in the patient's bathroom) to measure the contents. Discard used items in a designated container. Return unused items to storage.
17. Label the specimen.	Prepare a laboratory requisition, or accompany the specimen with a copy of the physician's orders (follow agency procedure). Label the specimen to correspond with the physician's order (see Volume 2, Unit 21, "Urine Elimination"). Make sure that the specimen is sent promptly to the laboratory for processing.
18. Record on chart.	Promptly enter information as to time, amount, color, actual procedure, whether specimen was collected, etc.

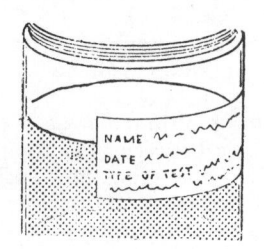

Charting example:

10:30 A.M. Catheterized for sterile urine specimen. 900 cc clear straw-colored specimen obtained. Sent with requisition to laboratory for culture.

J. Mishymoto, S.N.

ITEM 2: MALE CATHETERIZATION

Catheterization in the male is usually performed by the orderly, male nurse, or the physician. It may become necessary, however, for the female nurse to carry out the procedure. Recommended catheters for routine male catheterization are: 14-16 (French) olive-tip coudé (Tieman) or a Tieman-Foley.

Important Steps	Key Points
1. Wash your hands.	
2. Obtain and assemble equipment.	Sterile disposable catheter sets are in general use. The tray will include: a French catheter, antiseptic solution, cotton balls or pledgets for cleansing, lubricant, specimen bottle with cap and label, receptacle for waste urine, forceps, drapes, and sterile gloves.
3. Approach and identify the patient and explain the procedure.	This procedure may cause some embarrassment or anxiety for the patient; therefore, carefully describe the procedure. Assure him that he will not feel pain, but that he will feel the pressure of the catheter as it is inserted. Provide for privacy by drawing the curtains around the bed and closing the door.

URINARY CATHETERIZATION 213

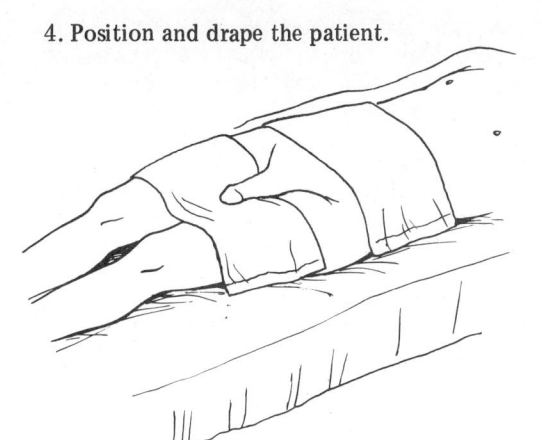

Important Steps	Key Points
4. Position and drape the patient.	Raise the bed to working height to avoid back strain. Lower the siderail on the side where you are working. Move the patient to the proximal side of the bed. Apply a bath blanket over the patient's chest and abdomen and fanfold the top bedding to his midthigh. The bath blanket will provide warmth and protect the patient's modesty. Call for assistance if needed; e.g., if the patient is unconscious and cannot hold his legs in position during the procedure. With the patient in the dorsal recumbent position, abduct his legs slightly and flex his knees. Place the treatment light for best focus on the genital area and allow yourself an adequate working area.
5. Prepare the catheter tray.	Open the catheter tray and place it on the bed at the patient's proximal hip. Refer to the unit on sterile technique for opening sterile packages. Remember to open the tray by grasping the outside of the wrapper with clean hands.
6. Put on sterile gloves.	Refer to Unit 1, "Aseptic Technique."
7. Prepare the work area.	Place water-resistant, sterile drape (shiny side away from you) under the patient's penis, over the bedclothes. Place a second towel (or drape) over the bath blanket just above the penis. The second drape may be fenestrated; in this case, the opening should be directly over the penis. Place the specimen bottle at one side of the tray (may be used later if you are obtaining a sterile urine specimen). Continue to reassure the patient, explaining each step.

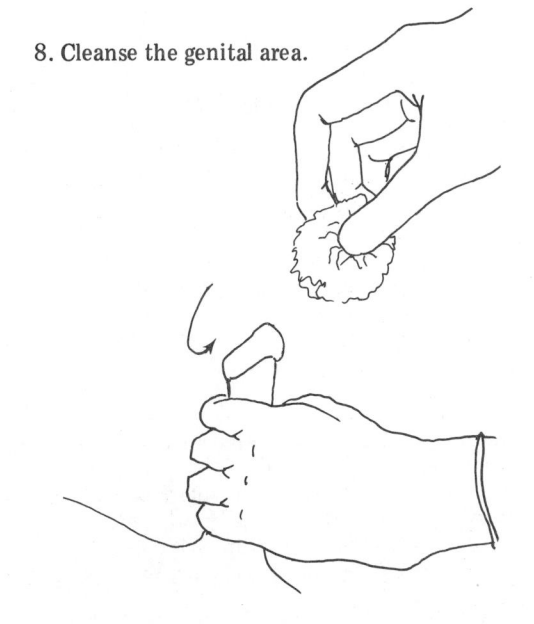

Pour antiseptic solution over cotton balls. Open the antiseptic lubricant package and express lubricant on a cotton ball. |
| 8. Cleanse the genital area. | With your left hand immediately behind the glans, gently but firmly grasp the penis between your third and fourth fingers. Spread the urinary meatus between the thumb and forefinger. (If you handle the penis too lightly, you may stimulate an erection; therefore, a firm pressure is indicated.) With your right hand (reverse hand positions if you are left-handed), pick up an antiseptic saturated cotton ball and cleanse the glans. Clean in a circular motion, moving toward the tip of the penis. Discard the cotton ball in the waste container. Pick up a second cotton ball and cleanse firmly but gently over the meatus. Discard the cotton ball in the waste container. |

Important Steps	Key Points
9. Pick up the catheter with forceps at least 4 inches from the tip.	Lubricate the catheter tip generously with a water-soluble lubricant. Use the forceps or your index finger and thumb, and avoid touching the tip end of the catheter.
10. Insert catheter.	Holding the penis in your left hand, draw it forward and upward (at 60° to 90° angle toward the legs), stretching it slightly. This action will straighten the urethra and make it easier to insert the catheter. Ask the patient to try to void; this relaxes the urethral sphincters. Insert the catheter slowly and gently about 7 inches. NOTE: A slight resistance may be felt as the catheter passes the internal urethral spincter; use a gentle constant pressure. Forceful pressure on the catheter at this point can cause a spasm of the spincter and make it impossible to insert the catheter. CAUTION: If you encounter resistance in the insertion, or if the catheter is not rigid enough, stop the procedure and call for the physician. There are often obstructions or strictures that may require special handling. *Under no circumstance use force to insert the catheter.* Hold the catheter with the left hand while collecting the urine. For support, you may rest your hand lightly on the patient's pubis.
11. Collect a specimen.	Follow Step 12 of the previous procedure if a specimen is needed.
12. Complete urine removal.	Withdraw no more than 1000 cc. Rapid withdrawal of urine may collapse the walls of the bladder and cause the patient to go into shock. Follow your agency procedure concerning the amount of urine that may be withdrawn at any one time.
13. Remove the catheter.	Take it out slowly and gently, slightly rotating it so that any residual urine left in the neck of the bladder will be removed. Place the used catheter on the tray. Dry and cleanse the genital area with a towel or cotton balls. Remove your gloves.
14. Remove the tray and make the patient comfortable.	Place the tray on a chair beside the bed. Replace the bed covers, remove the bath blanket and return it to storage (in the bedside stand or patient's closet). Discard the soiled blanket in the linen hamper or chute. Position the bed for the patient's comfort. If the linens were soiled during the procedure, be sure you change them so that the patient is clean and dry. Adjust the siderails, call light, and bedside stand for his convenience. Leave him comfortable, ask if there is anything else you can do, and tell him when you will return.

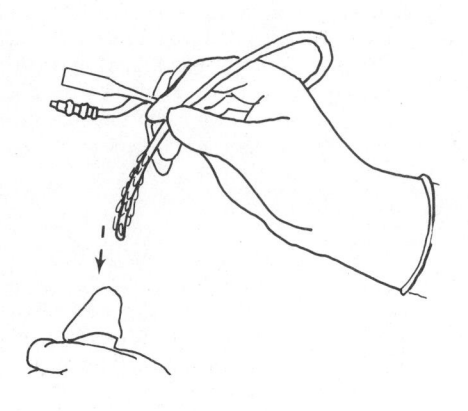

Important Steps	Key Points
15. Remove supplies from the room.	Empty the urine receptacle, noting the amount, color, and odor for later recording. The disposable waste receptacle on the catheter tray is usually calibrated for easy measuring. If it is not calibrated, use the graduate measure that is usually kept in the patient's bathroom. Discard used items in the designated container. Return unused items to storage.
16. Label the specimen.	Mark the specimen to correspond with physician's orders (see "Urine Elimination," Volume 2, Unit 21, for specifics). Prepare a laboratory requisition, or accompany the specimen with a copy of the physician's order (follow agency procedure). See that the specimen is sent promptly to the laboratory for accurate processing.
17. Record on the patient's chart.	Promptly note the procedure, enter information regarding the time, amount, color, actual procedure, by whom, etc.

Charting example:

2:30 P.M. Catheterized for sterile urine specimen. 650 cc slightly red cloudy urine obtained. No unusual odor noted. Sent to laboratory with requisition.

J. Nunn, Orderly

ITEM 3: INSERTION OF A RETENTION CATHETER

The most commonly used retention catheter is called the Foley catheter. It is sized like the French catheter (8 French to 30 French). In addition to the catheter size, the size of the balloon is also indicated on the distal end of the catheter, e.g., 14 Foley, 5 cc. The size of the balloon is dependent on the volume of water or air the balloon can hold. Common balloon sizes are 5 cc, 10 cc, and 30 cc. Other types of retention catheters are discussed in the section, Additional Information for Enrichment.

Three-way retention catheters are preferred because they permit a continuous rinsing of the bladder with various bacteriostatic solutions, e.g., 0.25 per cent acetic acid, neomycin or polymyxin.

If the catheter is too soft and pliable for ease of insertion through the long male urethra, a metal catheter guide (stylet) may be inserted through the lumen of the catheter to make the catheter more rigid for easier insertion. When the catheter is in place, the catheter guide is removed so that the urine can flow freely through the lumen. NOTE: Use of a catheter guide is limited to use by the physician or G.U. technician.

Most retention catheters are available on disposable catheter trays. The tray may or may not provide sterile drainage tubing and bag. You will follow your agency procedure when obtaining your supplies, i.e., request the drainage set separately if it is not included on the retention catheter set.

The closed system of urinary drainage is preferred. In the closed system, the catheter, drainage tubing, and drainage bag are one continuous unit. The unit is not separated at any point to remove urine because of the high probability of introducing organisms into the urinary bladder. Urine is removed from the closed system by draining it off through the drainage valve at the bottom of the drainage bag. Some research studies recommend the use of a 40 per cent formaldehyde solution added to the drainage bag to inhibit growth to bacteria in the stale urine. (Follow agency procedures, however.)

Another precaution that can be added to the closed drainage system is a plastic foam pad 2 inches in diameter, 1 inch thick, threaded on the Foley catheter to midway up the catheter and autoclaved as a total unit. After the catheter is inserted and the balloon inflated, the pad is pushed up to rest snugly against the urinary meatus. This helps to mobilize the catheter in the urethra. The pad is moistened several times daily with an antiseptic cream or solution to help maintain an antiseptic barrier at the external urinary meatus. NOTE: The distal end of the catheter drainage tube should always be above the urine level in the drainage bag. Otherwise, air bubbles moving through the tubing will carry bacteria up to the bladder. The bacteria grow in stagnant urine in the drainage bag and in columns of urine standing in the drainage tube.

The open urinary drainage system was used prior to the 1970's. This open drainage system could be disconnected at any point to remove the urine, e.g., at the catheter/tubing connection or at the tubing/drainage bag connection. After extensive laboratory research, it was found that many urinary tract infections occurred because of poor technique used in handling the open system of urinary drainage which permitted pathogenic organisms to be introduced into the urinary tract. Therefore, in recent years this system has become almost nonexistent.

There are important nursing considerations that must be carried out when a patient has an indwelling (retention) catheter in place:

1. Force fluids (unless contraindicted by the patient's condition or physician's orders). This assists in flushing bacteria and sediment out of the urinary system.

2. Accurate recording of the intake and output is vitally important as an indicator of kidney function. Any abnormal recordings (too much, too little, unusual color or odor) should be reported immediately to the physician. Levels of urinary output will vary within a 24-hour period, depending on the age of the patient.

Age	Amount
first and second day of life	15-60 cc
third to tenth day	100-300 cc
tenth day to 2 months	250-450 cc
2 months to 1 year	400-500 cc
1 to 5 years	500-700 cc
5 to 8 years	700-1000 cc
8 to 14 years	800-1400 cc
15 years +	1500 cc

3. The retention catheter and tubing are changed according to your agency's procedure, e.g., the catheter itself may be changed every 7 to 10 days, while the drainage tubing may be changed every 24 hours or prn.

4. Avoid contaminating the drainage system. Usually the urine is removed from the bottom opening of the drainage bag at the end of each shift or according to the physician's orders. The possibility of introducing organisms into the urinary system is greatly increased when the tubing is disconnected from the drainage bag; use the drain tube at the bottom of the drainage bag to release the urine.

5. Cleanse the genitalia and the area around the urinary meatus at least twice daily with the agency's antiseptic solution or mild soap solution to keep the catheter from becoming encrusted. Crusting around the urinary meatus is very uncomfortable and unsightly for the patient. In addition, it provides an excellent site for a urinary tract infection to begin.

Select a catheter according to the patient size. A common size for the adult patient is a 14 French with a 5 cc bag. The retention catheter tray set is similar to the plain catheterization tray except that in place of the plain French catheter, the Foley catheter is substituted and there is a prefilled syringe of sterile water to inflate the balloon. As mentioned previously, some retention catheter sets may include the drainage system also. If not, obtain the drainage system with the catheter set.

Follow Steps 1 through 7 of Item 1. When preparing the work area in Step 7, you must also test the balloon of the catheter to be sure that it does not have a hole in it. Therefore:

Important Steps	Key Points
7a. Test the balloon.	While holding the catheter valve in your left hand, pick up the prefilled syringe with the right hand and insert the tip of the syringe into the catheter valve. Push the plunger into the syringe with the palm of your right hand.
	If the balloon inflates and there is no visible leak, draw the water into the syringe by pulling out (back) on the plunger until the 8 cc of water is back in the syringe.
	If there is a leak in the balloon, it must be discarded and replaced. Draw water back into the syringe. Remove the syringe from the catheter valve and place it at one side for later use. Discard the leaky catheter and obtain a new one. After checking the new balloon, withdraw the syringe from the catheter valve and place it at the side of the tray until needed.

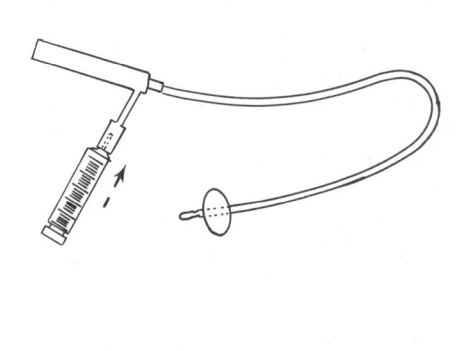

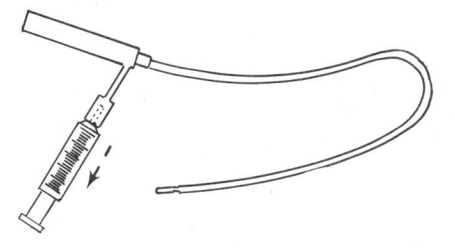

Proceed with Steps 8 through 15 of Item 1.

16. Insert the catheter an additional 1/2 to 3/4 inch.	This action will move the catheter inward, away from the urethral outlet at the base of the bladder. It is also more comfortable for the patient. If the catheter is left at the neck of the bladder, it will cause pressure and make the patient feel as though he must urinate.

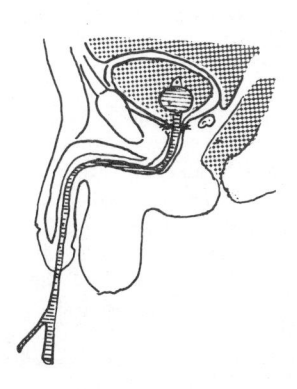

Important Steps	Key Points
17. Inflate the balloon.	Insert the tip of the prefilled syringe into the catheter valve. Inject water into the balloon by pushing the plunger into the barrel of the syringe with the palm of the right hand. Remove the syringe from the catheter valve and lay it at one side of the tray. There is a special valve that prevents the water from running out of the balloon when the syringe is removed. Gently pull on the catheter to see if it is anchored securely, then gently push back into the bladder about 1/2 inch.
18. Remove the protector cap or plug from the drainage tubing.	First be sure that the side drainage valve on the drainage bag is closed to prevent urine from leaking onto the floor. The cap on the tubing is removed by unscrewing, from right to left; the plug is removed by pulling straight out from the drainage tube. Attach the tubing to the free end of the catheter. Be sure it is securely attached.
19. Attach the metal hook to the bed frame.	Usually the hook is attached to the stationary part of the bed frame along the side of the bed, near the middle. The metal hook is the attachment for suspending the drainage bag so that it does not lie on the floor. The design of the hook may vary somewhat from product to product, but the purpose of the hook remains the same, to support the drainage bag.
20. Set the drainage bag into the support rest.	This will prevent the bag from being stepped on or kicked while you are taking care of the patient at the bedside.
21. Dry the genital area.	Remove the drapes from the patient; take off your gloves.
22. Remove the tray and make the patient comfortable.	
23. Secure the catheter.	Prevent tension or pulling on the catheter as the patient turns and moves in bed. Most disposable trays have a special catheter clip (clamp) that is used to attach the catheter to the bedding. The clip works much like a safety pin. If a catheter clamp is not available, a piece of tape can be placed around the catheter 12 to 18 inches from the urinary meatus. Make a slide loop with the tape so that a safety pin can be attached through the loop to the bedding. If a safety pin is used, you must be sure that you do not stick the patient and that you do not put the safety pin through plastic sheets (holes in the sheets may permit drainage to soak the mattress and make it unfit for future use).

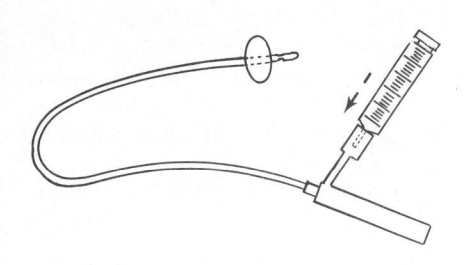

Important Steps	Key Points
	Tape may be secured (use nonallergenic tape) to the female patient's thigh as a further security measure. In any event, be sure that the tubing is free from kinking and that it permits free movement by the patient.

To secure the catheter in the male patient, it is best to tape the catheter to the lower abdomen so that the penis is pointing toward the head. This will prevent the formation of an abscess in the peno-scrotal angle. |
| 24. Remove supplies from the room. | Return unused items to storage. Discard used items in a designated receptacle. |
| 25. Record the procedure on the patient's chart. | Charting example:

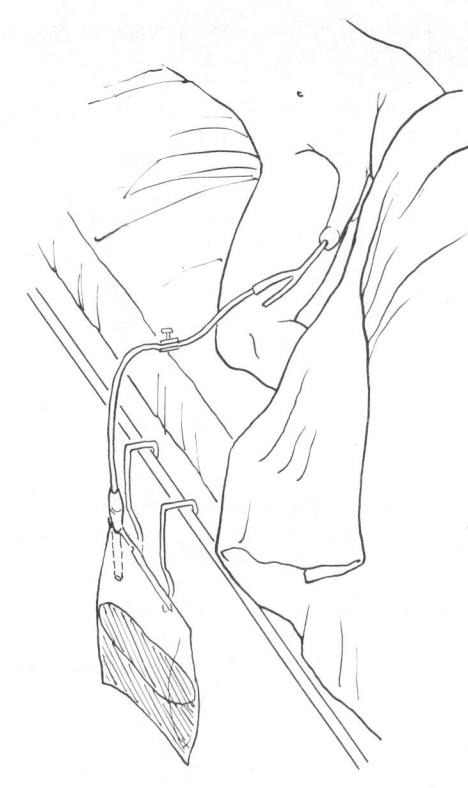

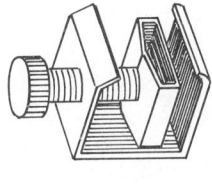

1:30 P.M. Foley catheter inserted and connected to drainage. Draining freely. Urine clear amber.

J. Sonntag, S.N. |

It has been reported by the University of Michigan Medical Center that intermittent self-catheterization techniques by selected paraplegics have obtained the following results:

1. It helps eliminate overdistention of the bladder wall with resultant ischemia.

2. It is socially more acceptable for a patient to catheterize himself.

3. The leg bag is eliminated.

4. It enables some improvement in sexual relations when the indwelling catheter is removed.

5. It is a suitable technique for use outside the hospital for both male and female paraplegics.

ITEM 4: REMOVAL OF A RETENTION CATHETER

To remove the retention catheter, untape the catheter from the thigh or abdomen. Follow Steps 1 through 7 of Item 1.

Important Steps	Key Points
8. Expose the meatus and cleanse with an antiseptic pledget.	See Step 8 in Item 1 for the female, or Step 8 in Item 2 for the male.
9. Deflate the balloon.	Insert an empty syringe into the catheter valve. Withdraw all of the solution into the syringe (5–8 cc). Lay the syringe to one side.
	If you cannot remove the solution to inflate the balloon, call the physician.
	Do not pull a catheter with an inflated balloon out of the bladder. This is extremely painful to the patient and also injures the delicate urethral mucosa.
	If the physician cannot deflate the balloon, the patient may need to have it removed surgically.
10. Remove the catheter.	Take it out gently and slowly, slightly rotating the catheter as you withdraw it to remove residual urine in the neck of the bladder.
	Place the catheter on the tray.
11. Cleanse and dry the genital area.	Use antiseptic cotton balls or towels which are provided. Remove your rubber gloves.
12. Remove the tray, catheter and tubing, and make the patient comfortable.	Discard soiled linens, replace the bed covers. Leave the patient comfortable. Adjust the siderails, call light and bedside stand for his convenience. Ask if there is anything else you can do, and tell him when you will return.
13. Take the supplies out of the room.	Empty the urine receptacle and note the amount, color and odor for recording on the chart. Discard used items in the designated container. Leave the work area neat and tidy.
14. Record on the patient's chart.	Note your procedures immediately. This recording is often omitted on the patient's chart and leads to much confusion and embarrassment if the case should be taken to court sometime in the future.
	Charting example:
	4:10 P.M. Foley catheter removed. 350 cc clear, yellow urine obtained. Immediately ambulated to the solarium.
	J. Nunn, Orderly

ITEM 5: CARE OF PATIENTS WITH CYSTOCATHS

The Cystocath is a sterile-packaged, disposable plastic unit used for bladder drainage following gynecological and bladder surgery (vaginal hysterectomy, vaginal repair, A and P repair, pan hysterectomy [total] and radical vulnectomy, suprapubic cystotomy, etc.). Its use is contraindicated for patients with a scarred or abnormal bladder, or who have vast hematuria with clotting after bladder surgery.

URINARY CATHETERIZATION

This method offers a number of advantages:

1. It seems to promote earlier spontaneous postoperative voiding.
2. Bladder infections are minimized because it is a closed system.
3. It is comfortable for the patient.
4. It provides for easy observation of the urinary drainage by the nursing personnel.
5. Patients can move about freely without the unsightly urinary drainage bag dangling for everyone to see.
6. It provides an easy system for collecting urine specimens and checking residual urine after the patient voids.
7. It provides an easy method for irrigation of the bladder.
8. It decreases urethritis from repeated urethral catheterizations of the patient (or use of the retention catheter).

The catheter insertion is the responsibility of the physician and is usually done in the operating room utilizing strict aseptic procedures.

The soft, flexible, special plastic catheter is introduced into the bladder through a special trocar-type needle that is inserted through the abdominal wall at the midline, 2 inches above the symphysis. (Slight variations in the insertion site may occur due to various types of abdominal operative incisions.) A section (approximately 10-12 inches) of the catheter remains on the outside of the abdomen.

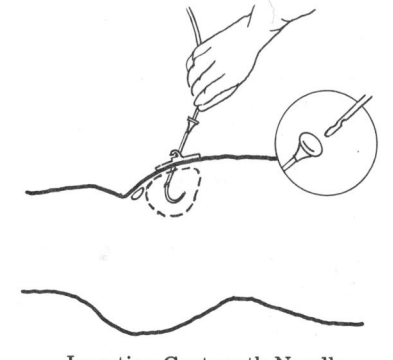

Inserting Cystocath Needle

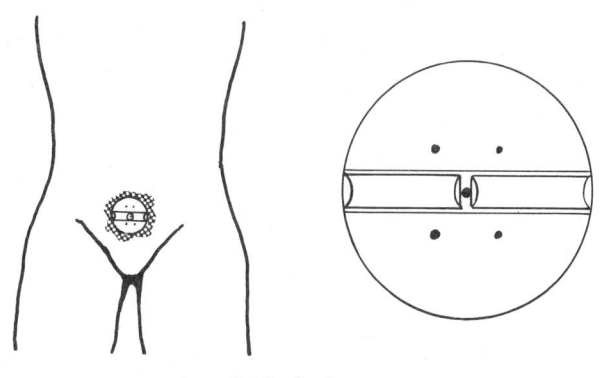

Body Seal

After the catheter is in place, the needle is slowly removed and discarded. The catheter is then secured in position with the special body seal.

A three-way stopcock is attached to the distal end of the catheter, and then the urinary drainage bag is attached to the other end of the stopcock. The catheter and urinary drainage tubing can then be taped to the patient's abdomen.

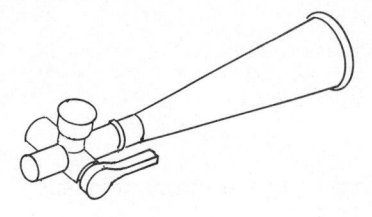

Three-way Stopcock

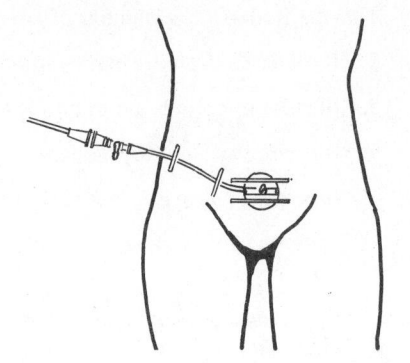

Complete Cystocath Set-up

The main nursing precautions to be used in caring for patients with Cystocaths are:

1. Prevent undue tension on the catheter.

2. Maintain the vent system to assure proper urine flow.

3. Utilize aseptic technique when obtaining a sterile specimen from the system.

4. Irrigate the catheter prn to maintain urine flow.

5. Stoppage of urine flow should be remedied by slightly withdrawing the catheter to free the proximal end from possible bladder wall attachment.

6. Avoid cutting the catheter (needle is withdrawn *before* the catheter is removed).

7. Utilize Sitz baths to help the patient void (after vaginal packing is removed or if the physician orders).

8. Establish a normal voiding pattern by closing the drainage system for alternating periods (e.g. 15 to 30 minutes q 4 hours throughout the day). Usually this procedure can be instituted on the third post-operative day if there are no contraindications.

9. Placement of a sterile dressing over the skin opening is required after removal of the catheter and body seal.

VI. ADDITIONAL INFORMATION FOR ENRICHMENT

Your instructor will give additional reading assignments if you are interested in learning more about patients who require urinary catheterizations.

Repeated research studies report that strict adherence to aseptic technique is mandatory to prevent your patient from developing a urinary tract infection.

Urinary catheterization was utilized in ancient times by the Egyptians. Recorded history indicates that in 3000 B.C. they were using bronze or tin catheters.

During the intervening years until 100 B.C., various materials were used to make catheters: wood, gold, iron, and the leaves of an onionlike plant. Before use, the practice was to lubricate them with various oils of the time.

The flexible catheter, made of woven silk, was developed by a German, Pikel, in the 1730's. A fellow countryman, Heister, developed a curved silver catheter.

In 1752 Benjamin Franklin made a catheter of catgut. During the last half of the 18th century, many people experimented with the use of rubber, which could be adapted for catheter use. However, it was not until the vulcanizing process was developed by Charles Goodyear in 1835 and continually improved upon until his death in 1860 that rubber became generally used for urinary catheters.

Continuing research has devised new materials for catheters such as silicones, Teflon, etc., which avoid tissue reaction or trauma. Science continues to make rapid progress in developing health care supplies and equipment that are more adaptable to patient and health personnel needs. The continuing improvements in the design of economical, disposable items afford greater security for patients, particularly in the area of infection control. Although manufacturers of health supplies, equipment, and pharmaceuticals are providing high levels of sterility in their products, it still remains the prime role of the health worker to adhere vigilantly to strict principles of asepsis in all activities that relate to patient care!

Following is a table of commonly used catheters. Study the table, and ask your instructor to provide a sample of each so that you can become familiar not only with the use of the catheter, but with its size, appearance, and feel.

COMMON URINARY CATHETERS*

Name	Description	Common Uses and/or Advantages
1. Robinson	Round, hollow-tip with two or more eyes. Also solid-tip with only one eye.	Obtaining urine specimens; relieving acute bladder retention.
2. Whistle-tip	Modified Robinson; oblique, beveled open end.	Providing more efficient drainage.
3. Hollow-tip (multi-eyed)	Three or more openings on each side of the tip.	Lavage of the bladder, especially in the presence of clots
4. Coudé (elbowed)	Modified Robinson; curved, with a rounded or bulbous tip with one or two eyes. Usually made of red rubber.	Providing easier passage in the tortuous male urethra, especially with enlarged prostate.
5. Hendrickson	Constructed with coiled stainless steel wire embedded in catheter wall.	With Toomey two-ounce syringe for forceful clot evacuation.
6. Foley (double or triple lumen)	Double lumen, with second lumen leading to inflatable balloon near tip. Tip may be straight or elbowed, with one or two eyes. Made of latex or plastic. Red latex is radiopaque, amber latex is not. (Silicone style is pictured.)	Most commonly used self-retaining catheter. Inflatable balloon prevents catheters from slipping out of bladder, thus giving patient freedom of movement. Most common balloon sizes are 5 cc and 30 cc. Provides continual drainage, particularly postoperatively. Aids in achieving hemostasis. Can be used as a cystostomy tube by inserting into the bladder, or as a nephrostomy tube by inserting into kidney pelvis.
7. Alcock	Foley catheter with four eyes, one situated at the distal end.	For bladder irrigation following prostatic resection.
8. Bunts	Foley catheter with opening along the shaft.	For instillation of anti-microbials in the urethra; to allow for more effective urethral drainage.
9. Emmett hemostatic (two-way or three-way)	Foley catheter with multi-eyed long tip distal to the Foley balloon.	Can be inflated in the prostatic fossa while extra long tip remains in the bladder for urine drainage.
10. Trahner	Double-balloon catheter with opening between balloons.	For diagnosis of lesions such as urethral stricture, diverticulum, or fistula. Catheter is inserted through urethra into bladder, two balloons are inflated, and urethrographic medium is injected to visualize entire urethra.

*From *RN Magazine*, April 1972, and reprinted with permission.

COMMON URINARY CATHETERS* (Continued)

Name	Description	Common Uses and/or Advantages
11. Councill	Foley catheter with open tip end to allow stylet with screw to protrude for attachment to threaded filiform.	When a stricture is present and catheter is to be left indwelling. After insertion, stylet and filiform are removed.
12. dePezzer (mushroom)	Straight or angulated large single channel with preformed tip in shape of mushroom. Some tips have open ends.	As a suprapubic tube.
13. Malecott (four-winged)	Large single channel with tip shaped as two or four wings that collapse into tube shape on traction. With body heat, wings collapse without trauma for removal.	As a nephrostomy tube. Inserted into cavity with straight catheter-guide stylet, removed after catheter is in place.

*From *RN Magazine*, April 1972, and reprinted with permission.

How is your catheter I.Q.?

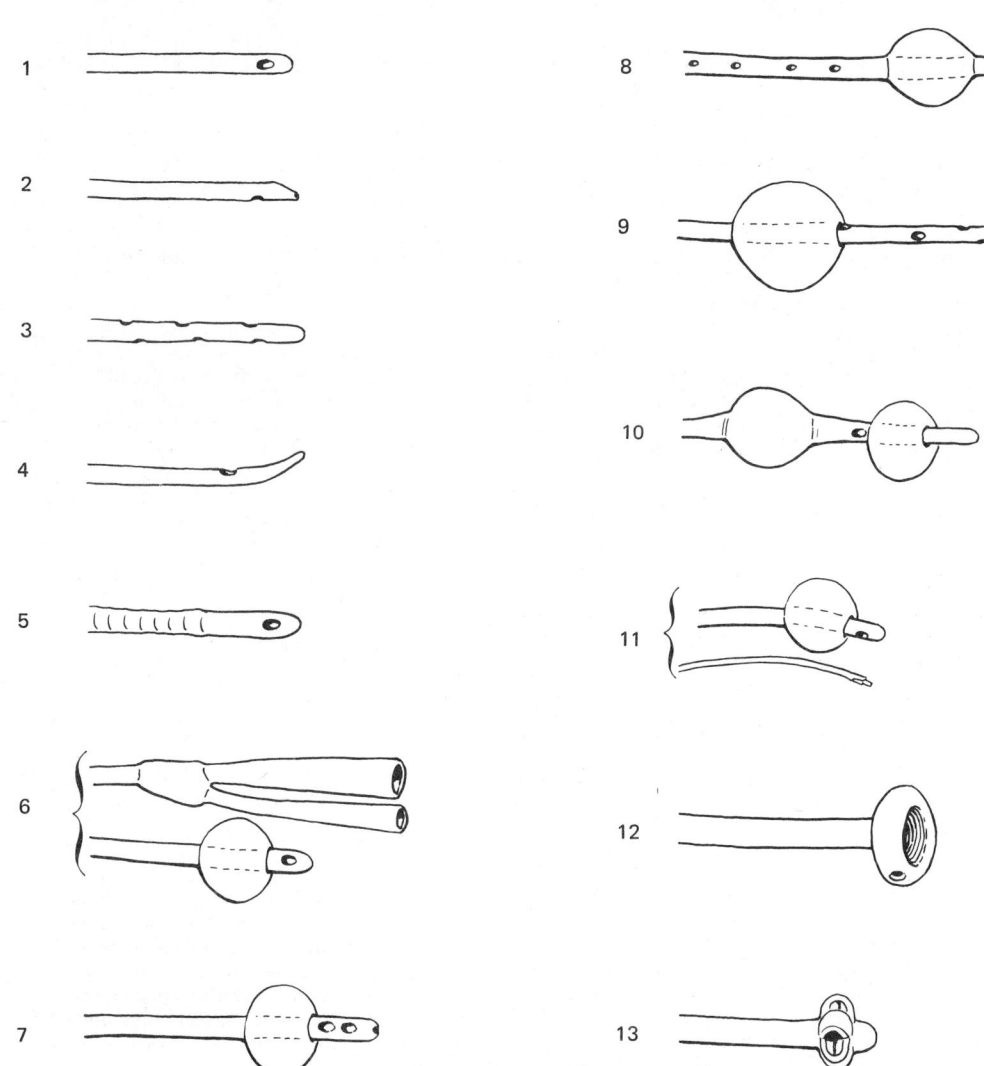

URINARY CATHETERIZATION

POST-TEST

Fill in the blanks:

1. Aseptic technique must be carried out during a urinary catheterization because _____
   _____.

2. Give at least four reasons for doing a catheterization.

   a. _____

   b. _____

   c. _____

   d. _____

3. Forcing fluids is a desirous activity in most cases of the patient with a retention catheter because _____
   _____.

4. The closed system of urinary drainage is the preferred method because _____
   _____.

5. Urine specimens are always obtained by catheterization. True ___ False ___

6. Excessive amounts of urine removal should be avoided because _____
   _____.

POST-TEST ANNOTATED ANSWER SHEET

1. The urinary bladder is a sterile cavity and the introduction of pathogenic organisms in the bladder must be avoided, p. 207.

2. Any of the following:

   Obtain sterile urine specimen; measure residual urine; insertion of a retention catheter to drain, irrigate or install a chemotherapeutic agent into the bladder; prepare a patient for a surgical procedure or delivery; keep bladder empty in the incontinent patient to avoid decubiti; maintain cleanliness of genitalia following surgical procedure or delivery, p. 207, 208.

3. The additional liquids assist in flushing (washing) bacteria and sediment out of the urinary tract, p. 216.

4. There is a limited possibility of contaminating the drainage system and introduction of organisms into the urinary tract, p. 215.

5. False, p. 208.

6. The bladder wall can collapse and put the patient in shock, p. 211.

URINARY CATHETERIZATION

PERFORMANCE TEST

Given a female patient 24 years old who is being prepared for a colostomy in the morning, you will catheterize her, obtain a sterile urine specimen, and leave the retention catheter in place.

Explain safety precautions to your instructor as you proceed.

NOTE: Catheterization may be performed on a student partner or a simulated model according to agency preference.

PERFORMANCE CHECKLIST

1. Wash hands.
2. Assemble equipment.
3. Identify patient.
4. Position and drape patient.
5. Prepare catheter tray (test balloon).
6. Put on sterile gloves.
7. Prepare sterile work area.
8. Expose meatus.
9. Clean genitalia.
10. Pick up catheter with forceps.
11. Insert catheter into meatus.
12. Obtain specimen.
13. Complete urine removal.
14. Inflate balloon and reposition catheter if needed.
15. Attach drainage tubing.
16. Place drainage bag in support rest.
17. Dry genital area and remove tray.
18. Make patient comfortable.
19. Secure catheter.
20. Remove used items.
21. Record activity on nursing record.

Unit 6

APPLICATION OF HOT AND COLD COMPRESSES, PACKS AND SOAKS

I. DIRECTIONS TO THE STUDENT

Proceed through this lesson. After you have finished, take the Post-Test and practice in the skill laboratory. When you feel that you are ready, make arrangements with your instructor to take the Performance Test.

II. GENERAL PERFORMANCE OBJECTIVE

Following this lesson you will be able to prepare and administer moist hot and cold compresses, packs and soaks.

III. SPECIFIC PERFORMANCE OBJECTIVES

Upon completion of this lesson you will be able to:

1. Assemble supplies and equipment necessary to correctly administer moist hot and cold compresses, packs and soaks.
2. Apply the various moist hot and cold applications using safety precautions to prevent injury to the patient and to yourself.
3. Discuss the purpose and objectives for the local application of heat and cold.
4. Discuss the various physiological effects of moist heat and cold treatments.

IV. VOCABULARY

Read the definitions of the terms listed below. Do not attempt to memorize them before proceeding with the lesson. Each term will be explained or defined again in the text. On completion of the lesson, however, you should know the correct definition of each term.

anoxia—deficiency of oxygen.
conduction—the passage of heat from molecule to molecule, as through a metal tube.
edema—a condition in which the body tissues contain an excessive amount of tissue fluid.
Hubbard tank—a special water treatment tank used in the Physiotherapy Department.
hypothalamus—the portion of the brain that controls visceral activities such as the maintenance of water balance, sugar and fat metabolism, regulation of body temperature, and the secretions from the endocrine glands.
hypothermia—body temperature below the normal limits.
suppuration—the process of pus formation.
vasoconstriction—the constriction or narrowing of the caliber (diameter) of the blood vessel.
vasodilation—the dilation or widening of the lumen of the blood vessels.
vasomotor—referring to muscular control of the blood vessel walls.
viscosity—relative resistance to flow; e.g., of a gummy substance.

V. INTRODUCTION

Dry and moist heat and cold applications have been employed therapeutically in homes and hospitals for many years. You have probably had occasion to apply a hot water bottle or an ice bag on top of a moistened wash cloth or towel during your lifetime. Not only do nurses employ these measures, but physiotherapists also utilize similar applications as part of rehabilitation treatments.

Although the choice of temperature and type of application to be used is usually determined by the physician, there are at least seven factors that you must consider if you are to select the application to be used:

1. The age of the patient. (The very young and the very old are particularly sensitive to changes in temperatures.)

2. The patient's general physical condition and the presence of other physiological problems.

3. The condition of the patient's skin (broken, infected, excessively dry, etc.).

4. Purpose of the treatment (cleansing, soaking, therapeutic, soothing).

5. Part of the body affected.

6. Length of time for the treatment (minutes, hours).

7. Availability of various types of equipment and supplies.

In addition to the above, an important physiological factor to consider in applying heat or cold applications is the status of the patient's circulatory system. You will recall from earlier units that heat is distributed through the body via the circulating blood. The amount of blood circulating depends on:

1. Cardiac output.

2. The integrity of the deep and superficial vascular system.

3. Amount of activity carried on by the patient.

4. The position of the patient (standing, lying down).

You will recall in your review of Unit 31: Assisting with Procedures, that the skin plays an important role in maintaining body temperature.

As the local and general needs of the body change, the blood vessels in the skin are capable of dilating to hold large amounts of blood, or constricting to convey small amounts of blood. Influenced by the hypothalamus, the vasomotor centers in the medulla oblongata send nerve impulses to constrict or dilate the blood vessels as the need arises. Although the depth of the receptors in the nerve endings varies, usually the cold receptors are superficial, whereas the heat receptors are located deeper in the skin. The receptors have great capability to adapt to heat or cold; however, it is important to remember that applications above 110°F (43.3°C) or below 40°F (4.44°C) can cause serious tissue damage.

Not only does tolerance for temperature changes vary with individuals, but it also differs in various parts of the body. Generally, the areas where the skin is thinner and not exposed (such as the mucous membranes) are more sensitive. Conversely, the exposed areas of the skin usually have thicker layers and are less sensitive (e.g., the palm of the hand or the sole of the foot).

Water is a better conductor of heat than air. Safety precautions must therefore be taken when applying moist heat to prevent tissue damage from a burn; this means correct temperature, and frequent checks of the patient's skin and vital signs. Another important safety factor is the duration of the treatment. The shorter the treatment, the greater the tolerance for the heat. The larger the area to which the heat or cold is applied, the less tolerant the skin is to extremes of temperature.

It is generally accepted that there are three types of sensory nerve endings that are stimulated by thermal (temperature) changes: warm receptors, cold receptors, and pain receptors. Remember that extremes in temperature stimulate the pain receptors.

APPLICATION OF HOT AND COLD COMPRESSES, PACKS AND SOAKS

LOCAL HEAT APPLICATION

When the skin becomes warm and pink, it is primarily the result of a moderate heat application. This process is known as *vasodilation*. The dilation of the subcutaneous vessels allows for increased blood circulation to the skin. This causes loss of heat to the environment. There is also an increased rate of blood flow, resulting from a decrease in the blood viscosity. Although the exact physiologic mechanism is unknown, heat also relieves pain produced by muscle spasm.

The local application of heat may be prescribed for the following purposes:

1. To relieve pain.
2. To reduce congestion.
3. To reduce inflammation or swelling.
4. To relieve muscle spasm.
5. To provide comfort.
6. To elevate the body temperature.
7. To decrease the blood supply in other areas of the body.

The accepted temperature ranges for application of heat are:

Fahrenheit		Centigrade
105°F to 115°F	very hot	41°C to 46°C
98°F to 105°F	hot	37°C to 41°C
93°F to 98°F	warm	34°C to 37°C

LOCAL APPLICATION OF COLD

When cold is applied, the skin becomes pale and cool; this is a result of the vasoconstriction (decrease in the lumen) of the cutaneous blood vessels. The cold receptors of the sensory nerve endings are stimulated and the body reacts to conserve heat. Do you remember what happened when heat was applied to the skin? _____ .

Which sensory receptors were stimulated with the heat application? _____

_____ .

In addition to vasoconstriction (which reduces circulation in the skin to conserve heat), there is a decrease in the tissue metabolism. Cold produces a topical anesthetic effect, and caution must therefore be used to prevent tissue burns. The patient himself is unable to distinguish potentially serious problems of the skin because of the local anesthesia he experiences.

Cold applications may be used to prevent edema resulting from sprains, strains, and contusions. Another widely accepted use is for hemorrhage. The cold application acts to constrict the blood vessels and decrease the blood flow. Cold is also used to reduce inflammation.

An important fact to remember is that prolonged use of cold has the same effect as heat applied for shorter periods of time. In other words, the immediate effect of cold applications is vasoconstriction, while the prolonged effect of cold application is vasodilation.

The physician usually will indicate the temperature to be used for cold applications, e.g., tepid, cool, cold or very cold.

Fahrenheit		Centigrade
80°F to 93°F	tepid	26.7°C to 33.9°C
65°F to 80°F	cool	18.3°C to 26.7°C
55°F to 65°F	cold	12.3°C to 18.3°C
below 55°F	very cold	below 12.5°C

Note: Colder temperatures may be tolerated if the area for application is small and the duration of the treatment is brief.

To help you understand the different physiological reactions that occur when heat or cold is applied for a SHORT DURATION, study the following chart comparisons:

Heat Applications	*Cold Applications*
Vasodilation of cutaneous vessels.	Vasoconstriction of cutaneous vessels.
Decreased heat production.	Increased heat production (by shivering).
Lowered blood pressure.	Elevated blood pressure.
Increased respiratory rate.	Increased respiratory rate.

ITEM 1: SOAKS

A *soak* is the direct immersion of a body part in warm water or in a medicated solution. Soaks are generally employed to aid in cleansing burns, to apply medication to an infected area, to aid suppuration and to increase circulation to a particular area of the body.

Tap water is generally used for soaks. The physician usually indicates the type of solution, the body area to be soaked, the temperature of the solution and the duration of the treatment. *Note:* If sterile technique is required, sterile solutions and sterile containers will then be utilized, and you will follow aseptic principles while carrying out the procedure.

The duration of the soaks (body, arm, foot, leg) is normally 15 to 30 minutes, administered several times a day.

Although the soak temperature is generally prescribed by the physician, it should be approximately 105°F (40.6°C) to 110°F (47.2°C). The body part is immersed gradually in the solution so that the patient may become accustomed to the temperature change. The container of solution should be placed near the patient to provide for his general comfort during the procedure and to assist in maintaining proper body alignment. If the whole body is immersed in the Hubbard tank, be sure the head and extremities are supported in a comfortable position. Check the temperature of the solution with a thermometer every 5 to 15 minutes so that an even temperature can be maintained throughout the soak. At the same time, observe the area to see if there are any untoward reactions occurring, such as extreme reddening, blistering excessive drainage, pain, and so forth. The warmth of the soak causes the skin to turn pink (owing to vasodilation of the superficial blood vessels) and the skin will be warm to the touch (as a result of increased stimulation of the heat receptors in the skin).

ITEM 2: APPLICATION OF HOT SOAKS

Important Steps	Key Points
1. Check the physician's order.	Make sure that there is a designation of the exact area to be treated, whether it is to be a sterile or nonsterile procedure, duration of the treatment, dosage, and type of medication to be added to the solution, if any.

APPLICATION OF HOT AND COLD COMPRESSES, PACKS AND SOAKS 231

Important Steps	Key Points
2. Assemble supplies and equipment.	Choose a container for the solution sufficiently large to accommodate the area to be soaked. In the case of a severe body burn, the patient may be taken to the Physical Therapy Department for soaking in the Hubbard tank. Wash your hands.
3. Approach the patient, identify him, and explain the procedure.	Read his Identaband. Explain what the procedure will consist of; e.g., immersing the limb, or body, in water to cleanse, provide comfort, treat with a medication solution, to soak loose dried dressings for easy removal, or whatever. Wash your hands.
4. Prepare the solution.	a. If your agency keeps the water in a heated storage unit, you should bring the solution to the room just before the treatment starts, in order to prevent initial cooling. b. If your agency utilizes a portable two--burner electric hot plate, place it carefully on the bedside stand. As a safety precaution, be sure that it is securely set on a flat surface so that it will not tip over or be too close to the patient. c. Pour the stated amount of solution (this will vary depending on the extremity to be soaked, as well as on the size of the container). d. Place the filled basin on the heating unit. e. Turn the heating unit on to "high."
5. Position the patient.	You can do this while the solution is heating to the prescribed degree. CAUTION: *Never* leave a child (or an elderly or confused patient) alone while you are heating the solution. You must provide for the patient's safety. He might inadvertently touch the heating element or overturn the basin and cause severe injury. Position the bed at a comfortable working height.

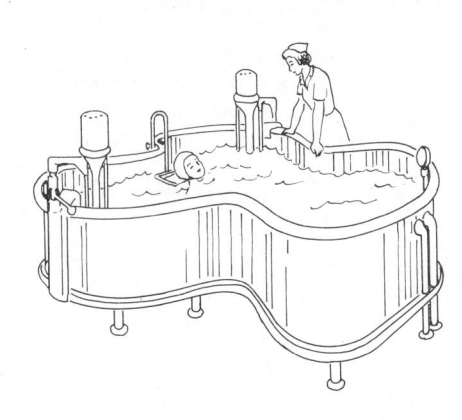

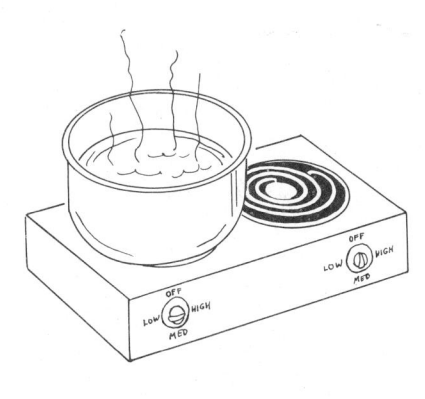

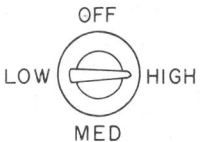

Important Steps	Key Points
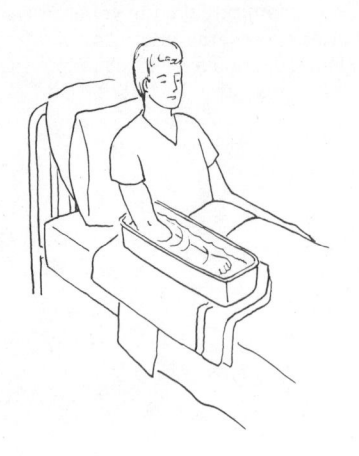	a. *Basin on bed:* If the soak basin is to be placed on the bed, it is best to have the bed flat to avoid spilling. Place a plastic sheet on the bed under the basin to protect the bottom bed linens from becoming wet or soiled. If the leg is to be soaked, position it comfortably and expose the limb so that it can be placed in the solution basin (the procedure is like placing the foot in a wash basin when giving a bedbath). If the arm is to be soaked, the patient, if he prefers, can be in a sitting position. Move him to the center of the bed so that there will be ample room to place the soak basin beside him during the procedure. If you place the soak basin on the bed for either the foot or arm, be sure to put a bath towel or plastic sheeting under the basin to protect the bed.
	b. *Basin on floor:* If it is a foot to be soaked, it may be more comfortable for the patient to be sitting in a chair. In that case, be sure that he is covered with a bath blanket to provide for privacy and warmth. Expose the foot that is to receive the treatment.
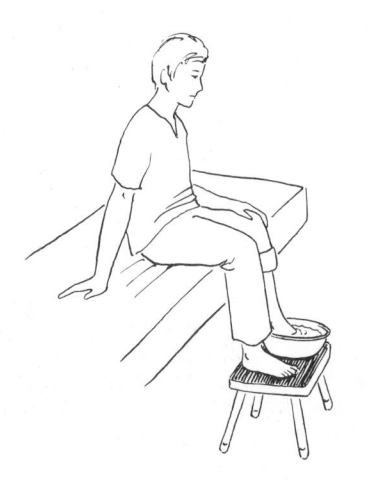	c. *Basin on footstool:* You may wish to lower the bed so that the patient can sit on the side of the bed with his leg hanging over the side. The soak basin can then be placed on a footstool. Select whichever approach is best for your patient. Another method for the soak is to take the patient to the Physical Therapy Department so that the limb can be immersed in a hydrotherapy tank made especially for soaking arms, legs, or the entire body.

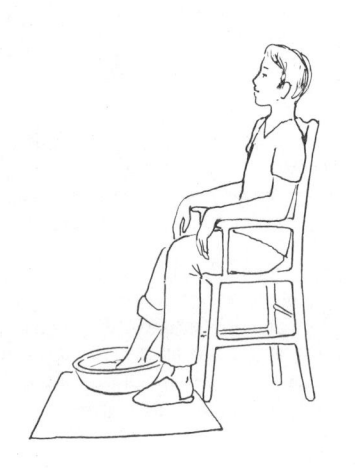

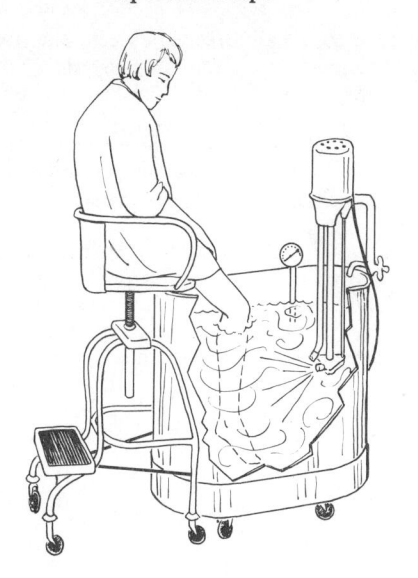

APPLICATION OF HOT AND COLD COMPRESSES, PACKS AND SOAKS

Important Steps | Key Points

Maintain good body alignment for the patient during the positioning and treatment. Place the soak basin so that it is comfortable for the patient, i.e., near the body and aligned with the length of the extremity.

6. Check the temperature of the heating solution.

You will need to do this with a thermometer every five to 10 minutes. When the temperature rises to the desired level (47.2°C or 115°F), turn the burner to "low."

7. Prepare the soaking site.

Drape the patient so that the area is exposed, but maintain his privacy and warmth. Remove soiled dressings and dispose of them in the designated container. Use the sterile technique that you learned in the Unit 1, Aseptic Technique.

8. Pour the heated solution into the container (soaking).

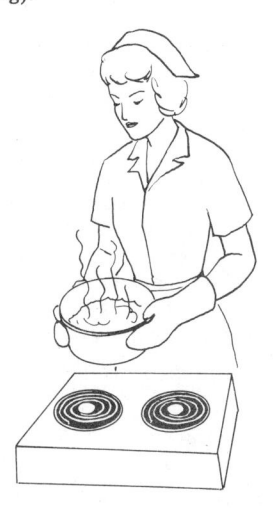

If medication is to be added to the solution, now is the time to add it. Be sure that it is mixed thoroughly with the solution. Remove the basin from the burner by picking it up with protective "hot mitts" to avoid burning your hands. A heavy bath towel may be used in place of the hot mitts. Pour the solution into the soaking container. Be careful not to splatter the patient or yourself—you could cause a burn. Also, a wet uniform can become a fomite for pathogenic organisms. Put the container back on the heater, add more solution and turn the control on "hot" (this will prepare the solution for the next application).

9. Recheck the solution temperature.

Do this before you place the limb in the soaking container to avoid burning your patient.

10. Lift the patient's limb into the soaking container.

Immerse the limb *slowly* to allow adjustment to the heat of the solution.

Important Steps	Key Points
11. Check the temperature of the solution regularly.	Every 5 to 10 minutes check to make sure that the temperature remains nearly constant throughout the treatment. Observe the patient's skin; if it becomes excessively red, remove the limb and let the solution cool. Remember that your observations must be recorded on the patient's chart at the end of the treatment.
12. Add more heated solution.	From your heating vessel, you may add solution prn to maintain the proper temperature of the soak. Pour it directly into the container as far away from the patient's skin as possible to avoid scalding or burning him.
13. Continue the treatment.	The prescribed treatment time must be completed (15 to 30 minutes). Continue to observe the patient's skin condition and vital signs (e.g., if patient becomes weak).
14. Remove the patient's limb from the soaking solution.	Support the limb as you remove it; refer to Volume 1, Unit 14, on positioning if you have forgotten how and why. Remove the soaking basin to the nearby table or bedside stand. Dry the limb thoroughly with the bath towel. If there is an open wound, pat dry around it, not directly on it. Observe the skin and wound area; does it look clean? Were crusts or purulent drainage removed? Does the skin area seem to be healing? Is it getting smaller?
15. Position the patient.	Remove the plastic sheeting; dry, neatly fold, and return it to storage. Leave the patient comfortably settled. Return him to bed, if necessary, or adjust the bed for comfort. Replace wet or soiled linen as needed. Straighten the bedding and fluff the pillow. Lower the bed to its lowest level, raise the siderails if indicated, place the call light and bedside stand within easy reach. Ask if there is anything he needs. Tell him approximately when you will return.
16. Return the supplies.	If the soaks are on a repeat cycle (4 times a day), you may leave the articles in the room. Be sure, however, that the basin has been removed from the electrical heating unit and is turned off. Be sure the heating unit is out of the patient's reach. Replenish the solution and medication supplies as needed. Leave the room orderly and ready for the next treatment.

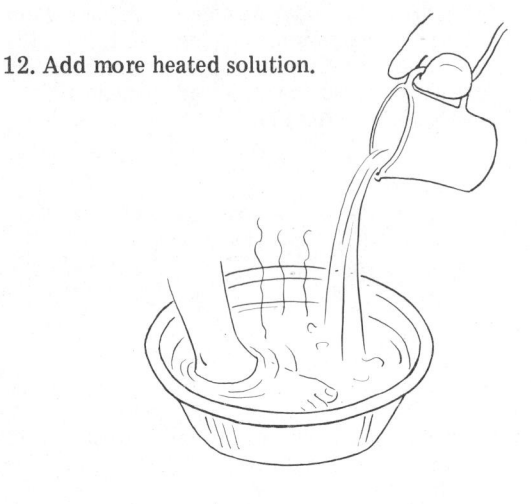

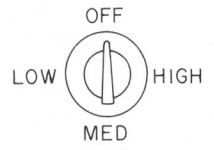

APPLICATION OF HOT AND COLD COMPRESSES, PACKS AND SOAKS 235

Important Steps	Key Points
17. Report and record.	Charting example: 8:10 A.M. Let foot soak in potassium permanganate solution 1:10,000 at 115°F for 20 minutes. Skin is healing well; wound measures 3 cm today. No complaints of pain. Is in cheerful mood. L. Domer, R.N.

ITEM 3: HOT COMPRESSES AND PACKS

The difference between a compress and a pack (foment) is in the material used and the body area on which it is used. A pack is usually applied to an extensive body area and consists of warm, moist flannel or similar material; a compress is normally applied to a limited body area and consists of warm, moist, gauze dressings. Because the principles involved are the same, these two procedures will be considered together.

Soaks differ from packs and compresses in that soaks are used for shorter periods of time and usually at lower temperatures.

Hot compresses and packs are applied at the hottest temperature the patient can tolerate without burning the superficial tissue. The material can be wrung out manually, with a clothes wringer, or with special handlers so that it does not drip on the patient when applied, yet it must remain moist enough to conduct the desired amount of heat.

Compresses and soaks usually cool off rapidly; therefore, the length of time they retain heat depends on the temperature of the solution, the thickness of the material, and the type of insulation used. Generally, they remain hot for 15 to 20 minutes, then have to be reheated and reapplied. Most of the treatments last for an hour and are administered three to four times a day.

ITEM 4: APPLICATION OF HOT PACKS AND COMPRESSES

Important Steps	Key Points
1. Check the physician's order.	Identify the area to be treated according to the order. Determine if there is need for medication; be sure to have appropriate medication, in correct strength, and in adequate supply. Note the duration and frequency of the treatments.
Assemble the equipment.	If you have an appliance that steams the packs or compresses, bring it to the room. A Hydrocollator is a commonly used piece of equipment. If this is not available, you will need material for the pack or compress, a heating unit, solution, thermometer, pickup forceps, towels and a plastic sheet.

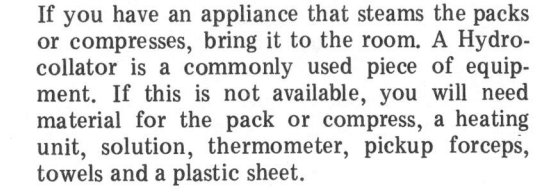

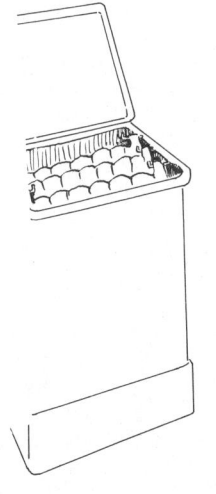

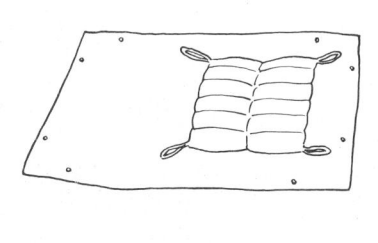

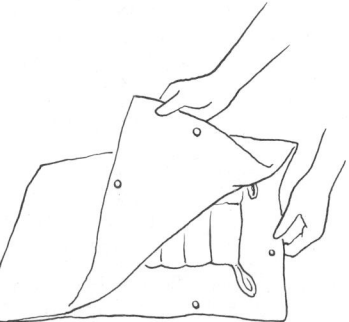

APPLICATION OF HOT AND COLD COMPRESSES, PACKS AND SOAKS

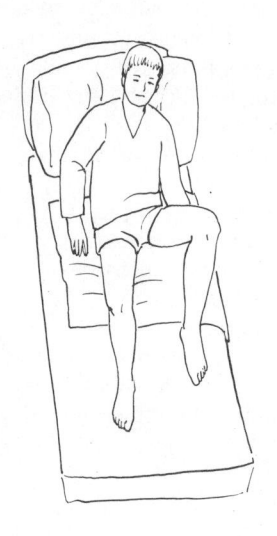

Important Steps	Key Points
3. Approach the patient, identify him, and explain the treatment.	Read his Identaband. Tell him, for example, that you will be putting the pack or compress over the area (leg, arm) three times a day for 15 minutes to aid in cleansing the wound and to provide comfort, as well as to assist in healing his wound more rapidly. Wash your hands.
4. Prepare the pack or compresses.	Immerse the material (gauze, flannel) in the solution contained in the basin on the heating element. Turn the unit to "hot."
5. Position the patient.	The best position for the patient is one that is more comfortable. It will vary somewhat depending on the location of the area to be treated. Drape the area so that it is exposed to afford easy application of the pack, keeping the patient covered for modesty and warmth. Place the plastic sheeting under the area to be treated.
6. Check the temperature of the solution.	Turn the heating unit to "low" when the solution has reached the designated temperature. Add medication to the solution if it has been prescribed.
7. Prepare the pack or compress.	Grasp the two lateral edges of the pack or compress with the two pickup forceps. Twist the pack or compress in opposing directions to wring out the excess solution; the forceps keep you from burning your hands.
8. Apply the pack or compress.	Place it directly over the area to be treated. You may have to fold the dressing so that it fits the area to be treated. Lay the pack on the wound slowly so that the patient can adjust gradually to the heat. Remember that the pack should be as hot as the patient can comfortably tolerate. Wrap the pack or compress in the plastic sheeting to concentrate the heat and hold it over the wound for as long a time as possible.

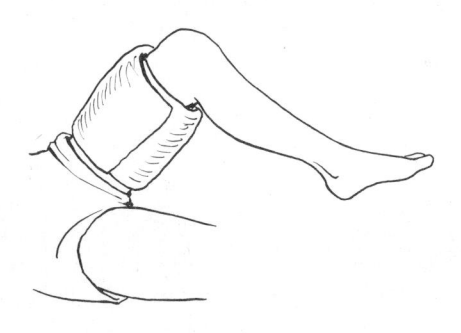

APPLICATION OF HOT AND COLD COMPRESSES, PACKS AND SOAKS

Important Steps	Key Points
9. Check the patient often.	Lift the edge of the pack at frequent intervals to see that the skin is not burning. If the patient is uncomfortalbe, you may have to unwrap the plastic to release some of the confined heat.
10. Start heating the second pack or compress.	Do this while the first pack is being applied to the patient. Be sure to turn the heater unit on. Pack #2 will be ready by the time pack #1 is cool and needs to be replaced. This provides for continuity of treatment so that treatment may be extended for the full amount of time, as prescribed. Remember that you must stay at the patient's bedside while the heating element is on if your patient is very young, elderly, or confused. This will prevent the patient from accidentally burning himself on the heating unit or by overturning the hot solution.
11. Remove the pack or compress.	Exchange packs if the treatment is to be continued; when the treatment is finished, discard the used gauze packs in the designated container. (The flannel pad may be reused if the dressing was not soiled. However, it is preferable to start each treatment with clean packs or compresses.) Pat the area around the wound dry. Remove the plastic sheeting and fold it for reuse at the next treatment. Store it in the designated place in the patient's room. Replace the bed linens and leave the patient comfortably positioned in the bed, in good alignment, and properly supported. Leave the call light and bedside stand within easy reach. Raise the siderails if indicated. Adjust the bed to its lowest height.
12. Take care of the equipment.	Turn off the heating element. Remove soiled packs or compresses and dispose of them in the incinerator. Replenish supplies (solution, gauze, flannel, medication, etc.) so that you are ready to begin the next treatment on time.
	Before you leave the patient's room, ask him if there is anything else you can do for him. Tell him when you will return. Then do so, or at least have someone else look in on him to see if he needs anything.

Important Steps	Key Points
	Leave the environment tidy, with lights and shades adjusted to meet the needs of the patient.
13. Report and record.	Record the time, area of application, temperature of the solution, duration of the treatment, and the appearance of the skin when treatment was finished.
	Charting example:
	8:00 A.M. Hot moist compress applied to the inner aspect of the left thigh at 115°F (46°C) for one hour. At the completion of the treatment the skin was pink and the wound looked clean. No evidence of suppuration present. Patient remarked that most of the pain was gone and the packs provided much comfort.
	L. Marion, R.N.

Recently appearing on the market are prepackaged sterile hot moist dressing systems. If your agency uses the prepackaged thermal systems, you should complete the In-service Program describing the procedure. The Curity Thermal Pack System is one example. Obviously this innovation will improve the moist compress technique. Keep alert for new systems on the market that can improve care for the patient.

ITEM 5: COLD COMPRESSES AND PACKS

Moist cold compresses are usually applied to smaller areas, and cold packs are reserved for the larger body surfaces, as with hot applications.

An ice compress generally consists of gauze or cloth material (wash cloths, towels, etc.) placed in a basin containing ice chips and a small amount of cold water. The compress is then wrung out to minimize dripping and placed on the designated body area.

Although ice chips may be inserted into the middle of the compresses and then applied directly to the patient, this becomes uncomfortable for the patient when the ice begins to melt. This practice, therefore, should be avoided.

Ice packs may be applied to a small area, or to the entire body to lower the body temperature. In the latter case, hypothermia blankets or pads may be used instead.

When ice packs are applied to an extremity, the arm or leg is wrapped in cloth (sometimes a face or bath towel) and the ice chips are packed around it; an additional layer of cloth is then placed over the ice to reduce the melting rate.

Ice packs and compresses remain effective for 15 to 20 minutes, depending on the environmental temperature and the patient's temperature. The patient will probably tell you when the ice has melted, and in some instances he may apply his own continuing cold packs after you have instructed him in the procedure. The skin must be observed frequently for impending tissue damage from prolonged vasoconstriction of the blood vessels, which over a period of time may lead to tissue necrosis resulting from lack of oxygen being carried to the tissues.

APPLICATION OF HOT AND COLD COMPRESSES, PACKS AND SOAKS

ITEM 6: APPLICATION OF COLD COMPRESSES AND PACKS

Important Steps	Key Points
1. Check the order.	Be sure that there is no change in the treatment order, or that it has not been discontinued.
2. Assemble the equipment.	The amount of ice chips you will need depends on the size and location of the treatment area. Bring the ice chips to the patient's room in a basin or bucket. Some agencies have an ice supply on each unit; others receive theirs from a Supply Department. If you are applying a small compress, a small metal basin filled with ice chips will usually be adequate. If the prescribed pack is a large one, however, a bath basin may be necessary. Plastic sheeting is usually needed for this treatment.
3. Approach the patient, identify him, and explain the procedure.	Read his Identaband. Explain that you will be applying a cold pack, where, and why; e.g., "The treatment will reduce the swelling in your arm and the pain should also decrease because the nerve endings in the subcutaneous skin are no longer being pressured by the increased fluid in the tissues," or, "Your physician has ordered the packs to be applied continuously until the swelling goes down." Wash your hands.
4. Prepare the pack or compress.	Place gauze or material in the basin filled with ice chips and enough water to nearly cover the ice chips. After the pack has been chilled (about 5 minutes), wring it as dry as possible to prevent ice water from dripping on the bed linens and running down the patient's arm.
5. Position the patient.	Expose the part to be treated so that modesty and warmth can be maintained. Drape the top bed linens so that the treatment area is exposed for easy application of the pack. Place plastic sheeting under the area to be treated to protect the bed linens from becoming soiled or wet. The patient should be positioned to keep the pack in place by the pull of gravity. Neither you nor the patient will then have to hold the pack in place throughout the treatment; e.g., if you are applying an ice pack to his eye, it would be best to have the patient in a dorsal recumbent position; if you are applying a pack to the upper part of his back, the patient should be in a supine position.

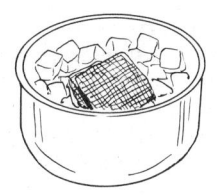

Important Steps	Key Points
6. Apply the pack or compress.	Place the wrung-out pack or compress directly on the prescribed site. Completely cover the area. If the pack or compress is applied to an extremity, you may wrap the plastic sheeting around the limb, covering the pack; this will reduce melting and evaporation.
7. Start cooling another set of packs or compresses.	This is done only if you exchange the packs and compresses. Otherwise, remove the pack or compress from the treatment area when it becomes warm, chill it by putting it back in the basin of ice chips, wring it out and reapply to the designated site.
8. Replenish ice chips as needed.	Usually during the treatment some ice will melt and the water must be discarded. You must check the basin of ice chips frequently so that the melted ice does not overflow onto the floor or stand. (You could easily slip and fall on the wet floor.)
9. Observe the patient.	Check the vital signs periodically as required by your agency if the treatment is to last for a long time; e.g., if the body is being packed in ice to bring down an elevated temperature. Peek under the edges of the pack or compress to see whether the swelling is decreasing, or if the bleeding has stopped. Look for decreasing signs of inflammation (skin red, pain diminished because the local pain receptors have become numb and thus produce a local anesthetic effect). You must remember, however, that there is danger of tissue necrosis from prolonged cold treatment because it decreases the amounts of oxygen and nutrients brought to the tissues. The skin itself may take on a bluish-white appearance because of the constriction of the blood vessels.
10. Terminate the treatment.	Stop at the designated time, or when contraindications occur (e.g., necrosis, excessive pain). Discard the pack or compress in the designated container. Empty the water basin and return it to the reprocessing room. Remove the plastic sheeting; if it is wet, dry it with paper towels from the patient's bathroom. Fold the sheeting and return it with the basin to storage or the reprocessing department.

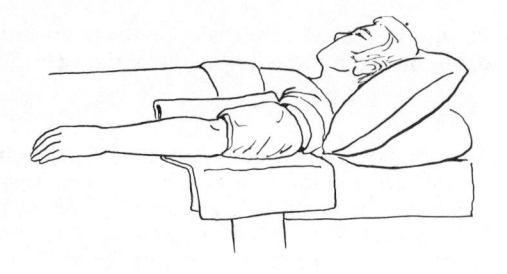

Important Steps	Key Points
11. Leave the patient comfortable.	Pat the skin area dry if necessary. Replace the bed linens if they are soiled or wet. Straighten the linens. Settle the patient comfortably but not in a position that is contraindicated by the orders. Lower the bed so that he can get in and out easily without falling. Raise the siderails if they are needed.
	Place the bedside unit and call light within easy reach, and ask the patient if there is anything else you can do. Tell him approximately when you will return.
12. Report and record.	Charting example:
	3:15 P.M. Cold pack terminated from left upper arm. Swelling has decreased markedly. Patient is comfortable. Skin cool to touch and slightly bluish-white.
	J. Board, R.N.

VI. ADDITIONAL INFORMATION FOR ENRICHMENT

Ask your instructor for further reading assignments regarding the treatment of patients who have been receiving soak, compress or pack applications.

A clinical experience in the Physical Therapy Department would be valuable to you; here you can see first-hand various hot and cold treatment modalities (methods).

242   APPLICATION OF HOT AND COLD COMPRESSES, PACKS AND SOAKS

POST-TEST

1. List five variables to be considered in the application of compresses, packs, and soaks:

   a. _____

   b. _____

   c. _____

   d. _____

   e. _____

2. Applications above __40__ °F and below __110__ °F can cause tissue damage.

3. Three types of sensory nerve endings that are stimulated by thermal change are:

   a. _____

   b. _____

   c. _____

4. The _____ of cutaneous blood vessels allows for increase in blood circulation in the skin.

5. The application of cold causes _____ of the cutaneous blood vessels.

6. List five purposes for the local application of heat:

   a. _____

   b. _____

   c. _____

   d. _____

   e. _____

7. The generally accepted range for a *hot* application is:

   __93__ °F to __115__ °F or _____ °C to _____ °C.

8. The duration of soaks is usually __15-30__ minutes.

9. The immediate effects of cold applications produce _____.

10. The generally accepted range for a *cold* application is:

    __55__ °F to __93__ °F or _____ °C to _____ °C.

True or False:

11. A pack is usually applied to small areas of the body. __F__

12. Soaks are most effective if they last over 30 minutes. __F__

13. The temperature of the solution used for soaks should be checked at least twice prior to patient application. __T__

14. The method used to lower the entire body temperature is called hyperthermia. __F__

15. The skin becomes cool and pale from the application of cold. __T__

APPLICATION OF HOT AND COLD COMPRESSES, PACKS AND SOAKS 243

POST-TEST ANNOTATED ANSWER SHEET

1. age of patient, patient's general physical condition, skin condition, purpose of treatment, part of body affected, treatment length, availability of supplies and equipment, p. 228.
2. 40°F to 110°F, p. 228.
3. warm receptors, cold receptors, pain receptors, p. 228.
4. vasodilation, p. 229.
5. vasoconstriction, p. 229.
6. relieve pain, muscle spasm, reduce congestion, inflammation or swelling, provide comfort, increase body temperatures, decrease blood supply, p. 229.
7. 93° to 115°F; 34° to 41°C, p. 229.
8. 15-30 minutes, p. 230.
9. vasoconstriction of cutaneous blood vessels, p. 229.
10. 55 to 93°F, or 12.5 to 33.9°C, p. 230.

True or False

11. F, p. 235.
12. F, p. 230.
13. T, p. 233.
14. F, p. 238.
15. T, p. 229.

PERFORMANCE TEST

In the skill laboratory with your partner, you will prepare, apply, and remove at least two of the following:

        Hot: compress, pack, or soak

        Cold: compress, pack, or soak

to the inner aspect of the lower right leg. You will assemble all of the supplies and equipment needed for the procedure before you begin. You will discuss the purpose, objectives, and physiological effects of hot or cold treatments.

PERFORMANCE CHECKLIST

APPLICATION OF HOT SOAKS

1. Check physician's order.
2. Assemble supplies.
3. Approach and identify the patient, and explain procedure. Wash hands.
4. Prepare solution, pour in appropriate amount of solution.
5. Position patient, and explain safety precautions.
6. Check temperature of solution.
7. Prepare application site.
8. Pour heated solution into soaking container.
9. Place limb into soaking container, and support limb.
10. Add heated solution prn to maintain correct temperature.
11. Continue treatment for stated time, observing patient's skin and general condition.
12. Remove limb from container and dry thoroughly.
13. Position patient. Remove supplies.
14. Return supplies to storage, or replenish as indicated.
15. Record treatment.

APPLICATION OF HOT PACKS AND COMPRESSES

1. Check physician's order.
2. Assemble equipment.
3. Approach and identify the patient, and explain the procedure. Wash hands.
4. Prepare pack or compress.
5. Position and drape the patient.
6. Check temperature of solution.
7. Prepare pack or compress. Wring out excess moisture.
8. Apply pack or compress slowly to allow for adjustment to the heat. Wrap with plastic to retain heat.
9. Check skin periodically throughout treatment. Start heating next application.
10. Remove pack or compress and discard.
11. Return or replenish supplies and equipment.
12. Leave patient comfortable and safe.
13. Record treatment.

APPLICATION OF COLD COMPRESSES AND PACKS

1. Check physician's order.
2. Assemble equipment and supplies.
3. Approach and identify the patient, explain the procedure. Wash hands.
4. Prepare pack or compress.
5. Position and drape the patient.
6. Apply pack or compress. Start another set of packs or compresses to cool.
7. Replenish ice chips prn.
8. Observe patient.
9. Terminate treatment, leave patient comfortable.
10. Return or replenish supplies or equipment.
11. Record treatment.

Unit 7

PHARYNGEAL SUCTIONING

I. DIRECTIONS TO THE STUDENT

This lesson pertains to the technique of suctioning the nose and throat and trachea. After completion of the lesson, take the Post-test and practice in the skill laboratory until you can successfully pass the Performance Test. Make an appointment to demonstrate to your instructor your ability to suction.

II. GENERAL PERFORMANCE OBJECTIVE

Following this lesson you will be able to suction the nose, throat, and trachea correctly and safely.

III. SPECIFIC PERFORMANCE OBJECTIVES

When you have completed this lesson, you will be able to:

1. Safely and correctly suction the nasal passageway.
2. Safely and correctly suction the throat.
3. Safely and correctly suction the pharynx.
4. Provide personal hygiene as required for the patient.
5. Provide safety measures for the patient while carrying out the suctioning procedure.
6. Instruct the patient and the family regarding suctioning.
7. Discuss with the instructor the indications for suctioning.
8. Provide a patent airway for the patient.
9. Describe the indications for nasal or pharyngeal suctioning.

IV. VOCABULARY

bronchioles—terminal ends of the bronchi.
bronchus (plural, bronchi)—one of two branches of the trachea.
cyanosis—slightly bluish, grayish, or dark purple discoloration of the skin due to a deficiency of oxygen (O_2) and an excess of carbon dioxide (CO_2) in blood; caused by gas or any condition interfering with the entrance of air into the respiratory tract, also by overdoses of certain drugs or any form of asphyxiation, or by inadequate oxygenation of blood from any cause.
cough reflex—An involuntary mechanism activated by irritation of a membrane in the respiratory system and producing a cough.
epiglottis—a leaf-shaped lid (pedicle) composed of fibrocartilage that protects the glottis when swallowing; food is shunted into the esophagus and air into the trachea per the action of the epiglottis.
expectorate—to cough up and expel mucus or foreign material from the throat or lungs.
glottis—the sound-producing apparatus of the larynx.

laryngopharynx—lower portion of the pharynx, extending from the cornua of the hyoid bone to the cricoid cartilage of the larynx.
larynx (voice box)—the enlarged upper end of the trachea, a musculocartilaginous structure lined with a mucous membrane.
mucous—resembling, or secreting, mucus (q.v.).
mucopurulent—consisting of mucus and pus.
mucus—a viscid fluid secreted by mucous membranes and glands; it consists of a mucin, leukocytes, inorganic salts, water, and epithelial cells.
mucous plug—a mass of mucus obstructing a portion of the respiratory tract.
naris—external opening of the nasal cavity; the "port of entry" for air. (Nostril)
nasopharynx—posterior nasal space; part of pharynx above the soft palate.
oropharynx—portion of pharynx behind the mouth, between the soft palate and upper portion of the epiglottis.
pharynx—throat, common passageway for food and air.
phlegm—thick mucus from the respiratory tract.
rib retraction—a characteristic action of deep chest inspiration, depressing the ribs and distal portion of the sternum, in permitting uptake of extra oxygen when there is respiratory distress, as in obstruction.
sensorium—a "center of all sensation" in the brain; also, collectively, one's total conscious activity.
stridor—harsh, high-pitched sound during respiration, resembling the blowing of the wind and caused by obstruction of an air passage.
suction—the act or capacity of sucking up by reducing the air pressure over part of the surface of a substance.
tenacious—adhering to, adhesive, retentive; e.g., tenacious mucus is mucus that adheres to the lining of the respiratory tract.
trachea (windpipe)—a four and one-half inch tube extending from the larynx to the bronchial tubes, lined with a mucous membrane and cilia, for continuous moistening and cleaning of the air.

V. INTRODUCTION

You will recall from Volume II, Unit 29, on "Care of Patients Receiving Oxygen Therapy" that regular breathing (respiration) is essential to life. Breathing is controlled by the respiratory centers located in the medulla and pons of the brain as well as by peripheral centers composed of clusters of chemosensitive cells known as carotid bodies and aortic bodies. Through the act of breathing in (inspiration), we take in air (which has 20.93 per cent oxygen (O_2) and 79.02 per cent nitrogen (N_2) and carry it to the respiratory system (nose, pharynx, larynx, trachea, bronchi, and lungs). The oxygen is absorbed into the circulatory system, which in turn carries it to all parts of the body. The oxygen content in the blood is a necessary chemical component upon which all tissues and living cells depend. Without oxygen some cells may die in as little as 30 seconds.

When oxygen is prevented from entering the blood stream in the proper concentration, steps must be taken to assist the patient in getting more oxygen into his system. Disease or obstruction in the respiratory tract prevent the proper intake of oxygen.

<u>Obstruction of the airway is one of the most common forms of respiratory failure</u>s and one which is most easily reversed. Obstruction of the air passages may occur in the following situations:

A. When there is an interference with the cough reflex, which would normally clear the air passage of mucus or foreign object in the throat, e.g., in patients with a depressed sensorium (resulting from a head injury, overdose of medications, or metabolic disturbance).

B. Increased mucus production resulting from various diseases, such as bronchitis, reaction to anesthesia, or certain medications.

C. Anatomical blockage of trachea due to edema, tumor, etc.

D. Damage to the ciliated lining of the pharynx.

Common signs and symptoms you may observe in your patient who is not getting enough oxygen are as follows:

A. He may comment that he "can't breathe" or he feels as though he is suffocating.

B. He will appear restless and irritable, anxious or frightened (he won't know why).

C. He will have decreased muscle coordination, slowed mental capacities, and possible disorientation. (Remember, *all* living tissue must have oxygen in order to continue proper functioning.)

D. He may become dyspneic (have difficulty breathing). He may have rib retraction if dyspnea becomes severe.

E. He may become cyanotic (bluish in color) as a result of diminished oxygen content in the blood.

F. He may increase the rate and depth of respirations to try to get enough oxygen from the air to supply the needs of the body. Stridor may be present. Rattling or gurgling sounds may be heard.

G. He may faint (syncope) or complain of vertigo (dizziness) caused by a lack of oxygen in the brain.

ITEM 1: NASOPHARYNGEAL SUCTIONING

Mucus that accumulates in the throat and mouth is usually expectorated. In patients whose sensorium is depressed, however, the cough reflex may be depressed or ineffective. Mechanical removal of the secretions must therefore be accomplished through the procedure called *suctioning*.

Mucus may also accumulate in the nostrils. If the patient is alert, he can blow his nose to clear the nasal passage. If he is unconscious, you will need to remove the secretions by suctioning. Before beginning the procedure, check and prepare supplies at the patient's bedside. Be sure all equipment is complete and in working order. Check the suction tubing to be sure that there are no holes in it and be sure the suction machine is plugged into the electrical outlet and turned on. Test the vacuum ranges on the pressure gauge by placing your thumb over the Y-connector or thumb control. Regulate the suction (vacuum) range for the patient, which is usually expressed in inches or mm of mercury.

This procedure generally is carried out using medical asepsis (clean technique). In specific cases aseptic technique may be required, e.g., in isolation or with patients in reverse isolation. If a sterile procedure is used, follow procedures learned in Unit 1, "Aseptic Technique," for gloving and using sterile supplies. The actual suctioning procedure will be as follows:

Important Steps	Key Points
1. Wash your hands.	Use germicidal soap.
2. Identify the patient and explain the procedure.	Reassure the patient, talk calmly, and move slowly and precisely. Connect suction tubing. Test patency of tubing by running some solution through it.
	Explain each step of the procedure to the patient so that he will be less fearful and more cooperative.

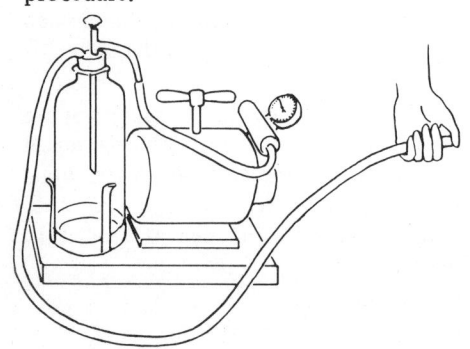

PHARYNGEAL SUCTIONING

Important Steps	Key Points
3. Position the patient.	Usually a semi-Fowler's position is most comfortable for the patient and permits an unobstructed view of the mouth and nose for correct suctioning. The dorsal recumbent position may also be used. However, the head should be turned toward you for ease in viewing the oral cavity.
4. Select the catheter. 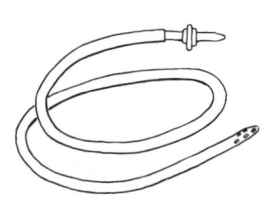	Usually a disposable plastic or rubber French catheter, size 12 to 14, is used. In some agencies catheters may be reprocessed and reused. Follow your agency's procedure. It will have either a glass Y-connector or a thumb control suction valve to control the negative pressure within the tubing (to draw the secretions through the tubing into the vacuum bottle). Select the size of the catheter according to the size of the nostrils and the amount of secretions to be removed. You may use a smaller size of catheter (8 to 12 French) for thin secretions; larger catheters (12 to 16 French) may be needed for the adult having thick secretions.
5. Measure the catheter for insertion.	On the catheter measure the distance from the tip of the nose to the tip of the ear (about 5 inches).
6. Insert the suction catheter. 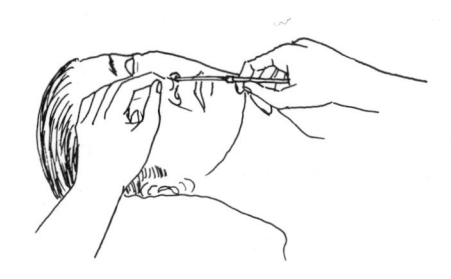	Insert it into the right naris about 3 to 5 inches. Generally, there are fewer septal deviations in the right naris. If you meet an obstruction, remove the catheter and try the left naris. If you find an obstruction here too, remove the catheter and call for assistance. Close the suction valve or open Y with your thumb. Moisten tip with water or water-soluble lubricant. NOTE: If patient's cough reflex is stimulated, remove catheter until coughing stops, then proceed.
7. Remove the catheter.	Remove slowly, using a rotating motion. Suction approximately 15 seconds at a time. (Keep thumb over suction control.) The rotating movement cleans the secretions on all sides of the nostril and prevents pulling on the mucous membrane. *Remember:* You are not only suctioning secretions, but also oxygen.

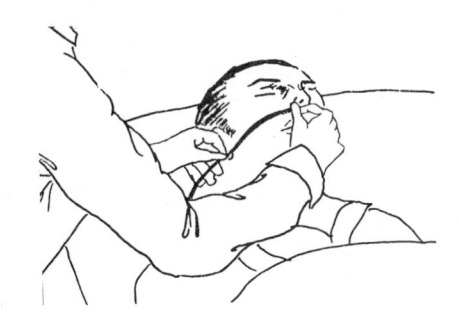

Important Steps	Key Points
8. Rinse the catheter.	Place distal end of catheter into container of irrigating solution (distilled water, saline, or whatever solution your agency uses). With the thumb over the suction valve or open Y, run solution through the catheter and tubing until the solution runs clear into the suction bottle of the suction machine.
9. Repeat suctioning of the right naris.	Repeat if indicated, then cleanse catheter as in Step 8 before proceeding.
10. Insert the catheter.	Insert into left naris about 3 to 5 inches. Close suction valve or open Y with thumb.
11. Remove the catheter.	Slowly remove the catheter using a rotating motion, keeping thumb over the suction control.
12. Rinse the catheter.	Rinse in cleansing solution until solution returns clear into the suction bottle.
13. Tell the patient to cough.	Instruct patient if he is alert. This will bring secretions up to the back of the nose and throat so they can easily be suctioned.
14. Reinsert the catheter into each naris.	This will remove additional secretions. *Remember: Suctioning periods should be brief. Permit your patient to rest between suctioning.* This is a very tiring, frightening procedure for the patient.
15. Remove the catheter.	Rinse the catheter as in Step 8. Observe the patient at all times for hypoxia. Talk calmly to him. Reassure him and inform him about each step. Place the catheter on the tray at the patient's side. Turn off suction machine.
16. Leave patient comfortable.	Fluff pillows, straighten and tighten linens, and change soiled bedding as needed. Give mouth care to keep the oral mucosa moist and eliminate halitosis.
	Leave the call light within easy reach of the patient. Adjust the bed for comfort and raise siderail if appropriate. Tell the patient when you will return.
17. Remove soiled items.	Replace suction catheter with clean catheter, ready for next use. You may need to suction in an emergency, so you should always be prepared. Empty the suction jar and replenish irrigating solution as needed.
18. Record on patient's chart.	Charting example:
	1:15 A.M. Nasopharyngeal suctioning employed. Large amounts of mucopurulent liquid obtained. Putrid odor. Cooperates readily.

M. Herrick, S.N.

ITEM 2: OROPHARYNGEAL SUCTIONING

Oropharyngeal suctioning (sometimes called mouth suctioning) is carried on as in the above procedure except that the catheter is inserted directly into the mouth instead of through the nose. The same precautions are followed in this procedure as for nasopharyngeal suctioning.

The gag reflex may be stimulated more easily with this procedure, which would make the patient cough violently. This is distasteful and irritating to the patient. The coughing and gagging with this type of suctioning may also cause a serious drop in the blood oxygen levels and may lead to cardiac arrest, particularly in the debilitated patient. For the unconscious patient you may need to depress the patient's tongue so that you have good access to the entire oral cavity. Sometimes tracheal suctioning is done expressly to initiate coughing so that the patient can bring up deep secretions without necessitating deep tracheobronchial suctioning. To remind yourself about the amount of oxygen you are withdrawing from the patient, hold your breath during the procedure. When you have a need to breathe, release the suction valve so that the patient can also take in some oxygen.

A firm metal suction tip may be used instead of the soft catheter. A common metal suction tip is called the Yankauer. Since it is rigid it does not coil up in the mouth. In addition, because it is rigid, you must insert it gently to avoid bruising or tearing the oral mucosa. Since it is not as flexible as the catheter, it may be difficult to reach pooled secretions in the posterior oral cavity.

Note: Do not interchange catheters. In other words, use separate catheters for nose, mouth, and pharynx.

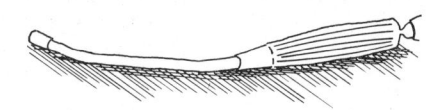

ITEM 3: BULB SYRINGE SUCTIONING

This procedure is carried out on infants to rid the nasal and oral passageways of secretions.

Important Steps	Key Points
1. Wash your hands.	
2. Identify the patient.	Check the identification band. This point is important with the infant since he cannot respond to questioning.
3. Position the infant.	Usually position in the dorsal recumbent position.
4. Select a syringe.	Take the syringe in your right hand. Cover the bulb portion with the palm of your hand.

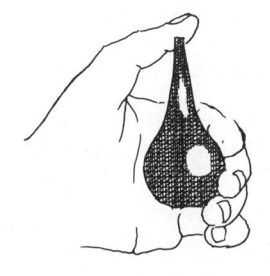

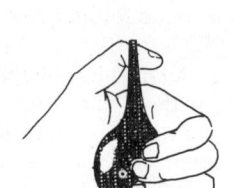

Important Steps	Key Points
5. Make a fist.	This will squeeze the bulb and express the air from the syringe.
6. Insert the tip in the external naris. (or mouth).	Be gentle; do not injure the delicate mucosa of the infant.
7. Release the bulb.	As the air returns to the bulb of the syringe, it will provide a sucking action, which will withdraw the secretions.
8. Express the secretions from the syringe.	When the bulb is fully inflated, remove the distal tip from the naris or mouth and make a fist over the bulb of the syringe. This will express the air and force the secretions out.
9. Dispose of the secretions.	Dispose on a gauze or in a basin, which is usually supplied as part of the bulb syringe set.
10. Rinse the syringe.	You may need to rinse the syringe. Use the same motion of closing your fist over the bulb. However, be sure the tip end is placed in the basin with water (or any solution your agency uses). Allow the bulb to expand and fill with water.
	Express the water into the waste basin by closing your fist over the bulb portion. Repeat suctioning as needed to keep the infant's respiratory passages free.
11. Store the supplies.	They are usually kept at the bedside. Clean and replenish items as needed. Empty waste basin in patient's bathroom, rinse it with cool water, and return it to the bedside for future use.
12. Position the infant.	Position him on his side for easy drainage of secretions from his mouth. You may have to prop the infant on his side by placing a rolled blanket at his back for support.
13. Record on patient's chart.	Charting example:
	7:10 A.M. Oral aspiration carried out, moderate amount of thin, clear mucus obtained. Breathing easier.
	T. Freeland, S.N.

ITEM 4: TECHNIQUES TO STIMULATE COUGHING

Mechanical stimulation of the trachea can be used to produce vigorous coughing and assist the patient to bring up deep bronchial secretions. If coughing can be stimulated, deep tracheobronchial suctioning may be avoided (this procedure is included in Unit 8, "Tracheostomy Care"). Deep coughing can prevent respiratory complications (obstruction, pneumonia, etc.).

A. External Mechanical Tracheal Stimulation

Important Steps	Key Points
1. Wash you hands.	
2. Approach and identify the patient, and explain the procedure.	It is extremely important that you explain what you are about to do so that the patient can fully cooperate. This is a disagreeable procedure for the patient and can be very painful if the patient is a recent post-op.
3. Place your fingers on patient's anterior neck.	Thumb and forefinger are placed on either side of the trachea. See the illustration.
4. Move your fingers up and down.	Using a firm, steady pressure, move from the prominences of the clavicle up toward the chin. Movement will be approximately 1/2 to 1 inch in length.
5. Talk to the patient.	Keep the patient calm and cooperative. The external irritation you are applying usually will trigger coughing. You should have the suction machine available if the patient cannot get up the secretions.

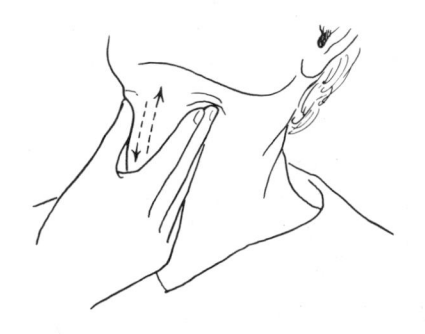

Important Steps	Key Points
6. Provide gauze or an emesis basin.	The emesis basin is for the patient to cough into. You may need to splint the patient's operative site with your hand or a pillow to minimize pain in the operative site. (If you have forgotten the procedure, review Volume II, Unit 23, "Collection of Sputum and Gastric Specimens, and Care of the Vomiting Patient."
7. Position the patient for comfort.	Reassure the patient to prevent the procedure from becoming too tiring or disagreeable. Leave the patient in a comfortable position. Replace siderails if indicated. Leave call light within easy reach. Offer a drink. Remember to keep the mucous membranes moist. Tell the patient when you will return.
8. Record on patient's chart.	Charting example: 10:15 A.M. Coughing was produced by external pressure over trachea. Large amount of thick mucopurulent secretion raised. Complained of being tired. Positioned for comfort in semi-Fowler's. M. Anderson, S.N.

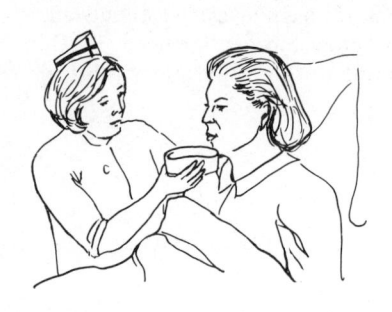

B. Forceful Exhalation to Induce Coughing

Important Steps	Key Points
1. Wash your hands.	
2. Approach and identify the patient, and explain the procedure.	You must gain cooperation from the patient. He must understand the procedure.
3. Instruct the patient to take a *deep* breath.	Talk quietly and calmly. Reassure the patient. Observe patient closely for anoxia.
4. Instruct the patient to breathe out *slowly*.	Talk to the patient. Ask him to breathe slower. Have him breathe out until all air is exhaled. The air flowing slowly through the trachea dries the tracheal mucosa, permitting a slight carbon dioxide build-up, which in turn seems to trigger the cough mechanism. The success of this effort depends on *forceful* exhalation of the air slowly over a period of time.

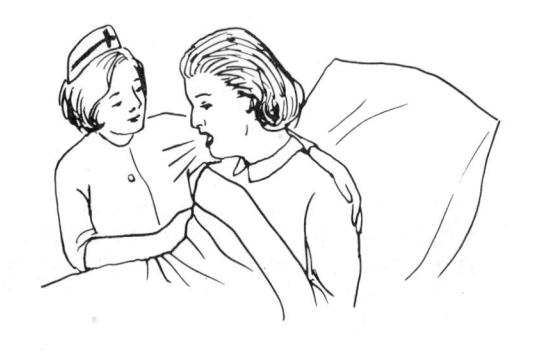

Important Steps	Key Points
5. Repeat Steps 3 and 4.	Usually the patient will need to practice this procedure, since normal exhalation is easiest for the patient. He will have to concentrate on forced, slow exhalations.
	Continue to reassure the patient and encourage him. Remind him of the more disagreeable alternative of mechanical stimulation of the trachea with a catheter. *Do not threaten the patient.* Explain the advantages of his voluntarily bringing up secretions versus the mechanical means which could be employed.
6. Collect the sputum.	Use a gauze or basin according to your agency's policy.
7. Leave the patient comfortable.	Observe the patient for change in color, rate and sound of respirations. Position the patient in comfort, e.g., semi-Fowler's position. Fluff pillows and tighten bedding. Leave call light within easy reach and adjust siderails if indicated. Tell the patient when you will return.
8. Record on patient's chart.	Charting example:
	11:30 A.M. Secretions were easily brought up using the deep breathing method to stimulate coughing. Small amount of clear, thin mucus was obtained.
	B. Kahn, S.N.

ITEM 5: PHARYNGEAL AND ENDOTRACHEAL SUCTIONING

Although this is a common procedure, it is one that does interfere with arterial oxygenation. The decrease in oxygen in the alveoli is directly proportional to the amount of suction (negative pressure) and the length of time the procedure takes. In other words, a high pressure and a lengthy suctioning time decrease the amount of oxygen measurably. If the patient is old or in a debilitated condition, the suctioning can set off cardiac arrhythmias or, at the extreme, cardiac arrest.

You can frequently determine the need to suction by the respiratory sounds. A coarse, heavy, rattling breathing sound indicates thick, tenacious mucus. A fine, light, bubbly sound (like air bubbling through water) indicates thin mucus, which accumulates in large amounts. The pulse rate can increase or decrease depending on the amount of respiratory tract obstruction.

Important Steps	Key Points
1. Check supplies to be sure they are available and in working order.	Be sure the suction machine (portable or wall-mounted) is connected to the electrical outlet. Suction setting:

Portable

Adult: 7 to 15 inches Hg (mercury)
Infant: 5 to 10 inches Hg (mercury)

Wall-mounted

Adult: 120 to 150 mm Hg (mercury)
Infant: 60 to 100 mg Hg (mercury)

PHARYNGEAL SUCTIONING

Important Steps	Key Points
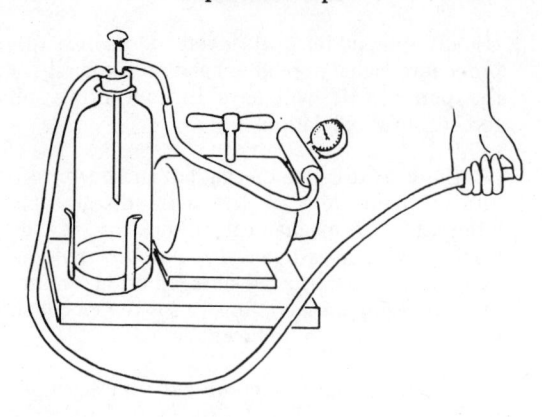 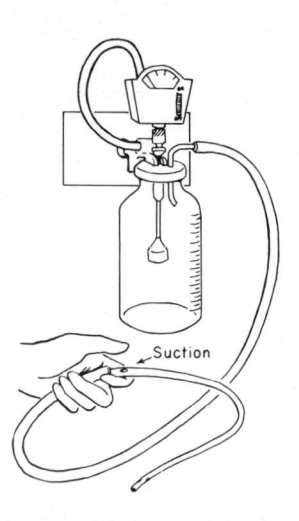	Check tubing to be sure there are no holes or kinks in it. Run solution through tubing to be sure it is clear. Open sterile catheter package, a package of 4 by 4 inch gauze, aspiration (suction) set, and sterile gloves on bedside stand.

Portable suction

Wall-mounted suction

2. Wash your hands.

Use germicidal soap and dry hands thoroughly.

3. Approach and identify the patient, and explain the procedure.

Explain the total procedure to the patient. Gain his cooperation. This is most important because these patients, if alert, are usually apprehensive.

4. Prepare the suction catheter.

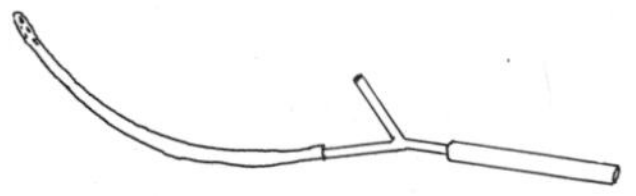

Using aseptic technique, remove catheter from the package and attach to Y-connection of the suction tubing. Leave catheter tip in sterile wrapping (remove catheter just far enough so that it can easily be attached to the suction tubing).

5. Position the patient.

Provide for privacy by drawing curtains or closing the door. Raise bed to working height. Unless contraindicated, have the patient sit in an upright position. Lower proximal siderail if appropriate.

6. Turn on the suction machine.

7. Wash your hands and put on sterile gloves.

Use aseptic technique.

Important Steps	Key Points
8. Pick up a sterile 4 by 4 inch piece of gauze.	Use your left hand. Ask the patient to stick out his tongue so that you can hold it. This prevents the tongue from falling into the back of the throat and shutting off breathing. Pulling the tongue out and straight forward also raises the epiglottis and permits easier insertion of the catheter.
9. Ask the patient to inhale.	With your right hand, grasp catheter between thumb and forefinger. While continuing to hold tongue securely with left hand, introduce catheter carefully toward the posterior of the mouth. Keep patient breathing evenly, no talking.
10. Introduce the catheter into the trachea.	At this point the patient will probably cough. Relax the tongue and ask the patient to breathe normally. NOTE: If the patient can bring up enough secretions from the coughing generated by the tracheal stimulation, the remainder of the procedure may not be needed.
11. Suction.	Place your right thumb over the open Y-connector; this creates a negative pressure in the catheter and draws the mucus up through the catheter. Aspirate for brief periods (5 to 10 seconds). Permit the patient to rest between suctionings to allow him to oxygenate again. Frequent catheter insertions are irritating to the tracheal mucosa. Introduce catheter carefully, and suction thoroughly but quickly.
12. Observe the patient throughout and after the procedure.	Be alert for color change, change in respiration, or increased belligerence or disorientation (which may be an indication of anoxia). Listen to changing breath sounds. As secretions are removed, the breathing should become quiet again.
13. Rinse the catheter.	Rinse as needed between suctionings to keep lumen open and free of secretions.

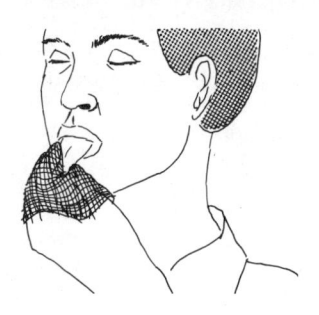

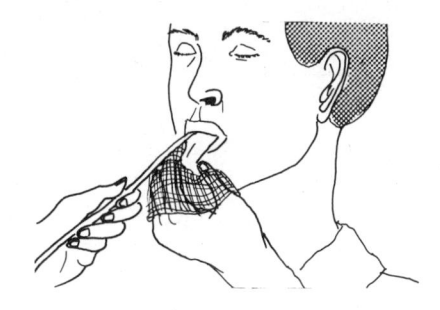

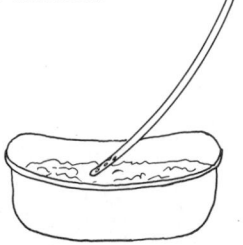

Important Steps	Key Points
14. Remove the catheter and gloves.	This should be done only after the patient's respiratory tract is clear.
15. Give mouth care.	This is comforting to the patient. It keeps the oral mucosa moist and helps eliminate halitosis. Dry mucosa can be a site for entrance of microorganisms.
16. Position the patient for comfort.	Leave the patient in a comfortable position; e.g., semi-Fowler's. Raise siderail if indicated. Fluff pillow and tighten bedding. Change soiled linens as needed. Place call light within easy reach. Tell patient when you expect to return.
17. Discard used items.	Replenish supplies as needed.
18. Record on patient's chart.	Charting example:

3:45 A.M. Tracheal suctioning done. Obtained small amount of clear, thin secretion.

J. Jones S.N.

POST-TEST

Indicate answers by circling the letters "T" for true and "F" for false.

T (F) 1. Sterile technique is essential for intratracheal suctioning.

T (F) 2. A "Y" connecting tube is not essential for suctioning secretions from the tracheobronchial tree.

(T) F 3. The upright position is recommended for the suctioning procedures.

T (F) 4. Mechanical stimulation of coughing always accompanies nasal suctioning.

(T) F 5. You should introduce the catheter as the patient inhales.

(T) F 6. You should connect the catheter to the Y-connector before inserting the catheter.

(T) F 7. Periods of aspirations must be brief (5 to 10 seconds).

T (F) 8. Mouth care is not essential after the suctioning procedure.

Fill in the blanks.

9. Enumerate five signs of airway obstructions:
    a. Pt. states he can't breathe.
    b. Restless, irritable, anxious, frightened.
    c. ↓ muscle coordination; disorientation.
    d. Dyspnea; rib retraction
    e. Cyanotic, ↑ pulse & respiration, syncope, vertigo.

10. Position indicated for suctioning the alert adult patient is Semi-Fowler's .

11. The decrease of oxygen in the alveoli during endotracheal suctioning is directly proportional to amt suction pressure , and to length of time suction catheter is in place .

12. Use of sterile normal saline would assist in cleansing catheter of secretions.

13. Determining the approximate depth to which the catheter is to be inserted is done by measuring the distance from the tip of the nose to the ear .

14. Indicate four physiologic malfunctionings in which normal removal of secretions is difficult and necessitates suctioning:
    a. Interference c̄ cough reflex .
    b. diseases (bronchitis) meds, anesthesia .
    c. Anatomical blockage of trachea (tumor, edema)
    d. Damage to ciliated lining of pharynx.

POST-TEST ANNOTATED ANSWER SHEET

1. F, p. 256.
2. F, p. 256.
3. T, p. 249.
4. F, p. 249.
5. T, p. 257.
6. T, p. 249.
7. T, p. 257.
8. F, p. 258.
9. a. States he cannot breathe, p. 248.
   b. Restless, irritable, anxious, frightened.
   c. Decreased muscle coordination, disorientation.
   d. Dyspnea, rib retraction.
   e. Cyanotic, increased pulse and respiration, syncope, vertigo.
10. Semi-Fowler's position, p. 249.
11. Amount of suction pressure, length of time the suction catheter is in place, p. 255.
12. cleansing the catheter of, p. 250.
13. nose; ear, p. 249.
14. a. interference with the cough reflex, p. 247.
    b. various diseases (e.g., bronchitis, certain medicines), anesthesia.
    c. anatomical blockage or trachea (e.g., tumor, edema).
    d. damage to ciliated lining of the pharynx.

PERFORMANCE TEST

1. Given a mannequin in the skill laboratory, you will correctly suction the oral cavity, the nares, or both.

2. Demonstrate the procedure for external irritation of the trachea to produce coughing.

3. Demonstrate on the laboratory mannequin the technique for tracheal suctioning.

PERFORMANCE CHECKLIST

1. Check time on nurses' notes and with charge nurse prior to starting procedure.
2. Obtain supplies and equipment.
3. Wash hands.
4. Explain procedure and reassure patient.
5. Provide privacy.
6. Position patient.
7. Adjust bed to working height.
8. Turn on suction machine.
9. Use aseptic technique if procedure is to be done aseptically.
10. Be able to determine approximate depth to which the catheter is to be inserted nasopharyngeally and oropharyngeally.
11. Adhere to specific time allotted for aspiration.
12. Be able to insert catheter via airway for oropharyngeal suctioning.
13. Provide mouth care.
14. Provide for patient's comfort and safety.
15. Wash hands.
16. Record significant observations on patient's chart.
17. Clean and replenish used items.

Unit 8

TRACHEOSTOMY CARE

I. DIRECTIONS TO THE STUDENT

Read this lesson carefully. It includes the care of the tracheostomy tube and the removal, cleaning and reinsertion of the inner cannula. After you have completed the lesson, take the post-test and practice in the skill laboratory. Demonstrate to your instructor your ability to care for the tracheostomy tube.

II. GENERAL PERFORMANCE OBJECTIVE

Following this lesson you will be able to care for the patient who has a tracheostomy tube.

III. SPECIFIC PERFORMANCE OBJECTIVES

Upon completion of this lesson, you will be able to:

1. Identify the different types of tracheostomy tubes and their component parts.
2. Provide a patent airway for the patient.
3. Discuss with the instructor the indications for a tracheostomy.
4. Provide the special personal hygiene required for the patient.
5. Eliminate hazards to the patient who has a tracheostomy tube inserted.
6. Suction the tracheo-bronchial tree without injury to the patient and without dislodging the tracheostomy tube.

IV. VOCABULARY

Read the definitions of the terms listed below. Do not attempt to memorize these definitions before proceeding with the lesson. Each term will be explained or defined again in the text. On completion of the lesson, however, you should know the correct definitions of these terms.

Adam's apple—laryngeal prominence of the voice box (larynx).
aphonia—loss of voice.
asphyxia—a decrease in the amount of oxygen (O_2) and an increased amount of carbon dioxide (CO_2) in the body as a result of some interference with respiration, which can cause unconsciousness and death.
bifurcation—a structure that divides off into two branches.
bronchi—the two subdivisions of the trachea.
bronchiole—a terminal end of the bronchi.
cannula—a tube or sheath enclosing a trocar or obturator such that when free of the trocar, it permits free flow of liquid from the body.
carina—point of division of the trachea into the two main bronchi.
cartilaginous—pertaining to or consisting of cartilage, which is a dense type of connective tissue forming part of the skeletal system. (Cartilage is firm and compact and can stand

much pressure or tension; it has no nerve or blood supply of its own. Cartilage is found in the septum of the nose, the trachea, larynx, knee joints, etc.)

cilia—microscopic, hair-like projections lining the respiratory tract. (Active motion of the cilia moves the air through the respiratory tract.)

copious—plentiful, excessive.

cuff—an encircling part; e.g., a tracheal cuff is an inflatable balloon cuff surrounding the distal portion of a tracheostomy tube, which when inflated provides a leak-proof ventilating system.

edema—a condition in which the body tissue contains an excessive amount of tissue fluid; it can be local or generalized.

endotracheal—endo=within; tracheal=trachea; e.g., endotracheal tube is one that is inserted into the trachea, usually through the nose or mouth, to provide an open airway in an unconscious or anesthetized patient.

erosion—an eating away (of tissue), or destruction (of tissues) at the surface layer.

esophagus—a 9-inch musculomembranous canal that extends from the pharynx to the stomach; an upper portion of the digestive system.

glottis—the sound-producing apparatus of the larynx consisting of two vocal folds.

halitosis—offensive (bad) breath.

hyoid—a bone at the anterior surface of the neck at the root of the tongue.

hypoxia (anoxia)—lack of an adequate amount of oxygen in inspired air; low O_2 content in the tissues.

larynx—the voice box, which rests on top of the trachea; an upper portion of the respiratory system.

lumen—the opening within a tube, blood vessel, or intestine.

obturator—anything that obstructs or closes a cavity or opening (e.g., tracheal obturator, a part of a tracheostomy tube set; it obstructs the outer cannula and is used for the initial insertion of the tracheostomy tube).

trachea (windpipe)—4 1/2-inch cartilaginous tube extending from the larynx to the bronchial tree.

trachelotomy—incision into the cervix (neck) of the uterus (womb).

tracheostomy—an incision into the trachea, usually made for insertion of a tube to overcome tracheal obstruction.

trocar—a sharp pointed instrument used with a cannula to pierce a cavity wall or for removing small pieces of tissue for microscopic examination.

sternum (breast bone)—the narrow flat bone in the middle of the anterior thorax to which the ribs attach.

stoma—a mouth or small opening; an artificially created opening between two cavities or passages, as in tracheostomy.

viscid—sticky, adhering, gummy.

V. INTRODUCTION

You will recall from your units on Volume 2, Unit 29, "Care of Patients Receiving Oxygen Therapy" and Volume 2, Unit 30, "Cardiopulmonary Resuscitation" that a patent (open) airway (trachea or windpipe) is essential for the preservation of life. Review these two units if you feel that you have forgotten the brief introduction to the anatomy and physiology of the respiratory system.

For this lesson we will concentrate on the trachea. The trachea is a 4½ inch tube that extends from the larynx downward and divides (bifurcates) at the distal end (carina) into the right and left bronchi. The trachea filters, warms, and moistens the air by means of the ciliated mucous lining. The trachea lies directly in front of the esophagus.

If you place your fingers *gently* in the hollow of the neck above the sternum and just below the Adam's apple (laryngeal prominence), you will find ridges. Do you feel them? These ridges are C-shaped cartilagenous rings (16 to 20 in number) which lie one above the other. They are embedded posteriorly in smooth muscle and are also separated by bands of smooth muscle. The cartilage provides stability for the trachea and prevents its collapse and resultant obstruction of the air flow. The intervening bands of muscles between the cartilages provide for flexibility so that the head can be bent and raised.

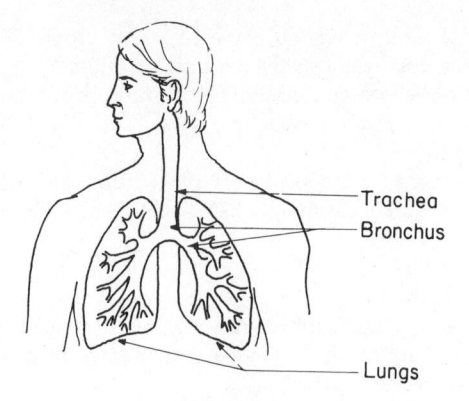

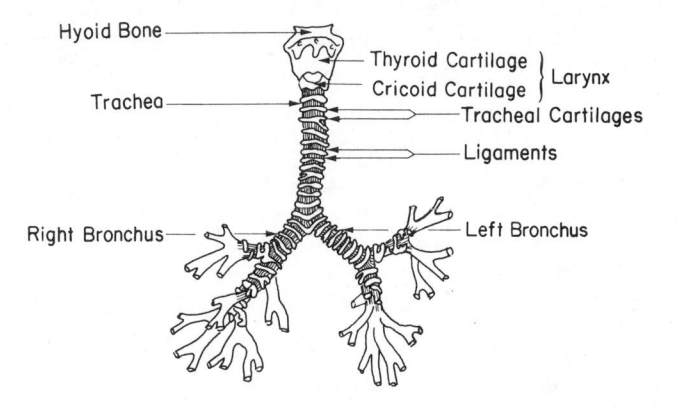

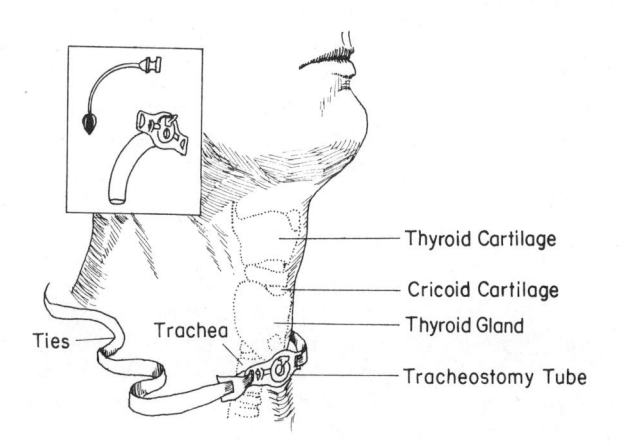

The hyoid bone, the thyroid cartilage, and the cricoid cartilage (see above diagram) provide prominent landmarks on the neck when a tracheostomy must be performed. A tracheostomy is a surgical procedure in which an opening is made into the trachea for the insertion of a tube through which the patient can breathe when he has a tracheal obstruction. A tracheostomy is performed when an endotracheal tube (which is passed through the nose or mouth) cannot be inserted or is contraindicated by the patient's condition, e.g., in a severely burned or unconscious patient who cannot tolerate the tube, or in a case of serious infection. Using aseptic technique, a horizontal incision is made (usually by the physician) in the neck just below the first tracheal ring. The curved tracheostomy tube with the obturator in place is inserted into the opening. After insertion, the obturator is removed so that the patient can breathe. The inner cannula (if there is one) is then inserted and locked into place. The tube is held in place by means of tapes which are tied snugly around the patient's neck.

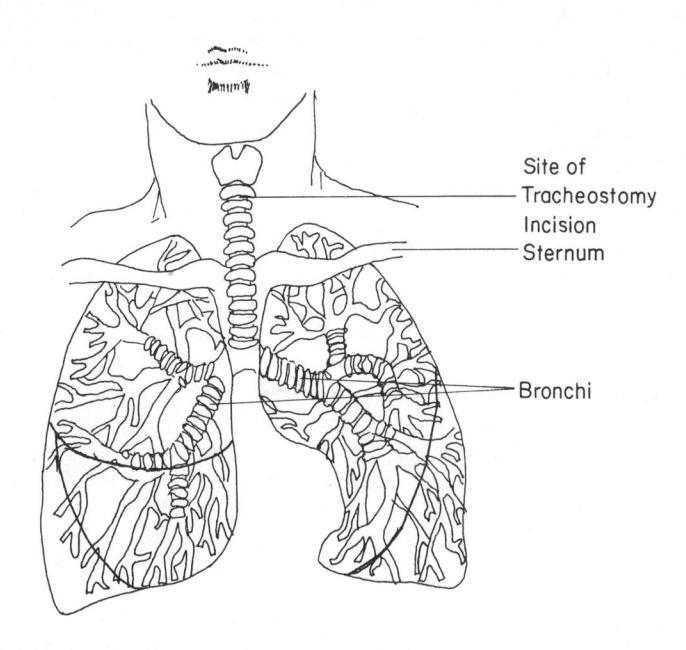

Site of Tracheostomy Incision
Sternum
Bronchi

A tracheostomy can be temporary or permanent, depending on the patient's condition. It can be done as a non-emergency procedure in the operating room or as an emergency procedure at the bedside, again depending on the patient's condition and the physician's wishes. A tracheostomy is done for the following reasons:

a) To establish and maintain a patent airway.

b) To remove secretions in the tracheobronchial tree when the patient is unable to cough adequately.

c) When a patient cannot tolerate an endotracheal tube.

d) To prevent aspiration of secretions in the unconscious or paralyzed patient.

e) To treat a patient who needs assisted ventilation (IPPB) and cannot tolerate an O_2 mask or catheter.

The patient who has a tracheostomy is usually very apprehensive, fearful of choking, and of being unable to breathe.

The tube resting in the trachea causes irritation to the tissues, which results in an increased production of secretion. The patient may be unable to clear his trachea of the secretions and therefore he must be suctioned frequently. Unless the secretions are removed promptly, the patient can be asphyxiated. Tracheal suctioning will be discussed later in this Unit. Because of the opening in the windpipe, the air is not forced up from the lungs past the vocal cords into the larynx—therefore, the patient cannot speak. Reassure him that he will be able to speak again when the tracheostomy tube is removed. Being unable to call for help when needed is very frightening. Reassure your patient that you will be observing him frequently. Be sure that his call signal is placed within easy reach. Sedatives to calm the patient are used with extreme caution because they depress the respiratory activity. The nurse must be in close contact with the patient to assist him to breathe easily. Placing the patient in a semi-Fowler's position, unless contraindicted, assists in breathing by permitting the lungs to expand fully and provides comfort because the abdominal contents cause less pressure on the diaphragm.

Frequently, magic slates are used so that the patient can write messages. You can also ask your questions in such a way that he can respond by nodding, moving his head, blinking his eyelids, etc. The <u>patient can talk briefly if the opening in the tracheostomy tube is covered with a finger while he speaks. This closes the tracheostomy tube and permits the air to flow over the vocal cords.</u>

Tracheostomy tubes are made of plastic, rubber, or metal. The rubber and plastic tubes are available plain or with inflatable cuffs that are attached around the distal portion of the tube. The cuffed tubes are preferred when the patient must be placed on an assisted ventilation machine (IPPB). The cuffed tube provides a closed system, assuring more complete ventilation.

Use of the inflated cuff requires alert and precise nursing care. The inflated cuff can decrease the blood supply in the trachea. If the cuff is not deflated at least every hour, the trachea can erode or necrose, causing a massive tracheal hemorrhage. Deflation of the cuff may cause some movement of the tracheostomy tube, which may in turn stimulate the cough reflex. This will bring secretions up so that they can be more readily suctioned. However, a forceful cough could dislodge or expel the tracheostomy tube. If this occurs, the opening in the trachea would quickly close and the patient would be unable to breathe. Therefore, as an emergency precaution, a tracheal dilator, a hemostat, and the obturator for the tracheostomy tube are usually kept attached to the head of the patient's bed so that the tracheostomy opening can be opened and the tube can be quickly re-inserted. (Although this is usually done by a physician, the nurse may need to do it in an emergency.) Tracheostomy tubes are sized according to the diameter of the lumen of the tube.

TABLE 8-1. COMPARISON OF TYPES OF TRACHEOSTOMY TUBES

	Plastic	Rubber	Metal (Silver)
Cost	Relatively inexpensive	Moderately priced	Costly
Sterilization	Cannot be resterilized	Can be sterilized several times	Can be sterilized an indefinite number of times
Consistency and Weight	Lightweight, soft; molds to trachea. Causes very little irritation to tracheal muscosa	Moderate weight, less pliable than plastic. Relatively comfortable	Rigid and heavy; causes tracheal irritation
Care	Easy to care for and dispose of	Easy to care for	More complicated; silver must be polished periodically
Wall Thickness	Large internal diameter	Medium internal diameter	Has smallest internal diameter of the three types
Ease of Connection to Assisted Devices	Easy	Comparatively easy in most products	Relatively difficult although some adapters may be available

Since there are differing size scales depending upon the manufacturer, you will obtain the correct tube according to your agency instructions. In any event, the sizing goes from smaller numbers to larger numbers. Size used is dependent upon the size of the patient's trachea; e.g., the infant size would be considerably smaller than that needed for an adult.

COMPONENTS OF THE TRACHEOSTOMY SET

Some tracheostomy sets are composed of three parts. (These parts *are not interchangeable* with another set.) However, the new plastic tubes usually consist of a single cannula.

A. *inner tube* (or *cannula*)

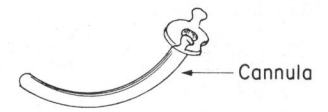

B. *outer tube*

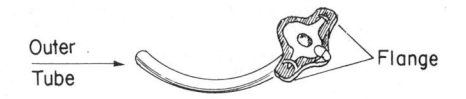

C. The *obturator* is an olive-shaped or bullet-tipped insert which fits the outer tube. It is used during the insertion of the tracheostomy tube to keep the distal end of the tube from tearing the tissue as it is inserted. In other words, the olive-shaped tip extends beyond the lumen of the tube at the distal end and provides a smooth, rounded surface during the insertion. The obturator is removed as soon as the tube is in place so that the patient can breathe; then the inner cannula is inserted and locked into place.

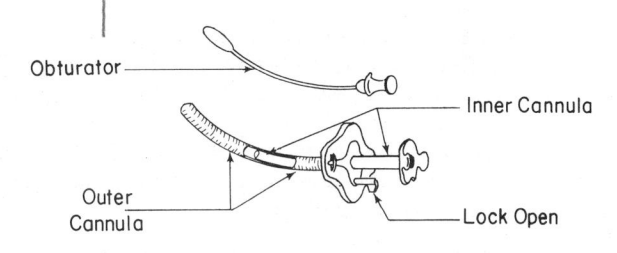

The tube is held in place with ties attached to the outer edges (flanges) of the tracheostomy tube and tied snugly around the patient's neck to keep the tube in place. A dressing is then placed underneath and around the tracheostomy tube to catch the secretions; this dressing is changed prn.

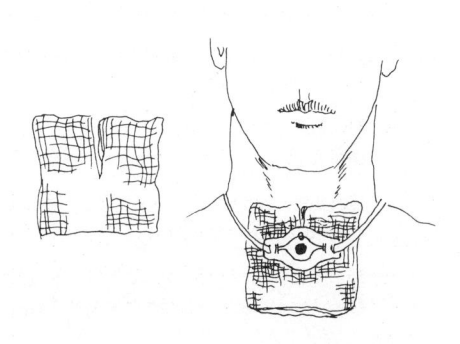

The following equipment is usually kept at the patient's bedside for routine and emergency care. Check your agency procedure for specifics.

1. An extra tracheostomy set and obturator (fited for the patient).
2. Tracheal dilator and/or hemostat to open tracheostomy incision if the tube is expelled.
3. Tracheostomy dressings and ties.
4. Rubber gloves.
5. Pipe cleaners or brush for cleaning the inner cannula.
6. Cleaning solution designated by your agency, e.g., hydrogen peroxide, 2 per cent solution of sodium bicarbonate, sterile saline.
7. Sterile distilled water.
8. Scissors (to cut neck ties in case of emergency).
9. Silver polish for the use of the metal tubes.
10. Suction machine and tubing with Y connector.
11. Sterile disposable suction catheters, usually whistle tip.
12. Medicine dropper.
13. Sterile container for irrigating solution.

Note: Obturator, hemostat, and tracheal dilator may be attached to the head of the bed for easy access in case of emergency. The patient should know that these items are there, and why. Letting the patient know that these extra items are readily available will help to relieve his apprehension and fright.

GENERAL NURSING MEASURES FOR THE TRACHEOSTOMY PATIENT

1. Provide a warm, moist environment for the patient. (Normally this is done as the air moves through the upper respiratory tract). Since the patient now breathes through his tracheostomy tube, the outside air should be warmed (about 80°F, or 28.7°C). Moisture can be provided by: keeping a moistened gauze over the tracheostomy opening, by continuous humidified O_2, by a humidifier, or by a croup tent (for a child). Moist mucous membranes assist in preventing infection and the development of mucopurulent plugs.
2. Maintain an extra sterile tracheostomy, for use in an emergency if replacement is needed.
3. Maintain a functioning suction machine with sterile suction catheter always available. A PATENT AIRWAY MUST BE MAINTAINED AT ALL TIMES TO PREVENT ASPHYXIATION OF THE PATIENT. (Disposable sterile packages containing a glove and suction catheter are available for this purpose.)
4. Keep the tracheobronchial tree free of secretions; careful suctioning must be done as often as needed.
5. Observe frequently for signs of hemorrhage or infection around the site of the incision.
6. Change patient's position frequently to provide comfort and also to prevent decubitus formation.
7. Maintain nutritional intake. Fluids can be swallowed by these patients, although at first they are afraid to try. Stand by and reassure the patient as he takes fluids

TRACHEOSTOMY CARE

slowly. (He may be on IV fluids the first few days). The physician will increase the nutritional intake gradually and the patient will be placed on a soft diet.

8. Give mouth care frequently throughout the day and night. Halitosis is frequent because of the dry oral mucous membranes. Patients are very sensitive to this. Dry mucous membranes also become the site for potential infections. Keep the oral cavity (and teeth) clean and moist.

9. Removal of the tracheostomy tube is done gradually over a period of time. The tracheostomy opening is plugged with a cork for increasing periods. When the patient can permit the plug to remain in for 24 hours, the tube is removed. The incision site is then pulled together with tape, and heals in a few days, after which no air will escape.

10. Give full instructions to the patient on the care and cleaning of his tracheostomy tube if he is discharged with the tube still in place. Many agencies will have a patient education program set up to teach the required care after discharge. Follow your agency procedure.

11. Be alert for the four most common tracheostomy complications that may occur immediately after surgery:

    a. Hemorrhage at the operative site, which can drown the patient if the excessive bleeding is in the trachea, or the bleeding within the tissue can cause enough pressure to obstruct the airway.

    b. Subcutaneous emphysema (O_2 in the subcutaneous tissue) or pneumothorax (introduction of air into pleural cavity, causing the lung to collapse).

    c. Aspiration of secretions or sanguineous secretions into the lung, which could cause pneumonia.

    d. Cardiac arrest due to anoxia during prolonged suctioning.

ITEM 1: CLEANSING THE INNER CANNULA

The inner cannula should be cleansed as often as needed to keep it free from tenacious secretions and crusts. Cleansing should be done quickly and effectively, since secretions will be forming on the outer cannula during this process.

Note: If the patient has a tube with an inflatable cuff, the cuff must be deflated before removing the inner cannula.

Important Steps	Key Points
1. Check the supplies at the patient's bedside.	Be certain that equipment needed for removal and cleaning of inner cannula is available. NOTE: Some agencies may provide a tracheostomy dressing tray. PLAN FOR THE UNEXPECTED—ALWAYS HAVE YOUR SUPPLIES AVAILABLE. REPLENISH SUPPLIES AS USED.
2. Wash your hands.	Wash thoroughly with germicidal soap, and dry hands well.

Important Steps	Key Points
3. Position the patient.	Provide privacy by pulling the curtain or closing the hall door. Position the bed at working height. Remember that maintaining proper body alignment prevents muscle strain for you and your patient. Lower the siderails if indicated. Place the patient in <u>semi-Fowler's position. A pillow under his head permits extension of the neck and facilitates removal of the inner cannula.</u>
	NOTE: When the patient is an infant, it will be necessary to restrain his extremities.
4. Identify the patient and explain the procedure.	Work calmly and efficiently. Remember that having a tracheostomy is a very traumatic experience. Since the patient is unable to talk and his respiratory energy is limited, a means of communication is important. In the immediate postoperative period, writing messages may be a way for the patient to communicate.
	A magic slate is helpful for this purpose, because the words can be erased promptly by raising the plastic cover and the tablet is ready for reuse.
	NOTE: If your agency recommends a sterile procedure, open sterile supplies and put on sterile gloves. Use strict aseptic technique throughout.
5. Suction the inner cannula, if necessary.	Explain each step clearly to the patient during the procedure. As he gets better, involve him in the care as much as possible.
6. Remove the inner cannula.	The outer cannula has a lock that secures the inner cannula. *The turn key (lock) must be unlocked for the removal.* With your left hand, hold the outer cannula securely in place by putting your left thumb and index finger in the neck plate of the tracheostomy tube. Turn the key 1/4 of a clockwise turn to unlock. When unlocked, remove the inner cannula gently by pulling it out toward you.
	NOTE: *Do not force removal.* Seek assistance if you have difficulty in withdrawing the cannula.
7. Place the inner cannula in the container.	Wash it thoroughly with cold distilled water to remove secretions and crusts. Avoid using warm water because it tends to coagulate the secretions. Cleanse the lumen with a moistened pipe cleaner or brush until it is meticulously clean. (Remaining foreign particles could cause irritation or infection.) If incrustations remain, it may be helpful to immerse the cannula in a separate basin filled with a hydrogen peroxide solution. Other solutions which may be used to loosen secretions are 2 per cent sterile sodium bicarbonate solution or a sterile normal saline solution. (Follow agency procedure.)

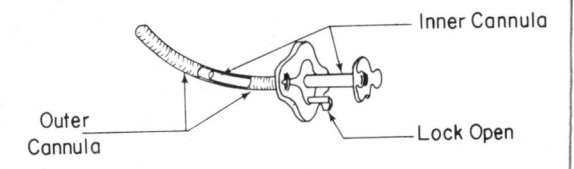

Important Steps	Key Points
	Careful handling of the metal tracheostomy tubes is extremely important. Because they are made of soft metal (silver), these tubes dent easily. A dented tube may not fit the trachea securely or may injure the tissue when the tube is being inserted or removed.
	NOTE: Each agency establishes the procedure for complete exchange of tubes (e.g., weekly); follow agency procedure.
8. Observe the patient carefully.	If he coughs while the inner cannula is out and secretions are brought up, wipe tracheal stoma with designated wipes.
	NOTE: DO NOT use facial tissues to wipe secretions since the lint from these tissues may be inhaled through the trachea and cause additional irritation or blockage to the respiratory tract. Be alert for clues of hypoxia: cyanosis, tachycardia, drop in blood pressure, dyspnea, change in behavior (increasing anxiety, demanding or belligerent attitude). Cyanosis will not occur until arterial oxygenation is less than 85 per cent. In other words, cyanosis is *not* an immediate sign of hypoxia.
9. Rinse and dry the inner cannula.	After a thorough cleansing of the inner cannula, rinse well with prescribed solution, e.g., sterile distilled water or saline. (Follow agency procedure.) REMEMBER: swiftness, with thoroughness, is emphasized because secretions can quickly form in the lumen of the outer tube and obstruct the patient's airway.
	When the inner cannula is meticulously clean, dry it with pipe cleaners or absorbent towels. REMEMBER: the tube must be totally dry; if not, the remaining drops of liquid could be inhaled into the bronchi, causing a violent cough reflex. This could dislodge the outer cannula or cause a irritation which could ultimately result in a type of pneumonia.
	CAUTION: Because there is a possibility of dropping the inner cannula on the floor, a second, sterile tracheostomy tube set should always be available at the patient's bedside to insert in case of emergency.
10. Reinsert the inner cannula.	With your left hand, aspirate the outer cannula with the catheter, if necessary. Hold the outer flange of the cannula with your thumb on one side and index finger on the other. With your right hand, insert the inner cannula into the lumen of the outer cannula. Lock in place by turning the key on the outer cannula 1/4 of a turn counterclockwise. Gently pull on the cannula to see if it is securely locked.
	NOTE: *Do not force.* Gentle insertion is essential to prevent discomfort for the patient.

Important Steps	Key Points
11. Change the dressing.	Cleanse around the tube with a solution and apply a prepared dressing or cut a gauze square as shown in the diagram. Place it under and around the outer cannula (from the bottom up) to catch secretions. This dressing should be changed as often as necessary. During the dressing change care must be taken to prevent the tube from dislodging or moving.
	NOTE: The tapes that hold the outer cannula securely in position may also be changed whenever they become soiled. Cut the tapes at the attachment point on the tracheostomy tube flange and pull them gently from under the patient's neck. Discard into waste container. Apply fresh tape (from dressing tray) by tying it to the flanges on each lateral side of the tracheostomy tube. Slit the end of the tape in half for about one inch; thread one side of the slit through the hole in the flange of the outer tube; tie securely. Repeat with the tape for the other side. Extend the tape ends under and around the patient's neck.
	Tie a secure knot slightly to one side of the neck so that the patient will not have to lie uncomfortably on the knot. Dexterity is needed in tying the tape to avoid dislodging the tracheostomy tube.
12. Give mouth care.	Check the oral cavity. Mouth care includes care of the teeth; use glycerin and lemon swabs or other technique practiced by your agency. The oral cavity becomes dry and frequently has a bad odor. Patients are very sensitive to this.
	NOTE: If the patient has excessive secretions in the mouth and is unable to expectorate, use oral suction to aspirate the secretions (refer to Unit 7).
13. Place the patient in a comfortable position.	Fluff and adjust the pillows; raise the siderails. Adjust the level of the bed as he desires and if indicated. Place the call light within easy reach. Tell him when you expect to return. Ask if there is anything else you can do.
14. Record the procedure on the patient's chart.	Note the time at which it was performed, length of time spent, nature of secretions (color and consistency), and, most importantly, the patient's reactions to the procedure. Record the patient's respiratory rate and color.
	Charting example:
	10:15 A.M. Tracheostomy tube aspirated. Mucus is serosanguineous and tenacious. Inner cannula cleaned and replaced. Procedure tolerated well. Color, respirations and pulse remained stable throughout. Patient cooperative.
	B. Agura, S.N.

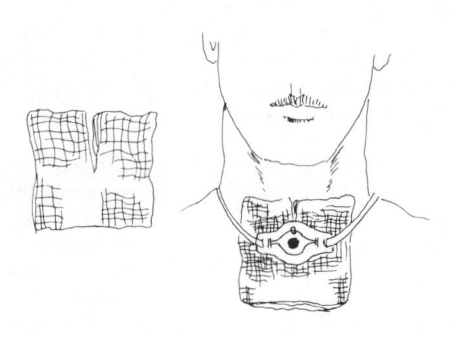

Important Steps	Key Points
15. Clean and replenish articles used from tracheostomy care tray.	Obtain supplies from central supply. Check finally to see that all items are available within easy reach in the event of an emergency situation.

ITEM 2: TRACHEOBRONCHIAL SUCTIONING

Aspiration of secretions following a tracheostomy is of prime importance in maintaining a patent airway. Patients lose their ability to cough effectively because they are unable to develop a high endobronchial pressure behind the closed glottis, a result of the introduction of the tracheostomy tube into the trachea. Therefore, even though the tracheostomy patient appears to be coughing adequately, he is usually less able to expel the tracheobronchial secretions than a person with an intact trachea.

If secretions are copious and seem to come from deep in the tracheobronchial tree, intra-tracheobronchial suctioning is indicated. However, if the secretions seem to be localized around the tracheostomy tube, then suctioning and cleaning of the inner cannula are indicated.

Before beginning the suctioning procedure, observe the patient's respirations (rate and quality). Note the breath sounds (refer to differentiation of breath sounds in Unit 7).

Tracheal suctioning will vary somewhat, depending on the individual patient. However, frequent suctioning ($\bar{q}$ 5 to 15 minutes) may be necessary for the patient with a new tracheostomy who has a large amount of secretions. However, as the incision heals and the patient's condition improves, the frequency of suctioning will decrease measurably.

Note: It cannot be overstressed that *the most critical activity you will carry out for the tracheostomy patient is that of maintaining a patent airway at all times.*

Important Steps	Key Points
1. Wash your hands. Approach and identify the patient.	Explain the procedure to help him understand what is going to happen so that he can cooperate with you. (Do this even though he appears unconscious.)
2. Position the patient.	Elevate the bed to working height. Lower the proximal siderail, if indicated. Move the patient to the proximal side of the bed for ease in working. Adults as well as children are usually most comfortable in the semi-Fowler's position; it enables the patient to breathe easier and gives you an unobstructed view of the tracheostomy tube.
	The infant patient is usually placed in a flat dorsal recumbent position. This prevents his head from falling forward and occluding the airway.
	A small pillow may be placed under the infant's neck and shoulders so that the anterior portion of the neck is slightly elevated for maximum exposure of the tracheostomy tube.
	For the very small infant, it may be necessary to restrain the extremities using the "mummy restraint" described in the unit on Intravenous Observation.

Important Steps	Key Points
3. Check and prepare supplies and equipment.	Be sure that all supplies and equipment are complete and in working order, e.g., suction machine, sterile suction catheters, containers with designated solution for cleansing catheter lumen of mucus, dressings, etc. Be sure that the suction machine is plugged into the wall outlet and turned on. Adjust the amount of suction by the gauge on the machine according to the doctor's orders.
	Sterile suction catheters are used for *each* suctioning. A disposable suction catheter is preferred. However, if reusable rubber catheters are used, they are used once only, then cleaned and resterilized.
	The catheter tips may be smooth and rounded (commonly called the Robinson catheter); or smooth with lateral opening on the tip end (commonly called the whistle tip catheter).
	There may be any number of eyes along the sides of the catheters. A thumb control valve may be built into the catheter, or a separate Y tube may have to be attached to the catheter and the suction machine.
	NOTE: If oral or nasal suctioning is also required, *separate catheters* are used to avoid cross-infection.
	Select a catheter that is 1/2 to 2/3 the size of the lumen of the tracheostomy tube for easy insertion without occluding the airway, yet with a lumen large enough so that mucus can be easily suctioned through it. The suction catheter may be part of the tracheostomy tray. Assemble a syringe with 5 to 10 cc of solution (normal saline or distilled water), which may be inserted into the trachea to liquefy mucus if it is too thick to pull through the suction catheter.
	Open the sterile gloves and sterile dressing tray.
	NOTE: If it is difficult to oxygenate the patient, give him 100 per cent O_2 (by mask or catheter) prior to suctioning.
4. Put on the sterile gloves.	Use aseptic technique. Handle the sterile catheter only with your gloved hand.
	NOTE: Some agencies may advise using only one sterile glove to handle the sterile supplies.
5. Test the patency of the suction catheter.	Place the proximal tip into the solution basin. Withdraw a few cc's of solution through the tubing. By placing your left thumb over the control valve or Y opening, the suction is started. Removing the thumb from the control stops the vacuum, and the water (or drainage) stops moving through the catheter into the vacuum bottle of the suction machine.

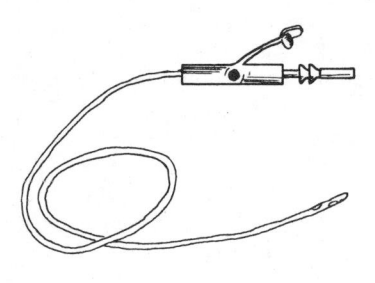

Important Steps	Key Points
6. Assess the patient's level of consciousness.	Make sure that the patient's tracheostomy tube is securely in place. If he is conscious, ask him to cough to expel the mucous plug. Wipe this from the opening with lint-free gauze.
7. Gently inject saline into the tracheostomy to liquefy the mucus.	The exact amount of solution needed may vary from 5 to 30 cc's (check your agency's procedure for recommendations).
8. Insert the catheter about 5 inches through the tracheostomy tube. 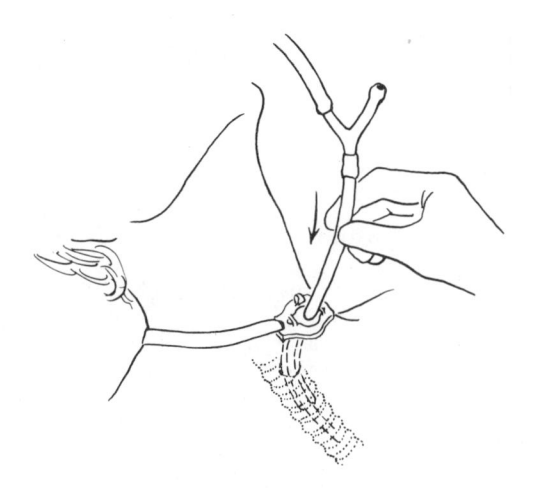	Ask the patient to breathe in while you insert the catheter, to help prevent a spasm or cough. Moisten the tip end of the catheter with water for ease of insertion. *Do not* put your thumb over the suction control during insertion. When the bronchus is reached, the cough reflex will be stimulated. Reassure your patient and continue to suction. CAUTION: If the patient coughs continuously, he may have a laryngeal spasm. *Immediately* remove your thumb from the suction control until he stops coughing. Then carefully proceed with suctioning.
9. Close the valve and gently withdraw the catheter (cleanse it if necessary). 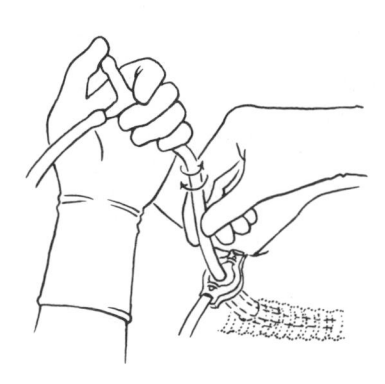	Close the valve by putting your left thumb over the suction control of the Y tube or the built-in suction control. Rotate the catheter gently and slowly between your right thumb and index finger. This permits the eyes in the catheter to dislodge mucus which may have collected on the inside of the tracheal tube. NOTE: If the catheter "grabs" the mucosa, take your thumb off the valve control and release the suction. Intermittent release of suction can help prevent damage to the tracheal mucosa. Do not repeatedly poke the catheter in and out of the tube; this could injure the tracheal mucosa. However, you may have to completely remove the catheter periodically to clear the lumen of secretions by sucking sterile water through the lumen. Hold the catheter in the trachea *no longer than 10 to 15 seconds.* Prolonged suctioning can produce hypoxia; remember that air as well as mucus is being suctioned.

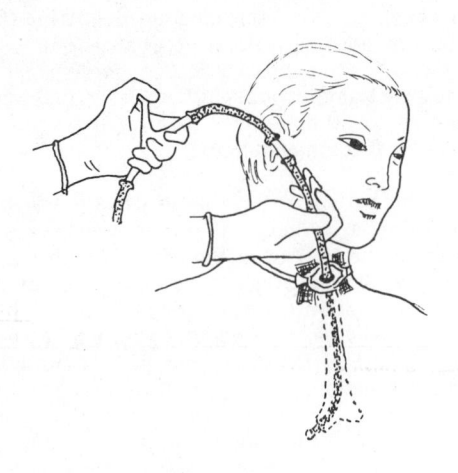

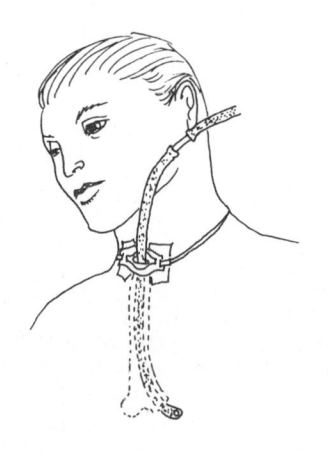

Important Steps	Key Points
10. Aspirate the *right* bronchus.	Permit the patient to rest at least 3 minutes between aspirations. Continue gentle insertion of the catheter to a depth of 8 to twelve inches to aspirate the bronchus. Withdraw the catheter about 1 cm to fill the tip of the catheter. Raise his right shoulder and chin, and turn his head to the *left*. Insert the catheter 1 to 2 cm, with your thumb on the suction control. Rotate the catheter 360 degrees as you carefully and gently withdraw it 1 to 2 cm. NOTE: Turn the patient's head *away from* the bronchus to be suctioned.
11. Aspirate the *left* bronchus.	Raise the patient's left shoulder, chin up, and turn his head to the *right*. Insert the catheter gently 1 to 2 cm with suction still on. Withdraw the catheter completely and gently, slowly rotating it 360 degrees. Clear the lumen of the catheter by drawing water through the lumen. Successive aspirations can be done only if the catheter is not contaminated.
12. Allow the patient to rest.	Suctioning is very tiring to the patient. Remember that you are suctioning off his air as well as the mucus secretions.
13. Dispose of the catheter.	Discard it in the waste container.
14. Remove your glove(s).	Discard in the waste container.
15. Change the patient's dressing.	This should be done only if it is soiled. Repeat the foregoing steps as necessary to keep the airway open.
16. Leave the patient comfortable.	Give mouth care as needed. (This may not be required with each suctioning, but is surely needed several times a day.) Place the patient in semi-Fowler's position, if he can tolerate it. Remove the soiled linens and replace with clean, dry linens, as needed. Put the call light within easy reach and raise the siderails, if indicated. Tell the patient when you expect to return.

Important Steps	Key Points
17. Record the procedure on the patient's chart.	Charting example: 4:15 P.M. Tracheo-bronchial suction carried out. Large amount of thick muco-purulent drainage obtained. No bleeding or signs of infection noted around incision site. Vital signs remained stable throughout procedure. Deep suctioning needed $\overline{q}$ 2 hours. D. Shaw, S.N.
18. Replenish used articles.	*Supplies and equipment should be replaced immediately.* An emergency may arise and you will not have time to obtain fresh supplies. Your thinking and advanced planning can forestall a fatal incident.

ITEM 3: INFLATION AND DEFLATION OF TRACHEAL CUFF

The cuffed tracheostomy tube (plastic or rubber) prevents air leaks around the tracheal opening and permits a closed system within which adequate ventilation may be maintained. Since the materials (especially the plastic) are lightweight, there is little pressure on the tracheal wall which could lead to erosion.

The tracheostomy tubes with cuffs are either single or double lumen. Cuffs may be attached to the tracheostomy tube by the manufacturer or packaged separately to be applied to the tracheostomy tube when needed. Because there are varying procedures (depending on the manufacturer), read the literature provided by the manufacturer before using. Obtain assistance if you are unfamiliar with the product. With the single lumen, the cuff is bonded (fixed) to the tube, but it is more difficult to keep clean than the double-lumen tubes and usually must be replaced every 48 hours. The double-lumen cuffed tube permits alternate inflation of the cuff sites, thereby avoiding prolonged pressure on the tracheal tissue at one site. The double-lumen cuff has decreased the possibility of the cuff ballooning over the distal end of the tracheostomy tube. These cuffed tubes can be kept in place from 2 to 4 hours. However, if tissue damage is caused by the pressure of the inflated balloon, the damaged area will be larger (because of the two balloons) and may be more difficult to repair.

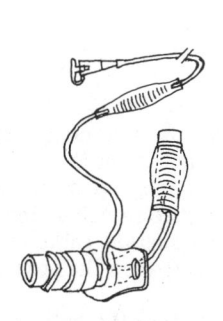

Single-lumen cuffed tube 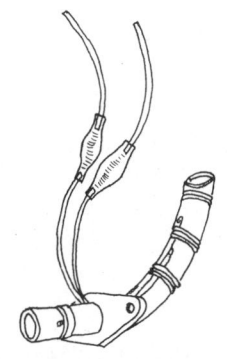   Double-lumen cuffed tube

Usually deflation and inflation of the cuff are carried on at regular intervals, e.g., every hour and prn. Tracheal aspiration is carried out before the procedure and is often done during a regular tracheal suctioning. Deflate the cuff before removing the inner cannula. The patient can eat with a tracheostomy tube in place. In this case, however, the tracheal cuff must be deflated during the meal.

Note: There is current research being carried on to ascertain the best method of inflating and deflating the tracheal cuffs with regard to the amount of inflation and the deflation interval. Thus, the above recommendations may be altered when new research findings become available.

Important Steps	Key Points
Follow steps 1 through 9 of Item 2: Tracheobronchial Suctioning (clearing upper airway).	
10. Have patient take several deep breaths.	This will prevent hypoxia from occurring while you deflate the cuff. Encourage the patient to breathe deeply before and during deflation of the cuff. Talk calmly and reassuringly to him to keep him from being apprehensive and to encourage his cooperation. Tell him exactly what you are doing. Be sure that the upper airway is free of secretions before you deflate the cuff. This will prevent aspiration.

If the cuffed tube is inserted (or slips) too deep, it can occlude the bronchi; if it rides too high, it may occlude the trachea.

Because the inflated cuff creates pressure on the tracheal wall with a resulting diminished blood supply or tracheal edema, the cuff should be deflated at least HOURLY. Unless the pressure on the tracheal wall is released periodically, tissue death (erosion or necrosis) may occur because of the lack of nutrients reaching the tissues via the blood stream.

Important Steps	Key Points
11. Deflate the tracheal cuff.	Do this with the tip of the 5 cc syringe inserted into the distal end of the inflation tube. (The plunger is entirely within the barrel of the syringe.) The syringe is usually a part of the tracheal suctioning tray. Withdraw 2 to 5 cc of air *slowly* into the barrel of the syringe. Keep the syringe attached to the tube. The slow action of withdrawing the air into the barrel of syringe pulls the air out of the balloon cuff and allows the secretions to be pushed up by positive pressure exerted from the bronchi.
12. Suction the lower airway.	Frequently the cough reflex will have been stimulated when the cuff pressure was released, thus bringing up more secretions. Be sure that the tracheobronchial tree is free of secretions. Put the suction catheter to one side until you have completed the next two steps.
13. Continue the cuff release for 3 to 5 minutes.	Be sure that the patient is ventilating properly during this deflation period.
	NOTE: Some patients cannot tolerate even this short a period without assisted ventilation. For these patients a cuff release of 30 to 60 seconds may be all that can be tolerated. Therefore, the cuff release should be done more frequently than every hour. (Follow agency procedure.)

Important Steps	Key Points
14. Inflate the cuff.	Push *slowly* on the plunger of the syringe to reintroduce the air into the balloon cuff. Introduce just enough air (2 to 5 cc) to create a leak-free system. Note the exact amount of air introduced for recording later on the chart.
	To check a leak-free system in the conscious patient, note his speech (e.g.: Does he have aphonia?) and whether air is coming from the oral cavity, nostrils, or from around the tracheostomy tube.
15. Remove and dispose of the catheter.	If the patient remains free of secretions, dispose of the catheter in a waste container. If he appears to have secretions, suction again and then dispose of the catheter.
16. Remove gloves, if used.	This will depend on agency procedure. Dispose in waste container.
17. Change dressing, if soiled.	Work carefully so as not to dislodge the tracheal tube.
18. Leave the patient comfortable.	Give mouth care as needed. Position him for comfort, probably in a semi-Fowler's position. Remove soiled linens and replace with fresh linens. Fluff pillow, straighten bedding, place call light within easy reach, and raise siderails if indicated. Tell patient when you expect to return.
19. Record on patient's chart.	Charting example:
	6 P.M. Tracheal cuff released for 5 minutes. Reinflated cuff with 4 cc air. No difficulty with respirations noted. Color and pulse remained stable throughout.
	H. Taub, S.N.
20. Replenish supplies immediately.	Emergencies can arise with tracheotomized patient, so that you must be prepared to act in *advance*. Always have supplies and equipment on hand and in working order.

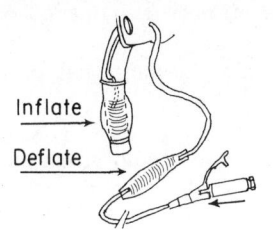

POST-TEST

Indicate in the column at the left whether the statements are true or false (mark T or F).

__T__ 1. The inner cannula should be completely dry after cleaning and prior to insertion.

__F__ 2. If you notice a dent on the metal inner cannula, you should go ahead and reinsert it.

__F__ 3. Facial tissues should be used to wipe off secretions.

__T__ 4. One should hold the outer cannula with one hand (thumb on one side and index finger on the other) while unlocking and removing the inner cannula.

__F__ 5. If the inner cannula has incrustations adhering to it and you cannot remove it by using plain water, you should reinsert it the way it is.

__F__ 6. One can take as long as one wishes while cleaning the inner cannula.

__F__ 7. It is in the realm of nursing responsibility to remove the outer cannula.

__T__ 8. One should always check to see that the tapes of the tracheostomy tube are tied securely around the neck.

Fill in the blanks.

9. Name the three main types of tracheostomy tubes:

   a. _Plastic_ b. _Rubber_

   c. _Metal_

10. Give two reasons why a tracheostomy might be indicated.

    a. _Establish & maintain open airway._

    b. _Provide easy access to suctioning the tracheobronchial tree._
    Prevent aspiration in unconscious patient.
    Treat a patient who needs assisted ventilation.
    When O₂ catheter or mask can't be tolerated.

POST-TEST ANNOTATED ANSWER SHEET

1. T, p. 271.

2. F, p. 271.

3. F, p. 271.

4. T, p. 270.

5. F, p. 270.

6. F, p. 271.

7. F, p. 266.

8. T, p. 272.

9. a. Metal, p. 266.

   b. Plastic

   c. Rubber

10. Any one of the following, p. 264.

    To establish and maintain an open airway.

    To provide easy access to suctioning the tracheobronchial tree.

    To prevent aspiration in the unconscious patient.

    To treat a patient who needs assisted ventilation.

    When oxygen catheter or mask cannot be tolerated.

PERFORMANCE TEST

In the classroom or skill laboratory, your instructor will ask you to perform the following activities without reference to any source material. You will need a simulated model to take the part of the patient.

1. Given an adult patient with a tracheostomy, you are to clean and reinsert the inner cannula, carefully do a tracheobronchial suctioning, deflate and inflate the tracheal cuff, and apply a clean dressing.

2. During the above procedure, you will discuss the indications for performing a tracheostomy and describe the reasons for using safety precautions during the procedure.

3. From a display, you will identify the various types of tracheostomy tubes as well as the parts of the tracheostomy tubes. You will describe the functions of each part of the tracheostomy tube to your instructor.

PERFORMANCE CHECKLIST

CLEANING THE INNER CANNULA

1. Check supplies and equipment.
2. Wash hands.
3. Position patient.
4. Identify patient and explain procedure.
5. Suction inner cannula.
6. Remove inner cannula.
7. Clean inner cannula.
8. Observe patient for signs of hypoxia, etc.
9. Rinse/dry inner cannula.
10. Reinsert inner cannula.
11. Change dressing.
12. Give mouth care.
13. Leave patient comfortable.
14. Record on chart.
15. Replenish supplies.

TRACHEOBRONCHIAL SUCTIONING

1. Wash hands and approach and identify the patient.
2. Position patient.
3. Check supplies and equipment.
4. Put on sterile gloves.
5. Test patency of catheter.
6. Assess patient's level of consciousness.
7. Inject saline to liquefy mucus.
8. Insert catheter 5 inches.
9. Close valve, withdraw catheter, and rinse catheter.
10. Aspirate right bronchus and rotate catheter 360 degrees.
11. Aspirate left bronchus and rotate catheter 360 degrees.
12. Allow patient to rest between suctioning.
13. Dispose of catheter.
14. Remove and dispose of gloves.
15. Change dressing.
16. Leave patient comfortable.
17. Record on patient's chart.
18. Replenish supplies.

INFLATION/DEFLATION OF TRACHEAL CUFF

1. Wash hands and approach and identify the patient.
2. Position patient.
3. Check supplies and equipment.
4. Put on sterile gloves, if indicated.
5. Test patency of catheter.
6. Assess patient's level of consciousness.
7. Inject saline to liquefy mucus.
8. Insert catheter 5 inches.
9. Close valve, withdraw catheter, and rinse it.
10. Ask patient to take deep breaths.
11. Deflate tracheal cuff.
12. Suction lower airway.
13. Maintain cuff release (3 to 5 minutes).
14. Inflate tracheal cuff.
15. Remove and dispose of catheter.
16. Remove and dispose of gloves.
17. Change dressing.
18. Leave patient comfortable.
19. Record on chart.
20. Replenish supplies.

Unit 9

APPLICATION OF TOURNIQUETS

I. DIRECTIONS TO THE STUDENT

You are to proceed through the lesson using this workbook as your guide. You will need to practice the procedures related to the use of the tourniquets for the various treatments and circulatory tests in the skill laboratory with a student partner or other persons. After you have completed the lesson and your practice, make arrangements with your instructor to take the Performance Test.

II. GENERAL PERFORMANCE OBJECTIVE

Upon completion of this lesson, you will be able to apply tourniquets for the treatment of pulmonary edema, and for the Trendelenburg and Perthes circulatory tests.

III. SPECIFIC PERFORMANCE OBJECTIVES

When you have finished this lesson, you will be able to:

1. Describe the indications for the use of tourniquets in treatment of pulmonary edema and diagnosis of circulatory disturbances.

2. Discuss with your instructor the main objectives of therapy for pulmonary edema and the diagnostic circulatory tests (Perthes and Trendelenburg).

3. Describe and employ safety precautions when using the various tourniquets.

4. Instruct the patient regarding the reasons for applying the tourniquets.

5. Correctly and safely apply the rotating tourniquet.

6. Correctly and safely apply the tourniquets for the Trendelenburg and Perthes circulatory tests.

IV. VOCABULARY

Read the definitions of the terms listed below. Do not attempt to memorize them before proceeding with the lesson. Each term will be explained or defined again in the text. On completion of the lesson, however, you should know the correct definition of each term.

alveolus (plural, alveoli)—air cell of the lung; pulmonary air space.
bronchus (plural, bronchi)—one of the two divisions of the trachea that branch into the lung and terminate in the bronchioles (bronchial tubes).
capillary—small blood vessel that carries blood and combines with arteries and veins to form the capillary system. Capillaries connect the smallest arteries (arterioles) to the smallest veins (venules).
dyspnea—difficult breathing that may result in air hunger.
edema—a condition in which the body tissues retain an excessive amount of tissue fluid.
embolism—an obstruction of a blood vessel by a foreign substance or blood clot (thrombus).
embolus (plural, emboli)—a mass of undissolved matter present in the blood or lymphatic system which may be solid, liquid, or gas.

hypoxia (anoxia)—deficiency of oxygen in the inspired air; reduced oxygen content or tension.

phlebitis—inflammation of a vein; also called thrombophlebitis.

phlebotomy (venesection)—a procedure for withdrawing venous blood (500-700 ml) to lower the venous pressure, thereby reducing the venous return to the heart.

saphenous veins—two veins of the leg, one short and one long.

subcutaneous—that which is beneath or introduced under the skin.

systemic circulation—the cycle of blood flow through the heart, out to the entire body via the entire arterial system, and the subsequent venous return to the heart.

thrombosis—the formation of a blood clot (e.g., coronary thrombosis, or blood clot in the heart muscle).

tourniquet—a constrictor used on an extremity to produce pressure over an artery for the purpose of controlling bleeding; also used to distend veins to facilitate a venipuncture or to give intravenous injections.

venesection (phlebotomy)—cutting an opening into a vein to remove blood.

venipuncture—puncture of a vein for any purpose (e.g., to give intravenous fluids or to withdraw blood for test purposes).

V. INTRODUCTION

In order to understand the various tourniquet procedures, it is necessary to review briefly the circulatory system within the heart and lungs, as well as the major circulation of the lower extremities.

The circulatory system refers to the heart, blood vessels, and lymphatic vessels, a closed system that carries the blood throughout the body (systemic) to provide oxygen, chemicals, and various nutrients to sustain the life of the cells and the tissues. It also functions to remove certain elements such as heat, CO_2, and various chemicals from the tissues, and to help combat infections.

The blood is propelled through the circulatory system by the pumping action of the heart. The circulatory system is composed of several parts. "Peripheral circulation" refers to the superficial blood vessels in the skin and subcutaneous tissues of the body. "Pulmonary circulation" refers to the flow of blood from the right ventricle of the heart to the lung, where it is oxygenated, and the return flow to the left atrium. "Portal circulation" refers to the flow of blood to the liver via the portal vein and then out of the liver via the hepatic vein into the inferior vena cava.

The average amount of blood in the normal adult (70 kg) is about 5 liters (5000 cc, 5 quarts, 10 pints); e.g., for a person weighing 132 pounds, 3 2/5 quarts, or 6 4/5 pints of blood; for a person weighing 70 kg or 154 pounds, 5 liters.

Blood is estimated to be about 7 per cent of the body weight and is normally slightly alkaline in reaction (pH 7.35). Arterial blood (which has been oxygenated) is bright red, whereas venous blood (which has lost much of its oxygen content as it returns to the heart) is usually dark red or almost black in color.

Blood is composed of a liquid called plasma (composing 55 per cent of the whole blood), in which are suspended red blood cells (RBC, erythrocytes), white blood cells (WBC, leukocytes), platelets (thrombocytes), and fat globules.

Blood is 22 per cent solid and 78 per cent water.

Normal values:

RBC 4,500,000/cu mm (female); 5,000,000/cu mm (male)

WBC 7000 to 8000/cu mm

Platelets 200,000 to 400,000/cu mm

The heart is a muscular pumping organ about the size of a closed fist. It is located just above the diaphragm and the stomach in the mediastinum between the lungs.

BREAST BONE
(STERNUM)

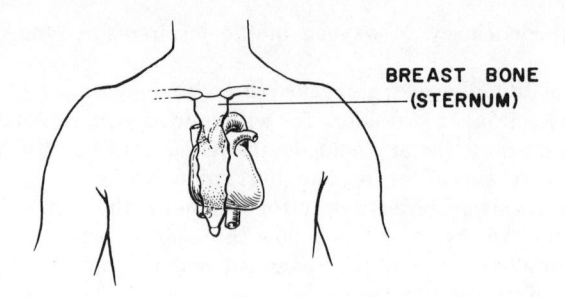

The heart is made up of muscle tissue called the *myocardium*, and is enclosed in a fibrous sac called the *pericardium*. The inner lining of the heart is called the *endocardium*.

There are four chambers of the heart; the upper chambers are called the right and left atria (*singular:* atrium or auricle), and the two lower chambers are called the right and left ventricles.

The *cardiac cycle* is the completed series of events of one heartbeat. The sequence of events in the cardiac cycle is regulated by a flow of electrical impulses initiated in the sinoatrial (SA) node. The electrical activity of the myocardium can be amplified and recorded as a tracing known as an *electrocardiogram* (ECG or EKG). The phase of the cardiac cycle in which the ventricles contract is known as *systole*; the phase in which the ventricles relax and dilate is known as *diastole*.

Blood from the entire body is brought by the collecting veins to the superior vena cava and the inferior vena cava (plural: *venae cavae*) and is emptied into the right atrium of the heart. It goes from the right ventricle to the lung (for oxygenation) via the pulmonary arteries and returns to the left atrium via the pulmonary veins. Blood leaves the left ventricle via the aorta and is circulated throughout the body through the arterial and venous systems. The smallest arteries are called arterioles and the smallest veins are known as venules. The blood vessels communicating between the arterioles and the venules are called capillaries.

There are small flaps or cuplike valves inside the veins that keep the blood from flowing backward within the vein. They assist in moving the blood toward the heart. Deficient valves in the veins cause varicosities.

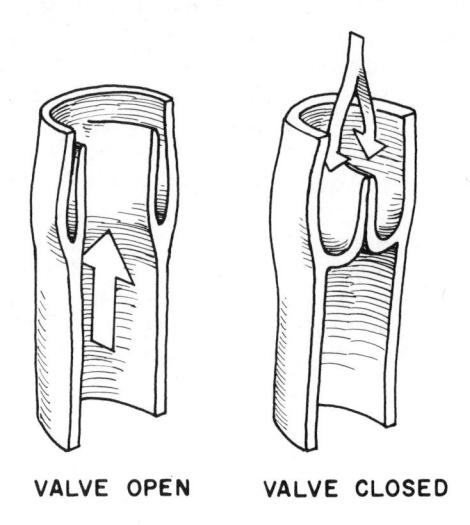

VALVE OPEN   VALVE CLOSED

Review the following diagrams to refresh your memory concerning the systemic circulatory system.

APPLICATION OF TOURNIQUETS

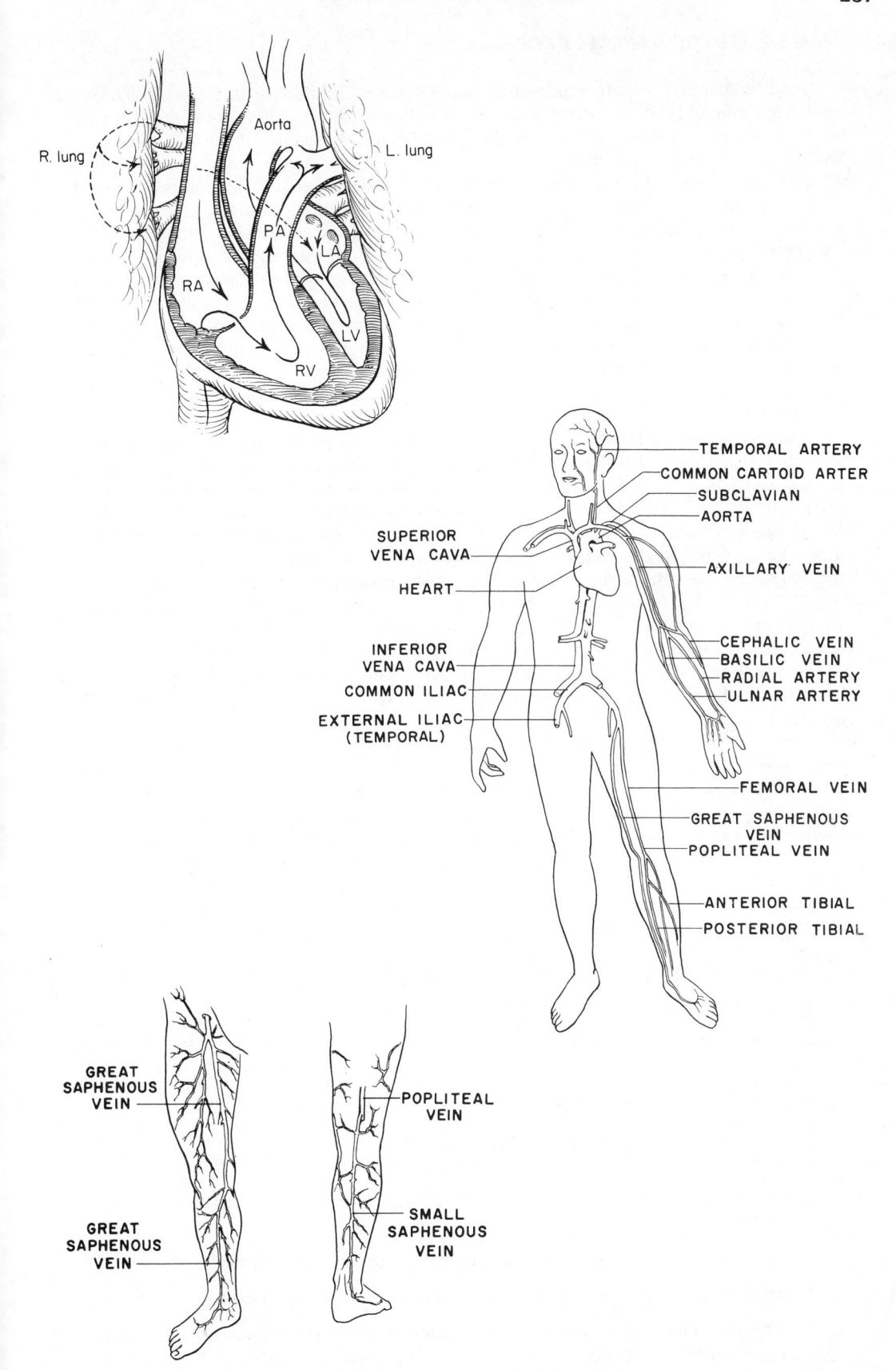

ITEM 1: ACUTE PULMONARY EDEMA

Acute pulmonary edema is one of the most common medical emergencies. Pulmonary edema is a clinical syndrome rather than a disease. It is most frequently seen in patients who have, or are suspected of having, left-sided heart failure. Weakening of the left ventricle is caused by such conditions as myocardial infarction (MI) or arteriosclerotic heart disease (ASHD), which make the left ventricle incapable of maintaining sufficient output of blood with each heart contraction. On the other hand, the right ventricle continues to pump blood toward the lungs. This imbalance between inflow on the right and outflow on the left side of the heart may have drastic results. The pulmonary capillaries and the alveoli become engorged because blood continues to flow to the lungs without being adequately pumped out into the systemic circulation by the left ventricle. Fluid, which is initially serous and then becomes sanguineous, escapes into the adjacent alveoli through the communicating bronchioles and bronchi, and is mixed with the air. Further, it is churned by the respiratory agitation up through the trachea and thus the fluid is pushed up out of the lungs and is discharged through the mouth and nose. This produces the moist breathing sounds known as the "death rattle."

The typical attack of pulmonary edema occurs at night after the cardiac patient has been recumbent for a few hours. Recumbency increases the venous return to the heart and favors reabsorption of edema fluid from the legs. Such a patient may experience extreme respiratory distress, and may prefer to sit with his arms extended in front of his body so that he can make maximal use of the accessory muscles or respiration. However, as the dyspnea progressively worsens, the cough becomes more severe and produces copious amounts of frothy sputum, sometimes blood-tinged. The patient is usually extremely apprehensive and may be pale and perspiring profusely. He may be cyanotic with cold and clammy skin. Respirations are rapid and deep or shallow; the pulse rate is rapid. The blood pressure may be elevated or it may drop to shock levels. The neck veins become distended because of the elevated venous pressure produced by the systemic venous constriction. The patient may begin to breathe noisily, nearly drowning from the blood-tinged fluid that is pouring into his bronchi and trachea.

These symptoms may subside within 15 minutes to several hours, but the situation constitutes an emergency and demands immediate intervention. Pulmonary edema also may occur in the post-operative or traumatized patient who has suffered severe blood losses and has been given large amounts of intravenous fluids and blood transfusions, thereby overloading the circulatory system. It can also occur in patients who have suffered a cerebrovascular accident (CVA or stroke) or following the inhalation of irritating gases such as ammonia.

Treatment for pulmonary edema must be given promptly and efficiently. The main objectives of the treatment are:

1. To reduce the right atrial backflow of systemic venous blood.

2. To increase the left ventricular outflow.

3. To calm the patient and make him as comfortable as possible.

The therapy that is usually initiated may include one or more of the following:

1. Morphine sulfate or some other respiratory depressant given to depress the respirations and help to lessen apprehension.

2. Oxygen administered by face mask or nasal catheter to combat the severe hypoxia that may result.

3. Mercurial diuretics to help decrease the edema and circulatory blood volumes.

4. Phlebotomy, or venesection, performed to lower the venous pressure.

5. Aminophylline to help reduce cardiac output and relax the blood vessel walls. It also relieves bronchial spasms.

6. Digitalization, usually started at once. Be sure to find out before administering the drug if the patient is already receiving a digitalis drug routinely (generally the case for the cardiac patient). If so, alert the physician before medication is administered. Serious complication such as digitalis poisoning can occur from overdosage.

7. Rotating tourniquets on the extremities are frequently used to retard the venous flow. The purpose of this technique is to produce a venous stasis in the extremities, which consequently relieves the venous blood return to the heart.

Types of Tourniquets

Electric pneumatic tourniquets are automatic machines that make use of four pneumatic cuffs with controlled pressure usually set at the patient's diastolic pressure. The machine has an automatic timer that releases one cuff and inflates another cuff at set time intervals so that three tourniquets are inflated at any given time. Authorities vary the time interval, ranging from 5 to 15 minutes, depending on the condition of the patient. Some physicians prefer a 5-minute rotating time interval because of the possibility of a venous thrombosis and subsequent pulmonary embolism with longer rotating time periods. Other physicians prefer a 15-minute rotating schedule.

The advantages of the electric pneumatic tourniquet are its precise operation and the fact that it frees health personnel to perform other life-saving procedures for the patient.

Four sphygmomanometer cuffs may be employed to carry out the procedure if the automatic device is not available. The cuffs are inflated manually, as though taking a blood pressure reading, to a point slightly above the level of the patient's diastolic pressure. The pressure, placment of the cuffs, and the rotation schedule are the same as for the automatic machine—5- to 15-minute intervals.

Four rubber tubing tourniquets (at least 2 feet long with an outside diameter of 5/16 to 1 1/2 inches) are tightened around the extremities to produce venous congestion without obliterating the arterial pulse. If this method is to be used, caution should be taken to prevent tissue damage by using padding (such as an ABD pad) over the skin before placing and tightening the tourniquet. You must remember that for the patient to receive maximum benefit from this procedure, the tension on each extremity must be correctly applied so that the correct amount of venous obliteration is maintained. The timing, placement, pressure, and rotation of the tourniquets follow the same schedule as above, i.e., three of the four extremities are compressed at all times while the fourth extremity is free of a tourniquet.

Principles of Applying Tourniquets

Tourniquets are placed as high on the extremity as possible and are tied just tight enough to produce venous stasis (usually at the point of the diastolic reading for the patient). Be sure that the tourniquets do not completely obliterate the arterial vessels, or the extremities will suffer from anoxia and death to tissues will result. If rubber tourniquets are used, the tourniquet is tightened so that the nurse's finger can be placed between the tourniquet and the padding, and an arterial pulse can be felt in the extremity with the tourniquet tied. If the pulse cannot be felt, the tourniquet should be removed immediately and reapplied. At the stated intervals (5 to 15 minutes), the fourth tourniquet is tied and the next tourniquet is untied (rotation is in a clockwise or counterclockwise direction, e.g., left arm, left leg, right leg, right arm, left arm, etc.). It is helpful to post the rotation time schedules at the head of the bed so that you can keep the rotation accurate and on time.

When the procedure is terminated, the tourniquets are removed one at a time, in rotation. *Never remove all the tourniquets simultaneously.* To do so would suddenly increase the volume of the circulating blood and would cause an excess of blood to return to the heart and lungs, producing another episode of pulmonary edema. Follow the release procedure on the following page.

290　　　　　　　　　　APPLICATION OF TOURNIQUETS

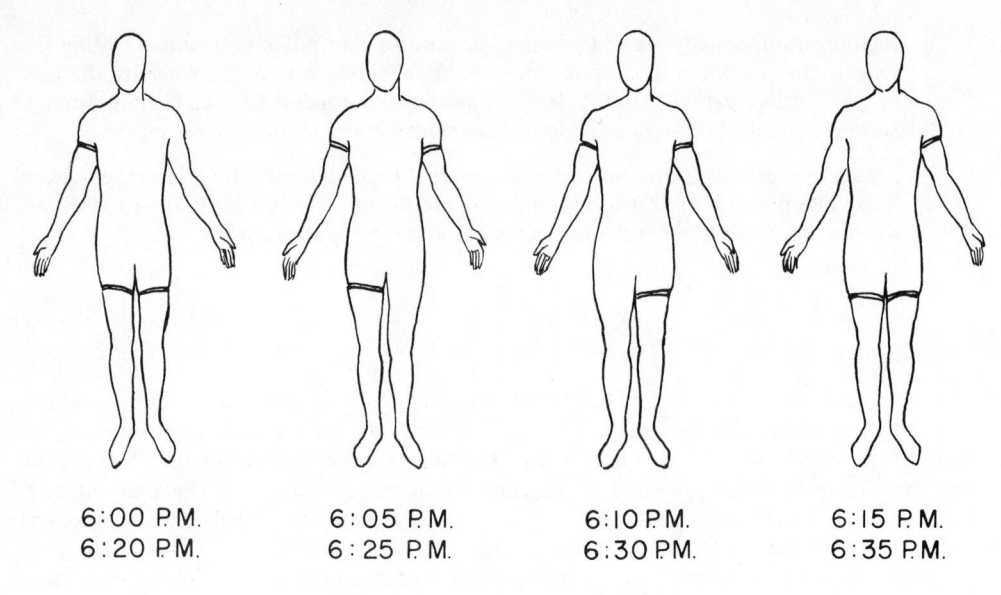

6:00 P.M.　　　6:05 P.M.　　　6:10 P.M.　　　6:15 P.M.
6:20 P.M.　　　6:25 P.M.　　　6:30 P.M.　　　6:35 P.M.

Time Compression and Release of Tourniquets

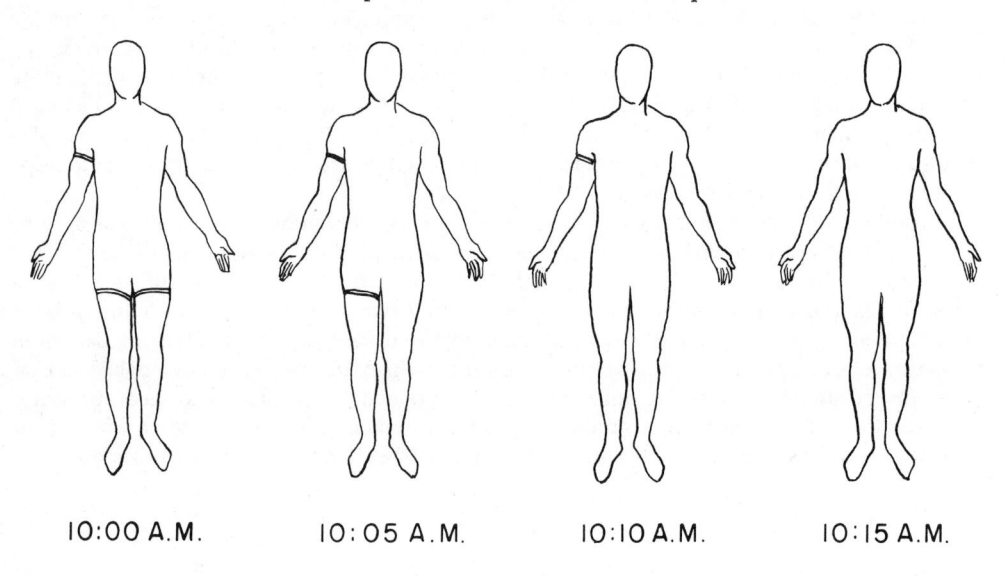

10:00 A.M.　　　10:05 A.M.　　　10:10 A.M.　　　10:15 A.M.

Important Steps	Key Points
1. Check supplies at bedside.	Sometimes an impending pulmonary edema may be anticipated and emergency equipment may already be in the room.
	Check the electric tourniquet to see that it is plugged into the electrical outlet and inflate the cuff to be sure there is no leak. This should also be done with the cuffs of the sphygmomanometer; check them to see that there is no leak when inflated. If rubber tourniquets are used, be sure that four are available and that they are long enough to encircle the patient's extremities. Also be sure that pads are available for use under the rubber tourniquets to prevent injury to the skin.

APPLICATION OF TOURNIQUETS

Important Steps	Key Points
2. Note the time of the emergency.	Wash your hands. Call for assistance if you are alone in the room. The emergency cart and additional assistance will arrive momentarily.
3. Observe the patient.	Write your observations on a note pad so that you can remember details and sequence of events for later recording on the patient's chart.

    a. Note the rate and nature of respirations (e.g., dyspnea, apnea, hyperpnea, Cheyne-Stokes, etc.).

    b. Note the pulse rate and volume (increased, decreased, strong, weak, thready, bounding, etc.).

    c. Note the blood pressure (if dropping, it may denote approaching shock, etc.).

    d. Note the patient's posture (sitting upright, on the side of the bed, with his arms extended, etc.).

    e. Note if he is coughing (wet, dry, persistent, bringing up secretions); this may indicate lung congestion.

    f. Note the type of secretions, if any (frothy, blood-tinged, mucoid).

    g. Note the color and feel of his skin (cyanotic, pale, cold, clammy, edematous).

    h. Note signs of fatigue on minimal movement. (This may be due to the impaired circulation which has deprived the muscle tissue of its needed O_2 and nutrients. This also may indicate that the metabolic wastes are not being removed by the blood because of the circulatory stasis. These wastes then accumulate in the tissues, decreasing the muscle tone and creating fatigue much like that of athletes who have been exercising vigorously for a period of time.)

    i. Note whether the patient's veins are distended due to the increased venous pressure from the sluggish circulation.

    j. Listen to the patient's complaints of "feeling pressure" or having a "heavy feeling" due to the deficiency of O_2 in the circulation. (This is usually more pronounced when the patient is in the dorsal recumbent position.)

    k. Look for edema. (It is usually the "pitting" or "dependent" type; i.e., when you press the ankle tissue with your thumb and then remove it, the thumb print remains in the tissue.)

APPLICATION OF TOURNIQUETS

Important Steps	Key Points
	Prolonged edema can cause fluid to back up into the portal system, causing the excess fluid to filter out into the abdominal cavity and create a condition called *ascites*. When large amounts of edematous (ascitic) fluids are withdrawn from the abdomen, the patient frequently looks very emaciated. This is caused by the deprivation of nutrients in the muscle tissue resulting from the sluggish circulatory flow.
4. Reassure the patient.	Stay with the patient at all times. The situation is usually one of emergency, and the patient is likely to be very apprehensive and fearful of impending death.
	Tell your patient that you or someone else will be with him at all times. Answer his questions directly; this in itself often decreases the anxiety perceptibly. Putting the patient into high Fowler's position or starting O_2 may make him breathe more easily. *Listen carefully* to find out what is causing his fear; e.g., "What will happen to my family if I die?" Tell him you will keep them informed about his progress and that you will have a social worker meet with the family to make financial plans or do whatever the patient thinks may be necessary.
	Some patients can relax better if members of the family are in the room; others want to be alone. *Listen* to your patient to find out what he desires. Keep the environment quiet and clean. Often the evening and night hours cause increased apprehension. Be sure that someone remains with him and that you or some other nurse sees the patient at frequent intervals, possibly every 30 to 60 minutes.
5. Explain the tourniquet procedure.	Tell him that the purpose of the rotating tourniquet is to decrease the blood flow to the heart and lungs so that the impaired heart can handle the blood flow that is now circulating more efficiently. The procedure is stopped as soon as the heart can once again take over its full job. Explain that there will be some discomfort and a tingling sensation in the extremities when the tourniquets are tied. The extremity will also appear cyanotic because of the restricted blood flow, but this is done purposely to help relieve the burden on the heart. You should explain this to family members, too, if they are present, so that they will not be upset.
6. Position the patient.	Lower the siderails. Adjust the bed to the most comfortable working height. An upright position (Fowler's) is more comfortable for the patient since it allows for gravitational pull on the thoracic and abdominal contents, permits maximum expansion of the lungs, and increases the amount of O_2 that gets into circulation.

APPLICATION OF TOURNIQUETS

Important Steps	Key Points
	When the patient lies in the dorsal recumbent position, the body fluids pool near the spine and put more pressure on the major vessels in the body, inhibiting the blood flow and decreasing O_2 to the body tissues. This is very uncomfortable.
	Extending the patient's arms away from the body also facilitates maximum expansion of the chest. Support his arms on pillows as you learned in Unit 16 in Volume 1 on positioning the patient. Another method of increasing comfort is to support his arms and head on a pillow that has been placed on an overbed table in front of the patient. The patient may believe he can breathe better while sitting on the edge of the bed or in a chair. Permit him to do so, if at all possible. However, because of his weakened condition, take safety precautions to assure that he will not fall.
	Have someone stand by for support; use restraints to hold him securely in bed or in the chair. Remove or loosen constricting clothing so that he can breathe more easily.
	NOTE: <u>Do not pull curtains around the bed or close the windows—this could make the patient feel as though he were suffocating.</u> (Of course, you must be sure that the patient is not in a draft and that his privacy is maintained.) Opening or closing of windows is not required in air-conditioned agencies.

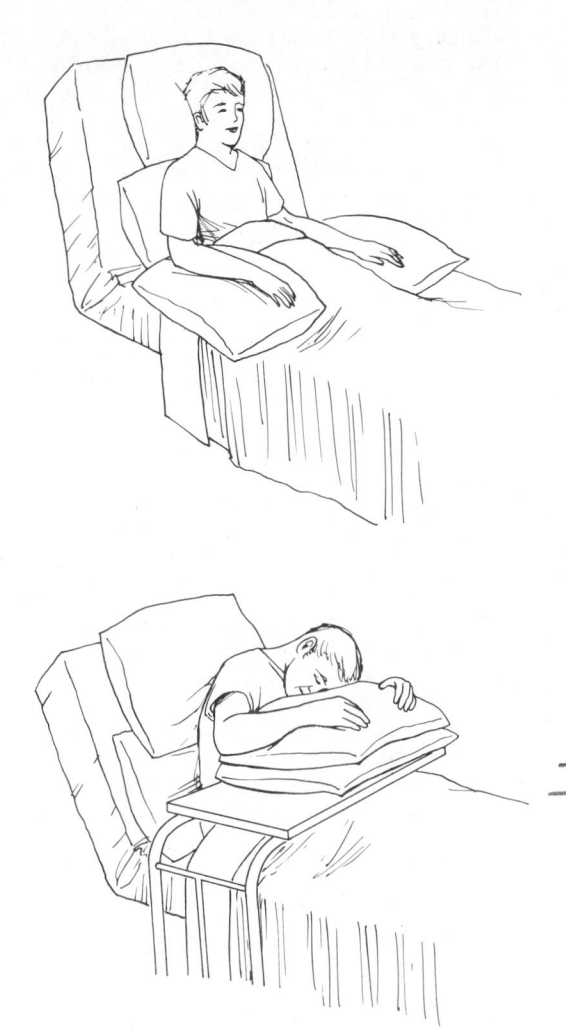

7. Apply the tourniquets.

   a. Automatic.

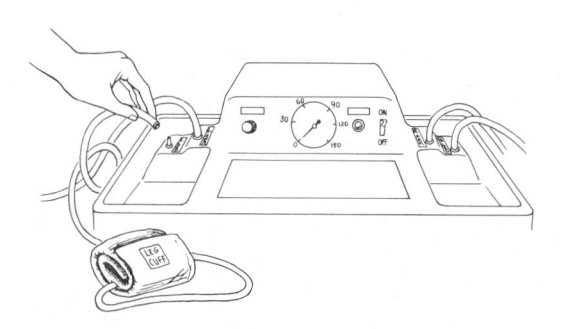

Connect the machine to electricity and then attach the cuffs to the electrical machine. Apply the four cuffs, one at a time, to each of the extremities. Apply directly to the skin, on the arms, above the elbow, and on the legs above the knees. Attach the connecting tubes of each cuff to the machine. Set the desired pressure on the machine (usually at the patient's diastolic reading); set the timing dial as prescribed by the physician; e.g., to rotate timing at 5- or 15-minute intervals. Thus one tourniquet set at a 15-minute interval would be kept on an extremity for a total of 45 minutes, then released for 15 minutes and reinflated again for a continuing time. Remember that only one extremity is untied at a time.

The machine automatically inflates and deflates the cuffs in clockwise rotation at the prescribed time intervals.

Important Steps	Key Points
b. Sphygmomanometer cuffs.	The application is the same as above in terms of placement, rotation, and timing. However, there is a cuff for each extremity, and the deflation, rotation, and inflation must be done manually. The procedure usually requires one person to be responsible for this activity, while someone else assists the physician or carries out the other therapeutic measures.
c. Rubber tourniquets.	The application is the same as in step b. However, with this least desirable method, it is difficult to maintain a precise degree of constriction on all three extremities simultaneously. There is no actual gauge by which you can read the precise diastolic pressure. The rubber tourniquet is applied around the extremity and over padding to prevent pinching or injury to the skin, and is then tied with a figure-8 knot pulled snugly. Do not obscure the peripheral pulse. If there is no pulse, release the tourniquet immediately and reapply.
8. Observe the patient.	Continue to watch the vital signs regularly and make observations as described in Step 3, i.e., respiration, pulse, blood pressure, etc. Observe the patient's reaction to the treatment and record what you see on the note pad. Continue to reassure him. When the symptoms subside and the physician determines it is time, the tourniquets can be removed.
9. Remove the tourniquets.	Take them off one at a time in continuing rotation, at the prescribed time intervals. Removing all the tourniquets at one time would overwhelm the circulatory system and produce a repetition of the cardiac failure; the rotating tourniquet process would then have to be started again.
10. Make the patient comfortable.	Remove used supplies and equipment, and return them to storage or discard as indicated. Sponge the patient if needed to relax and cleanse him after a period of profuse diaphoresis and expectoration of fluids. Change the bed linen. Give him a backrub to relax him further and help him rest after this tiring procedure. Position the bed comfortably in moderate Fowler's. Raise the siderails; place the call light and bedside stand within reach.

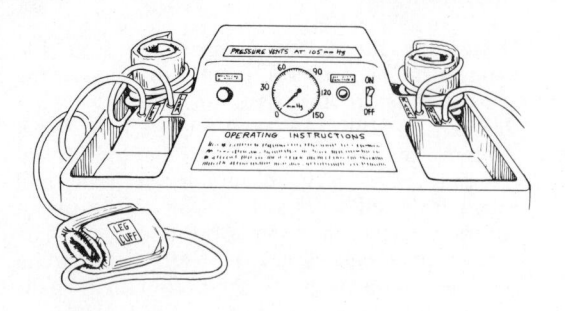

Important Steps	Key Points
	Ask if there is anything else he needs, and tell him approximately when you will return. Remove articles as necessary to leave the room tidy. Replenish supplies, so that all will be ready if the emergency arises again.
11. Record on the chart.	You have been keeping notes of the activities on your note pad; transfer them to the patient's record promptly. Report to your charge nurse on the current status of the patient.

An interesting note in the November 12, 1971 issue of *Medical World News* reported that doctors at Hadassah-Hebrew University Hospital in Jerusalem used the pneumatic tourniquet on an extremity to treat chronic osteomyelitis by diverting the peripheral blood into the bony circulation while giving antibiotics under pressure distal to the site of infection. In the test, all signs of infection disappeared by the seventh day.

ITEM 2: TRENDELENBURG AND PERTHES CIRCULATORY TESTS

Both the Trendelenburg and the Perthes circulatory tests are used to assist the physician in making the diagnosis of varicose veins. Varicose veins are abnormally distended, swollen, knotty, or lengthened superficial veins. They are most commonly found in the lower extremities, but they can also occur in other parts of the body. The normal blood flow in the veins is directed toward the heart, and the flow of the blood in the veins is prevented from reversing itself by a series of small cup-shaped valves. The malfunction of these valves in the veins may be due to disease such as phlebitis or to a long-standing distention caused by pressure on the veins in such conditions as pregnancy or obesity, or there may be a hereditary weakness of the vein wall. The exact cause of varicosities is unknown; some authorities believe that there is a deficiency of calcium in the walls of the blood vessel, and others believe there may be a vitamin C deficiency.

It is estimated that 50 per cent of all women over the age of 40 have varicose veins, while 25 per cent of all males over 40 have this condition. The individual's occupation may be a contributing factor; those whose work requires them to stand many hours, such as dentists, beauticians, nurses, elevator operators, barbers, printers, teachers, etc., seem to have a greater incidence of varicosities than those people who are engaged in more sedentary occupations.

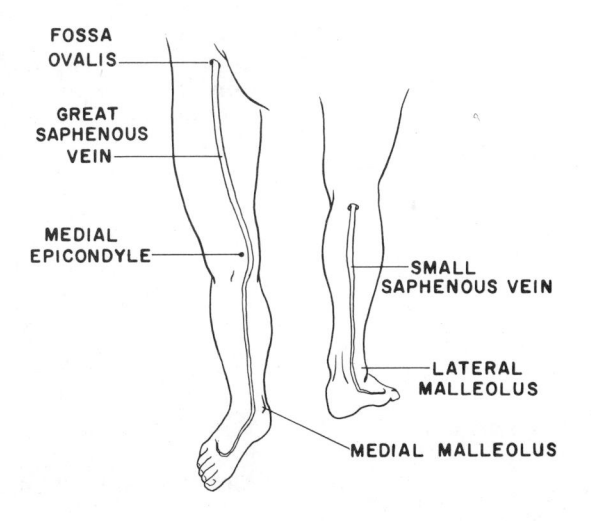

The veins most commonly affected in the lower extremities lie in the subcutaneous fatty tissues, especially the long saphenous vein. The great saphenous veins emerge from the femoral canal and run down the anteromedial aspect of the lower extremity to the medial side of the foot. The small saphenous vein emerges from the popliteal fossa behind the knee, runs down the posterior aspect of the calf of the leg, and curls under the lateral malleolus. The malleoli are the protuberances on the medial and lateral aspects of the ankle, the medial being part of the end of the tibia, the lateral part of the end of the fibula.

Symptoms resulting from venous congestion are: fatigue of the leg muscles, a heavy feeling or cramp of the legs at night, disfigurement to the extremity by large swollen veins. If the varicose veins are not treated, chronic inflammation of the veins may follow with a resulting vein ulceration and ultimate hemorrhage. Among women, the symptoms seem to intensify during menses.

The Trendelenburg test, also known as the Brodie-Trendelenburg, is used to test the competance of the valves in the long and short saphenous veins.

Trendelenburg Test

Important Steps	Key Points
1. Wash your hands.	
2. Approach the patient, check his Identaband and explain the procedure.	Tell him that a rubber tourniquet will be used around the leg to constrict the superficial veins. The entire test will take approximately 15 to 30 minutes per leg. The patient may feel some discomfort and tingling sensation in his leg while the tourniquet is in place. The tourniquet will be applied at several positions along the leg to determine the exact location of the pathology. It is first applied while he is lying down; then he will be asked to stand beside the bed. The veins will then be closely observed for their pattern of filling. (The way in which the veins fill indicates the competency of the valves in the vein.)
3. Assemble the equipment.	A pneumatic tourniquet, a Penrose drain, or a plain rubber tube (2 feet long with outside diameter of 5/16 to 1 1/2 inches) may be used.
4. Position the patient.	Lower the siderails, if used. Adjust the bed to a comfortable working height. Have the patient lie in a dorsal recumbent position and elevate one extremity 65°. This eases the emptying process of the veins by utilizing gravity. To speed up the process, you can stroke the leg from the ankle to the thigh (the direction of the blood flow returning to the heart).
5. Apply the tourniquet.	When the veins appear to be collapsed, apply the tourniquet around the upper thigh. Tighten it so that the superficial veins are constricted, but not the deep veins. You should still be able to feel a pedal pulse.
6. Have the patient stand beside the bed.	Observe and note the time the tourniquet is applied, and the time that it takes to fill the veins *below the tourniquet*.

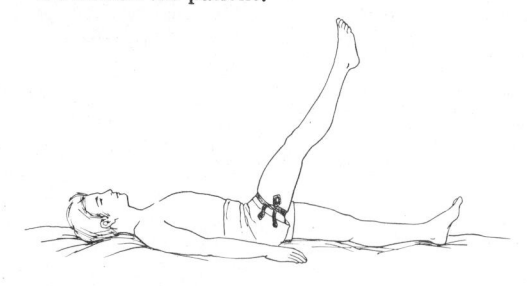

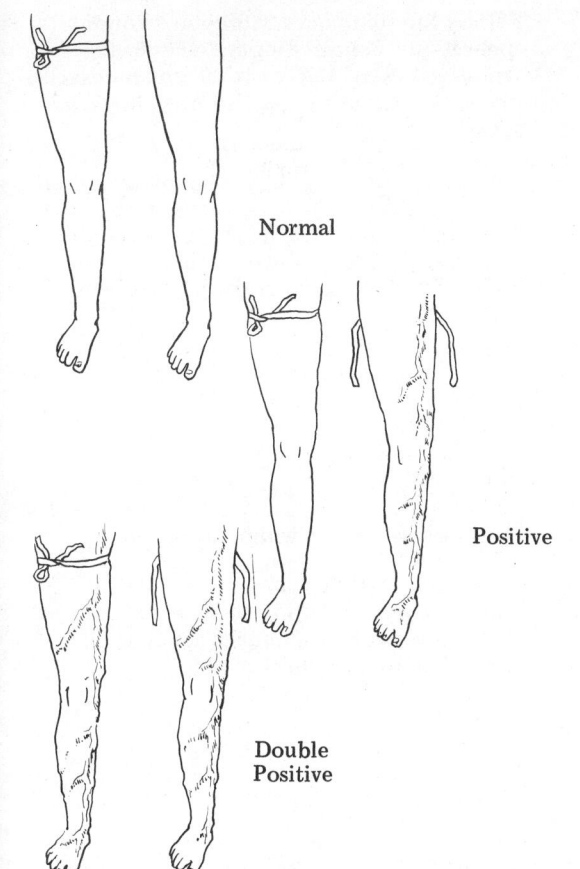

APPLICATION OF TOURNIQUETS

Important Steps	Key Points
Normal	The test is considered NORMAL if the veins fill slowly when constricted and when the tourniquet is released. The results are thus negative, indicating the competence of the saphenous and communicating veins.
Positive	The test is considered POSITIVE if the veins fill slowly when constricted, but fill rapidly above the tourniquet when released.
Double Positive	The test is considered to be DOUBLE POSITIVE when there is rapid filling during compression and an increased blood flow above the tourniquet on release. This indicates incompetence in both the saphenous veins and the femoral communicating veins.

TABLE OF TRENDELENBURG TEST RESULTS (See above)

	Veins Filling	Time	Test Indications	Interpretation
Tourniquet ON (Constrictive)	Remain empty or fill slowly	20–30 sec.	Negative	Communicating valves are adequate, and deep veins are patent
	Fill rapidly	5–15 sec.	Positive	Communicating valves are inadequate, or deep femoral system is not patent
Tourniquet OFF (Release)	Column of blood falls downward; veins fill rapidly	1–10 sec.	Positive	Incompetent valves in upper saphenous system
	Veins fill slowly		Negative	Competent valves in upper saphenous system

The illustrations on this page were adapted from original printings by Frank H. Netter, M.D. from the CIBA COLLECTIONS OF MEDICAL ILLUSTRATIONS. Copyright by CIBA Pharmaceutical Company, Division of CIBA-GEIGY Corporation. All rights reserved.

Important Steps	Key Points
7. Remove the tourniquet.	Release the tourniquet within 60 seconds after application. Follow Steps 5 and 6 above at various levels of the leg to determine exactly where the varicosity lies. Record observations at each level.
8. Position the patient for comfort.	Following the examination, position the patient as he desires. Raise the siderails, if indicated. Place the call light and bedside table within easy reach. Ask if there is anything else he needs. Tell him approximately when you will return.
9. Remove supplies and equipment.	Leave the room neat; return supplies for reprocessing.
10. Report the record.	Write the time and type of procedure, and describe results. Charting example: 9:30 A.M. Trendelenburg test done by Dr. Kuni. The veins filled within 25 seconds at each of the 5 levels of tourniquet application. Ambulatory in room following test. J. Kahn, R.N.

Perthes Test

A subjective tourniquet test, the Perthes circulatory test is used to diagnose an obstruction of the deep veins and the adequacy of the valves in the communicating veins. This test also determines the effectiveness of a saphenous ligation. The temporary constriction of the saphenous vein by tourniquet has the same effect as a saphenous ligation.

Important Steps	Key Points
1. Wash your hands.	
2. Approach the patient, check his Identaband and explain the procedure.	Explain that this test is required to determine the patency (openness) of the deep (femoral) veins in the leg, and the valves in the communicating blood vessels between the deep and superficial vessels. These are small cup-like valves located at specific distances within the vein which keep the blood flowing toward the heart. The test will take approximately one half hour per leg. There will be some discomfort and a tingling sensation in the extremity while the tourniquet is on. It may appear cyanotic (bluish) because of the stasis of the blood flow while the tourniquet is in place.
3. Assemble supplies and equipment.	A tourniquet, writing pads and pens, and a marking pencil to outline the veins while they are engorged are all required items.

APPLICATION OF TOURNIQUETS

Important Steps	Key Points
4. Position the patient.	Adjust the bed to a comfortable working height. Lower the siderails as indicated. Assist the patient to a standing position beside the bed. This will permit easy observation of the veins as they fill with blood.
5. Apply the tourniquet.	Apply at the midthigh. Secure it tightly enough with a figure-8 knot so that it will not loosen while the patient is vigorously walking for 5 minutes. Do not obscure the pedal pulse, however.
6. Observe the veins after exercise.	a. If the veins are *empty* (or collapsed) below the tourniquet, the deep veins are *patent* (open) and the communicating valves are *competent*. This condition is called *normal*. The exercise has forced the blood into the deep veins and onward through the systemic circulation.
	b. If the veins remain *unchanged*, this indicates *incompetence* in the valves in both the saphenous and the communicating veins. Remember, if the vessels are competent, the blood flow would be redirected into the deep vessels.

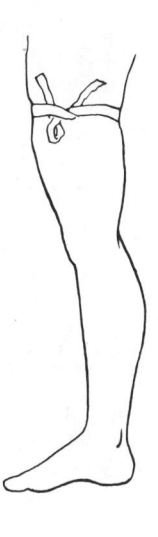

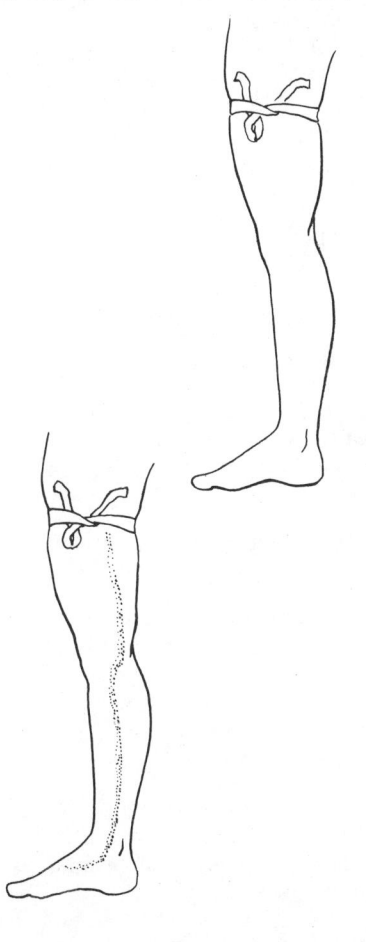

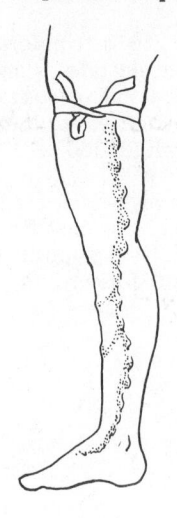

APPLICATION OF TOURNIQUETS

Important Steps	Key Points
	c. If the veins *increase in size and are painful*, the indication is that the deep veins are *occluded*. NOTE: Some physicians may want to outline the veins with the marking pencil to serve as a guide when surgery is performed.
7. Remove the tourniquet.	Loosen it after 5 minutes.
8. Position the patient for comfort.	Assist him back to bed. Raise the siderails if indicated. Place the call light and bedside stand within easy reach.
9. Report and record.	Charting example: 10:45 A.M. Perthes test done on left leg by Dr. Kuni. The veins become very distended, tortuous and painful. After outlining the veins with marking pencil, the tourniquet was removed. Patient was returned to bed and made comfortable. J. Kahn, R.N.

VI. ADDITIONAL INFORMATION FOR ENRICHMENT

Symptoms of inadequate circulation in the lower extremities can be treated in a variety of ways:

1. Bedrest with elevation of the extremity for significant periods of time (days).

2. The use of an Ace bandage or an elastic stocking may provide temporary relief. Note: the stocking should be made to fit the patient's precise measurements reaching from toes to just below the knee. It is preferable to have the heel covered by the stocking.

3. Another temporary treatment may be the use of sclerosing medications injected directly into the offending vein.

4. For a more permanent cure of the chronic varicosities in the main saphenous trunk, a surgical procedure can be performed in which the pathologic vein is ligated (tied off with surgical material called a suture) and/or stripping (removal) of the distal portion of the saphenous vein from the groin to the ankle by means of a surgical instrument called a vein stripper is done. This procedure is done only if the deep vessels are working properly and can take over the entire circulation of the extremities.

You will learn more about the exact surgical procedure when you progress through the operating room experience.

If you have further questions, ask your instructor to give you additional reading assignments or observation experiences in the surgical or cardiac clinics.

POST-TEST

1. Name the main objectives of the therapy in pulmonary edema.
   a. ↓ rt. atrial backflow of systemic venous blood.
   b. ↑ left ventricular outflow
   c. Calm & comfort patient

2. Name the different types of equipment used in the rotating tourniquet procedure.
   a. Electric pneumatic tourniquet
   b. Sphygmomanometer cuffs
   c. Rubber tubing

Indicate in the blank space provided by marking a T or F if statement is true or false, respectively.

3. __F__ When terminating the rotating tourniquet procedure, all tourniquets are removed simultaneously.

4. __F__ Tourniquets are applied below the knee and below the elbows on the extremities for the rotating tourniquet procedure.

5. __T__ A safeguard check when applying a rubber tourniquet is to be able to feel the arterial pulse in the tied extremity.

6. __F__ Rubber tourniquets can be applied directly to the patient's skin.

7. __T__ A safety measure used in the rotating tourniquet procedure is a preliminary check to see if there are leaks in the blood pressure cuff.

8. __T__ If an electrical rotating tourniquet is employed in the treatment of pulmonary edema, it is important to check the functioning of electrical plugs before use.

9. __F__ Confronted with an emergency, the nurse should always concentrate on the procedure and later reassure the patient.

10. __F__ The recumbent position is recommended for the rotating tourniquet procedure.

11. __T__ If the patient states that he can breathe better while sitting in a chair, you should allow him to do so.

12. __T__ In an effort to decrease the patient's apprehension, tight clothes should be loosened when the patient is in pulmonary edema.

Complete the following:

13. Trendelenburg and Perthes circulatory tests are used to assist in making the diagnosis of ___varicose veins___.

14. Name at least three contributing factors to the development of varicose veins:
    a. Disease; pregnancy; obesity
    b. Hereditary weakness; occupation
    c. Vitamin or Ca++ deficiency.

15. The symptoms of venous congestion in varicose veins are:
    a. _Fatigue of leg muscles_
    b. _Heavy feeling & leg cramps at night._
    c. _Disfigurement by swollen vessels_
16. If varicose veins are not treated, the occurrence of phlebitis may lead to _vein ulceration_ which in turn may cause _hemorrhage_.
17. The specific purpose of the Trendelenburg circulatory test is _test competency of the valves in the saphenous veins._
18. The specific purpose of the Perthes circulatory test is _obstruction of the deep veins & adequacy of valves in the communicating veins._

POST-TEST ANNOTATED ANSWER SHEET

1. a. to reduce right atrial backflow of the systemic venous blood;
   b. to increase left ventricular outflow;
   c. to calm and comfort the patient, p. 288.
2. a. electric pneumatic tourniquet;
   b. sphygmomanometer cuffs;
   c. rubber tubing, p. 289.
3. F, p. 289.
4. F, p. 289.
5. T, p. 289.
6. F, p. 289.
7. T, p. 290.
8. T, p. 290.
9. F, p. 292.
10. F, p. 292.
11. T, p. 293.
12. T, p. 293.
13. varicose veins, p. 295.
14. a. disease;
    b. pregnancy, obesity;
    c. hereditary weakness;
    d. vitamin or calcium deficiency;
    e. occupation, p. 295.
15. a. fatigue of the leg muscles;
    b. heavy feeling or leg cramps at night;
    c. disfigurement by swollen vessels, p. 296.
16. vein ulceration, hemorrhage, p. 296.
17. test competency of the valves in the saphenous veins, p. 296.
18. obstruction of the deep veins and the adequacy of the valves in the communicating veins, p. 298.

PERFORMANCE TEST

In the skill laboratory, your instructor will ask you to apply one of the following tourniquets on your partner.

1. Rotating tourniquet for treatment of pulmonary edema.
2. Application of tourniquets for the Trendelenburg circulation test.
3. Application of tourniquet for the Perthes circulation test.

You should be able to discuss the signs and symptoms of pathology that the above procedures are used for, and also to explain what the signs and symptoms indicate.

PERFORMANCE CHECKLIST

ROTATING TOURNIQUETS

1. Check supplies (there must be no leaks; proper electrical current). Wash hands.
2. Note time of emergency and observe patient (you should be able to describe at least seven signs or symptoms which the patient presents and the significance of each).
3. Explain procedure to patient; check Identaband.
4. Position patient correctly and use good body movement for self.
5. Apply tourniquets correctly and safely. Discuss application and release sequence.
6. Remove tourniquets in proper sequence.
7. Leave patient comfortable and safe, and room neat.
8. Record activity accurately.

TRENDELENBURG TEST

1. Wash hands, check Identaband, and explain procedure.
2. Assemble equipment.
3. Position patient, using correct body movement.
4. Apply and remove tourniquet properly.
5. Discuss interpretation of various test results.
6. Leave patient comfortable and safe, and room neat.
7. Record activities correctly.

PERTHES TEST

1. Wash hands, check Identaband, and explain procedure.
2. Assemble equipment.
3. Position patient, using correct body movement.
4. Apply and remove tourniquet at appropriate time interval.
5. Discuss various interpretations of vein responses that can occur in the test.
6. Leave patient comfortable and safe, and environment neat.
7. Record observations accurately.

Unit 10

INSERTION OF NASOGASTRIC AND GAVAGE TUBES

I. DIRECTIONS TO THE STUDENT

Read this lesson carefully because it is quite complex. You will need to study every detail in order to become knowledgeable about insertion and use of the various types of gastrointestinal (g.i.) tubes.

II. GENERAL PERFORMANCE OBJECTIVE

At the completion of this unit you will be able to employ the correct techniques for inserting gastrointestinal tubes, tubes used for special feedings, and special laboratory tests.

III. SPECIFIC PERFORMANCE OBJECTIVES

When you have finished this unit, you will be able to:

1. Assemble equipment and insert the various kinds of gastrointestinal tubes without injury to the patient.
2. Feed a patient via a nasogastric, a gastrostomy, or an enterostomy tube.

IV. VOCABULARY

Read the definitions of the terms listed below. Do not attempt to memorize these definitions before proceeding with the lesson. Each term will be explained or defined again in the text. On completion of the lesson, however, you should know the correct definitions of these terms.

burette—a graduated glass.
Cantor tube—a single long tube used for intestinal decompression. It has a mercury-weighted balloon at its distal tip to assist in stimulating peristalsis and moving the tube into the intestine. It is inserted through the nose and down the digestive tract to the intestine; the proximal end of the tube is connected to a suction machine.
decompression—removal of air or drainage from a wound, cavity, or passageway.
distention—the state of being stretched out or bloated; e.g., the abdominal cavity may be distended with gas or fluid.
enterostomy(enter- = intestine; -ostomy = mouth)—a surgical operation to make a permanent or temporary opening through the abdominal wall into a part of the intestinal tract. This opening is used when feeding patients who may have a carcinoma in the digestive tract above the surgical opening.
esophagus—the muscular tube in the digestive tract that connects the oral cavity with the stomach. It is located directly behind the trachea (windpipe).
Ewald tube—a specific rubber tube with a large lumen (opening) passed through the mouth and down the esophagus to the stomach to withdraw stomach contents for various laboratory examinations; useful in diagnosis of disease.
flatus—expulsion of gas (air) rectally; if gas is expelled orally, it is called burping or eructating.

gag reflex—an involuntary (*not* controlled by the will) retching or vomiting action caused by stimulation of certain nerve endings in the back of the throat which, in turn stimulate the vomiting center in the brain.

gastric—pertaining to the stomach.

gastrostomy (*gastro-* = stomach; *-ostomy* = mouth)—a surgical operation making a temporary or permanent opening through the abdominal wall into the stomach. A tube is inserted into the opening and the patient may be fed in this manner. This procedure may be done for a carcinoma in the upper digestive tract.

gavage—feeding through a tube inserted into the stomach. The tube is inserted through the nose and down the esophagus to the stomach.

Jutte tube—special rubber gastrointestinal tube that has a fine wire tip over the distal end.

lavage—washing out of a cavity (e.g., gastric lavage is washing out of the stomach contents and is used in emergency cases, such as that of a child who has swallowed a poisonous fluid).

Levin tube—a long plastic or rubber single-lumen tube inserted through the nose or mouth to the stomach and used to drain off stomach fluids and/or to keep the stomach decompressed (free of gas).

medulla—lower portion of the brain stem, the enlarged portion of the top of the spinal column inside the cranium.

Miller-Abbott tube—the most common double-lumen g.i. rubber tube used to drain or decompress the small intestine. It has an inflatable rubber bag on the distal end which helps stimulate peristalsis (involuntary wave-like motion of digestive tract) when in the small intestine. It is inserted through the nose down the esophagus, through the stomach, and into the intestine. The proximal end of the tube is connected to a suction machine.

nasogastric tube—a rubber or plastic tube inserted through the nose down to the stomach.

nausea—inclination or desire to vomit.

peristalsis—involuntary wave-like motion of the digestive tract that moves food through the digestive tract (alimentary canal).

Rehfuss tube—a gastrointestinal drainage tube that has a small metal tip on its distal end. It is inserted through the nose down to the intestine.

V. INTRODUCTION

Gastrointestinal intubation is the insertion of a specified tube through the nose or throat, into the stomach or intestine. The primary reasons for this relatively common procedure are:

1. To drain the stomach or intestinal tract by means of some kind of suction apparatus. It is used to prevent postoperative vomiting, to prevent postoperative obstruction (blocking) of the intestinal tract, and to prevent gas formation in the stomach or intestine after an operation.

2. For diagnosis (to identify a disease, to determine the cause of a pathological condition).

3. To wash out the stomach contents; e.g., after taking a poison.

4. To provide a route for feeding one who is unable to take food by mouth.

There are usually three markers (black rings) on the distal end of each of the tubes to indicate how far the tube has been inserted: 1 band = stomach; 2 bands = pylorus; 3 bands = duodenum.

ITEM 1: LEVIN TUBE

This is the most commonly used tube for gastric (stomach) intubation and suction. It is designated to empty (decompress) the stomach of its contents (food, blood, gas, or other drainage).

The Levin tube (plastic or rubber) is about 3 feet long; its tip is solid, but there are a number of holes along the side of the tube for the first 6 to 9 inches. The other end of the tube is open and is usually connected to one of several types of suction equipment (to be discussed later in this Unit).

The Levin tube is also used for gavage feedings (see Item 6).

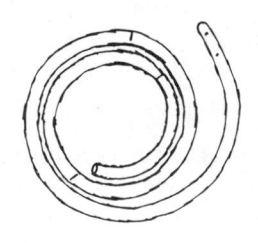

Insertion of Gastric Tube for Drainage Purposes

The most common one used for this purpose is the Levin tube.

Important Steps	Key Points
1. Prepare the required equipment.	Wash your hands and clear a place for the equipment on the bedside stand.
	If a *rubber Levin tube* is used, you will need to cool it and make it stiff for insertion through the nose by placing it in a pan of chipped ice until thoroughly chilled (15 to 30 minutes).
	Generally, the *plastic Levin tube* is now used. It is stiff enough for insertion and will not have to be chilled. However, if for any reason it is not stiff enough, it can also be chilled in a pan of chipped ice. Assemble an emesis basin, tissues, a lubricant for the tip of the tube (to ease insertion), a 20 to 50 cc aspirating syringe, some adhesive tape, and a fresh glass of water.
	In some agencies, you will obtain these items separately for the patient; in other agencies a special tray may be ordered that would include the tube, lubricant, and aspirating syringe.
2. Approach the patient, explain what you are going to do, and enlist his cooperation. Wash your hands.	Check the identification bracelet to be sure you have the correct patient.
	The patient may be in pain and very frightened. You need to help reassure him that you will be gentle with him and will tell him exactly what is being done; e.g., the purpose of passing the tube is to prepare for some gastric studies, a means of feeding, to relieve distention in the stomach caused by gas, bleeding, etc. Explain that the passage of the tube is painless but that it may cause gagging as it passes down the back of the throat. However, tell him to breathe deeply and he will be less likely to be nauseated.

Important Steps	Key Points
3. Position the patient.	Usually the Fowler's position is assumed if possible. This enables the tube to move down the digestive tract with the help of gravity. It is also easier for the patient to spit out vomitus if this becomes necessary. The patient may be in the supine position, however, if his condition warrants it.
4. Give a basin and tissues to the patient.	Hand the emesis basin and tissues to the patient if he is able to handle them. Otherwise, place the emesis basin close beside his face with the tissue near the pillow.
5. Measure the tube for insertion distance.	Measure from the patient's nose to the proximal earlobe and then down to the umbilicus (navel). This is roughly the distance from the lips to the stomach. Mark this distance on the tube by placing a piece of tape at that point.
6. Take a working position and lubricate the tips of the tube.	Stand at the right side of the patient; the tip end of the tube will be grasped in the right hand, and the left hand will hold the remaining tube. (Reverse hand positions if you are left-handed.)
	Lubricate the tip end of the tube in water; this moistens the tube and permits easier insertion. If the tube should get into the lung, the water on the tip end of the tube is less likely to irritate the lung tissue than would an oil-base lubricant. (Follow your agency procedure.)
7. Instruct the patient to open his mouth, and hand him a glass of water.	Tell the patient to swallow a mouthful of water as you pass the tube down the esophagus to the stomach (bend his head forward so his chin rests on his neck). If the patient is unable to hold the glass of water and emesis basin, you may need to have someone assist you.

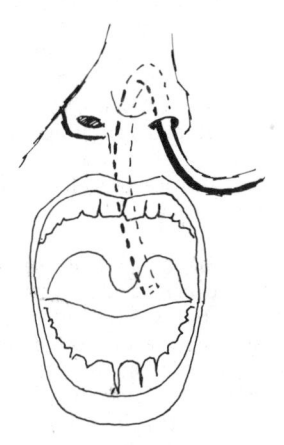

The tube is passed in one of two ways:

Through the mouth: Pass the tube over the top and middle of the tongue toward the back of the throat.

Through the nose: Pass the tube gently up one nostril. (Use the nostril that seems to be free of blockage or obstruction. Each side of the nose will have to be tested; usually one side is easier to use.) You can check the position of the tube as it passes down the back of the patient's throat; ask him to open his mouth, and then you can hold down the back of his tongue with a tongue depressor. Rotate the tube very gently and slowly between your index finger and thumb of the dominant hand for ease of insertion.

INSERTION OF NASOGASTRIC AND GAVAGE TUBES 311

Important Steps	Key Points
8. Push the tube into the patient's stomach.	Use a slow, gentle but firm motion. If the tube is pushed too fast, it will stimulate the nerve endings in the back of the throat and they in turn will stimulate the center in the medulla that causes the patient to vomit. Continue to remind him to swallow water as the tube is passed; then set up peristalsis in the esophagus. He may prefer to suck on ice chips (if permitted) rather than to drink water. Try to keep the patient relaxed by talking quietly and reassuringly. (Take your time; do not hurry the patient.)
9. Check to see if the tube is in his stomach.	You will have reached the tape mark you have put on the tube. Since the stomach always has a little gastric juice in it, it is relatively simple to check whether the tube is in the stomach. Apply the aspirating syringe to the exposed end of the tube; pull the plunger back. This action should pull the gastric juice up through the tube into the syringe. If gastric juice is not obtained, it must be determined whether the tube is in the trachea (the breathing passageway that lies directly in front of the esophagus). Aspirate the contents into the emesis basin.
10. Test to see whether the tube is in the trachea.	The patient may become apprehensive at this point. You can reassure him that all is well and that the procedure will be finished soon. The free end of the tube is placed in water; if it bubbles, this usually indicates that it is in the lung and must be removed at once. OR Ask the patient to hum (he will *not* be able to hum if the tube is improperly placed because it would go between the vocal cords). Therefore, *if he can not hum,* the tube is in the lung and should be removed at once. If the patient becomes cyanotic (blue) or dyspneic (has difficulty breathing), the tube is probably in the trachea. *It must be removed immediately.*
11. Secure the tube to the patient's face with adhesive tape.	When it is determined that the tube is in the stomach, the exterior tip of the tube is taped to the patient's face. Usually the tip of the tube is taped on the forehead; this will keep the tube out of the patient's way as he moves about.

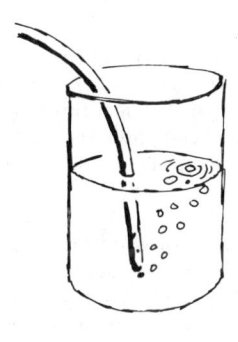

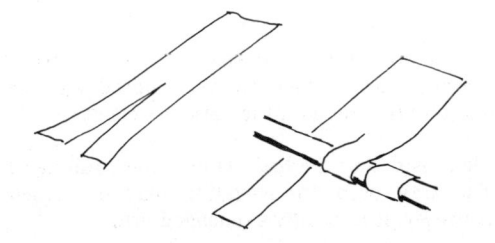

UNIT 10

Important Steps	Key Points
12. Attach the free end of the tube to the suction machine.	The doctor may order a suction machine (to pull out contents from the stomach in order to keep it free of gas and drainage) to be attached to the tube. He will instruct whether he wants continuous or intermittent (off-and-on) suction and will indicate the degree of pull he wants. The tube is pinned with a safety pin around the tube, securing it to the patient's gown. This provides the patient with the opportunity to move about without dislodging the tube. Plenty of room should be provided for the patient to move about freely without pulling on the tube. This tube may also be used for gastric feeding.
13. Prepare to irrigate the tube.	Irrigation of the tube is done to keep the lumen (opening) of the tube open to permit clear passage for drainage through the tube. Irrigations are usually ordered at stated intervals or prn (whenever necessary). Besides keeping the lumen open, this prevents gas from accumulating in the stomach, which causes considerable discomfort to the patient.
a. Assemble irrigating equipment.	Obtain a clean aspirating syringe, irrigating solution, and a receptacle for returned solution (an emesis basin will suffice).
b. Disconnect the tube from the machine and draw up the irrigating solution.	Disconnect the Levin tube from the suction machine and then secure the distal end of the tube to the machine in its holder. Hold the Levin tube between the middle fingers of your left hand; also hold the plunger of the syringe between your index finger and thumb. With your right hand, pull the plunger of the syringe and draw up 15 to 30 cc of irrigating solution.
c. Attach a filled syringe to the free end of the Levin tube and then irrigate.	Inject 10 to 15 cc of solution slowly into the tube. Pull back on the plunger to withdraw fluid. Work *gently* and *slowly* to prevent injury to the sensitive mucous lining of the stomach. The process of injecting and withdrawing solution is repeated until the lumen is clear. NOTE: If fresh bleeding is apparent, the procedure will be stopped *immediately*. The doctor must be notified at once if he is not present.
d. Observe the contents of the irrigating solution.	The color, odor, consistency, and amount (absence or excess) must be noted and accurately recorded on the patient's chart.
e. Remove the syringe from the tube and attach the tube to the suction machine again.	Clean and tidy the bedside unit and equipment. The tray used for irrigation may be reused. However, it is usually exchanged prn.

INSERTION OF NASOGASTRIC AND GAVAGE TUBES   313

Important Steps	Key Points
14. Leave the patient comfortable.	Because the process of draining the patient's stomach continues over a period of time, he usually is NPO (since everything he would take by mouth would come right back through the tube). The patient therefore loses tissue fluids rapidly and becomes dehydrated. Thus it is important for him to receive intravenous feedings to replace liquid and chemical losses.

There are two other helpful means of unclogging the tubing which are essential to follow:

a. Gently moving the tubing in and out slightly.	Occasionally one of the eyelet openings at the distal end of the tube adheres to the wall of the stomach; by pulling the tube away from the lining of the stomach, the tube is permitted to drain fully again.
b. Gentle "milking action" of the tube may free the blocking.	Hold the tube securely in place while milking. Some thick material may stop up the lumen of the tube between the nose and the drainage bottle. Gently squeeze the tubing between your palm and fingers. Move gently and carefully along the tubing in this manner until suction is restored.
15. Report and record.	Note the completion of treatment with a description of the stomach contents.

Charting example:

10:30 A.M. Levin tube inserted. Tubing irrigated with NaCl solution, solution returned clear. Many gas bubbles noted. Patient felt relief immediately. Attached to low suction.

A. Brown, R.N.

One of the most uncomfortable aspects of this procedure is the constant irritation caused by the tube at the back of the throat. Therefore, the doctor may permit the patient to suck on ice chips or throat lozenges or hard candy to keep his throat, as well as the tube, slightly moist.

The nose may also become tender, sore, and cracked; good hygiene must be given not only to the nose but also to the throat. Frequent opportunities to cleanse his mouth are comforting to the patient as well as an excellent way to prevent infections from the tube's continuing irritation.

Because the patient is usually very ill and apprehensive, you must keep his environment quiet, clean, tidy, and well-ventilated. The patient often is hypersensitive to odors, so his room and belongings must be kept immaculately clean and sanitary. Unsavory stimuli in his environment can cause him to become nauseated and vomit.

Answer his light promptly. Check on him frequently.

ITEM 2: REMOVAL OF GASTROINTESTINAL TUBES

Important Steps	Key Points
1. Approach and identify the patient; explain what you are going to do.	"The tube is being disconnected because you are doing so well."
	Wash your hands.

UNIT 10

Important Steps	Key Points
2. Position the patient.	Usually the semi-Fowler position is best, although any position in which the patient is most comfortable is acceptable.
3. Untape the tube from the patient.	
4. Remove the tube slowly.	Talk quietly to the patient as you rotate the tubing very gently between your index finger and thumb of your dominant hand.
	If you pull the Levin tube out too quickly, the patient will gag.
5. Discard the used tubing.	Put it in a designated container.
6. Make the patient comfortable.	Remove the tape marks from his skin with a tape remover solution, if necessary.
	Give him oral hygiene. Tidy the linens, fluff the pillows. Position the patient for comfort.
	Leave drinking water, bedside stand, and call light within easy reach.
	Tell him when you expect to return.
7. Return the equipment.	Take it to the processing room.
8. Report and record.	Charting example:
	10:30 A.M. Levin tube removed. Oral hygiene given. Patient left comfortable and ready to take a nap.
	A. Brown, R.N.

ITEM 3: INSERTION OF INTESTINAL TUBES FOR DRAINAGE PURPOSES

Miller-Abbott Tube

This is a long double-lumen rubber tube used for draining the small intestine. One of the lumens supplies an air-passage to inflate the balloon at the distal end of the tube. The inflated balloon in the small intestine stimulates peristalsis (the wave-like movement of the digestive tract).

The procedure for inserting this tube is the same as the procedure for insertion of the Levin tube.

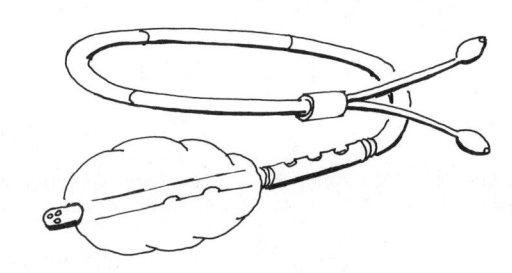

INSERTION OF NASOGASTRIC AND GAVAGE TUBES

Important Steps	Key Points
1. Inflate the balloon.	This must be done after the tube reaches the stomach. A sterile syringe and needle is used to inject 5 to 10 cc of air (or mercury) into the outlet connecting the air passageway to the balloon. The inflated (and weighted, if mercury is used) tube then passes into the small intestine by peristaltic action of the digestive tract.
2. Place the patient in a *right Sims* position.	This makes the passage of the tube faster and easier by helping the peristaltic action and gravity to move the tube from the stomach to the small intestine.
	The *tube should not be secured* until it finally rests in the small intestine. This can be determined by the ring markings on the outside of the tubing as well as the appearance of the drainage. When the tube reaches the intestine, it is attached to a suction machine. The tube is secured to the patient's face with adhesive tape and/or pinned to his gown to permit freedom of movement.
	Removal of this long tubing should be done slowly—a few inches every 5 minutes or so. Rapid removal can stimulate the gag reflex and the patient may vomit unnecessarily. The same precautions are observed when using this method as for patients using a Levin tube.

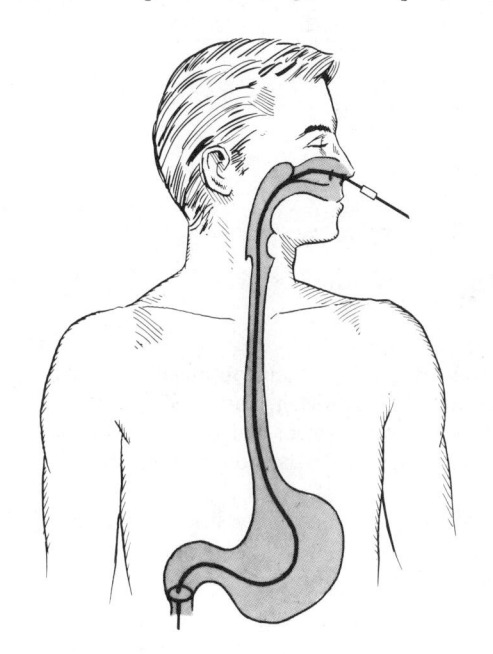

Cantor Tube

This is another type of intestinal drainage tube. It has a small inflatable bag sealed to the distal end of the tube. Before insertion of this tube through the nose, the inflatable (balloon) bag is injected (with needle and syringe) with 5 to 10 cc of mercury. This will make the tip end of the tube somewhat bulky for insertion, and therefore it must be well-lubricated. The principal of operation is the same as for the Miller-Abbott tube. The proximal end of the tube is attached to a suction machine.

The drainage holes in the tube are proximal to the balloon bag.

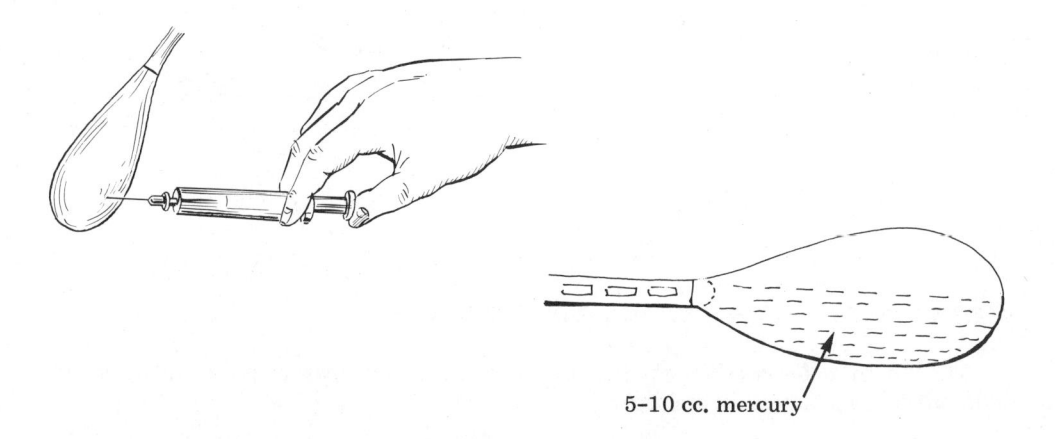

5-10 cc. mercury

Harris Tube

This is another long single tube used for intestinal suction and drainage. It is similar to the Cantor tube, except that the inflatable balloon is tied to the distal end of the tube (it has 4 cc of mercury in it). The holes that allow the drainage to be sucked into the tubing are proximal to the balloon bag. The well-lubricated tube is inserted through the nose using the Levin tube procedure.

The nursing care and observation of the equipment and drainage are the same as for the other patients with gastrointestinal suction and drainage.

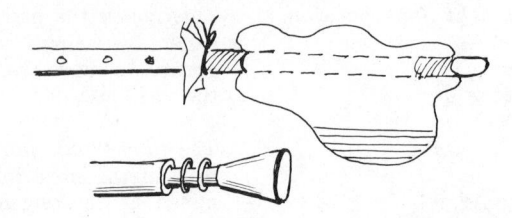

ITEM 4: INSERTION OF TUBE FOR REMOVAL OF GASTRIC CONTENTS FOR DIAGNOSTIC STUDY

Each agency has available a gastric analysis tray, which is usually obtained from the supply department. Items found on the tray would include: a stomach tube (Levin, Rehfuss, Jutte, or Ewald); a tube clamp; lubricant; towel; aspirating syringe; and several specimen bottles (the number will vary depending on the examination to be done). Your agency laboratory manual would give the specifics.

The various tubes mentioned above are named in your vocabulary list. If you have forgotten what they are, review the vocabulary before proceeding with the lesson.

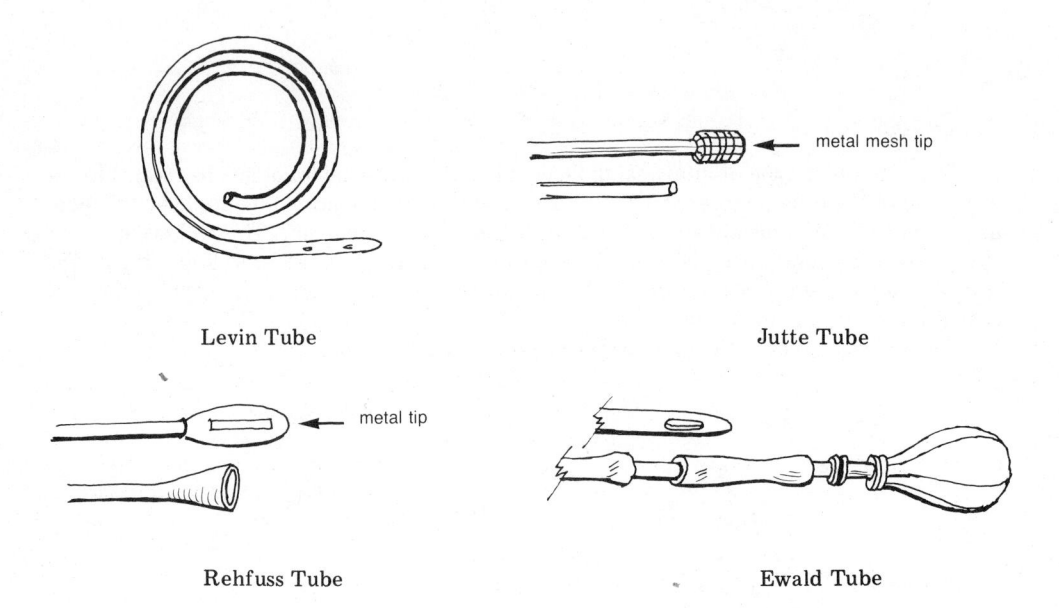

Levin Tube

Jutte Tube ← metal mesh tip

Rehfuss Tube ← metal tip

Ewald Tube

ITEM 5: INSERTION OF TUBE FOR GASTRIC ANALYSIS

The procedure for insertion of a tube for gastric analysis follows the procedure described in Item 1 for gastrointestinal drainage.

INSERTION OF NASOGASTRIC AND GAVAGE TUBES

Important Steps	Key Points
1. Wash your hands and prepare the equipment.	Obtain a gastric analysis tray from Supplies. Assemble the equipment for easy access on the bedside stand. Place it conveniently near the patient's head (on the side you are working).
2. Approach and identify the patient; explain the procedure.	Explain that a tube will be inserted through the nose or mouth (note agency preference). Although the passage of the tube is painless, some people gag when the tube passes down the back of the throat. Slow, deep breathing and swallowing help to minimize gagging.
3. Position the patient.	
4. Give a basin and tissues to the patient.	
5. Measure the tube for insertion distance.	
6. Take a working position and lubricate the tip of the tube.	
7. Instruct the patient to open his mouth, hold a glass of water, and swallow a mouthful.	
8. The tube is pushed slowly, gently, but firmly into the stomach.	
9. Check to see whether the tube is in the stomach.	
10. Insert an aspirating syringe into the proximal end of the tube.	Do this by pulling back on the plunger. Withdraw at least 10 cc of gastric contents.
11. Place a specimen in a labeled specimen jar.	Each specimen jar must be labeled with the patient's name, room number, hospital number, time, date, and whether it is specimen #1, #2, or whatever. The number and times that specimens are to be collected will depend on the purpose of the test. Check your laboratory manual for the specific requirements of your agency. You will take care of the specimen. If you do not remember the procedure for labeling and recording of a specimen, refer to Volume 2, Unit 21, "Urine Elimination" and Unit 22, "Bowel Elimination."
12. Make the patient comfortable.	The tube may be left in temporarily until all needed specimens have been collected; then it will be removed. Reassure the patient; ask if there is anything needed. Be sure to check this patient frequently because he may become quite apprehensive. Also, the tube is very annoying and irritating.
13. Return supplies and equipment.	When the procedure is complete, tidy the work area so that it is neat and clean. Return all used supplies to the proper place.
14. Record on the patient's chart.	Note the time, amount, color, and consistency of the specimen.

Important Steps	Key Points
	Charting example:
	6:30 A.M. Gastric specimen obtained via the Ewald tube. Specimen #1 contained 10 cc foul-smelling, dark-brown liquid. Odor somewhat like feces. Specimen to laboratory stat.
	A. Brown, R.N.
15. Send or take specimen to laboratory.	Include physician's order and/or the laboratory requisition with each specimen. Specimens must go to the laboratory at once for correct interpretation.
	NOTE: To remove the tube, follow the procedure in Item 2.

ITEM 6: SPECIAL FEEDING METHODS VIA THE GASTRIC, GASTROSTOMY, AND ENTEROSTOMY TUBES

Gastric gavage is a feeding given through a tube inserted either through the mouth or nose and into the stomach. Insertion and removal of this tube follows procedure outlined in Items 1 and 2. Patients who receive this type of feeding are unable to take foods orally (by mouth). Patients of any age may be fed in this manner, from the very small infant to the elderly geriatric patient.

The feeding can be given continuously over a 24-hour period by means of a special Murphy drip method, or it can be given at prescribed intervals, e.g., qid, four times a day, or q4h (every four hours).

Gavage feedings are specially prepared formulas made in the Diet Kitchen. They vary in nutritive value, and therefore the physician prescribes not only what caloric value he wants but also the volume of fluids and frequency to be given in a 24-hour period. The determination will depend on the patient's disease, age, and weight.

Recent research studies at Yale University noted that insertion of the gavage tube in the premature infant ("preemie") causes profound cardiorespiratory changes in the infant. The extreme change seemed to occur when the tube was inserted to a depth of 5 inches, although the pulse returned to normal rate within 24 seconds. Further research will determine the exact technique that will minimize detrimental physiological responses in such infants when a gavage tube is inserted.

The gastrostomy feeding may also be used. In this case a small incision is made in the upper left abdominal wall directly into the stomach. A gastrostomy tube (catheter with a large lumen) is inserted about 3 inches into the opening. The area is sutured (sewn) to close the surgical wound and also to secure the catheter to prevent it from slipping out of the incision. In about 10 days the wound is healed and the tube can be taken out and reinserted prn.

Remove the tube by withdrawing slowly as you rotate the tube between the index finger and thumb of your dominant hand. This prevents the lumen of the catheter from adhering to the stomach wall. Discard used supplies. Cover gastrostomy opening with sterile dressing.

The *enterostomy* (surgical formation of a permanent opening into the intestine through the abdominal wall) may be used as a method of feeding when the patient is unable to be fed through the stomach because of advanced carcinoma (cancer) of the stomach or major gastric surgical procedures or complications. The feeding tube is inserted into the stoma and the technique of feeding follows exactly as for the gastrostomy feeding. If you have forgotten what a stoma is, review the unit on bowel elimination.

You will be responsible for the initial insertion of the tube; you or an assistant will be responsible for giving the periodic feedings. You must demonstrate concern, support, and also demonstrate the ability to perform the task easily, correctly, and quickly.

INSERTION OF NASOGASTRIC AND GAVAGE TUBES

Important Steps	Key Points
1. Wash your hands and prepare the equipment.	The tray for the feeding procedure can be obtained from the supply department. The formula (feeding) is obtained from the Diet Kitchen. It is usually then stored in the refrigerator on the nursing unit, although it is ordered daily, like any other diet. Take the equipment to the patient's bedside and place it conveniently on the bedside stand or overbed table.
2. Approach and identify the patient, explain what you are going to do, and enlist his cooperation.	Some of the patients receiving this type of feeding may be unconscious, and therefore will not be able to cooperate. But explain the procedure to him anyway. Read your patient's identification bracelet to be sure you have the correct patient.
3. Position the patient.	Use the same position as that for the gastric intubation procedure for the gavage. However, for enterostomy and gastrostomy feedings, the patient should be in a dorsal recumbent position.
4. Hand the basin and tissues to the patient.	You can do this only if the patient is conscious. The procedure is the same as in gastric intubation, Item 1.
5. Measure the tube for insertion.	This is the same as Step 5 of gastric gavage procedure.
	The gastrostomy and enterostomy tubes are inserted directly into the special openings in the abdomen. These tubes are usually 12 to 18 inches long.
6. Insert tube.	Follow previous procedure.
7. Pour an ounce of water at room temperature into a funnel, syringe, or burette.	The funnel, syringe, or burette is attached to the free end of the tube. The water is used to make sure that the tube is open.
	NOTE: If the tube is inserted each time it is used, this step would be omitted.
8. Pour warmed formula (105°F) into the equipment.	Formula should be given slowly. Gravity pull will draw it into the stomach.
	You can regulate flow by raising and lowering the receptacle as demonstrated in the adjacent diagram.

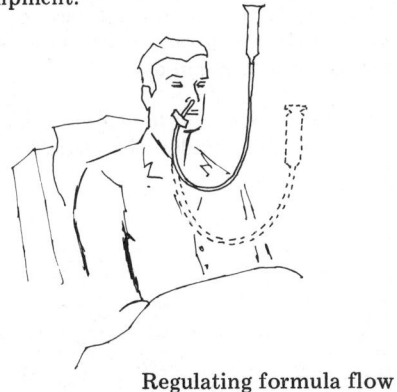

Regulating formula flow

Important Steps	Key Points
9. Maintain the level of formula slightly above the neck of the syringe.	If you allow the formula level to fall below the neck of the syringe, air will enter the tubing and then the stomach. This can cause great discomfort because of distention of the stomach.

Continue adding formula to the syringe until the prescribed amount is given. |
| 10. Pour 1 to 2 ounces of water into the syringe to clear the tube. | When the formula feeding is finished, pour in fresh water to clear the tube. Again, be sure to keep the liquid above the neck of the syringe to prevent air bubbles from collecting in the system or in the patient's stomach. (This step would be eliminated if the tube were removed after each feeding.) |
| 11. Clamp the tubing.

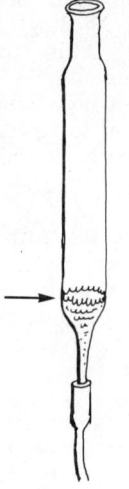

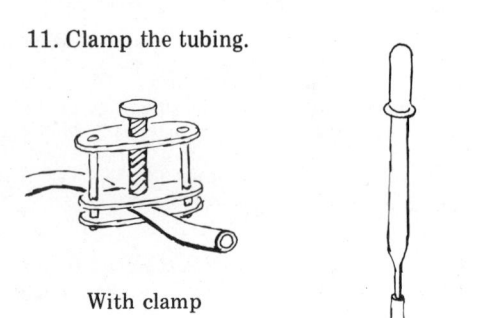

With clamp

With medicine dropper | If tubing is removed, clamp it tightly between your right index finger and thumb to prevent the tube from dripping as it is removed. Pull the tubing out slowly and gently to prevent gagging.

If the tubing is left in, close it (with the clamp or medicine dropper that comes on your tray) before removing the funnel, syringe, or burette to keep backflow of the formula from soiling the patient's gown or linen. |
| 12. Secure the tubing.

Secure under bandage | *For gavage:* Secure the end of the tube with tape to the patient's forehead as you did in Item 1. Be sure to avoid irritating the skin area and to keep it clean and dry.

For gastrostomy and enterostomy: Secure the end of the tube under the dressing on the abdomen. |

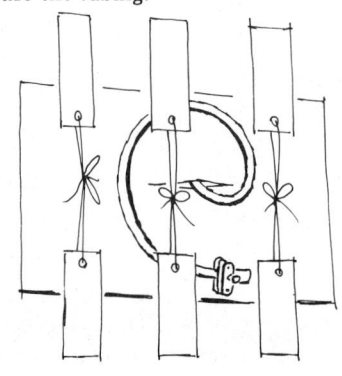

INSERTION OF NASOGASTRIC AND GAVAGE TUBES

Important Steps	Key Points
13. Give oral hygiene and nose care (for gavage only).	If tubing is left in, be sure that the nose is kept moist, clean and free from crusts. Sometimes the tubing is left connected to a large flask, which may be hung on an IV pole at the head of the bed.
14. Make the patient comfortable.	A person undergoing this procedure needs extra reassurance, kindness, and patience. It is possible that he will have to be fed by this means for a long period of time.
You may need to teach the patient and his family how to accomplish this feeding procedure. Be sure to stress the *safety* technique of checking to make sure that his tube is not in the lung. Stress the importance of cleanliness of the equipment, the patient, and environment to his peace of mind as well as a preventive measure against infection.
Be sure to tell the patient when you expect to return, and then keep your word.
15. Record on the patient's chart.	Note the amount of formula, how taken, and any other comments about the patient's reaction.
Charting example:
8:00 A.M. Gavage tube inserted and 200 cc formula taken without difficulty.
A. Brown, R.N.
NOTE: Gavage, gastrostomy and enterostomy tubes are removed as described in Item 2.

Remember the following considerations when caring for patients with gastrointestinal tubes:

1) Demonstrate kindness, gentleness, and quiet concern for their comfort.

2) Give meticulous and frequent oral hygiene and nose care.

3) Provide for freedom of movement, as much as possible, by securing the suction tubing to the clothing and/or skin to permit maximum activity.

4) See that the patient does not lie on the tubing; do not permit the tubing to be kinked because the suction will stop, as will the fluid drainage.

5) Observe, report, and record the insertion of the gastrointestinal tubes accurately. Report and record various tube feedings promptly and completely. (Follow examples given at the end of each Item in this lesson.)

These patients will provide a challenge to nursing care. They will often relax better if you give an extra back-rub, straighten or change bed linens prn. Your quiet, observant attention to details when caring for such patients can hasten their recovery.

VI. ADDITIONAL INFORMATION FOR ENRICHMENT

Your instructor will provide you with a list of reading materials if you wish to learn more about the subject of gastrointestinal tubes for decompression, diagnostic tests, cleansing, or feeding.

Review *Nursing Skills for Allied Health Services*, Volume 2, Unit 25, "Care of the Patient with Gastrointestinal Tubes", to refresh your memory on the various types of suction equipment used with the various gastrointestinal tubes.

INSERTION OF NASOGASTRIC AND GAVAGE TUBES 323

POST-TEST

Complete the following statements.

1. List four reasons for insertion of a gastrointestinal tube.

    (a) _____

    (b) _____

    (c) _____

    (d) _____

2. Name the four common tubes used in a gastric analysis examination.

    (a) _____ (c) _____

    (b) _____ (d) _____

3. List at least four nursing measures you would use in caring for patients with a gastrointestinal tube.

    (a) _____

    (b) _____

    (c) _____

    (d) _____

POST-TEST ANNOTATED ANSWER SHEET

1. (a) To prevent postoperative vomiting, intestinal obstruction, gas formation

    (b) For diagnosis

    (c) To wash out stomach (lavage), p. 308.

2. (a) Levin tube

    (b) Rehfuss tube

    (c) Jutte tube

    (d) Ewald tube, p. 316.

3. (a) Demonstrate kindness, gentleness, comfort.

    (b) Give oral hygiene and nose care.

    (c) Provide freedom of movement.

    (d) Maintain open lumen so fluid will continue to drain. Observe, record, and report contents of drainage, pp. 313, 321.

PERFORMANCE TEST

1. Given a patient with a feeding tube, you will assemble the equipment, prepare the patient (or the mannequin, Mrs. Chase), and give a feeding of 50 cc of water following the procedure outlined in the lesson, maintaining safety precautions. You will practice recording the activity on the nurse's notes. Your instructor will select a patient with a gastrointestinal, gastrostomy, or enterostomy tube.

2. You should be able to explain safety precautions that must be observed while inserting a gastrointestinal tube or when feeding a patient who has a gastrointestinal tube in place.

PERFORMANCE CHECKLIST

GAVAGE

1. Wash hands and prepare equipment.
2. Approach and identify the patient.
3. Position the patient (Fowler's).
4. Hand emesis basin and tissue to patient.
5. Pour 1 ounce water, room temperature, into funnel to check that tubing is patent.
6. Pour warmed formula (105°F) into syringe.
7. Regulate flow by raising and lowering the feeding tube.
8. Keep level of formula above neck of syringe to prevent air from entering the stomach.
9. Continue giving formula until prescribed amount is given.
10. Pour 1 to 2 ounces of water to clear tube.
11. Clamp tube; remove funnel from tube.
12. Secure distal end of tube.
13. Give oral hygiene and nose care.
14. Leave patient comfortable (position in good alignment with call cord and bedside stand nearby, and tell patient when you will return).
15. Chart activity.

Unit 11

SMEARS AND CULTURES

I. DIRECTIONS TO THE STUDENT

You are to proceed through this lesson using the workbook as your guide. In the skill laboratory or in the clinical area you will practice obtaining a smear or culture.

Please read the following paragraphs carefully. They will tell you exactly what you will be expected to know. If you feel that you have sufficient knowledge and skills to do the performance test accurately without further study of the lesson, please discuss this with your instructor. The skills required in the test must be performed without the use of reference materials.

II. GENERAL PERFORMANCE OBJECTIVE

To demonstrate the procedure for obtaining a smear or culture using medical asepsis or aseptic technique as required.

III. SPECIFIC PERFORMANCE OBJECTIVES

Upon completion of this lesson, you will be able to:

1. Take a smear (vaginal, cervical, urethral, rectal).
2. Take a throat or wound culture.

IV. VOCABULARY

Read the definitions of the terms listed below. Do not attempt to memorize them before proceeding with the lesson. Each term will be explained or defined again in the text. On completion of the lesson, however, you should know the correct definition of each term.

biopsy—excision of a small piece of tissue for microscopic examination.
cauterization—destruction of tissue by burning with electricity or a chemical.
colposcopy—a gynecological examination that utilizes the colposcope to examine the fornices of the vagina and cervix; it magnifies the cervix 13 times so that abnormalities may be seen.
conization—coring or removal of the mucous lining of the cervical canal and its glands by means of cutting with a high-frequency current.
culture—a mass of organisms growing in a laboratory culture medium.
curettage—scraping of a cavity (e.g., uterine curettage).
cytology—science of cell life and cell formation.
dysplasia—abnormal growth or development of tissue.
histology—study of microscopic structure of tissue.
incubation—the period of culture development.
inoculate—to inject the organisms of a disease into the body or onto culture media.
introitus—any aperture (opening) in the body (e.g., the external orifice of the vagina).
Papanicolaou (Pap) smear—a laboratory test to determine cancer, especially uterine or cervical cancer.
smear—material spread on a microscopic slide (e.g., vaginal smear).

speculum—a tubular instrument inserted into a body passage for inspection or medication (e.g., vaginal speculum).

stenosis (stricture)—narrowing of a passage or orifice (e.g., cervical stenosis).

surgical sound—an elongated instrument for exploring body cavities surgically; used for diagnosis or treatment (e.g., uterine sound).

tenaculum—sharp, hooklike, pointed instrument with slender shank for grasping or holding a part (e.g., uterine tenaculum).

V. INTRODUCTION

Smears and cultures are two laboratory procedures utilized to determine the type and presence of various organisms so that appropriate treatment can be instituted to cure the infection or disease.

The material obtained for the smear or culture can be taken from any body opening (natural, accidental, or surgical): the eye, ear, nose, throat, vagina, urethra, rectum, wounds, etc.

For the purpose of our discussions, the most common sites for obtaining smears or cultures will be described.

General steps for obtaining a smear are as follows:

1. First, the health worker will swab the area that is infected, or diseased, to obtain secretions containing the offending organism.

2. Wipe the specimen on a glass slide so that it can then be visualized under a microscope to identify the specific organism. The glass slide is held between the thumb and the index finger of the non-dominant hand. The applicator is grasped at the distal end with the dominant hand (holding it between the thumb and index finger). Starting toward the right of the slide, roll the applicator across the slide toward the left. *Do not touch* your thumb or fingers with the contaminated cotton-tipped applicator. Spread the material from the applicator onto the slide in an even manner, using a moderately heavy downward pressure on the slide. This will place the maximal number of cells on the slide with minimal destruction of cells.

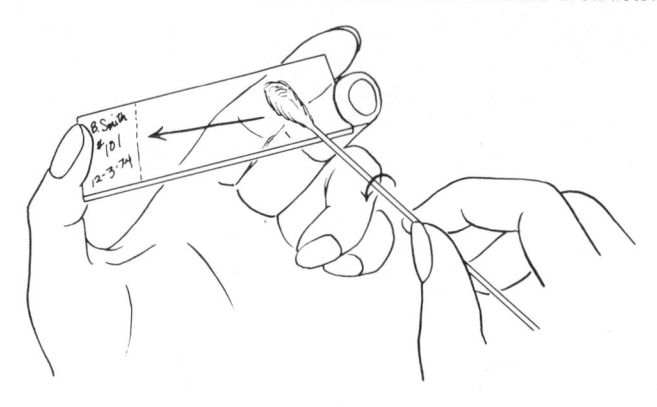

3. Fix the smear by spraying it with a specially prepared fixative, by immersing it in an alcohol solution, or by passing it quickly through the flame of a Bunsen or alcohol burner. (Agency procedure should be followed.)

4. Incubate the smear for a prescribed time (24 to 72 hours) at 37°C or room temperature. Excessive heating of the smear would kill the organisms.

5. Read the smear at various intervals to observe the growth of the colonies of organisms. Some growth can be observed by the naked eye; however, definitive identification of the specific organism is done by viewing the slide under the microscope. Various staining procedures are used in the laboratory to identify specific organisms.

SMEARS AND CULTURES

Vaginal, cervical, endocervical, and rectal smears and cultures are used for cytologic tests that assist physicians and nurse practitioners to make various diagnoses of gynecologic disorders, e.g., cervical cancer, endocervical cancer, maturation index (which indicates estrogen levels), and the presence of veneral disease, among other conditions.

Frequently, the Papanicolaou (Pap) smear is done at the same time as other tests. The Pap smear is a periodic screening device used to detect uterine or cervical cancer. If the Pap report comes back positive, further examination must be done to make the final diagnosis, e.g., biopsy, curettage, colposcopy, conization of the cervix, or various staining procedures.

Cytology classifications are reported as:

Class I—Normal or negative (there is a 10 to 20 per cent chance of being false negative).

Class II—Some atypical cells present (a result of inflammation).

Class III—Dysplasia present (follow-up is needed).

Class IV—Cancer in situ (parabasal cells affected).

Class V—Invasive cancer (deep layers of cells affected).

Pap smears should not be collected from the menstruating woman because the blood cells produced during that period can obscure the microscopic readings. The Pap smear should not be done within six weeks of having had the cervix cauterized, or for a longer period following radiation therapy, because the cervical cells are distorted by these procedures.

ITEM 1: VAGINAL, CERVICAL, OR RECTAL SMEAR AND CULTURE

Important Steps	Key Points
1. Assemble supplies and equipment.	Arrange them on a clean towel on a solid surface (table or Mayo stand), which can be placed near the patient. The required items include: 3 sterile applicators, 2 Ayer tongue blades, 2 frosted-end glass slides, Thayer-Martin culture plate, fixative, bivalve vaginal speculum, sterile glove(s), dressing forceps, and sponge.

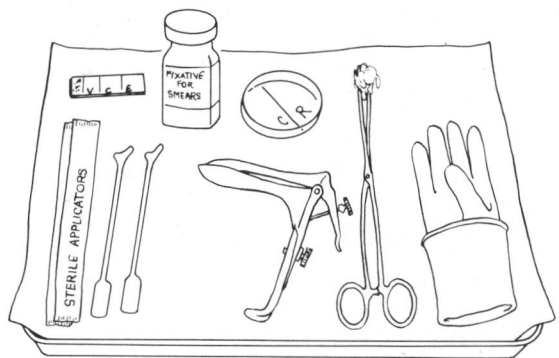

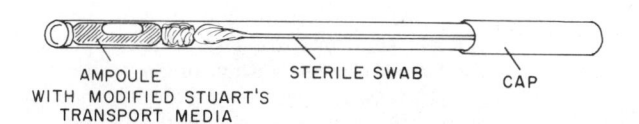

Important Steps	Key Points
2. Identify the slides and culture plate.	Mark the slides and culture plate according to agency procedure. Be sure that there are no fingerprints or powder on the clean slide.

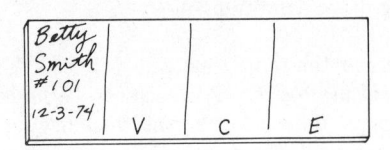

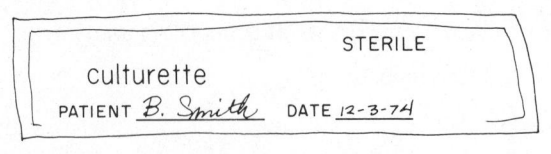

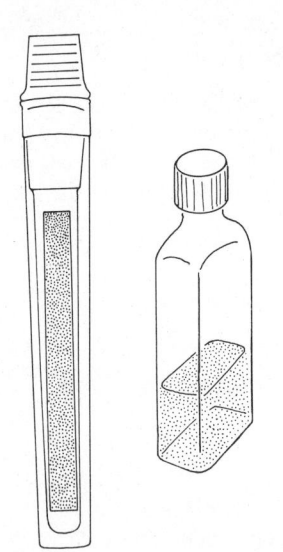

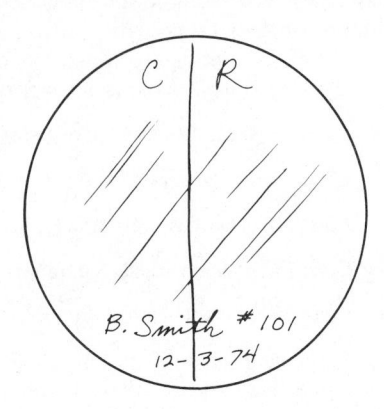

NOTE: More expensive media preparation can be used, e.g., Transgrow bottles or Clinicult (Smith, Kline and French). The Transgrow bottle is generally used if the specimen must be mailed to a laboratory. |
| 3. Wash your hands, approach the patient, and explain the procedure. | Introduce yourself and identify the patient (check her Identaband or chart). Explain that you will be taking a secretion sample from the cervix and vagina for laboratory examination to determine the cause of the pain, discharge, or whatever. |
| 4. Position and drape the patient for vaginal examination. | Be sure that she is as comfortable as possible. The buttocks should be at the edge of the table nearest the lowered foot-section.

Position the examining light for maximum visualization of the perineal area, while not obstructing access to the patient. |
| 5. Insert middle fingers into the patient's vagina. | Inspect the perineum for abnormalities (color, discharge).

Palpate Bartholin's glands and surrounding tissue to detect abnormal firmness, which could indicate cervical cancer. With your gloved hand, apply light pressure with the middle fingers on the posterior fourchette (vaginal wall muscles). |

Important Steps	Key Points
6. Ask the patient to relax "here."	The patient usually is able to relax the vaginal musculature where she feels the light pressure of your fingers. This will make it easier for you to insert the vaginal speculum.
7. Insert the bivalve vaginal speculum in an oblique plane.	Use the ungloved hand (some individuals may prefer to wear sterile gloves on both hands).
	Inserting the speculum in an oblique plane will avoid injury to the sensitive anterior structures.
	Do not lubricate the speculum because you cannot get a clean or live specimen for the smear or culture if it is contaminated with a lubricant. Some agencies may use warm water as a lubricant so that the speculum can be inserted more easily.
8. Direct the speculum posteriorly.	Direct it over the fingers.
9. Turn the speculum to the horizontal plane.	This should be done when the short upper blade is just in front of the cervix.
10. Remove your fingers.	The downward pressure on the vaginal fourchette will continue with the weight of the speculum secured in the open position.
	If you are manually maintaining the speculum in the open position, make sure that you continue the downward pressure on the vaginal fourchette to assure continued muscle relaxation.
11. Lift the anterior speculum blade.	Depress the thumb lever on the speculum.
12. Position the opened blades around the cervix.	Settle the completely opened blades so that the cervix is positioned between the opened blades.
13. Secure the blades in position.	Tighten the screw on the speculum, or simply hold the blades apart during the short procedure.
14. Remove the cervical mucous plug.	Use an applicator, if necessary.
15. Take a vaginal smear.	With the first spatula, scrape the vaginal pool with moderate pressure at the point marked "X" in the diagram.
	Keep the material on the blade.

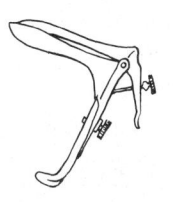

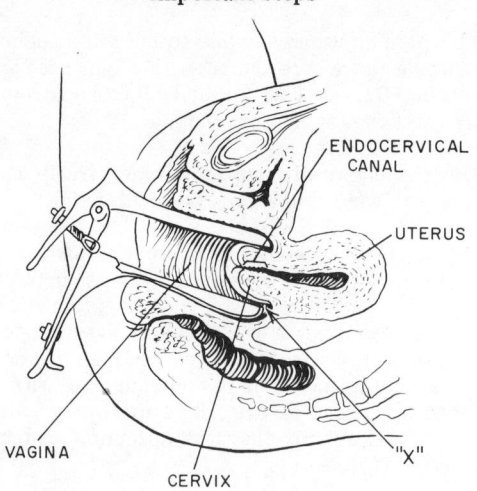

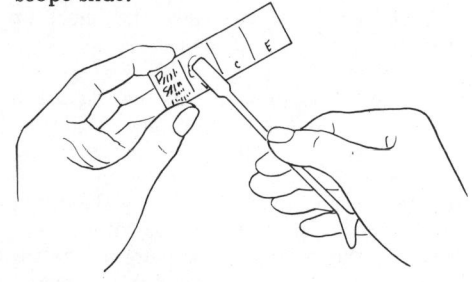

Important Steps	Key Points
	NOTE: You will have to determine which end to use (short or long), depending on the size and shape of the cervix, which will vary among your patients.
16. Spread the vaginal smear on the microscope slide.	On the section marked "V", spread the material evenly and moderately thin so that cells can be visualized under the microscope. If you spread the material too thickly, individual cells cannot be visualized very easily.
17. Take a cervical smear.	With moderate pressure, scrape the squamate columnar junction (SCJ) with the opposite end of the Ayer spatula. Rotate the spatula around the cervix so that cells can be picked up from all parts of the cervix. The SCJ is the point at which the red, irregular columnar epithelium of the endocervix meets the smooth, flat, pink squamous tissue of the cervix.

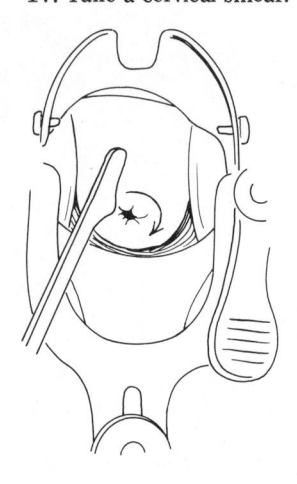

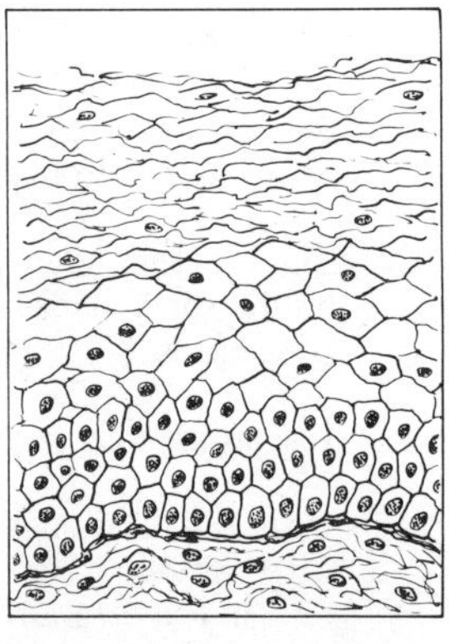

STRATIFIED SQUAMOUS EPITHELIUM OF THE ECTOCERVIX AND VAGINA

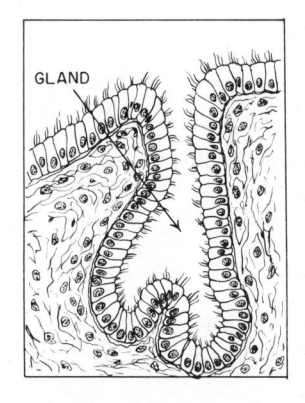

COLUMNAR EPITHELIUM OF THE ENDOCERVICAL GLANDS

SMEARS AND CULTURES

Important Steps	Key Points
18. Spread the cervical smear on the slide.	Apply the contents of both sides of the spatula on the section of the slide marked "C."
	Again, spread the material evenly and moderately thin.
19. Take an endocervical smear.	Using a sterile applicator, insert it into the cervical os, rotating it completely around the os so that all sides are touched and assuring that the maximal number of cells will be obtained.
	Be sure that the cotton is saturated. This usually takes 10 to 20 seconds.
20. Spread the endocervical smear on the slide.	Roll the applicator on the section of the slide marked "E."
	NOTE: Some agencies may do all three smears; some may do only the vaginal and cervical. Follow your agency procedure for making the slide and taking the smears.
21. Spray or immerse the slide in fixative immediately.	This must be done within four seconds to prevent drying and death of cells.
22. Take another endocervical smear.	Using the second sterile applicator, again saturate the cotton thoroughly by rotating the applicator in a 360° circle, touching all sides of the cervical canal.

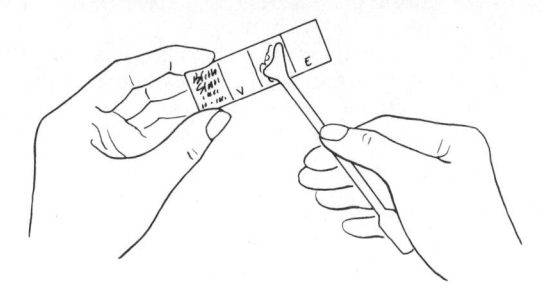

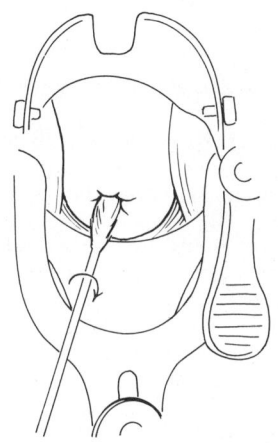

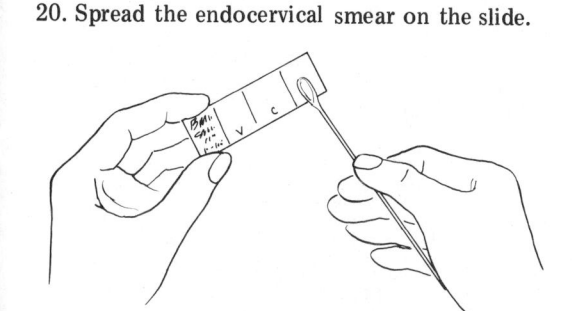

Note: The next two specimens (Steps 22-43) may be done separately from the first three smears. (Follow your agency procedure.)

23. *Remove the top of the culture plate*, and put it upside down on a flat surface.

Important Steps	Key Points
24. Inoculate the culture plate.	Roll the applicator in a "Z" pattern on the side of the culture plate marked "C" (cervical).
	NOTE: The culture medium that is most often used is the Thayer-Martin chocolate base media. It is very reliable and economical.
25. Discard the applicator.	Put it into the designated container.
26. Remove the vaginal speculum.	While continuing to maintain downward pressure on the vaginal fourchette, (a) unscrew the thumb lever and withdraw the speculum slowly and carefully; (b) inspect the vaginal mucosa for color, inflammation, or growths; and (c) close the speculum blades carefully and turn them in a oblique direction, within one inch of the introitus. Be careful to avoid catching the cervix, vaginal mucosa, or pubic hair in the speculum as you remove it.
27. Insert the third cotton applicator into the rectum.	Gently twirl or roll the applicator in a 360° circle around the inner anal wall at a depth of one inch.
	Saturate the cotton with secretions. Take at least 10 to 20 seconds so that you can obtain as many organisms as possible.
	If feces appear on the applicator, discard it and use a clean applicator.
	NOTE: The two sites (cervical and rectal) in steps 22 and 27 are recommended so that you can be assured of obtaining the *Neisseria gonorrhoeae* organism. Sometimes a woman may have douched just before the examination and will have washed the cervical organisms away; therefore the rectal specimen is required.
	NOTE: Some agencies may prefer to do a cervical and urethral culture. Use the same technique as above, except that the applicator is inserted in the urethral opening and then the medium is inoculated on the side marked "U."
	For the male, a sterile bacteriologic loop may be used to gently scrape the mucosa.
	NOTE: An additional culture specimen should be obtained from the pharynx of homosexual men when gonorrhea is suspected.

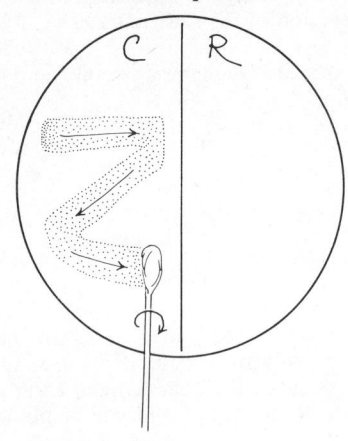

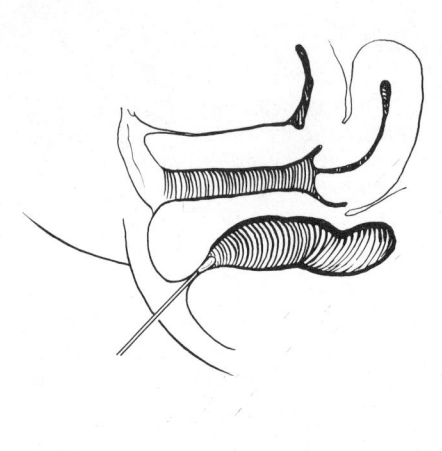

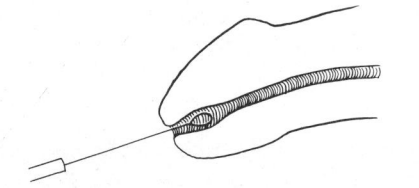

SMEARS AND CULTURES

Important Steps	Key Points
28. Inoculate the culture plate.	Roll the applicator lightly in a "Z" pattern on the side marked "R" (rectal). Discard the applicator and replace the cover on the culture plate.
29. Reposition the patient for comfort.	Dry the perineum and rectum, if needed. Raise the foot of the examining table. Take the patient's legs out of the stirrups and lower them out on the table. Help her as needed. If the patient is being seen in an office or clinic, she will probably be told to dress and wait for the doctor or nurse practitioner to return.
30. Obtain a wire loop to cross-inoculate the medium.	Take the loop from the holder (which may be kept in the examining room or the laboratory area). Heat it until it is red hot to destroy any unwanted organisms. If these organisms are not destroyed, you could expect a contaminated growth of organisms in the culture media.
31. Cool the loop momentarily.	This will prevent destruction of the organisms that were inoculated on the media.
32. Remove the plate cover.	Place it upside down on a flat surface.

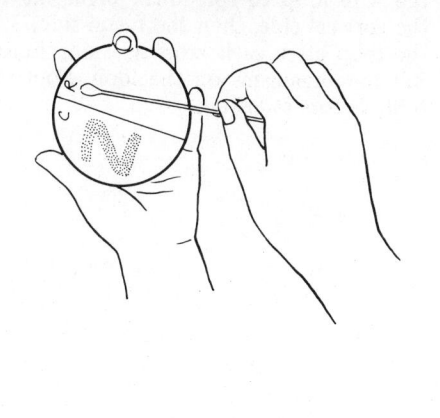

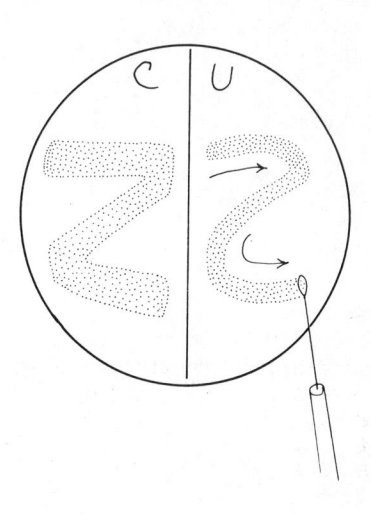

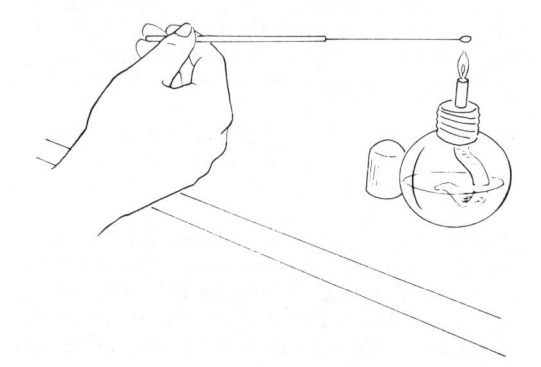

UNIT 11

Important Steps	Key Points
33. Cross-streak the inoculated media.	With moderate pressure, criss-cross the Z with the wire loop to spread the organism (first on the cervical side, then the rectal side). Reflame the loop after each cross-streaking in order to kill the organisms on the loop. Cool momentarily before streaking.
34. Reflame the loop and return to storage.	Flaming kills all organisms that were picked up on the loop during the streaking process. This must be done before returning the wire loop to storage. Store with the loop extended up out of the container so that the delicate wire is not damaged.
35. Replace the cover on the culture plate.	Be sure that it is correctly labeled with the patient's identification.
36. Put the culture plate in a "candle jar" immediately.	A tightly closed gallon jar with a candle burning in it seems to remove the O_2 from the air; the flame will go out when the O_2 is depleted. The candle must be relit each time a culture plate is put in or removed from the jar. Since the gonococcus organism is partly anaerobic, it grows best in a 3 per cent CO_2 atmosphere. NOTE: *Store the culture plate with the media on the top side of the plate.* In this way, moisture that may collect in the plate during the incubation period will not drip down on the medium while the growth of the organisms takes place.
37. Incubate the culture plates.	Record the tests on the chart. Keep them at a temperature of 35°–36°C (or room temperature) for at least 24 hours. (Follow your agency's procedure for specific time.)

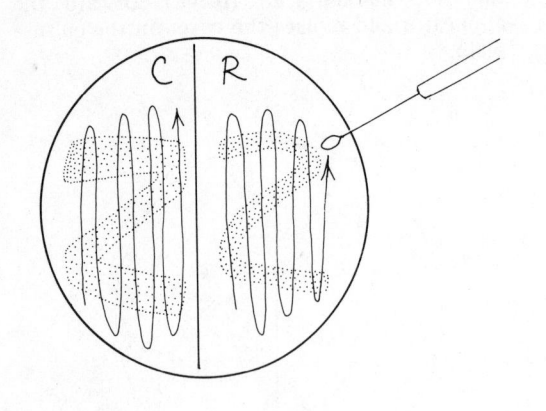

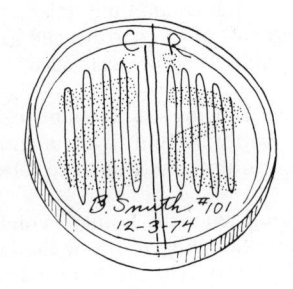

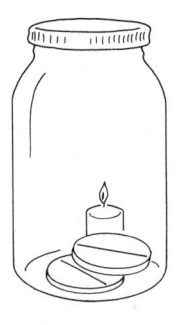

SMEARS AND CULTURES

Important Steps	Key Points
38. Mix a dye solution.	Use the amount of potassium hydroxide (KOH) powder that can be picked up on the tip of a toothpick and mix it in a test tube with 2 to 3 cc sterile water. The mixed solution must be used within 12 hours of preparation; if not, it must be discarded because of the chemical changes that take place.
39. Open the culture plates after 24 hours.	Use aseptic technique to avoid contamination of the medium with other organisms. Check for growth of organisms. If there is no obvious growth, incubate for another 24 hours.
40. Roll a sterile applicator across the growth on the medium.	Collect as much organism growth on the cotton as possible. Use a gentle touch. *Do not destroy the culture medium.*
41. Place a drop of the KOH solution on the cotton applicator.	Use the medicine dropper stored in the mixed solution. If the applicator turns red, it is an indication that the gonorrheal organism is present. Discard the applicator.
42. Return the covered culture plate to the covered candle jar.	Incubate for an additional 24 hour period to bring out more growth, particularly if only a few cells were obtained. Some agencies recommend flooding the entire plate with 10 per cent potassium hydroxide solution (KOH) to be sure that no colonies were missed.
43. Discard the culture plate.	Put it into a tightly closed container to minimize the putrid odor from the media plates.
44. Record the procedure on the patient's chart.	10:30 A.M. Vaginal, cervical, endocervical, rectal smears taken. Specimens sent to lab. Z. Solinski, R.N.

There are some "do-it-yourself" Pap test kits available for those women who cannot get to a clinic or who are unwilling to see their physician. These tests have limited value, since the history and physical examination are equally important.

ITEM 2: VAGINAL SMEARS FOR TRICHOMONAS VAGINITIS AND MONILIAL VAGINITIS

Two common vaginal infections, trichomonas vaginitis and monilial vaginitis, are also diagnosed by means of vaginal smears. First, follow Steps 1 through 13 above.

Important Steps	Key Points
14. Place a small mount of saline on a slide.	Mix 10 per cent potassium hydroxide (KOH) with the saline (KOH is *not* used if you are trying to obtain the *Trichomonas* organism; use only saline).
15. Take a vaginal smear.	Saturate a cotton-tipped applicator with discharge from the vagina.

UNIT 11

Important Steps	Key Points
16. Dip the saturated applicator into the solution on the slide.	Discard the applicator.
17. Put a coverglass on the slide.	Center it over the depressed section in the middle of the slide, and examine immediately under the microscope. Look for the branching arms of the fungus of the monilial organism, or for a moving flagellated organism if the *Trichomonas* organism is present. NOTE: The coverglass is a thin glass disc that covers a mounted object on the glass slide so that movement of live cells can be observed when viewed through a microscope.
18. Record the procedure on the patient's chart.	Charting example: 10:30 A.M.: Vaginal smear for *Trichmonas* taken; specimen examined under microscope. Trichmonas vaginitis visualized. Sent home with prescription. L. Sumi, R.N.

ITEM 3: IRRIGATION PROCEDURE FOR OBTAINING ENDOMETRIAL CELLS

A recently introduced technique to obtain endometrial cells has begun to replace the minor D and C (dilatation and curettage of the cervix) surgical procedure, which requires anesthesia and hospitalization. The disposable suction-type irrigation device is called the Gravlee Jet Washer, developed in the late 1960's by Dr. L. Clark Gravlee. This procedure can be done in an outpatient clinic or in a physician's or nurse practitioner's office. It is an accurate, convenient method to detect early endometrial carcinoma.

Important Steps	Key Points
1. Assemble the required supplies and equipment.	Arrange them on a clean tray for the purpose of collecting a Pap smear of the cervix and vagina, as described in the previous Item. To these items add a sterile, disposable Gravlee Jet Washer double-cannula tip assembly and a 30 cc syringe, uterine tenaculum, and uterine sound.
2. Wash your hands, approach the patient, and explain the procedure.	Introduce yourself and identify the patient (check her Identaband or chart).
3. Position and drape the patient for vaginal examination.	The buttocks should be at the edge of the table, feet in the stirrups. Lower the foot section of the table. Position the examination light for maximal visualization while permitting unobstructed access to the perineal area.
4. Take a vaginal and a cervical smear.	See Item 1, Steps 15 through 18.
5. Grasp the cervix with the tenaculum.	Apply pull (or traction) to straighten the endocervical canal as much as possible.

SMEARS AND CULTURES

Important Steps	Key Points
6. Introduce the sterile uterine sound into the uterine cavity.	Insert it gently, straight through the cervical os until an obstruction is felt (the top of the uterine cavity). This will determine the depth and the angle of the uterine cavity. Sometimes introduction of the sound may cause painful uterine contractions, and therefore a mild analgesic may be used before the procedure is started. If the sound cannot be introduced because of stenosis of the cervix, the procedure should be terminated. It is contraindicated in a stenotic cervix because of the danger of perforation. *Extreme caution* must be taken to avoid uterine wall perforations with the sound.
7. Pick up the cannula and adjust its stopper. 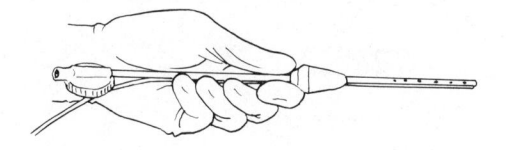	Bend the cannula to conform to the angle of the uterine cavity. Place the stopper at the approximate depth of the cavity.
8. Fill the reservoir. 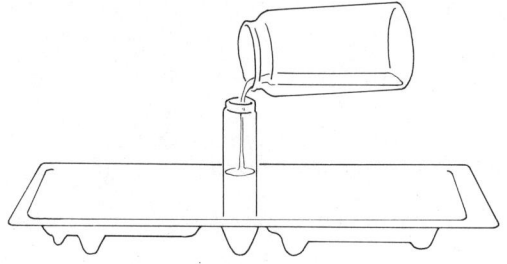	Pour in 30 cc normal saline.
9. Attach the reservoir to the washer tip. 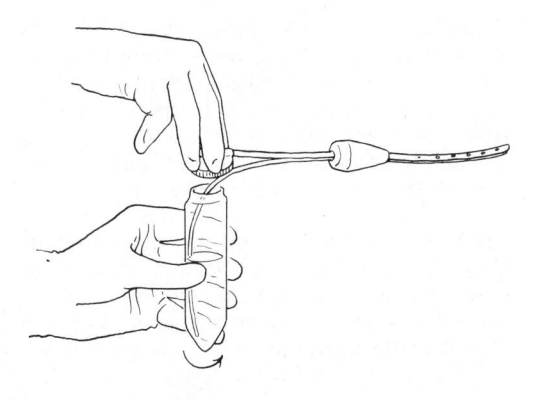	There are two cannulas arranged vertically, one on top of the other. Because the tips break easily, they should be bent *laterally*. Bend the small tube into the reservoir. You may need to rotate the cannula laterally when you place it in the reservoir.
10. Screw the reservoir firmly into the cap.	Continue to hold the reservoir in a vertical position with the non-dominant hand, turning the reservoir counterclockwise until it is secured to the cap.

UNIT 11

Important Steps	Key Points
11. Introduce the cannula tip into the uterine cavity.	Insert to the depth of the preset stopper (Step 7). To facilitate insertion, the tip can be rotated in an arc to the point at which the saline would spill out of the reservoir.
	The stopper should be resting firmly against the cervical os, forming a sealed cavity. To make sure that the seal is tight, a small amount of lubricant may be applied around the stopper.
12. Attach the 30 cc syringe to the Luer-lok on the reservoir cap.	The plunger of the syringe should be completely forward in the barrel.
13. Draw solution into the syringe.	Withdraw the plunger with a slow, even pull until the syringe is filled, and a negative pressure is established in the uterine cavity.
	While this solution is being drawn into the syringe, normal saline is drawn from the reservoir through the smaller cannula into the uterus. The saline seems to bathe the endometrial cavity and dislodge cells and tissue fragments. The solution re-enters the larger cannula and returns into the collecting syringe.
	The negative pressure in the uterine cavity closes the fallopian tubes so that uterine contents will not spill into the abdominal cavity. No more than 4 1/2 cc saline occupies the uterine cavity at any time.

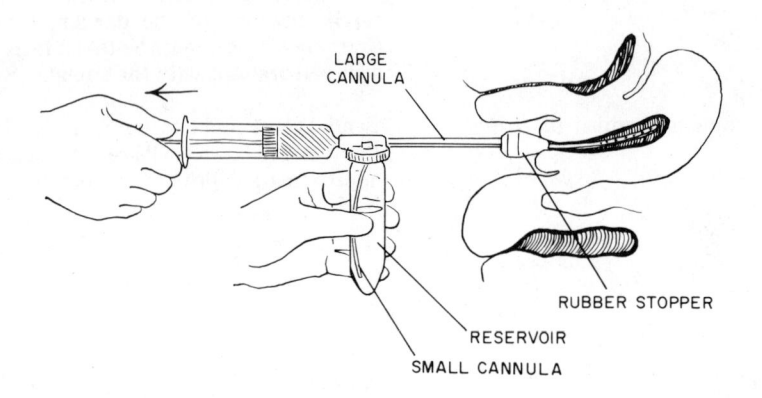

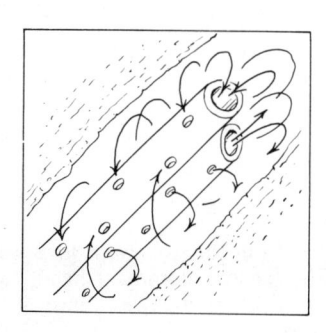

Important Steps	Key Points
14. Disconnect the syringe from the reservoir cap.	*Expel the contents* into the empty reservoir through the opening on the top of the cap. Disconnect the syringe and lay it aside.
15. Unscrew the cap from the reservoir.	Expel any remaining tissue on the jet tip into the reservoir. Then discard the cap assembly.
16. Screw on the closed cap securely.	This will prevent loss of the specimen during transportation to the laboratory.
17. Label the reservoir bottle.	Mark the appropriate patient identification (date, time, patient's name, identification number, etc.).
18. Remove the vaginal speculum.	See Item 1, Step 26, above.
19. Reposition the patient.	Give her directions for getting dressed and returning for further examination.
20. Record procedure.	

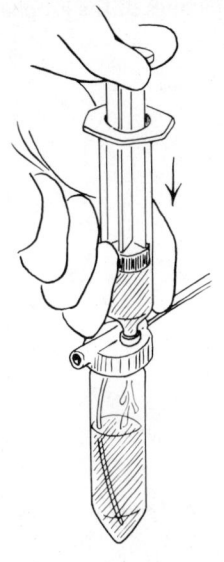

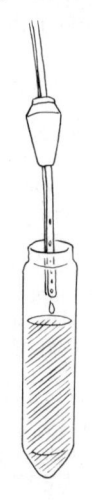

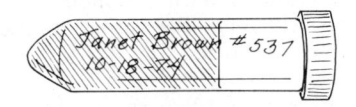

ITEM 4: THROAT CULTURE

The throat (pharynx) is that portion of the respiratory tract that extends from the arch of the palate (roof of the mouth) to the glottis and superior openings of the esophagus. The front of the neck is also sometimes called the throat.

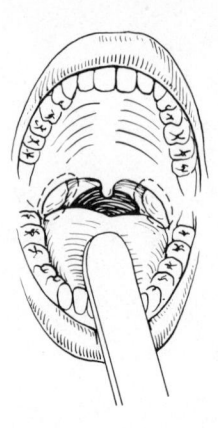

The throat is a frequent location for infections, among them staphylococcus, streptococcus, and pneumococcus.

Various types of culture tubes may be prepared with media so that specific organisms can be grown, e.g., staph tubes for staphylococci; monitubes for *Candida albicans*, hemolytic tubes for hemolytic streptococci, staphylococci, or pneumococci, and S. S. tubes for salmonella or shigella, etc.

Important Steps	Key Points
1. Assemble the supplies and equipment.	Arrange them on a Mayo stand: laryngeal mirror, tongue depressor, culture tube(s), and applicators.
2. Wash your hands; approach and identify the patient.	Explain that you are going to wipe the inside of the throat with a cotton-tipped applicator to obtain a specimen for laboratory examination.
3. Position the patient.	He should be in a chair facing you.
	Position the examination light over your left shoulder so that the throat can be seen with maximal illumination.
4. Depress the tongue with a tongue blade.	Ask the patient to open his mouth and say "Ah." This will relax the throat muscle and minimize the gag reflex.
5. Remove the sterile applicator from the culture tube.	NOTE: The culture tubes can be prepared in your laboratory, and there are also commercially prepared culture tubes such as the Culturette.
	a) Open the cap of the culture tube (unscrew and lay the cap upside down on a flat surface, or open the paper package containing the culture tube).
	b) Remove sterile applicators from the package or culture tube.

SMEARS AND CULTURES

Important Steps	Key Points
6. Swab the site with the sterile applicator.	Make a downward swipe along one of the tonsillar areas (right or left). Go as deep as you can before the patient gags. Keep the tongue depressed.
7. Remove the applicator gently.	Put it in the test tube, and replace the culture tube cap.
8. Take a second applicator and swab the opposite tonsillar site.	Use a firm, quick, downward stroke.
9. Remove the applicator quickly.	Keep the tongue depressed. Then place the applicator in a test tube and replace the cap. Remove the tongue blade. Discard into designated container.
10. Reposition the patient for comfort.	
11. Label each culture tube and prepare it for transfer to the laboratory.	Mark the patient's name, identification number, date, physician's name; include the completed request for examination. Send to the laboratory at once.
12. Record the procedure on patient's chart.	Charting example: 3:15 P.M. Throat culture taken. Specimen sent to laboratory with requisition. L. Sumi, R.N.

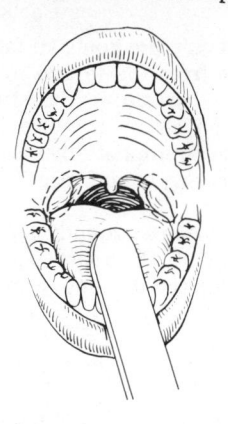

ITEM 5: WOUND CULTURE

Wound cultures are taken to determine the specific organism that is causing the infection. The culture can be obtained from a wound in any location.

Review the procedure for changing a sterile dressing in Unit 1, "Aseptic Technique."

Important Steps	Key Points
1. Assemble the supplies and equipment.	Put them on a flat working surface near the patient. You will need sterile culture tube(s) and sterile applications, a dressing tray, an antiseptic for cleansing around the wound, and a waxed paper bag for disposal of the soiled dressing. NOTE: If you are obtaining the culture from a patient in isolation, you will need to follow the isolation procedure with regard to mask, gown, gloves, etc.

SMEARS AND CULTURES

Important Steps	Key Points
2. Wash your hands.	
3. Approach and identify the patient.	Explain that you are going to take a sample of the drainage from the wound so that it can be sent to the laboratory for study. This will enable the physician or nurse practitioner to prescribe the appropriate medication to kill the organisms causing the infection.
4. Prepare the environment.	Draw the curtains around the bed to assure privacy, and close the doors to avoid drafts. Get tape ready for the dressing. Expose the wound site.
5. Remove the soiled dressing.	Use forceps or rubber gloves as indicated. Review Step 5 in "The Changing of Soiled Dressing" in Unit I, "Aseptic Technique," p. 44. Discard the soiled dressing into the waxed paper bag.
6. Inspect the wound.	Note the degree of healing, the presence of infection, pus, necrosis, putrid odor.
7. Cleanse the area around the wound.	Review Step 8, Unit I, "Aseptic Technique," page 44, for details.
8. Drape the wound site.	Review step 9 in Unit I, "Aseptic Technique," page 45, for details.

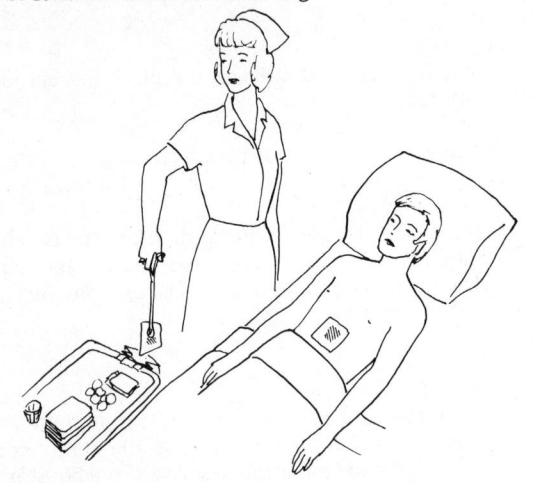

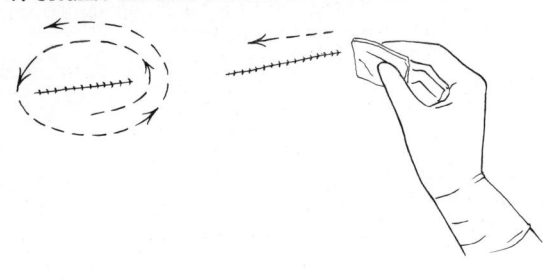

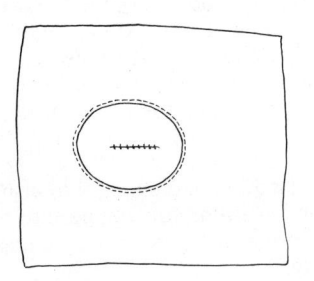

SMEARS AND CULTURES

Important Steps	Key Points
9. Swab the wound with the sterile applicator.	After opening the sterile applicator package or culture set and removing an applicator, make one wipe across the infected part of the wound. Be gentle so that you do not hurt the patient or destroy the cells causing the infection. *Do Not Wipe across the wound more than once with the same applicator.* If more material for culturing is needed, take another applicator.
10. Place the applicator in the culture tube.	NOTE: Follow your agency procedure for using a designated culture tube to obtain the specific kind of organism that is suspected. Close the cap on the culture tube to avoid contaminating other objects and to prevent any excessive drying of the material that would kill the organisms.
11. Set the culture tube aside.	It must await labeling and sending to the laboratory.
12. Apply the sterile dressing.	Then remove the drapes and discard along with the forceps or gloves in the designated container.
13. Secure the dressing retainer.	Use tape, gauze, etc.
14. Reposition the patient for comfort.	Leave the call light and bedside stand within easy reach.
15. Label the culture tube.	Mark the patient's name, date, and identification number. Complete the request form and send the tube to the laboratory.
16. Remove the soiled items.	Leave the room neat and tidy. Replenish the dressing supplies as necessary.
17. Record the procedure.	Charting example: 10:30 A.M. Abdominal dressing changed. Suture site cleansed with alcohol 70. Wound contained a moderate amount of thick, yellow, purulent drainage. No odor. Culture was taken of drainage and sent to laboratory with requisition. There were no complaints of pain. L. Domer, R.N.

VI. ADDITIONAL INFORMATION FOR ENRICHMENT

Continuing epidemiologic research develops new laboratory tests that can be utilized to ascertain various types of infecting organisms. This knowledge can assist in determining the appropriate chemical or therapeutic treatment. Ask your instructor for additional assignments if you are interested in particular tests.

POST-TEST

1. Smears and cultures are cytologic tests which aid in diagnosis. Name at least four diseases or conditions that can be determined by these tests.

2. What is the "Pap smear"?

3. Additional examinations are indicated if a Pap smear report returns positive. Name at least four other procedures that are likely to be done before a final diagnosis is made.

4. Why are cervical and rectal cutures for gonorrhea taken in the female?

5. Name two common vaginal infections that are diagnosed by means of a vaginal smear.

6. What is a "D and C"?

7. Name three common throat infections.

POST-TEST ANNOTATED ANSWER SHEET

1. Cervical cancer, endocervical cancer, maturation index, venereal disease, pp. 327, 335.

2. A cytologic test to detect uterine or cervical cancer, p. 327.

3. Biopsy, curettage, colposcopy, conization of the cervix, various staining procedures, p. 327.

4. Douching prior to the vaginal examination often washes away the cervical organisms, p. 332.

5. Trichomonas vaginitis, monilial vaginitis, p. 335.

6. A surgical procedure in which the cervix is dilated and curettaged, p. 336.

7. Staphylococcus, streptococcus, pneumococcus, p. 340.

PERFORMANCE TEST

In the skill laboratory or in the clinical setting you will be asked to perform at least three of the following procedures: vaginal, cervical, endocervical, urethral or rectal smear, throat or wound culture.

PERFORMANCE CHECKLIST

VAGINAL, CERVICAL, ENDOCERVICAL, AND RECTAL SMEARS AND CULTURES

1. Assemble supplies and equipment.
2. Identify slides and culture plate.
3. Wash hands, approach patient, and explain procedure.
4. Position and drape for vaginal examination.
5. Insert fingers into vagina and ask patient to relax.
6. Insert vaginal speculum.
7. Position and secure blades around cervix.
8. Remove fingers.
9. Remove mucous plug.
10. Take vaginal smear and spread on slide.
11. Take cervical smear and spread on slide.
12. Take endocervical smear and spread on slide.
13. "Fix" smear.
14. Take an endocervical smear and inoculate culture plate.
15. Discard applicator and remove vaginal speculum.
16. Take rectal smear and inoculate culture plate.
17. Reposition patient for comfort.
18. Obtain and heat wire loop. Cool loop.
19. Remove culture plate cover and place upside down on flat surface.
20. Cross-streak inoculated media (cervical, rectal).
21. Reflame loop and return to storage.
22. Replace cover on culture plate and check identification marks on plate.
23. Place plate in candle jar.
24. Store plate with media on top side of plate.
25. Incubate plate for designated time.
26. Inspect culture plate for growth.
27. Open culture plate and roll sterile applicator across the media growth.
28. Drop KOH solution on applicator tip; check for signs of gonorrheal organism.
29. Discard applicator.
30. Return culture plate to covered candle jar for additional incubation, if needed.
31. Discard culture plates and record on chart.

VAGINAL SMEAR FOR TRICHOMONAS VAGINITIS AND MONILIAL VAGINITIS

1. Follow Steps 1 through 9 above.
2. Place saline on slide (add KOH, if testing for monilial vaginitis).
3. Take vaginal smear and dip applicator tip in solution on slide.
4. Put coverglass on slide, center over depressed area on slide, and examine slide under microscope.
5. Record.

SUCTION-IRRIGATION PROCEDURE FOR OBTAINING ENDOMETRIAL CELLS

1. Assemble supplies and equipment.
2. Wash hands, approach patient, and explain procedure.
3. Position and drape for vaginal exam.
4. Take vaginal and cervical smear.
5. Grasp cervix with tenaculum and introduce uterine sound to test angle and depth of uterus.
6. Pick up cannula and adjust rubber stopper.
7. Fill reservoir with saline.
8. Attach reservoir to washer tip and secure to cap.
9. Introduce cannula tip into uterine cavity so that rubber stopper rests securely against cervical os.
10. Attach 30 cc syringe to reservoir cap.
11. Draw solution into syringe.
12. Disconnect syringe from reservoir cap and expel contents into reservoir.
13. Expel remaining tissue from jet tip into reservoir.
14. Discard cap assembly.
15. Screw on closed cap and label reservoir.
16. Remove vaginal speculum and reposition the patient.

THROAT CULTURE

1. Assemble supplies and equipment.
2. Wash hands, identify patient, and explain procedure.
3. Have patient seated facing you.
4. Depress tongue with tongue blade; ask patient to say "Ah."
5. Swab tonsil area with sterile swab (top to bottom on one side).
6. Place applicator in culture tube.
7. Swab opposite tonsil site and place applicator in culture tube.

8. Reposition patient.
9. Label culture tube and send to laboratory.
10. Record on chart.

WOUND CULTURE

1. Assemble supplies and equipment.
2. Wash hands, identify patient, and explain procedure.
3. Prepare environment and expose the wound site.
4. Remove soiled dressing and discard in waxed bag.
5. Inspect wound for healing.
6. Drape and cleanse wound site.
7. Swab wound with applicator and place applicator in culture tube.
8. Apply dressing and retainer.
9. Reposition patient for comfort.
10. Label culture tube and send to laboratory.
11. Leave room tidy.
12. Record procedure.

Unit 12

SKIN TESTS, IMMUNIZATIONS, AND OTHER PROPHYLACTIC AGENTS

I. DIRECTIONS TO THE STUDENT

You are to proceed through this lesson using the workbook as your guide. In the skill laboratory or in the clinical setting, you will practice giving and reading skin tests.

II. GENERAL PERFORMANCE OBJECTIVE

You will be able to demonstrate the procedure for giving a skin test and accurately reading the reaction.

III. SPECIFIC PERFORMANCE OBJECTIVES

Upon completion of this lesson, you will be able to:

1. Correctly apply a patch test.
2. Correctly perform a scratch test and read the results.
3. Correctly perform a tuberculin test and interpret the results accurately.

IV. VOCABULARY

Read the definitions of the terms listed below. Do not attempt to memorize them before proceeding with the lesson. Each term will be explained or defined again in the text. On completion of the lesson, however, you should know the correct definition of each term.

acquired immunity—immunity developed through life by contracting and recovering from a disease, or by having been passively immunized by injections of various antibody preparations or human immune serum globulin ("gamma globulin").
allergen—a substance that induces symptoms of an allergy.
allergy—heightened or greatly-increased sensitivity to a specific substance which, in similar quantity, is harmless to the average person.
anaphylactic shock—acute hypotensive collapse, sometimes briefly preceded by rash or angioedema and/or airway obstruction resulting from exposure (by inhalation, ingestion, or injection) to a foreign substance.
anaphylaxis—a hypersensitive state of the body caused by exposure to foods, medications, chemicals, pollens, animal danders, insect venoms, foreign sera (DPT, tetanus, etc.) and virus vaccines; it may be a local or systemic condition.
antibody—a substance that incites immunity (antagonism to invading bodies).
antigen—an immunizing agent that, when innoculated into the body of a susceptible person, may produce antibodies.
attenuated—diluted, made less virulent.
blastomycin—a skin test to determine the presence of blastomycosis.

coccidioidin—a sterile broth filtrate of a culture of *Coccidioides immitis* injected intracutaneously as a test for coccidioidomycosis (Valley fever, San Joaquin Valley fever).
Dick test—a test in which a small amount of scarlet fever toxin is injected intracutaneously to determine susceptibility to scarlet fever.
distributive care—area of concentration in nursing practice involved with prevention of disease and maintenance of health; it is largely directed toward continuous care of persons not confined to health care institutions.
evanescent—not permanent, of brief duration.
extrinsic—coming from without, outside.
histoplasmin—a sterile broth filtrate of a culture of *Histoplasma capsulatum*, injected intracutaneously to determine the presence of histoplasmosis.
hypersensitivity (allergic response)—abnormally increased sensitivity to a given agent; immunologically the definition is applied to four types:

> Type I: Immediate hypersensitivity.
> Type II: Intermediate hypersensitivity.
> Type III: Delayed hypersensitivity.
> Type IV: Cytolytic or cytotoxic response.

immunity—state of being resistant to a disease; immunity may be natural or acquired.
immunization—becoming immune or the process of rendering a patient immune.
intrinsic—coming from within, inside.
Mycobacterium tuberculosis—the causative agent of tuberculosis, most commonly pulmonary, in man.
natural immunity—the resistance of the normal body to infection, in contrast to specific acquired immunity.
prophylaxis—the prevention of disease; preventive treatment.
purpura—a condition characterized by purplish blotches beneath the skin due to hemorrhage; a serious symptom of disease.
reactors—persons who are sensitive to tuberculin.
Schick test—an intracutaneous skin injection to measure immunity to diphtheria.
skin tests—a method of determining the presence of certain antibodies.
systemic—pertaining to the whole body.
tuberculin—a biological product containing certain products of *Mycobacterium tuberculosis*.
urticaria (hives)—a skin eruption characterized by the appearance of pale, evanescent wheals often attended by severe itching.
vaccine—any substance for active inoculation against an infectious disease.
wheal—more or less round, evanescent elevation of the skin, white in the center, pale red on the periphery, accompanied by itching.

V. INTRODUCTION

Inflammation is a dynamic process that involves both cellular and vascular responses to tissue injury or to the introduction of an injurious agent into the body.

The body's inflammatory response either neutralizes or destroys the affecting agent. It goes further to assist in repairing the damaged tissue by bringing vital nutrients to the cells.

Pathogens are the extrinsic agents of inflammations. Intrinsic agents of inflammations can be caused by various factors such as: presence of either minimal or excessive amounts of normal substances within body fluids; limited removal of the end-products of cell metabolism; loss of oxygen and nutrients to the cells; and presence of abnormal substances in the blood and tissues. The combined action of the intrinsic and extrinsic substances that are present when tissue is injured is called the *antigen-antibody complex.*

Immunity from an infectious disease is based on the ability of the individual's own antibody mechanisms to combine with the foreign antigen to neutralize or prevent bacterial action. Although the antigen-antibody reaction is usually due to a foreign substance that is inhaled, ingested or injected, some persons develop an *autosensitive* reaction. Thus, the individual's own antigen is altered by chemical changes within his body and he becomes allergic to his own antigen. However, recent research indicates that many previously-described "autoimmune reactions or conditions" may have exogenous causes. Antibody production is reported to be the activity of the plasma cells and lymphocytes. Some antibodies circulate freely within the blood stream, while others are contained in specific blood cells within the body.

Hypersensitivity (allergic response) is an inflammatory condition caused by an antigen-antibody reaction. It is an unfavorable body response when the individual has not built up an appropriate antibody defense to the inciting agent. In other words, a hypersensitive state exists when the body has failed to produce enough antibodies in response to a specific antigen either to dilute the effectiveness of or destroy the allergen.

The severity of the allergic reaction, therefore, depends upon two factors: the amount of antigen (or allergen) present and the degree of sensitivity built up in the antibody system to deal with that allergen.

Allergic reactions take one of three forms:

1. *Local skin or mucous membrane reaction*, in which local hyperemia, edema, hemorrhage, necrosis or hives may appear.

2. *Systemic reaction*, in which there is generalized edema, swollen lymph glands, inflammation of the joints, malaise, fever, bronchiolar constriction and purpura.

3. *Anaphylactic shock*, a severe reaction in which there is vascular collapse and resultant cerebral hypoxia. There may be associated edema and/or contraction of the smooth muscle of the respiratory tract. In case of severe shock, immediate action must be taken or the patient may expire within minutes. The exact mechanism of anaphylactic shock is not understood. However, it is a major responsibility of the nurse to be aware of the possibility of this condition whenever a patient takes in a foreign agent (whether it be inhaled, ingested or injected). The signs of anaphylactic shock must be quickly recognized, and life-saving remedies instituted at once. The required nursing measures will be discussed later in this module.

Hypersensitive (allergic) reaction is a normal response to an unusual stimulus. It serves to alert the health worker to the patient's sensitivity and mandates immediate close observation and care following the allergic response.

There are four types of allergic reactions:

1. *Immediate:* An urticarial wheal quickly appears at the site of injection or anaphylactic shock.

2. *Intermediate:* This occurs within 30 minutes to a few hours and is commonly known as the *Arthus reaction.*

3. *Delayed:* A cellular antigen-antibody response that usually occurs within 72 hours. It takes time for cells to accumulate at the injection site in order to interact with the injected substance, e.g., tuberculin test.

4. *Cytolytic or Cytotoxic response:* Body tissues either serve as a target or provide the antigen for a direct encounter with humoral antibody, e.g., intravascular transfusion reaction, erythroblastosis fetalis due to Rh sensitization.

Emergency treatment of anaphylactic shock includes: 0.01-0.05 ml of aqueous epinephrine injection; oxygen; CPR; IV aminophylline (50 mgm per 25 pounds of body weight); and other measures.

The rapidity with which an allergic reaction takes place is directly related to previous contact with the antigen and the production of antibodies, to recovery from a specific disease, or to successful vaccination. Some antibodies do not seem to be retained, e.g., the common cold. The reason for this is unknown at this time.

Very young infants, aged persons, or those who are in poor health do not generate antibodies rapidly, and therefore these three types of patients need extra nursing care to prevent undue exposure to detrimental antigens.

Antigenic substances do not promote antibody formation in everyone. Some people develop a sensitivity to certain drugs: aspirin, penicillin, codeine, X-ray dyes, etc. At the present time, no positive skin test can be elicited from those who are allergic to these substances. One current theory is that such substances act as haptens, i.e., they are immunologic only when combined with a protein, often one belonging to the host, to form a complete antigen.

Other, as yet unknown, mechanisms may play an important role in susceptibility to these and other chemical compounds, such as hydrocarbon fumes, oxides of sulfur, nitrogen, etc. The nurse must, therefore, be constantly aware of the patient's allergies. Information about allergies should be elicited from the patient during the intake history, and should then be recorded on the chart and Kardex for all health workers to see and observe.

Epidemiologic control of infectious disease has been due largely to the development of vaccines that stimulate antibody reactions that, in turn, provide active or passive acquired immunity. The use of antitoxins (substances containing antibodies from the serum of an actively immunized animal) has also served as a control. Antibodies have likewise played a very large role in decreasing mortality and have also served to control infectious diseases. Vaccines (chemical substances) are manufactured in three general classes: (1) With living organisms (e.g., live measles and rubella vaccine). (2) With killed viruses (e.g., rabies vaccine) or bacteria (e.g., pertussis). (3) With toxins or other products thrown off by growing bacteria (e.g., tetanus toxoid).

Little is known as to why there are varying periods of immunity. Recovery from measles (rubeola) and mumps usually provides a long-lasting immunity, while recovery from a cold appears to give almost no immunity.

The skin and mucous membranes serve as the body's first line of defense against infection. The second line of defense is the development of antibodies, which are specific proteins produced in some body cells as a response to a specific antigen.

Antibodies are produced and transported in gamma globulin. As cells come into contact with foreign protein, they become sensitized to it. In turn they produce a chemical substance (antibody) that dilutes or destroys the foreign protein.

It is possible to strengthen the body's natural defense against disease-producing organisms through immunization. By injecting into the body small numbers of weakened (attenuated) or specific dead organisms, or modified toxins from bacilli or viruses, a long-term antigen-antibody reaction can be produced in someone who has not had the disease. Such acquired immunity is a common and highly effective method to prevent disease.

Periodic repeat injections (booster doses) are given over various time intervals to maintain levels of protection. The booster dose is usually one tenth the strength of the initial inoculating dose.

There are vaccines for diphtheria, pertussis, tetanus, poliomyelitis, measles (rubeola), rubella, mumps, influenza, smallpox, rabies, tuberculosis, cholera, yellow fever, typhoid, Rocky Mountain spotted fever, typhus, and plague (listed in order of frequency of use).

Note: Smallpox and tuberculosis vaccines are unique in that the immunizing agent is not the specific organism producing the human disease, but a similar organism that produces antibodies cross-reactive with viral or bacterial antigens of the true disease. Smallpox (variola) is immunized against by the vaccinia (cowpox) virus. Tuberculosis immunization utilizes BCG (bacille Calmette-Guérin), a bovine tuberculosis bacillus. Smallpox vaccine is now contraindicated except for travel to a few foreign countries outside the Western Hemisphere. The incidence of fatal complications from vaccination now far outweigh the risks of contracting smallpox. The use of paratyphoid vaccine was discontinued a number of years ago because of the lack of demonstrable effectiveness. Typhoid vaccine effectiveness has also been questioned and it may likewise be discontinued in the future.

Antitoxins are substances that are formed in response to the toxins produced by certain organisms. The antitoxin neutralizes the effects of the toxin produced by the pathogen. Tetanus antitoxin is a common antitoxin.

Passive immunity is a temporary means of supplementing the body's defense mechanism, thereby sparing the person from having the actual disease. Temporary protection is a measure utilized for those who have been exposed to a disease but have no known natural or acquired immunity. The injection is given before the disease starts, usually only to individuals who would suffer acutely if the disease were contracted, as in the case of an adult exposed to a childhood disease.

Temporary protection is obtained by using antitoxins and immune animal or human serum globulin. Gamma globulin is widely used when no specific substance is available to protect the individual from the disease to which he has been exposed.

Human immune serum globulin (HISB) preparations currently available include: (1) Pooled HISG (this is what most people mean when they say "gamma globulin"); it is commonly given for prophylaxis against infectious hepatitis and can also be used to prevent or modify measles. Some preparations are specifically titered for measles antibody content. (2) Tetanus immune serum globulin (TISG); e.g., Hypertet. (3) Mumps immune serum globulin. (4) Vaccinia immune serum globulin for treatment of smallpox vaccination; not effective against smallpox.

Some people are allergic to horse serum, and therefore biological substances that are suspended in horse serum (e.g., rabies antisera) should not be given to sensitive individuals. Rabies antisera may be replaced by HISG. Tetanus antitoxin is not given these days because of the high incidence of reaction. Since there is such a low incidence of reaction to gamma globulin, it is preferred. Prior to giving the antisera, an intradermal skin test should be given to ascertain the sensitivity of your patient. If there is no "hive reaction" after 20 minutes, the rabies antisera may be safely given. Always follow the medication brochure that is enclosed with the preparation.

The nurse's role in immunization involves teaching the public about the advantages of immunization and encouraging them to participate in their local Public Health Immunization Programs. In teaching the public, you should be able to give them information about communicable diseases; why immunization is desirable; when a booster shot is indicated; and what makes the program safe. Your local Public Health Agency can provide any information you need on immunization and prophylactic programs. Get to know your Public Health Nurse. You should be aware that your Public Health Agency requires the reporting of certain communicable diseases and keeps in contact with patients who have tuberculosis and venereal diseases. It is essential for you to become familiar with your local regulations. (See an example of a local regulation in Section VI, Additional Information for Enrichment, at the end of this Unit.)

Allergens can take many forms, e.g., house dust, animal danders, mold spores, plant pollens, drugs, and a myriad of other chemicals, foods, and pathogenic organisms.

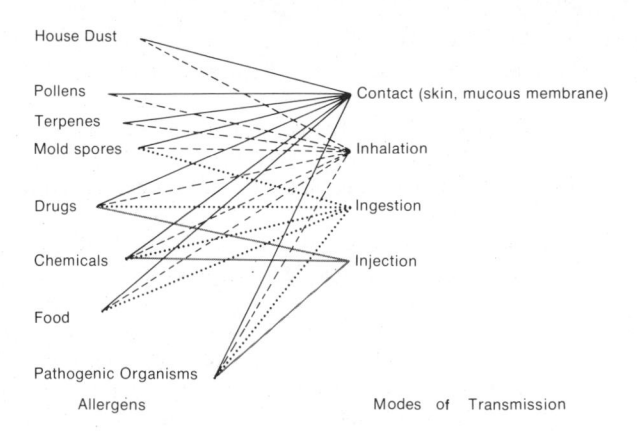

```
House Dust
Pollens                          Contact (skin, mucous membrane)
Terpenes
Mold spores                      Inhalation
Drugs                            Ingestion
Chemicals                        Injection
Food
Pathogenic Organisms
    Allergens                    Modes of Transmission
```

Hypersensitization (desensitization) is a treatment modality in which hypersensitive individuals are given multiple injections with extracts of their specific allergens in order to reduce their sensitivity to those substances. Usually this treatment must also be coupled with an avoidance of the substance.

HYPERSENSITIVITY REACTIONS

1. **Anaphylactic Shock.** When an allergen is taken in by a *sensitized person*, the reaction can range from mild to severe—so severe, in fact, that death can occur within minutes.

Symptoms of anaphylactic shock include: urticaria, bronchiolar constriction, edema, and finally, circulatory collapse. Circulatory collapse can occur as the initial symptom, however.

Anaphylactic shock can take place at any time. One of the critical roles nurses play when administering a drug is the observation of the patient for a short time (perhaps 15 minutes) after the drug has been given. This must be done to watch for signs of anaphylactic shock and, if necessary, to administer immediate, life-saving treatment.

Remember your CPR procedure and call for assistance:
1. Clear the airway and maintain ventilation; give O_2 if requested by physician.
2. Overcome circulatory collapse by administering IV solutions to expand the decreased blood volume (usually 1000 cc of 5 per cent glucose in water).
3. Give epinephrine to combat the allergic response.
4. Give $NaHCO_3$ to combat the allergic response.

If the patient does not respond to the above steps, a tracheostomy may be required to overcome the obstruction of the air passageway due to laryngeal edema.

Monitor the patient's vital signs at regular intervals and keep him warm.

Many anaphylactic shock reactions can be avoided if an allergic history can be ascertained from the patient before giving a medication. This is particularly essential when giving immunization and skin tests.

Some allergic individuals wear a Medic-Alert identifying bracelet or a "dog-tag" chain or a similar device. Unfortunately, many do not wear such bracelets or chains. If there is a medical identification tag present, HEED IT! Failure to do so may complicate the patient's problem because you may inadvertently give treatment that is contraindicated in his particular care, or there may be harmful delay in administering the correct treatment. Failure to observe specified precautions may result in legal liability if there is an unfavorable outcome.

Patients who do wear the identification tag or bracelet assist the health worker, both in preventing allergic responses by avoiding substances to which he is allergic, and in helping the health worker to correctly treat a reaction that has already occurred. However, you must always remain aware that a serious allergic reaction can occur in any patient.

2. **Serum Sickness.** Serum sickness is a hypersensitivity reaction that occurs several days after injection of a foreign serum *in a nonsensitive person*. Antisera for botulism, gas gangrene, snake bite and rabies are frequently sources of hypersensitive reactions. Symptoms of serum sickness that appear in seven to ten days include fever, arthralgia, urticaria, and lymph node enlargement.

Complications may arise in a severe case of serum sickness, among them: optic neuritis, carditis, bronchial neuritis, periarteritis nodosa, nephritis, and Guillain-Barré syndrome. Treatment of the complications is symptomatic.

With today's emphasis on preventive medicine, one type of serum sickness could be prevented by giving tetanus toxoid or TIG immunization, negating the need to give tetanus antitoxin. Prevention is a major role for the alert nurse.

3. **Atopy.** Atopy is the term used to designate a clinical state leading to development of eczema, hay fever, asthma, and non-seasonal allergic rhinitis. It is genetically determined and probably environmentally mediated. Specific atopic diseases are not inherited *per se* (e.g., a father may have hay fever and the daughter eczema; a grandfather may have asthma, the son may be asymptomatic and the grandson may develop hay fever, etc.).

Nurses should be alert to allergic patients since very often they develop secondary problems that may produce a clinical illness.

4. **Autoimmunity.** This is another hypersensitivity reaction in which the individual becomes sensitive to his own body cells or tissues. There are at least 14 mechanisms which have been demonstrated or are plausible explanations for the auto-allergic state. There are two main theories:

a. They occur as a result of an altered, cross-reacting, or isolated auto-antigen.
b. They are abnormal immunologic reactions.

Considerable research is being conducted to determine the etiology of the auto-immune hypersensitivity. It is important to continue reading current journals for the latest developments in theories on auto-immunity.

Nursing responsibilities for the allergic patient include:

1. Knowledge of the patient's specific allergy or allergies.
2. Separation of the patient from the offending antigen as much as possible.
3. Relief of symptoms as they occur (hives, edema, etc.).
4. Helping the patient to increase his tolerance by administering small, increasing doses of the antigen; this will aid in desensitizing the patient to the offending antigen.
5. Psychological support of the patient and his family until the allergy can be minimized and coped with.

Because there is continuing development in the field of immunizations and allergies, it is necessary for each nurse to maintain current knowledge to assure safe care to every patient.

ITEM 1: MUCOUS MEMBRANE TESTS

Allergens may be applied to the mucous membranes of the conjunctiva, the nose, and bronchi.

A drop of the allergen is dropped into the lower fornix of the eye (Step 5, Item 10, Instillation of Eye Drops, Unit 4, pg. 181).

Nasal and bronchial membrane tests merely require the patient to "sniff" or inhale the noxious allergen.

Many patients object to these tests and they are used only on a selective basis.

ITEM 2: THE PATCH TEST

The *Patch Test* was used in the 1930's and 1940's to detect tuberculosis. However, it has been proved unreliable for that use and is no longer so used. Today the patch test is most often used to diagnose contact (skin) allergy, and determine the etiologic agents.

Important Steps	Key Points
1. Assemble the supplies.	
2. Wash your hands.	
3. Approach and identify the patient.	
4. Explain the procedure.	
5. Cleanse the skin.	Wash the site where the test is to be given; be sure the skin is free of cuts or eruptions. The anterior forearm or the upper back adjacent to the spinal column are frequent test sites. The forearm is the preferred site for adults and the back is the preferred site for children.
6. Attach impregnated dressing.	A drop or two of the specified allergen has been applied to the 1 cm gauze dressing. It usually has a plastic (or similar material) backing to avoid leaking or wetting of the dressing with the allergen.

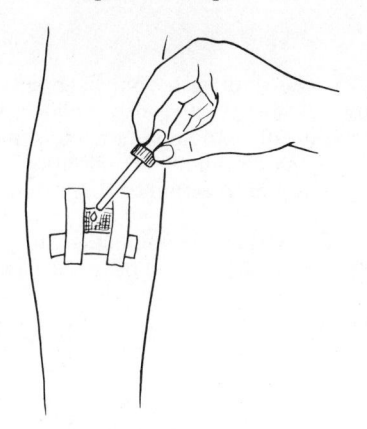

SKIN TESTS, IMMUNIZATIONS, AND OTHER PROPHYLACTIC AGENTS 355

Important Steps	Key Points
	The dressing is held in place with tapes. Some dressings are prepared for application and resemble square adhesive bandages.
7. Instruct the patient.	The patch is kept in place for varying lengths of time, according to the allergen being used (minimum: 24 hours). More often it is left in place for 48 hours. The patient may remove the patch earlier if intense itching occurs. He should call his physician at once for further directions. The patient should avoid wetting or scratching the test site until the patch is removed to keep from dispersing the allergen over a wide area.
8. Record the test.	Mark it on the patient's record.
9. Read the test.	Remove the patch at the specified time interval: 24, 48, 72 hours, or whatever. The *reaction is negative if erythema is not present*. However, the site should be observed daily for two weeks because a delayed reaction could occur. A *positive reaction is one in which erythema and/or vesicles are present*, depending on the specific allergen used.
10. Instruct the patient.	Tell him when to return. Leave the treatment room neat and tidy.

11. Record the reaction on the patient's chart.

ITEM 2: THE SCRATCH TEST

The *Scratch Test* is a series of tests primarily used for detecting the causative agent in inhalant allergies, such as dusts, danders, molds, and pollens. Scratch test kits come in various sizes, with varying numbers of antigens. Some physicians maintain multiple dose vials of antigens for the common local allergies instead of using the test kits, which often include antigens that are not needed for the patient. Complete or partial testing may be done as indicated by taking a careful history of the patient.

Important Steps	Key Points
1. Assemble the supplies.	Use a commercially prepared kit with needles for each test, antigen solution (in a capillary tube or bottle), and a basin for soap and water.
2. Wash your hands.	

356 SKIN TESTS, IMMUNIZATIONS, AND OTHER PROPHYLACTIC AGENTS

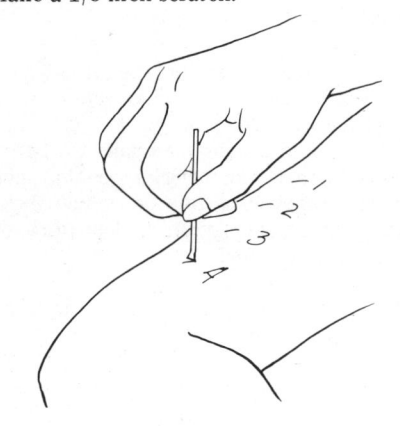

Important Steps	Key Points
3. Approach and identify the patient.	
4. Explain the procedure.	"I am going to wash your back with soap and water. Then I will gently scratch your back with a needle and apply a drop of medicine on the scratch. In about 30 minutes I'll read the results of your reaction to the various tests."
5. Ask the patient to strip to the waist.	Give him a short examining gown, and explain that the opening should be in the back.
6. Position patient face down on the examining table.	Expose his back. (The arm may be used.)
7. Wash his back (or arm).	The skin must be thoroughly cleansed and then dried. Place the basin, towel, and water to one side for later disposal after the procedure. Keep the patient from being chilled.
8. Write test numbers on sections of the skin to correspond with the antigen numbers.	Use washable ink. Each antigen has a number; this prevents incorrect readings because the antigen number corresponds with the exact numbered section on the skin. The numbers should be placed about 2 inches apart. Mark as many sites as you need for the tests.
9. Make a 1/8 inch scratch.	Use a separate needle for each scratch; a 26 gauge needle may be used. *Do NOT penetrate the skin;* just the dermal layer.
10. Place a drop on the scratch.	The antigen solution will bathe the cells in the deeper layers by seeping through the tear in the dermis.
	a). If the solution is in a capillary tube, break it in two and let the solution drop on the scratch.
	b) If the solution is in a bottle, dip the tip end of a toothpick into the bottle so that a drop of solution adheres to the toothpick. Let the solution drop on the scratch. Use a new toothpick or medicine dropper for each solution.

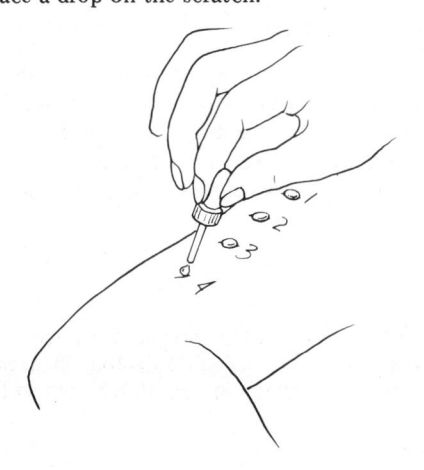

Important Steps	Key Points
11. Allow the solutions to "set".	This usually takes about 30 minutes. Be sure that the patient is not chilled during this time. Leave the back or arm exposed to the air.
12. Wipe the excess solution from the back.	
13. Read the results.	NEGATIVE: No change in the skin. POSITIVE: A wheal appears. They are designated as slight (1+), moderate (2+), or marked (3+). NOTE: The results may be read again in 24 hours to check for delayed reaction.
14. Permit the patient to dress.	Tidy the room. Give the patient instructions; e.g., "Return to my office within 24 hours (or 48 hours) for a delayed reading of the tests," or "I will check the sites again tomorrow to see if there are any other changes."
15. Record the results on the patient's chart.	

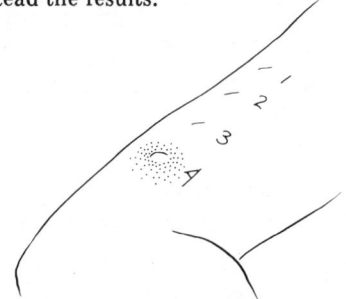

ITEM 3: METHODS OF TUBERCULIN SKIN TESTING

Tuberculin is a biological product used for skin testing and is indispensable in the control of tuberculosis. OT(old tuberculin) was developed by Dr. Robert Koch in Germany in 1890. It was used as a successful diagnostic tool for tuberculosis until the 1940's. Dr. Florence Seibert of Philadelphia developed PPD (purified protein derivative) in 1940. It is purer than OT, more specific for diagnosing tuberculosis, and there are fewer cross-reactions.

The test is based on the fact that infection with *Mycobacterium tuberculosis* produces sensitivity to certain products of this organism, which are contained in the culture extracts called "tuberculins." (*Note:* This is a statement from the American Thoracic Society.)

The tuberculins are prepared by several pharmaceutical firms and are available commercially in various dilutions. It is, therefore, imperative that you know your product. Follow the informational brochure that accompanies the drug package.

Tuberculin testing is a first step in a series to confirm that a patient is infected with the tubercle bacilli and may have clinical tuberculosis.

A positive tuberculin denotes that there is an infection, but does not signify the presence of active disease.

Follow-up of a positive tuberculin test includes: careful history, physical examination, chest X-rays, smears and cultures of sputum and/or gastric fluids, and placement on a chemotherapy program.

Tuberculin testing of persons who have close contacts with the positive reactor is essential. These people must be put on a chemoprophylaxis program.

There are three methods used for tuberculin testing:

1. Multiple puncture applicators (tine, Mono-vacc, Heaf or Sterneedle)

2. Injection by Jet gun or Hypospray.

3. Mantoux intradermal injection.

A. The Tine Test

The *Tine test* is a screening test for tuberculosis. A preparation of concentrated OT is used.

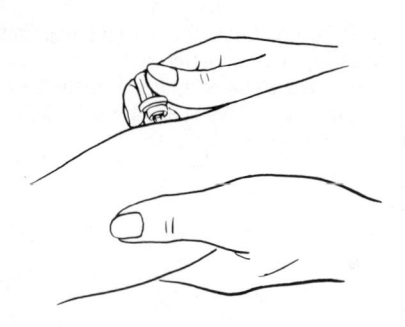

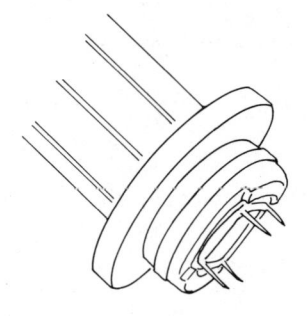

Important Steps	Key Points
1. Assemble the supplies.	An alcohol pledget and a tine set are required.
2. Wash your hands.	
3. Identify the patient.	Ask him to be seated.
4. Explain the procedure.	
5. Expose the right forearm.	Cleanse the arm with alcohol pledget, then discard pledget into a designated container.
6. Puncture the forearm.	
7. Instruct the patient.	Tell him to return for inspection of the site in 48 or 72 hours. Follow agency procedure.
8. Record the test.	Mark it on his record.
9. Read the reaction.	Inspect the test site in 48 to 72 hours. NEGATIVE TEST: Nothing has appeared on the skin except the puncture sites. POSITIVE TEST: Presence of reddish, raised indurations of 2 mm or larger around one or more of the puncture sites. NOTE: All positive reactions except vesiculating reactions should be retested using the Mantoux technique.
10. Record the time and the results.	Mark them on the patient's record.

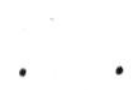

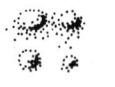

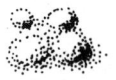

SKIN TESTS, IMMUNIZATIONS, AND OTHER PROPHYLACTIC AGENTS

B. The Mono-Vacc Test

The *Mono-vacc test* is another screening test for tuberculosis. A liquid OT is used on the special puncture instrument.

Important Steps	Key Points
Follow Steps 1–5 in the procedure for the tine test above.	
6 Puncture the forearm.	
7. Instruct the patient.	Ask him to return for inspection of the site in 3 or 4 days.
8. Record the test.	
9. Read the reaction. 2 mm 5 mm 7 mm 10 mm	Mark the patient's record. NEGATIVE TEST: Nothing observed on the skin. POSITIVE TEST: A palpable induration from 1–10 mm; there may be some local erythema, but the induration is the positive criterion. NOTE: All positive reactions except vesiculating reactions should be retested using the Mantoux technique.
10. Record the results.	Mark the time and the reaction.

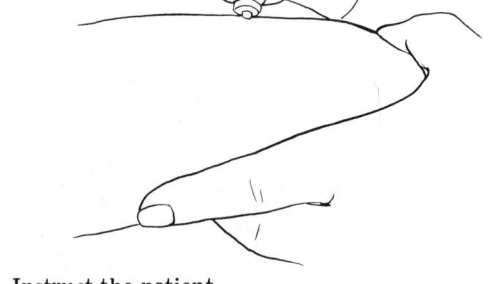

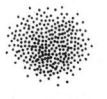

The Tine Mono-Vacc tests have both advantages and disadvantages. Note the following:

Advantages	*Disadvantages*
Simple procedure.	Uses OT.
No equipment necessary.	Highly concentrated, less pure product.
Convenient to use in any location.	Many false positive reactions.
Less frightening.	Multiple punctures with unmeasured dose.
Good for screening out non-reactors.	Verification with Mantoux is necessary.
	Expensive.
	Results difficult to interpret.

C. *Heaf or Sterneedle Test*

The Heaf test also screens for tuberculosis. Liquid PPD is used on a special instrument.

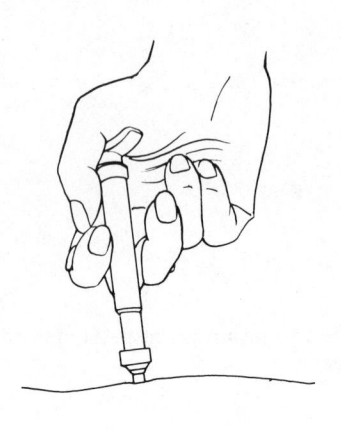

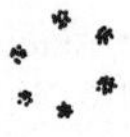

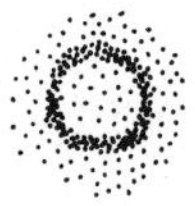

Important Steps	Key Points
Follow Steps 1-5 in the procedure for the Tine test above.	
6. Puncture the forearm.	
7. Instruct the patient.	Ask him to return for site inspection in 2 to 7 days (follow your agency procedure).
8. Record the test.	Mark it on the patient's record.
9. Read the reaction.	When the patient returns to the office at the designated time, inspect the test site.
GRADE I	GRADE I: There are discrete palpable indurations around at least four puncture points. Erythema is present.
GRADE II	GRADE II: There is a coalescence of the indurated points to form an edematous ring.
	GRADE III: There is more extensive induration forming a coin pattern measuring 1 cm in diameter.
GRADE III	GRADE IV: Extensive induration with possible sloughing of the center.
	NOTE: All positive reactions, except vesicular and sloughing reactions, should be retested using the Mantoux technique.
10. Record the reading.	Mark the time and results on the patient's record.

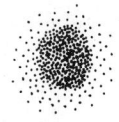

SKIN TESTS, IMMUNIZATIONS, AND OTHER PROPHYLACTIC AGENTS

The Heaf or Sterneedle test also has both advantages and disadvantages:

Advantages	*Disadvantages*
No training necessary.	Highly concentrated solution used.
Less frightening.	Multiple punctures with unmeasured dose necessary.
Good as a screening tool.	Verification with Mantoux is necessary.
Classification is according to Grades I, II, III, IV rather than measurement.	Difficult to interpret reaction.
	Frequent false positive reactions occur.

D. Jet Gun or Hypospray Tuberculin Test

The injection by the Jet gun or Hypospray is used when tuberculin testing is done on a massive scale because it is a painless and rapid way to test large numbers of people. The testing material is driven intradermally by high pressure *without a needle*. The gun delivers 0.1 ml 5 TU (tuberculin units) of PPD tuberculin.

Important Steps	Key Points
Follow steps 1–5 of the tine test procedure.	
6. Place the distal injection tip of the gun on the patient's forearm.	Be sure to hold firmly against the skin while supporting the patient's arm.
7. Pull the trigger.	Inject the tuberculin.
8. Remove the gun.	Put it aside.
9. Instruct the patient.	Tell him to return in 48 to 72 hours. Follow your agency's procedure.
10. Record the test.	
11. Read the reaction.	POSITIVE REACTION: Palpate the margins of induration. Measure (with a millimeter ruler) the transverse diameter of the induration at the point where the needle entered. The reading is recorded in mm of induration. A positive reaction for TB infection is indicated when the induration is 10 mm +.

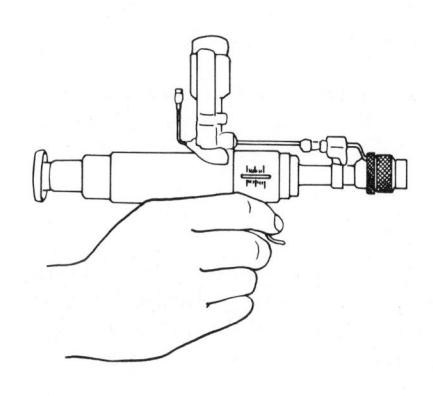

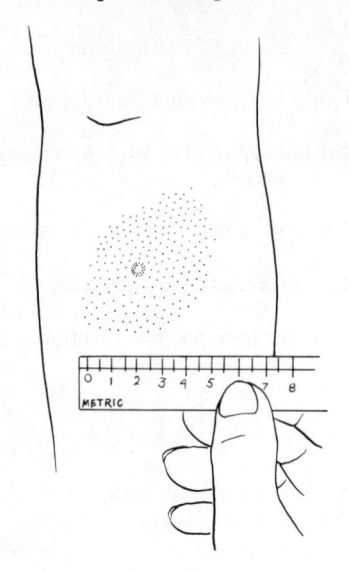

362   SKIN TESTS, IMMUNIZATIONS, AND OTHER PROPHYLACTIC AGENTS

Important Steps	Key Points
	DOUBTFUL REACTION: 5-9 mm induration.
	NEGATIVE REACTION: 0-4 mm induration.
	NOTE: *Induration*, not erythema, is the key to the positive reaction.

The advantages and disadvantages of the Jet gun (Hypospray) test are:

Advantages	*Disadvantages*
Speedy.	Machine can jam.
Easy to operate.	Unmeasured quantity of antigen injected.
Painless.	Small reaction if solution is lost.
Given superficially.	Machine is heavy to hold.
Best using PPD 5 TU.	Some retesting with needle may be necessary.
Good screening tool.	

E. *Mantoux Test*

The Mantoux test is an intradermal injection of tuberculin with a needle and syringe. It is a *definitive test* for diagnosis of tuberculosis, and is the *preferred technique*. The dose is 0.1 ml of PPD tuberculin containing 5 tuberculin units (TU). A tuberculin syringe with a 26 or 27 gauge blunt beveled needle is used for the injection.

Important Steps	Key Points

(Follow the intradermal technique described in Unit 2, "Preparation and Administration of Medications, pp. 106, 107.)

1. Assemble your supplies.	Needle, syringe, and tuberculin are needed.
2. Wash your hands.	
3. Identify the medication.	Compare the medication with the order.
4. Cleanse the vial stopper.	Wipe it with an alcohol pledget.
5. Assemble the needle and syringe.	

SKIN TESTS, IMMUNIZATIONS, AND OTHER PROPHYLACTIC AGENTS 363

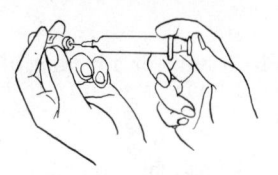

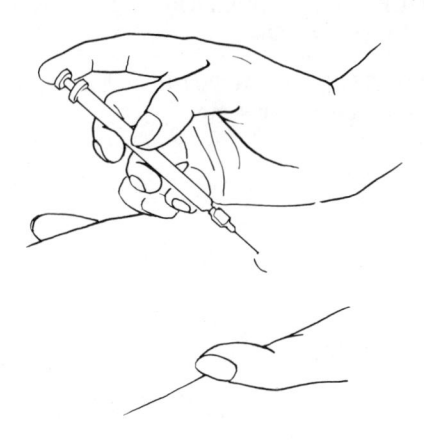

Important Steps	Key Points
6. Pick up the vial and insert the needle.	
7. Withdraw the tuberculin into the syringe.	
8. Remove the needle from the vial.	Place the vial to one side.
9. Explain the procedure to the patient.	
10. Cleanse the injection site.	Use an antiseptic pledget.
11. Pick up the syringe.	Expel air bubbles.
12. Grasp the patient's forearm to be injected.	While standing in front of the patient, turn his anterior forearm upward, facing you. Grasp the arm on the posterior side, toward the middle of the forearm. With your non-dominant thumb on one side of the arm and your index finger on the other side, pull the anterior skin taut. (See Item 6, Step 7, Unit 2, Pg. 106.)
	An alternative method for holding the syringe is utilized by many allergists: Hold the syringe barrel between the thumb and third, fourth and fifth fingers. This will permit you to stabilize the syringe while you inject the solution with the index finger pushing inward on the plunger.
13. Insert the needle.	With the bevel of the needle facing upward, insert the needle through the skin at an angle almost parallel to the skin (10 to 15 degrees). Insert the needle so that only the bevel penetrates the skin. Avoid hair follicles.
14. Inject the solution slowly.	If you have inserted the needle correctly, a small circular bump (wheal) that is blanched (white) will appear on the skin.
	Observe the patient for unusual reactions (such as shock).
15. Withdraw the needle.	Place to one side.

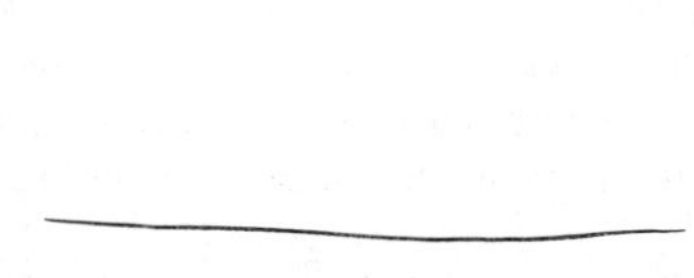

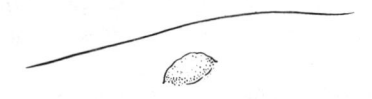

UNIT 12

Important Steps	Key Points
16. Position the patient for comfort and safety.	Have him lie down if he feels faint or ask him to sit a few minutes to be sure that no unusual effects occur.
17. Instruct the patient.	Ask him to return for a reading of the reaction in 48 to 72 hours, according to your agency's procedure.
18. Record the test.	Note it on the patient's record.
19. Read the reaction.	When the patient returns in 48 to 72 hours, inspect the injection site. Look for erythema. Palpate the margin of the induration, if needed. Measure (with a millimeter ruler) the transverse diameter of the indurated area at the point where the needle entered. The reading is recorded in mm of induration.
	POSITIVE REACTION: Tuberculosis infection is indicated when the induration measures 10+ mm. The induration, not erythema, is the key to the positive reaction.
	DOUBTFUL REACTION: The induration measures 5-9 mm.
	NEGATIVE REACTION: The induration measures less than 4 mm.
20. Record the reaction.	

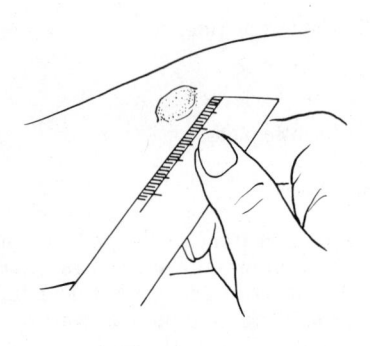

The advantages and disadvantages of the Mantoux test are:

Advantages	*Disadvantages*
Measured dose.	Training required to administer.
Pure product used.	Training necessary to read test.
Measurable reaction.	
Results more reliable.	

Skin tests can be done with other antigens, but are generally used for investigative purposes. They are frequently employed to assist in making a differential diagnosis. Three common fungal antigens used for differential diagnosis are: coccidioidin, histoplasmin, and blastomycin.

Survey chest X-rays are no longer advocated to locate persons with tuberculosis. Most persons infected with tuberculosis have negative chest X-rays.

The positive tuberculin skin test demonstrates that an infection is present. Every positive reactor is a potentially active tuberculosis patient. Positive reactors are placed on one year of chemoprophylaxis with isoniazid (INH) to reduce tuberculosis morbidity. The highest incidence of tuberculosis occurs in men over 25.

For further current information, call your local Public Health Department or Lung Association.

SKIN TESTS, IMMUNIZATIONS, AND OTHER PROPHYLACTIC AGENTS 365

VI. ADDITIONAL INFORMATION FOR ENRICHMENT

Your instructor can give you additional reading or practical assignments if you are interested in pursuing your studies in immunizations and allergies.

The following sample chart is included for your information. Since there are minor variations in practice around the country, check with your local Public Health Agency for your recommended program. The sample chart is used by permission of the County of Los Angeles Department of Health Services, Community Health Services.

County of Los Angeles Health Department

Recommendations

for

Use of Common Immunizing

and Other Prophylactic Agents

G. A. HEIDBREDER, M.D., M.P.H.
HEALTH OFFICER

Revised July 1972

76R199G-B-71 (rev. 5-72)—6/72

IMMUNIZATION PROCEDURES

General Information for Health Department Personnel: Active immunizing agents should not be given to persons ill or febrile during the previous 24 hours. However, presence of mild non-febrile upper respiratory illness is not a contraindication to immunization. Read the product description and directions provided by the manufacturer in the package insert. Record pertinent vaccine lot numbers. No product may be used beyond its expiration date.

Health Department personnel should report any unusual reactions in writing to the Immunization Project, Division of Acute Communicable Disease Control, 313 North Figueroa (Room 634), Los Angeles 90012, describing the reaction and providing the name, manufacturer, and lot number of the suspect product. Any defective vaccines and associated diluents, preloaded syringes, etc., should be forwarded immediately to the Immunization Project, under refrigeration if necessary, accompanied by an explanatory note. Refer reports of unusual reactions or defective products occurring outside the Health Department to the Food and Drug Administration, 1521 West Pico, Los Angeles 90015, or to the manufacturer.

Simultaneous Administration of Different Vaccines.

(1) Killed or inactivated vaccines, such as DTP, Td, typhoid and influenza vaccines may be given simultaneously during a single visit, and may be combined with one live virus vaccine such as measles, measles-rubella (MR), or polio. Separate syringes must be used.

(2) Live virus vaccines may be administered simultaneously only in certain specified combinations. Smallpox and poliomyelitis vaccines may be administered simultaneously. Licensed combined vaccines for measles-rubella (MR) and measles-mumps-rubella (MMR) may be administered in accordance with the manufacturer's recommendations. The individual vaccine strains licensed in combined form for protection against measles, mumps and rubella may be given by separate injections at the same time. In all other routine circumstances, live virus vaccines should be administered separately with an intervening interval of approximately one month. In unusual circumstances (such as concurrent outbreaks of measles and polio) the relevant live virus vaccines should be given on the same day; an interval of two days to two weeks should be avoided because interference between the vaccine viruses is most likely then.

Immunization for Foreign Travel. Many countries may require yellow fever, smallpox or cholera immunization for entry. These requirements change from time to time. The United States Public Health Service recommends that travelers be immunized against diphtheria, tetanus, and measles (if susceptible), and in addition recommends poliomyelitis and typhoid vaccines for travelers to certain countries.

The County of Los Angeles usually does not provide immunization for travel. Smallpox and cholera immunizations must be validated by the County Health Department, however, unless the immunizing physician possesses the State Uniform Stamp approved by the United States Public Health Service. Certificates can be validated between 8:00 a.m. and 4:30 p.m. at any of the Health Centers and most subcenters listed on the last page of this booklet.

Tuberculosis and Immunization. Certain viral infections, live viral vaccines and administration of corticosteroids all may depress or suppress reactivity to tuberculin for as long as 4 weeks. If tuberculin testing is contemplated, the test should be done before administration of these vaccines, or deferred for 4-6 weeks.

Repeating a Basic Series: There is no maximum interval between doses of any antigen. It is not necessary to restart a series if more than the usual interval has passed since the last dose.

IMMUNIZING AGENTS	PRIMARY IMMUNIZATION SCHEDULE	BOOSTER SCHEDULE	COMMENTS AND CONTRAINDICATIONS
Diphtheria and Tetanus Toxoids and Pertussis Vaccine (DTP)	**For children six weeks through 6 years:** First: 0.5 ml IM Second: 0.5 ml IM 4-6 weeks later. Third: 0.5 ml IM 4-6 weeks later. Fourth: 0.5 ml IM 1 year later.	Fifth dose DTP: 0.5 ml IM at time of school entrance.	If history of severe reaction, may reduce subsequent doses by 50% and add an extra dose. Or, smaller doses of individual antigens may be given. Under 1 year of age, preferable site is anterolateral thigh. After last booster, use adult Td at 10-year intervals.
Tetanus and Diphtheria Toxoids, Adult Type (Td)	**For children 7 years and older and adults (if no primary series of DTP):** First: 0.5 ml IM Second: 0.5 ml IM 4-6 weeks later. Third: 0.5 ml IM 6 months-1 year later.	0.5 ml every 10 years for life.	Preferable for children 7 and older because of adult sensitivity to diphtheria toxoid. Adsorbed toxoids superior in efficacy for both primary and booster immunization. Use Td instead of tetanus toxoid for wound management (q.v.).

IMMUNIZING AGENTS	PRIMARY IMMUNIZATION SCHEDULE	BOOSTER SCHEDULE	COMMENTS AND CONTRAINDICATIONS
Influenza Virus vaccine, bivalent (inactivated).	3 months or over if indicated. 2 doses 6-8 weeks apart or as specified by manufacturer. Begin in September and complete by mid-November for all age groups.	Yearly, as specified by manufacturer. Primary series must be repeated when vaccine strains change.	Recommended for persons with chronic debilitating conditions, including cardiovascular and respiratory disease and chronic metabolic disorders. May be considered for persons with other chronic diseases or for persons providing essential community services. Contraindication: Allergy to vaccine components. See package insert for details.
Measles virus vaccine, live, attenuated.	12 months or over. 0.5 ml subcutaneously. If obsolescent "Edmonston" low-passage vaccines are used, immune serum globulin is administered by separate syringe in opposite arm. Dosage of ISG is critical. See package insert for details.	Not established.	Fever and rash may occur 5-12 days after vaccination. Contraindications: Altered immune states, including leukemia, lymphoma, and generalized malignancy; radiation, steroid, alkylating agent or antimetabolite therapy; severe febrile illness; untreated active tuberculosis; dysglobulinemia; pregnancy; hypersensitivity to vaccine components (see package insert). Persons previously immunized only with killed measles vaccine or those immunized before 10 months of age should be revaccinated with live measles vaccine. Those who received ISG with live measles vaccine should be individually evaluated for revaccination.
Rubella virus vaccine, live.	For children one year to puberty: 0.5 ml subcutaneously. May be given in special circumstances to postpubertal females. When immunization of postpubertal females is considered, susceptibility should be established by HI test, pregnancy should be ruled out before vaccination, and reliable precautions should be taken against pregnancy for two months following vaccination.	Not established.	Contraindications: Pregnancy; altered immune states, including leukemia, lymphomas, or generalized malignancies, or treatment with steroids, alkylating agents, antimetabolites or radiation; severe febrile illness; allergy to vaccine components. See package insert for details. Rash, arthralgia, or transient arthritis can occur following immunization. Arthralgia more frequent following vaccine prepared in dog-kidney tissue cultures, and after administration to adult females.
Measles and Rubella virus vaccine, live.	For children 12 months to puberty only: 0.5 ml subcutaneously.	Not established.	Contraindications: Pregnancy; altered immune states (see Measles Vaccine above); untreated active tuberculosis; concurrent febrile illness; allergy to vaccine components (see package insert). Not to be given to postpubertal females. May be given to children previously immunized against either measles or rubella, or where history of previous immunization is unclear.
Measles, Mumps, and Rubella Virus Vaccine, live.	For children 12 months to puberty only: 0.5 ml subcutaneously.	Not established.	Same as for Measles-Rubella vaccine above.

IMMUNIZING AGENTS	PRIMARY IMMUNIZATION SCHEDULE	BOOSTER SCHEDULE	COMMENTS AND CONTRAINDICATIONS
Mumps virus vaccine, live.	**Recommended for all susceptible individuals over 12 mos. of age.** 0.5 ml subcutaneously.	Not established.	Contraindications: Altered immune states, including leukemia, lymphoma, generalized malignancy; radiation, steroid, or antimetabolite therapy; concurrent illness; hypersensitivity to vaccine components. Refer to package insert for further details.
Poliovirus vaccine, live oral, trivalent (Sabin vaccine, OPV).	**For children 6 weeks through 18 years.** See package insert for dosage. First: 1 dose orally. Second: 1 dose orally 6-8 weeks later. Third: 1 dose orally 8-12 months later. If circumstances do not permit the optimal interval between the second and third doses, the third dose may be given as early as 6 weeks after the second.	A dose of trivalent OPV recommended at time of school entry. **Need for additional boosters not established.**	May be given at same time as killed vaccines. Contraindications: Altered immune states, including leukemia, lymphoma or generalized malignancy; therapy with steroids, alkylating agents, antimetabolites, or radiation. Not recommended routinely for adults in the United States. Unimmunized adults at special risk because of possible exposure to a case, or travel to endemic areas, should be immunized with OPV as indicated for children.
Typhoid vaccine (killed)	**6 months through 9 years:** First: 0.25 ml subcutaneously. Second: 0.25 ml subcutaneously 4 weeks later. **10 years or older:** First: 0.5 ml subcutaneously. Second: 0.5 ml subcutaneously 4 weeks later.	0.25-0.5 ml subcutaneously or 0.1 ml intradermally every 3 years.	Recommended for persons chronically exposed to case or carrier, or to community outbreak; travel to highly endemic areas. Intradermal boosters yield fewer systemic reactions. Do not use acetone-killed or dried vaccine intradermally.
Vaccinia virus vaccine, active (live), dried or liquid form.	Primary immunization: **12 months or older.** Multiple pressure methods. (Dried vaccine must be reconstituted.) Sites: Outer aspect of arm over deltoid or triceps; **not** over scapula nor on thigh. Primary vaccination successful if vesicle appears within 7 days. Revaccination successful if vesicle or induration with ulcer or crust appears within 7 days. If unsuccessful, repeat with reliable vaccine lot. No dressing.	All persons on exposure to case. Every 3 years for high-risk groups.	**Not to be given routinely in the absence of special indications.** Vaccination recommended for persons at special risk of smallpox exposure, such as health personnel, travelers to endemic countries, and military personnel. Avoid vaccination during pregnancy. Contraindicated when patient **or household member** has eczema or other forms of chronic dermatitis, when patient has agammaglobulinemia, generalized malignancy, including leukemia and lymphoma, or is receiving steroid, antimetabolite or radiation therapy.

SKIN TESTS, IMMUNIZATIONS, AND OTHER PROPHYLACTIC AGENTS

IMMUNE SERUM GLOBULIN (GAMMA GLOBULIN)

Immune Serum Globulin (Gamma Globulin): For passive immunization against various diseases. Administered intramuscularly.

1. **Normal immune serum globulin,** for passive immunization against particular diseases.

   a. Infectious hepatitis: For household contacts, ISG should be given as soon as possible after known exposure. Its prophylactic value decreases as time increases after exposure. The use of ISG more than 5-6 weeks after exposure is not indicated.

   Guidelines for ISG Prophylaxis of Infectious Hepatitis for Acute Exposure

Person's Weight (lb)	ISG Dose (ml)*
up to 50	0.5
50-100	1.0
over 100	2.0

   *Within limits, larger doses of ISG provide longer-lasting but not necessarily more protection.

   0.06-0.11 ml/kg (0.03 ml/lb) every 4-6 months for prolonged intensive exposure such as travel to endemic areas. May prevent icteric hepatitis, but does not protect against anicteric hepatitis.

   b. Measles: 0.25 ml/kg (0.1 ml/lb) within 6 days of exposure for susceptible infants and children (6 mos. to 3 yrs. of age). Should be followed by live virus rubeola vaccine 3 months later unless contraindicated. Alternatively, live measles vaccine can usually prevent disease if administered within 2 days after exposure.

   c. Rubella: Not recommended. Adversely affects diagnostic tests for rubella.

2. **Specific immune serum globulins:**

   a. Tetanus immune globulin (TIG): 250 U. for wound prophylaxis; 3,000-6,000 U. for therapy. See "Wound Management."

   b. Vaccinia immune globulin (VIG): For severe generalized vaccinia, eczema vaccinatum, vaccinia necrosum, ocular vaccinia, accidental exposure with extensive skin disease to vaccinia. Available commercially. For those unable to purchase this product, it is also available through Dr. Paul F. Wehrle, Dr. John M. Leedom, or Dr. Allen W. Mathies at LAC-USC Medical Center (Area Code 213, 225-3115).

   c. Pertussis immune globulin: Value not established.

   d. Mumps immune globulin: Value not established.

3. **Non-human antisera:**

   a. Diphtheria antitoxin (equine origin): 10,000 U. for unimmunized contacts only if daily observation not possible; 20,000 to 120,000 U. for therapy. Screen for horse serum allergy before use.

   b. Tetanus antitoxin (equine or bovine origin): See "Wound Management." TIG is preferable.

   c. Rabies antiserum: See "Guide for Post Exposure Rabies Prophylaxis."

   NOTE: Any type of immune serum globulin may cause biological false positive STS and TPI tests for syphilis. Smallpox vaccination may cause false positive STS. These agents should therefore be used with caution while a diagnosis of syphilis is being considered.

WOUND MANAGEMENT

Wound Management. Available evidence shows that complete primary immunization with tetanus toxoid provides long-range protective antitoxin levels. Additionally, protective antitoxin develops rapidly in response to a booster dose in persons who have previously received at least two doses of tetanus toxoid. Therefore, passive protection with TIG or antitoxin need be considered only when the patient has had less than two previous injections of tetanus toxoid or when the wound has been untended for more than 24 hours.

The following table is a conservative guide to active and passive tetanus immunization at the time of wound treatment or debridement.

Guide to Tetanus Prophylaxis in Wound Management

History of Tetanus Immunization (Doses)	Clean, Minor Wounds Td	Clean, Minor Wounds TIG	All Other Wounds Td	All Other Wounds TIG
Uncertain	Yes	No	Yes	Yes
0-1	Yes	No	Yes	Yes
2	Yes	No	Yes	No[1]
3 or more	No[2]	No	No[3]	No

[1] Unless wound more than 24 hours old.
[2] Unless more than 10 years since last dose.
[3] Unless more than 5 years since last dose.

Combined tetanus-diphtheria toxoids (Td) should be used instead of tetanus toxoid.

If passive immunization is used, TIG is preferable to animal antitoxin because of longer protection and freedom from side reactions. For wounds of average severity, 250 units should be administered at a site separate from that used for accompanying Td. If TIG is unavailable, equine or bovine tetanus antitoxin may be used with proper precautions against serum sensitivity. The recommended dose is 3,000 to 5,000 units.

GUIDE FOR POST-EXPOSURE RABIES PROPHYLAXIS

RATIONALE OF TREATMENT—Every exposure to possible rabies infection must be individually evaluated. In Los Angeles County, as in the rest of the United States, the following factors should be considered before specific antirabies treatment is initiated:

Species of biting animal involved: Carnivorous animals (especially skunks, foxes, coyotes, raccoons, dogs, and cats) and bats are more likely to be infective than other animals. Bites of rabbits, squirrels, chipmunks, rats and mice seldom, if ever, require rabies prophylaxis.

Circumstances of the biting incident: An *unprovoked* attack is more likely to mean that the animal is rabid. (Bites during attempts to feed or handle an apparently healthy animal generally should be regarded as *provoked*.)

Extent of exposure: The likelihood that rabies will result from an exposure varies with the nature and extent of the exposure. Two categories of exposure should be considered:

Bite wounds: Any penetration of the skin by teeth.

Non-bite wounds: Scratches, abrasions, or open wounds.

Vaccination status of the biting animal: A properly immunized animal has only a minimal chance of developing rabies and transmitting the virus.

Presence of rabies in the region: If adequate laboratory and field records indicate that there is no rabies infection in a domestic species within a given region, local health officials may be justified in taking this into consideration in any recommendations concerning antirabies treatment following a bite by that species.

POST-EXPOSURE ANTIRABIES GUIDE

The following recommendations are only a guide. They should be used in conjunction with knowledge of the animal species involved, circumstances of the bite or other exposure, vaccination status of the animal, and presence of rabies in the region.

Animal and Its Condition		Treatment	
Species	Condition at Time of Attack	Kind of Exposure	
		Bite*	Non-Bite*
Wild Skunk, Fox, Raccoon, Bat	Regard as Rabid	S + V[1]	S + V[1]
Domestic Dog	Healthy	None[2]	None[2]
	Escaped (unknown)	S + V	V
	Rabid	S + V[1]	S + V[1]
Cat			
Other	Consider individually—See "Rationale of Treatment"		

*See text definitions   V: Rabies Vaccine (14 doses)   S + V: Antirabies Serum + Vaccine (21 doses)
[1] Discontinue vaccine if fluorescent antibody (FA) tests of animal killed at time of attack are negative
[2] Begin S + V at first sign of rabies in biting dog or cat during holding period (10 days)

LOCAL TREATMENT OF WOUNDS—Immediate and thorough local treatment of all bite wounds and scratches is the most effective means of preventing rabies. Experimentally, the incidence of rabies in animals has been markedly reduced by local therapy alone.

First-aid treatment to be carried out immediately: Copious flushing with soap and water, or with ethyl alcohol (43% or higher).

Treatment by or under the direction of a physician:

1. Thorough flushing and cleansing of the wound with soap solution or quaternary ammonium compounds such as benzalkonium chloride, cetrimonium bromide, or di-methyl-benzyl ammonium chloride. All traces of soap should be removed before applying quaternary ammonium compounds because soap neutralizes their activity.

2. If antirabies serum is indicated and the site permits, 50% of total dose may be infiltrated around the wound. As in all instances in which horse serum is used, a careful history should be taken and tests for hypersensitivity performed.

3. Suturing of wound is not indicated if there is a high likelihood that the biting animal is rabid.

PREVENTION OF EXPOSURE TO RABIES—Avoiding exposure to animals susceptible to rabies is the surest way to control this disease. Control measures include avoiding contact with all carnivorous wildlife, immunization of domestic pets, and keeping pets and children under control to avoid unnecessary biting incidents.

REFERENCE:

1. Committee on Immunization, Infectious Disease Soc. of America., *J. Inf. Dis.*, 123:227-40, Feb. 1971.
2. USPHS Advisory Committee on Immunization Practices, Center for Disease Control, *Morbidity and Mortality Weekly Report*, Vol. 21, No. 25, June 24, 1972.

SKIN TESTS, IMMUNIZATIONS, AND OTHER PROPHYLACTIC AGENTS

HEALTH DISTRICTS
COUNTY OF LOS ANGELES HEALTH DEPARTMENT

Health District	District Health Officer	*L.A. Exchange	*Other
ALHAMBRA	ELLEN POYET, M.D.		
Health Center—612 W. Shorb St., Alhambra		283-9021	
**Rosemead Subcenter—7865 E. Emerson Pl., Rosemead		573-9300	289-6101
BELLFLOWER	EARL W. KENDRICK, M.D.		
Health Center—10005 E. Flower Ave., Bellflower			866-7011
**Hawaiian Gardens Subcenter—22101 Norwalk Blvd., Hawaiian Gardens			420-2420
*Lakewood Subcenter—5110 N. Clark Ave., Lakewood		773-2822	866-9061
Norwalk Subcenter—12360 E. Firestone Blvd., Norwalk			864-7755
CENTRAL	MILTON R. COHEN, M.D.		
Health Center—241 N. Figueroa St., L.A.		625-3212	
COMPTON	PAUL WERMER, M.D.		
Health Center—300 E. Rosecrans Ave., Compton		636-8191	639-6010
*Avalon Subcenter—215 Sumner Ave., Catalina Island			Avalon 185
North Enterprise Subcenter—638 E. El Segundo, L.A.			532-6000
EAST LOS ANGELES	JANE SHIELDS, M.D.		
Health Center—670 S. Ferris Ave., L.A.		261-3191	
Maravilla Subcenter—929 N. Bonnie Beach Pl., L.A.		264-6910	
EAST VALLEY	ROBERT S. ROCKE, M.D.		
North Hollywood Health Center—5300 Tujunga Ave., N. Hollywood		877-9530	766-3981
Pacoima Subcenter—13300 Van Nuys Blvd., Pacoima			899-0231
Tujunga Subcenter—7747 Foothill Blvd., Tujunga			352-1417
EL MONTE	MARTIN D. FINN, M.D.		
Health Center—3550 N. Eastmont Ave., El Monte		686-2510	444-7751
Baldwin Park Subcenter—14247 E. Morgan St., Baldwin Park			962-3341
La Puente Subcenter—15930 Central Ave., La Puente			968-3711
GLENDALE	MARY E. SEDDON, M.D.		
Health Center—501 N. Glendale Blvd., Glendale		245-1831	244-6511
Burbank Subcenter—1101 W. Magnolia Blvd., Burbank		849-3353	842-2171
HARBOR	FRANK PACINO, M.D.		
San Pedro Health Center—122 W. 8th St., San Pedro			547-4461
Wilmington Subcenter—612 W. "E" St., Wilmington			835-5641
HOLLYWOOD-WILSHIRE	WILLIAM BURKE, M.D.		
Health Center—5205 Melrose Ave., L.A.		464-9121	
West Hollywood Subcenter—621 N. San Vicente, West Hollywood		655-7780	652-3090
INGLEWOOD	PHILIP KANI, M.D.		
Health Center—401 W. Manchester Blvd., Inglewood		678-1241	677-2161
Lawndale Subcenter—14614 S. Grevillea Ave., Lawndale		776-5747	675-0345
**Westchester Subcenter—9100 Sepulveda Eastway, L.A.		757-9171	645-4444
Imperial Heights Subcenter—10616 S. Western, L.A.			

Health District	District Health Officer	*L.A. Exchange	*Other
MONROVIA	ANSEL ZEHM, M.D.		
Health Center—330 W. Maple, Monrovia			359-2581
Altadena Subcenter—2490 Lake Ave., Altadena			797-8704
Azusa Subcenter—150 N. Azusa Ave., Azusa			334-1201
NORTHEAST	LAWRENCE H. COSGROVE, M.D.		
Health Center—2032 Marengo St., L.A.		225-5971	
Utah Subcenter—131 South Utah St., L.A.		266-0704	
POMONA	HERBERT MEEHAN, M.D.		
Health Center—750 S. Park Ave., Pomona		967-1411	714/623-6811
Citrus Subcenter—1435 W. Service, W. Covina		686-1010	338-8461
SAN ANTONIO			
Health Center—6538 Miles Ave., Huntington Park		583-1751	
Bell Gardens Subcenter—6912 Ajax Ave., Bell Gardens		773-1861	861-7278
**Downey Subcenter—10924 La Reina St., Downey			
SAN FERNANDO	DOROTHY McVANN, M.D.		
Health Center—604 S. Maclay Ave., San Fernando			365-4661
Antelope Valley Subcenter—44855 N. Cedar Ave., Lancaster			805/948-4615
Valencia Subcenter—23747 W. Valencia Blvd.			805/255-1171
SOUTH	PAULINE ROBERTS, M.D.		
Health Center—1522 E. 102nd St., L.A.		564-6801	
Florence-Firestone Subcenter—8019 Compton Ave., L.A.		583-6241	537-0030
SOUTHEAST	RICHARD WILCOX, M.D.		
Health Center—4920 S. Avalon Blvd., L.A.		231-2161	
SOUTHWEST	HAMPTON P. DESLONDE, M.D.		
Health Center—3834 S. Western Ave., L.A.		731-8541	
TORRANCE	RICHARD DEAR, M.D.		
Health Center—2300 Carson St., Torrance		775-7221	320-6010
**Redondo Beach Subcenter—217 Beryl St., Redondo Beach		772-4221	376-2401
**Villa Carson Subcenter—23233 S. Avalon Blvd., Wilmington			830-5342
WEST	GEORGE PRICHARD, M.D.		
Health Center—2509 Pico Blvd., Santa Monica			829-2911
Culver City Subcenter—4150 Overland Blvd., Culver City		870-7462	837-1251
**Malibu Subcenter—23525 Civic Center Way, Malibu			456-3381
Venice Subcenter—905 Venice Blvd., Venice			821-3484
WEST VALLEY	DEAN W. GILMAN, M.D.		
Health Center—14340 Sylvan St., Van Nuys		873-5674	787-3350
Canoga Park Subcenter—7107 Remmet Ave., Canoga Park			340-3570
WHITTIER	A. C. NEISWANDER, M.D.		
Health Center—7643 S. Painter Ave., Whittier		723-3381	698-6251
*Santa Fe Springs Subcenter—9255 Pioneer Blvd., Santa Fe Springs			692-1278
Pico Rivera Subcenter—6336 S. Parsons Blvd., Pico Rivera		699-0461	

*IF NO ANSWER AT SUBCENTER, CALL HEALTH CENTER

**International Certificates of Vaccination for travel are not validated at these subcenters.

UNIT 12

POST-TEST

1. Name the three routes by which antigens can enter the body.
2. What causes hypersensitivity (allergic reaction)?
3. Name two factors that determine the severity of the allergic reaction.
4. Name the three forms that an allergic reaction can take.
5. Describe the mechanism of anaphylactic shock.
6. Antibodies are produced and transported within what solution in the body?
7. How are antitoxins formed?
8. Describe anaphylactic shock.
9. Name one advantage, and one disadvantage, of the Medic-Alert bracelet.
10. Name four hypersensitive reactions.

POST-TEST ANNOTATED ANSWER SHEET

1. Inhalation, ingestion, or injection, p. 349.
2. An antigen-antibody reaction, p. 350.
3. The amount of allergen that is present, and the degree of sensitivity within the individual, p. 350.
4. Local reaction, systemic reaction, anaphylactic shock, p. 350.
5. The mechanism cannot be described because it is not yet understood, p. 350.
6. Gamma globulin, p. 357.
7. They are substances formed by the body in response to toxins that are produced by certain organisms, p. 351.
8. It is an immediate reaction to an antigen taken in by a sensitized person; it may be mild, or severe to the point of death within minutes. Symptoms include: urticaria, bronchiolar constriction, edema, and circulatory collapse, pp. 350, 352.
9. The Medic-Alert is a reliable device for alerting health workers to the presence of allergies if the patient wears the bracelet. The major disadvantage is that most people do not wear the Medic-Alert bracelet, p. 353.
10. Anaphylactic shock, serum sickness, atopy, auto-immunity. pp. 352, 353.

SKIN TESTS, IMMUNIZATIONS, AND OTHER PROPHYLACTIC AGENTS

PERFORMANCE TEST

In the skill laboratory or the clinical setting you will perform at least two of the following procedures: the Patch Test, the Scratch Test, the Tine Test, the Mono-Vacc test, the Heaf or Sterneedle test, the tuberculin Hypospray, or the Mantoux test.

PERFORMANCE CHECKLIST

THE PATCH TEST

1. Assemble supplies.
2. Wash hands.
3. Identify the patient.
4. Explain the procedure.
5. Cleanse the skin.
6. Apply impregnated dressing.
7. Instruct the patient.
8. Record test on chart.
9. Read the test.
10. Record reaction.

THE SCRATCH TEST

1. Assemble supplies.
2. Wash hands.
3. Identify patient.
4. Explain procedure.
5. Expose back and have patient lie face down on table.
6. Wash back.
7. Write test numbers on skin.
8. Make 1/8 inch scratch.
9. Place one drop of antigen solution on each scratch.
10. Allow "setting" time.
11. Wipe off excess solution.
12. Read and record results.
13. Have patient dress.

TINE, MONO-VACC, OR HEAF TEST

1. Assemble supplies.
2. Wash hands.
3. Identify patient.
4. Explain procedure.
5. Expose forearm and cleanse.
6. Puncture forearm.
7. Instruct patient.
8. Record test.
9. Read reaction.
10. Record reaction (time and response).

JET GUN OR HYPOSPRAY TUBERCULIN TEST

1. Assemble supplies.
2. Wash hands.
3. Identify patient.
4. Explain procedure.
5. Expose forearm and cleanse.
6. Place injection tip against arm, pull trigger, and inject tuberculin.
7. Instruct patient and record test.
8. Read and record reaction.

MANTOUX TEST

1. Assemble supplies.
2. Wash hands.
3. Identify medication.
4. Cleanse stopper.
5. Assemble needle and syringe.
6. Withdraw tuberculin into syringe and withdraw needle.
7. Explain procedure.
8. Cleanse injection site.
9. Grasp and support forearm to be injected.
10. Insert needle and inject solution so that wheal appears.
11. Withdraw needle.
12. Position patient for comfort.
13. Instruct patient and record test.
14. Read and record reaction.

Unit 13

ASSISTING WITH SOMATIC PSYCHIATRIC THERAPIES

(Electroconvulsive and Insulin Coma)

I. DIRECTIONS TO THE STUDENT

Read this lesson carefully because it is complex and detailed. Your instructor will probably give you some outside reading assignments, which will supplement the information in this unit.

After you have finished and have practiced the activities in the skill laboratory, make arrangements with your instructor to take the Performance Test.

II. GENERAL PERFORMANCE OBJECTIVE

Upon completion of this Unit you will be able safely and correctly to assist the physician in giving electroconvulsive shock and insulin coma treatments to your patients.

III. SPECIFIC PERFORMANCE OBJECTIVES

When you have finished this Unit, you will be able to:

1. Assemble supplies and have the electroconvulsive therapy (ECT) equipment in working order to prepare for giving ECT treatment.
2. Prepare the patient physically and mentally for the ECT or insulin coma treatment.
3. Prepare the patient for placement of the electrodes.
4. Test the electrodes for conduction.
5. Insert the mouth gag prior to beginning the ECT treatment without injuring the patient.
6. Observe and record the patient's vital signs and levels of consciousness following the somatic treatment.
7. Discuss the two methods for terminating the insulin coma treatment.

IV. VOCABULARY

Read the definitions of the terms listed below. Do not attempt to memorize these definitions before proceeding with the lesson. Each term will be explained or defined again in the text. On completion of the lesson, however, you should know the correct definitions of these terms.

Ambu resuscitator—a portable breathing system that has a face mask and a breathing bag.
ameliorative—tending to improve or moderate a condition, or to otherwise make it less severe.

anxiety—a state of tension or distress akin to fear, but produced by a threatened awareness of unacceptable feelings rather than by an external danger.

Babinski reflex—a reflex movement of the foot when the lateral aspect of the sole of the foot is stroked. Pathologic if the toes fan out and up; the normal response is downward curling of the toes.

conduction—the act of conveying an electrical impulse.

convulsion—sudden involuntary, spasmodic occurrence of muscle contractions and relaxations. **clonic convulsion,** convulsion with alternating contractions and relaxations. **tonic convulsion,** contraction that is maintained over a period of time (minutes) before relaxation occurs.

cranial—pertaining to the part of the skull that encloses the brain.

defibrillator—a machine (apparatus) used to counteract fibrillation of the heart by applying electrical impulses (with electrodes) to the heart or chest.

depression—a pathologic, psychological state brought on by feelings of loss and/or guilt; it is characterized by sadness and lowered self-esteem, and may vary in intensity from mild to severe.

electroconvulsive therapy (ECT)—commonly called electric shock therapy (EST), a form of treatment in which an electric current is administered to the brain to effect an artificial convulsive seizure. It is used in the treatment of some mental illnesses such as depression and schizophrenia.

electrode—a metal disc that serves as a conductor to contact a part of the patient's body (in this unit, the temporal area of the cranium) when an electrical current is administered to the patient's body.

electrode paste—a specially prepared ointment that serves as a conductor of the electrical current. It is applied to the electrode in the EST.

emergency cart—a mobile cart (or table) that contains emergency supplies and drugs. (Each agency establishes the contents and locations for its emergency cart.)

epilepsy—an illness in which episodic disturbances of consciousness may occur and in which convulsions may occur.

fibrillation (cardiac)—inefficient, irregular contraction of individual muscle fibrils (of the heart).

flaccid—relaxed, flabby, having absent or defective muscle tone.

grand mal—a typical generalized convulsive attack in an epileptic patient, with or without coma.

hormone—a chemical substance (originating in an organ or gland) that is conveyed through the blood or lymph to another part of the body, stimulating or inhibiting its activity or secretion.

hypersalivation—excessive and abnormal production of saliva.

hypersensitivity—excessive or abnormal sensitivity to a given agent, e.g., pollen, drug.

hypoglycemia—a condition in which there are abnormally decreased amounts of sugar (glucose) in the blood.

insulin—a pancreatic hormone (secreted by the islets of Langerhans) that is essential for carbohydrate metabolism. A synthetic (manufactured) insulin is also available for use in treatment of certain patients (e.g., diabetic; insulin coma).

insulin coma—a psychiatric treatment in which increasingly large doses of insulin are given daily to produce unconsciousness and a severe hypoglycemic reaction. (Usually 30 to 40 doses must be given to produce the desired result. However, coma can and does occur with a *single dose.*)

insulin shock—metabolic condition resulting from an overdose of insulin resulting in hypoglycemia.

intercostal—between the ribs (e.g., intercostal muscles or the outer layer of muscles between the ribs).

involutional melancholia—a severe depression related to "change of life."

level of consciousness—level of awareness or of perception; in psychiatry it refers to conscious, preconscious, unconscious.

manic depressive psychosis—a psychosis characterized by alternating states of depression and excitement.

myotonic twitching—simple tonic muscle spasms.
pancreatic—referring to the pancreas, a gland lying behind the stomach and draining into the duodenum.
perception—process of being aware of sensory impressions.
petit mal—a mild form of epileptic attack, a momentary loss of consciousness, without convulsions.
primitive movement—regression to early stages of behavior development, e.g., thumb-sucking.
psychoneurosis—a mild to moderately severe illness of the personality; there is a conflict between conscious and unconscious wishes.
psychosis—a serious illness of the personality involving major impairment of the ego structure. Serious maladjustments to life may occur.
pupillary reaction—the closing and opening of the center of the iris (colored part of eye) as a response to light.
schizophrenia (dementia praecox)—(Greek "split mind" or "split personality.") one of the major functional psychoses.
singultus (hiccups)—spasmodic, periodic closure of the glottis following spasmodic lowering of the diaphragm, causing a short inspiratory cough.
somnolence—prolonged drowsiness or condition resembling a trance; sleepiness.
temporal region or area—the area of the head referred to as the "temples," located laterally to the eyes and just above the ears.
torsion spasm—spasm characterized by a turning of a part of the body, especially at the pelvis.
tranquilizer—a drug that acts to reduce tension and anxiety with relatively little effect on alertness.
trigeminal pain—pain in the distribution of the fifth cranial nerve (trigeminus); may be facial pain, and also of the scalp, jaw, tongue, and eye.

V. INTRODUCTION

Somatic therapies for the treatment of mental illness, that is, treatments given to the body (soma) versus treatment to the psyche (mind), have been with us since earliest times. Various treatments for mental illness through the ages have included such somatic remedies as drugs, trephinement, bloodletting, leeches, electric shock, etc. In early times these treatments were thought to cure mental illness. However, nowadays they are considered merely ameliorative; that is, they may moderate the condition, but they do not affect the source of the disturbance. Modern-day treatments are individualized according to the need of the specific patient and his specific mental illness.

Somatic therapies came into common use in the 1930's and 1940's. At that time the most popular somatic therapies included insulin coma, Metrazol shock, electric shock, psychosurgery, and chemotherapy. The current therapies include: (1) pharmacological agents; (2) electric shock; and (3) insulin coma.

The somatic therapies require the services of highly skilled and knowledgeable nurses. Somatic therapy is often carried on in conjunction with appropriate psychotherapy.

National recognition of the problem of mental health did not take place until after World War II when large numbers of servicemen were discharged because of psychiatric disabilities. Many men were rejected for armed service because of serious psychiatric illness.

During their service experience, many servicemen came in contact with psychiatrists for the first time. They began to see mental health as part of the total health problem. When they returned to civilian life, they accepted treatment for mental illness as they accepted other medical treatment. Thus, the bias against psychiatric treatment began to lessen and mental health began to be regarded as part of the total health picture.

In 1946, the Federal Government authorized the formation of the National Institute of Mental Health (NIMH) under the auspices of the National Mental Health Act. A three-pronged program was established that included (1) training of psychiatric personnel, (2) support for psychiatric research, and (3) provision of financial aid to states for developing mental health programs.

Under the stimulus of the National Mental Health Act, nursing education programs began to incorporate psychiatric nursing and psychiatric principles in basic nursing programs. (Although some schools were doing this prior to the existence of the Act, after its establishment more emphasis was placed on the application of principles of mental health to all facets of nursing care.)

Mild depression and mild euphoria are experienced by everyone periodically throughout life. Only when these moods become severe or prevent functioning do individuals need the assistance of the psychiatrist and the somatic therapies.

Patients are given careful and thorough physical and mental examinations before being started on any somatic therapy. The examination usually includes an electroencephalogram (EEG) to ascertain the brain's activity and the electrocardiogram (ECG) to determine the cardiac status. These tests are used to determine whether the patient's physical or mental status contraindicates the utilization of a somatic therapy.

Hospitalized patients who have severe psychiatric disorders require skillful nursing care. It is extremely important not only to maintain a physically safe environment for the patient, but one in which the patient can achieve optimum psychological support. Skill in giving quality general nursing care to these patients is as important as their psychiatric care. In other words, these patients need the same general care as medical-surgical patients (proper diet, fluid intake and output, rest, activity, cleanliness, exercise, etc.).

These patients have a need to communicate. Listen to what the patient is saying. Be friendly, attentive, and supportive. Answer his questions directly and simply. He may forget what you say because he is anxious. You may need to repeat the same information several times. Be kind, understanding, and supportive to the patient at all times. Various methods of handling patients can be determined in group discussion. When a plan of action for the patient is determined (e.g., firmness or flexibility), it must be carried out by each member of the health team.

ITEMS NEEDED IN THE TREATMENT ROOM

Contents of Emergency Cart

a. Cardiac/respiratory drugs.

b. Tracheostomy tray.

c. Endotracheal tray.

d. Ambu resuscitator.

e. ECG scope.

f. Defibrillator.

g. Oxygen tank or oxygen wall setup.

h. Oral suction machine or wall-mounted suction.

Contents of the Physician's Tray

a. Acetone (used to cleanse the skin).

b. A selection of 2 cc, 10 cc, and 20 cc syringes.

c. A selection of needles, No. 21 and No. 22.

d. Alcohol sponges.

e. Tourniquet.

f. Adhesive bandages.

g. Sterile water for injection.

h. Anectine (keep refrigerated until 15 minutes prior to ECT treatment).

Contents of General Shock Treatment Tray

    a. Alcohol sponges or acetone (used to cleanse the skin).

    b. Supersaturated salt solution (used as an abrasive to prepare a conductive skin surface).

    c. Cotton balls (used with acetone to cleanse the temporal area of dirt and grease so that a good contact can be made with the electrode).

    d. Electrode paste (applied on the temporal areas and the surface of the electrodes to increase conductivity).

    e. Padded tongue depressors (used in emergency to prevent patient from biting his tongue).

    f. Rubber mouth gag (used to keep the jaws open during the treatment so that the patient will not swallow or bite his tongue during and after the treatment).

    g. Airway (may be inserted after the treatment, during recovery).

ITEM 1: ELECTROCONVULSIVE SHOCK THERAPY (EST OR ECT)

In 1938 Doctors Ugo Cerletti and Lucio Bini introduced electric shock therapy in Rome, Italy. This form of treatment is used in the treatment of depressions, such as manic depressive psychosis, involutional melancholia, psychoneurotic depression, and certain types of schizophrenia.

The "classical method" of shock treatment used by Doctors Cerletti and Bini differed from the brief stimulus shock treatments that are in use today. With today's method, there is greater control over the electrical voltage, amperage, and wave patterns. Less severe seizures are produced.

Electroshock therapy (EST) is administered by a highly qualified team of experts (psychiatrist, nurse, and sometimes an anesthetist). It is necessary for all involved health personnel to understand the nature of the treatment, the mechanisms of action, the procedures, the objectives of the treatment, and the use of drugs to complement the procedure (before, during, and after).

Personnel often have anxiety about the treatment and consequently have difficulty handling the questions, fears, and unusual behavior of patients who receive EST. Before you assist in the care of these patients, you should have an opportunity to verbalize your fears and apprehensions (perhaps in a seminar) with the psychiatrist and other members of the health team with whom you will be working. If you do not clear up your apprehensions, you may transmit them to the patient.

After a patient has received a series of treatments, he often becomes very anxious about further treatments. You must be patient, supportive, and understanding at all times. Reassure him that you will remain with him throughout the treatment and while he recovers. Assure him that his anxiety will decrease as he improves. Encourage him to talk with other patients about their feelings about the treatments (some agencies have developed group discussions for this). Let him know that his fears are shared by many others and are natural for patients receiving EST. Tell him he may experience temporary confusion, but that his mind will become clear again within a short time (a few hours to a week after the treatment). Amnesia concerning the treatment itself may remain indefinitely.

There are many theories about the effect of EST. One theory is that the EST "deconditions" the patient; that is, it interferes with the neural pathways of new behavior and permits older, healthier behavior to become more prominent. Another theory states that the treatment is viewed by the patient as punishment and thus relieves the patient of unbearable guilt feelings.

EST is used in combination with chemical therapies (psychotropic drugs) and psychotherapy. Each modality (method) of the therapy seems to reinforce the other aspects of the treatment, making the patient's recovery more rapid. The EST's are given two or three times a week for three to ten weeks, depending on the needs of the individual patient.

General preparation of the patient who is scheduled for EST usually follows the guidelines outlined below:

A. The Night Before the Treatment

Important Steps	Key Points
1. *Obtain written consent* for the treatment.	Follow your agency's procedure. (See sample consent form at the end of this unit.) Refer to Volume 2, Unit 34, "Preparation of Consents, Releases and Incidents," if you must refresh your memory on the legal implications of writing consents. Patients are admitted to private agencies voluntarily. Therefore, they may sign their own consent forms. If the patient was admitted under court order or if he is a minor, then the legal guardian must sign the consent for the patient.
2. Obtain the required EEG and ECG laboratory work, and chest X-rays as ordered or established by your agency's policy.	These examinations are usually ordered before beginning the series of treatments to determine if there are any physiologic conditions that would contraindicate the use of the ECT. The reports should be on the patient's chart *before* the series of treatments begins.
3. Tell the patient about the examination, what he can expect, etc.	Answer his questions directly and clearly. Continually reassure him. For example:

Patient	Nurse
"Will I die?"	"No, this treatment does not use a lethal dose of electricity."
"Will it cure me?"	"It's one means of treatment. Most of the work of cure will need to be done by you with your therapist."
"Does it hurt?"	"The whole treatment is painless, except for the injection of the medicine, which will be given in a vein in your arm. However, you may have some mild muscle discomfort after the treatment. A warm bath and routine exercise will help to minimize the muscle discomfort."
"Can I be electrocuted?"	"No, the amount of electricity used for the treatment will not electrocute you. It is a very small amount of electrical current."

Important Steps	Key Points
4. Inform the patient that he will be NPO after midnight.	NPO is required a minimum of six hours prior to treatment. As you will recall from Volume 2, Unit 33, "Preoperative Care of a Patient," this is done to minimize secretions in the respiratory and digestive tracts. (Remember to cancel or hold his breakfast.)

B. The Morning of the Treatment

Important Steps	Key Points
1. Wash your hands, approach and identify the patient.	Answer any questions he may have.

Important Steps	Key Points
2. Remove bobby pins and other metal objects from the hair.	The metal could serve as a conductor when the electrical current is discharged and result in a burn.
3. Remove foreign objects from mouth.	Remove dentures, chewing gum and other foreign objects from the mouth to avoid the possibility of aspiration during the procedure.
4. Remove nail polish from fingers and toes (as agency prescribes).	This is done so that the color of the nailbeds can be easily observed for symptoms of cyanosis during treatment and recovery. You may need to give nail care since these patients are frequently depressed and may neglect their personal hygiene.
5. Remove jewelry and valuables (contact lenses, watches, rings, etc.).	This prevents loss during the treatment. Also, the electric current will magnetize a watch. Place jewelry and valuables in a place designated by your agency (e.g., valuables envelope).
6. Give preoperative medication.	Give at the designated time (usually 15 to 45 minutes before the treatment). Usually a barbiturate and a secretory depressant (e.g., Nembutal or Seconal given orally and atropine given subcutaneously) are used.
7. Check treatment room supplies and equipment.	NOTE: Some agencies may take the patient to the operating room for the treatment. If this is done, the patient will usually be given a general anesthetic.

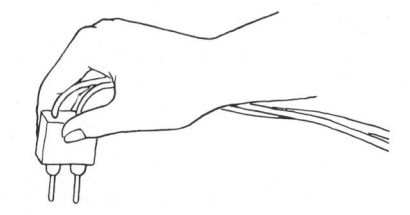

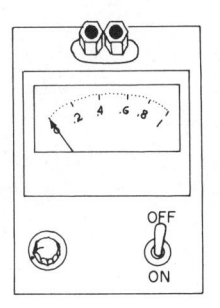

However, the following steps must be carried out whether the treatment is given in the operating room or in a treatment room.

a. *Attach electrodes* to the testing machine and check to be sure the electrodes are conducting.

b. *Assemble the EST machine* (see p. 382). Attach the electrodes to the machine. Be sure that the machine is plugged into the electrical outlet. Be sure that the machine is grounded (may be a part of your electrical system).

c. Have the *emergency cart* and *physician's* and *general shock treatment trays* ready for use. Be sure that all of the supplies are available as stipulated in the list of items given earlier.

d. Be sure that the *oxygen and suction equipment* is ready for use (attach the oxygen tubing to the outlet or to the oxygen tank and make sure that the tank has sufficient oxygen in it to give the treatment). Attach the oxygen catheter or mask to the tubing.

e. Be sure that the *ECG machine* is connected to the electrical outlet and is filled with tracing paper.

Important Steps	Key Points
	f. Be sure that the *cardioscope and defibrillator* are connected to the electrical outlet. Test to be sure that they are in working order. Make certain that these machines are also grounded.
8. Return to the patient's room.	Have the patient void before the EST is administered. An empty bladder will prevent incontinence when he loses consciousness during the treatment (with a resulting relaxation of the sphincter muscles). The Anectine injection may also relax the sphincter muscles.
9. Dress the patient in a hospital gown or pajamas.	This will prevent soiling, loss, or damage to his personal property during the treatment and recovery periods.
10. Transfer the patient to a stretcher.	The stretcher will be covered with a conductive rubber sheeting and grounded to prevent possible skin burn when the electrical current is discharged. Place the patient in a supine position and cover him with a bath blanket to provide warmth and protect his modesty. A small pillow may be placed under the head for comfort (it will be removed during the treatment). Be sure to attach the safety straps lightly across the thighs to keep him from falling off the stretcher, and from injuring his arms and legs as the stretcher goes through doorways. Continue to reassure your patient. Speak calmly and with confidence.

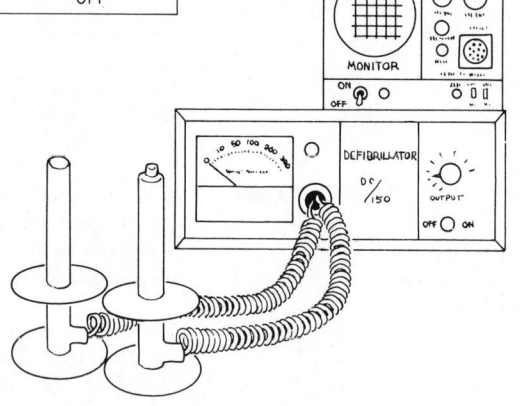

ASSISTING WITH SOMATIC PSYCHIATRIC THERAPIES

Important Steps	Key Points
11. Take the patient to the treatment room.	Continue to reassure him that you will remain through the treatment and recovery. (Some agencies assign a health worker to stay with the patient before, during, and after the treatment. Follow your agency's procedure.)

C. Assisting with the Treatment

Important Steps	Key Points
1. Place the stretcher in the proper position.	Lock the wheels so that the stretcher will not move during the treatment. Center the stretcher so that the spotlight (portable or overhead) can easily be directed to the work site.
2. Cleanse the patient's temporal areas for placement of electrodes.	*Bilateral:*

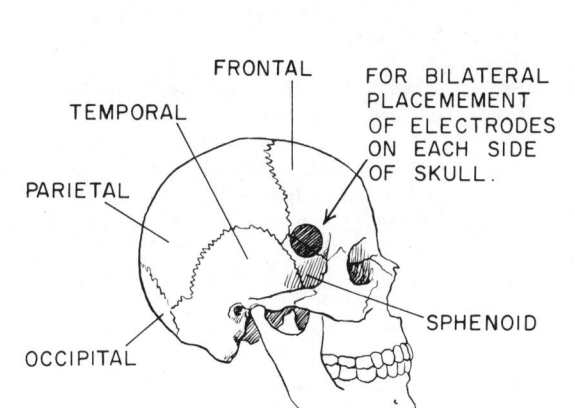

Wipe the temporal areas with acetone-saturated cotton balls or alcohol sponges. These chemicals will help dissolve surface grease and will provide a medically clean site for applying the electrodes. Discard the cotton balls or sponges in a designated waste container.

Next, rub the temporal areas with cotton balls saturated in a concentrated salt solution until the solution acts as an abrasive to provide a rough skin surface that permits a better contact surface for the electrode.

NOTE: The *bilateral temporal* placement of the electrodes is the most common method. Side effects may last up to 6 weeks.

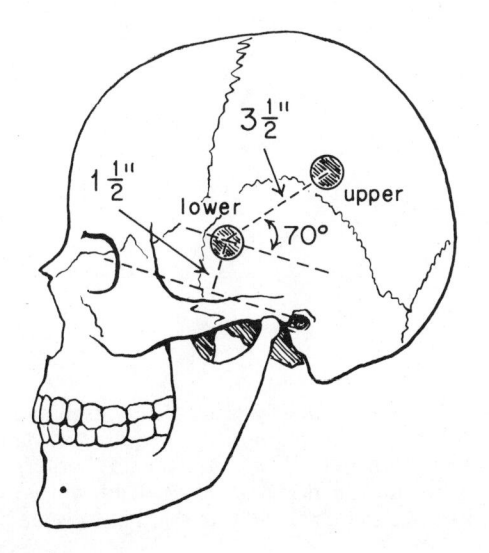

Unilateral:

The *unilateral* electrode placement puts the electrodes in two locations in the same hemisphere of the brain (either in the temporal or parietal area, according to the physician's choice). The unilateral is the preferred method because it produces far less confusion and less organicity (loss of memory, regression). The effect is much like a light stroke with a temporary organic change. Side effects may last up to 6 to 8 weeks.

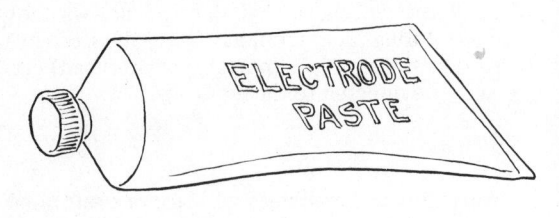

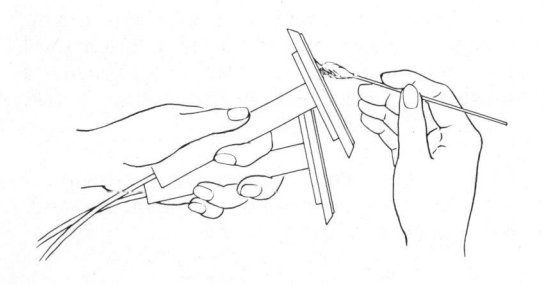

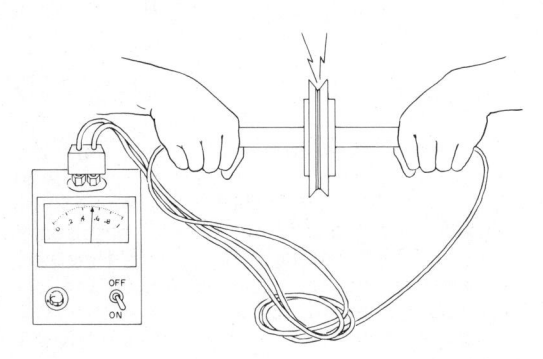

Important Steps	Key Points
3. Repeat electrode site cleansing.	Again cleanse the temporal (parietal) areas with acetone-saturated cotton balls to remove all traces of the salt. (Salt is not a conductor.) The second acetone application gets deeper into the crevices of the skin to remove any residual grease.
4. Apply electrode paste to the electrode sites (temporal or parietal).	The paste usually comes in a tube. Spread about 1/4 inch of paste on each of the temporal areas. Rub the paste thinly but thoroughly into the skin with the cotton-tipped applicator so that the area is evenly covered with a thin film of paste (the paste is very sticky). This improves the conduction of the electrical current (by decreasing the resistance) and prevents burning of the skin. The paste also has an emulsifying agent that assists in breaking down any remaining skin surface oils, which could increase resistance to the electrical current. If the paste is applied too thickly, it will permit the electrode to slip and an improper connection will result.
5. Apply electrode paste to the electrode.	Spread about 1/8 inch of paste on each electrode. Spread it evenly over the contact surface of the electrodes with the cotton applicator. When the electrode comes in contact with the skin surface, the prepared areas make a smooth, even contact and provide for maximum conduction of the electrical current. Sparsely applied paste either on the skin or electrode decreases the effects of a full, even contact surface, and could seriously impair the full effect of the electrical current conduction. Be sure that both surfaces are covered thinly and evenly with electrode paste.
6. Test the electrode conduction (with testing apparatus if used in your agency).	With the electrodes attached to the test conduction apparatus, the nurse puts the electrode plates together to ascertain if an electrical current is available. (The usual reading will vary from 0 to 1.0 ampere.)
7. Attach electrodes to the electroshock machine in the designated outlets.	You have previously plugged the machine into the wall electrical outlet. Turn on the Master Power Switch (lower right-hand corner) to warm up the machine. A red light will go on near the switch to indicate that power is on.

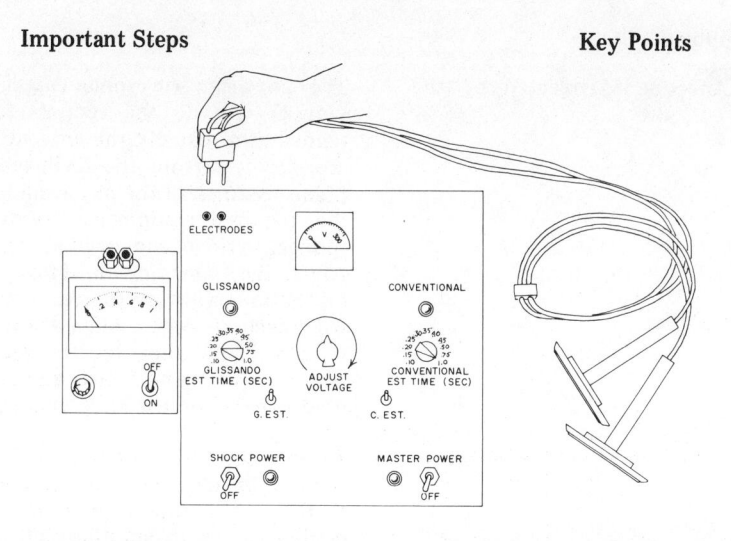

ASSISTING WITH SOMATIC PSYCHIATRIC THERAPIES

Important Steps   **Key Points**

8. Insert the rubber mouth gag.

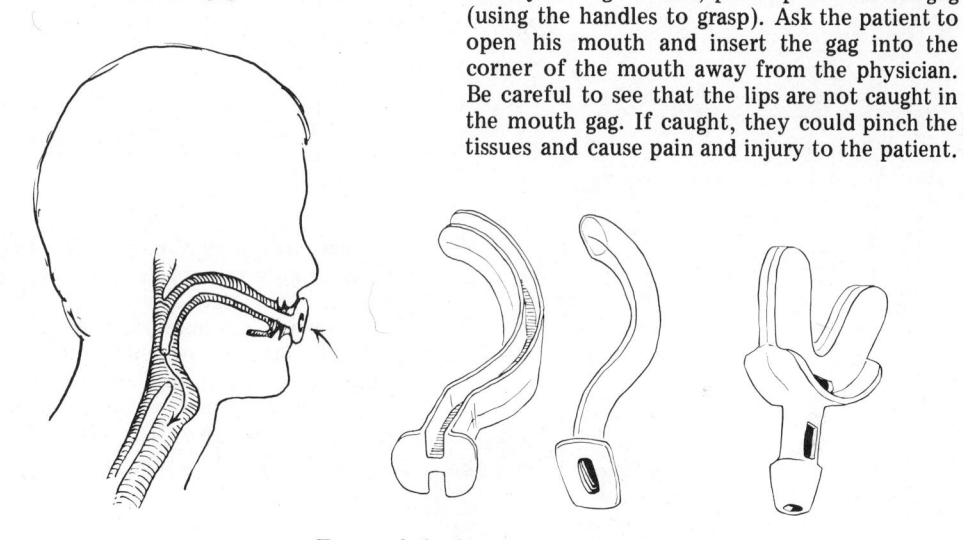

   With your right hand, pick up the mouth gag (using the handles to grasp). Ask the patient to open his mouth and insert the gag into the corner of the mouth away from the physician. Be careful to see that the lips are not caught in the mouth gag. If caught, they could pinch the tissues and cause pain and injury to the patient.

Types of airways.

9. Place the oxygen mask over the patient's face.

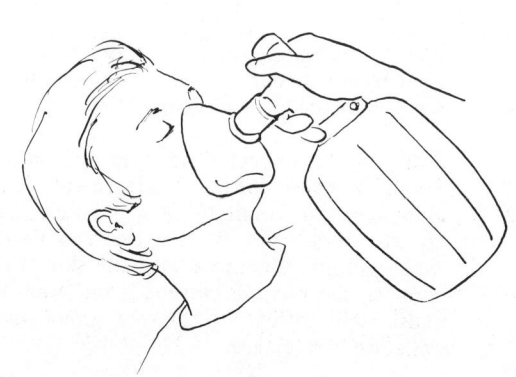

   Give the oxygen for 2 to 3 minutes. This will help decrease the apprehension of the patient and also provide a high oxygen content in the circulatory system. Continue to reassure him and stay close by. While you are reassuring the patient, the physician will prepare the arm to administer the Anectine intravenously.

Important Steps	Key Points
10. Intravenous Anectine is injected by the physician.	The physician (in some cases the anesthesiologist) will do the venipuncture in an extended arm. Usually the antecubital area in the arm farthest from the EST machine is used. Stand by to assist the physician by handing him the required equipment (tourniquet, alcohol sponge, syringe and needle, Anectine bottle). After the Anectine injection, the patient's respirations will vary (decrease or cease), and he will become very relaxed for one to two minutes, depending on the amount of drug administered. (The actual amount of Anectine used is based on the kilograms of body weight.)
11. Observe the patient for respiratory arrest.	At this time, the nurse must be alert to give oxygen as needed. Anectine is not an anesthetic, but a muscle relaxant often used in conjunction with anesthesia. It should be used only by skilled physicians.
	Cardiac arrhythmias may occur; therefore, an EKG monitoring machine is valuable in permitting appropriate treatment by the physician to reverse abnormal heart action. A cardiac defibrillator must be ready for use in case of fibrillation. In case of cardiac arrest, staff must be prepared to perform external cardiac massage (see Volume II, Unit 30, "Cardiopulmonary Resuscitation.")

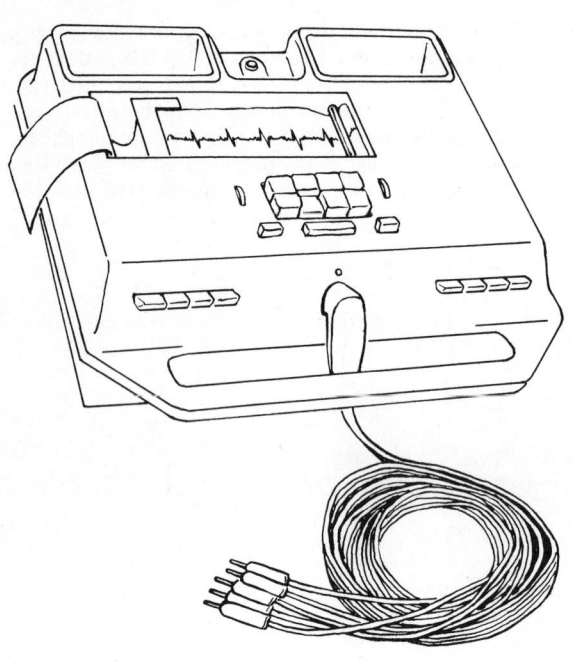

Portable EKG machine.

12. Place yourself beside the patient.	NOTE: Be sure to remove your watch so that it will not become magnetized during transmission of the electrical current.
	You will be expected to hold the electrodes firmly in place during the treatment. A severe skin burn can result if there is an air space at the electrode's site. Be sure that the electrodes make complete contact with the skin. Also, as soon as the electric current is initiated, it will cause the patient to have a grand mal, or epileptic-like seizure.

Important Steps	Key Points
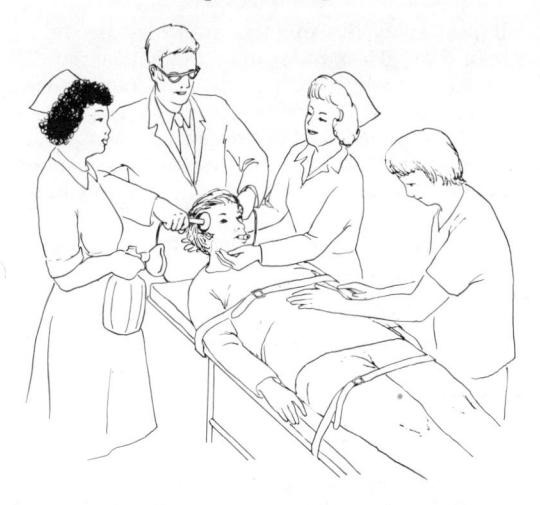	While standing at the head of the patient on his left side, one health worker will support the patient's head by putting his left hand under the neck, with his right hand supporting the jaw in a closed position. There should be a health worker standing at each side of the stretcher to prevent the patient from hitting himself during the shock. The seizure movement should be guided, but should not be inhibited. Because of the relaxation induced by Anectine, the strength of the convulsions is lessened and there is little likelihood of a vertebral fracture, although it was rather common in the early days of EST.
13. The physician will administer shock.	He depresses the lower left-hand Power Switch to give the prescribed voltage.
	The physician repeats the shock if necessary. Usually only one shock is given. However, if the physician did not get an adequate response, an increased dosage may be indicated.
14. Replace the electrodes on the machine.	Turn off the Master Power Switch. Do not put electrode surfaces together. (This could cause a spark and possible explosion.) Turn the patient's head to one side so that saliva will not be aspirated. (You may need to suction the saliva if there is an excessive amount. Otherwise, wipe his face clean with gauze or tissue.) You may need to give a little oxygen if the patient does not spontaneously breathe deeply. Generally, oxygen will be given by mask for about one minute or until the diaphragm restores the respiratory movement.
15. Replace the mouth gag with the airway.	When the patient begins to spit out the mouth gag, insert the rubber airway to prevent him from swallowing his tongue; this provides an open airway for his breathing. Set aside the mouth gag for cleaning at a later time. Oxygen can be administered with the airway in place if it is needed.
16. Check vital signs before returning the patient to his room.	If signs are stable, release the locked wheels on the stretcher and take the patient to his room or recovery area.
17. Move the patient to his bed.	Usually this can be done after a period of five to 30 minutes. Move the patient carefully; you will need assistance. He will be very drowsy and relaxed. Be sure to use good body mechanics for yourself and the patient. Place him in the supine position, with his head turned to one side to facilitate saliva drainage. Cover him with bedding, and remove the bath blanket.

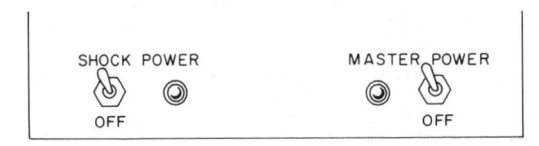

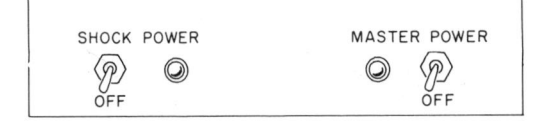

Important Steps	Key Points
18. Continue taking vital signs.	Repeat every five minutes until they are stable, then every 15 minutes until the patient is fully awake (usually 15 minutes to four hours). Someone should be in constant attendance until the patient is fully responsive. With some medication, e.g., Brevital, the patients respond rapidly and are ambulating within a half hour.
19. Permit the patient to sleep.	The sleep patterns vary—patients may sleep 30 to 60 minutes or longer.
20. Observe the patient.	This period (30 minutes to four hours) may be one of confusion for the patient, and he may be hyperactive because of the toxic effect of the treatment. Protect him from injuring himself. Reassure him that his strange feeling (loss of sense of reality) is a normal reaction to treatment and will disappear within the next few hours or days. Orient him to time, place, and person, e.g., "Mr. Jones, you are back in your room and it is now 10:30 in the morning." Or, "Here is your shoe, John. Can you put it on or shall I help you?"
21. Involve the patient in ward activities.	As soon as possible, order a meal for him and be sure that he eats, usually within an hour. He can be permitted to ambulate as soon as his sensorium (mind) becomes clear.
22. Go back to the treatment room.	Clean the room and replenish supplies.

23. Record on the patient's chart.	Charting example:
	
	8 A.M. Anectine _____ cc given IV by Dr. Chow.
	
	8:03 A.M. ECT given in treatment room (or operating room) by Dr. Chow with the assistance of Mr. Jackson, orderly, Miss Kanimura, N.A., and Miss Domer, R.N.
	
	Generalized tonic activity occurred for 10 seconds with a grand mal seizure. Incontinent at time of seizure. Minimal cyanosis observed and oxygen given by mask. BP 120/80, P. 92, R. 16.
	
	          L. Domer, R.N.
	
	8:15 A.M. Returned to bed via stretcher. Alert mentally and verbally. BP 120/80, P. 84, R. 16. Color pink. Sensorium clear. Breakfast ordered.
	
	          L. Domer, R.N.
	
	8:45 A.M. All of general diet eaten. Was very hungry this morning. Wants to take short nap.
	
	          L. Domer, R.N.
	
	NOTE: In this progress note the physician will record voltage used in treatment.

ITEM 2: INSULIN THERAPY

By 1937 Manfred Sakel's insulin hypoglycemic therapy for schizophrenic psychoses had been utilized in a number of hospitals in the United States and Canada. The first institution in this country to use insulin therapy was Creedmore State Hospital in New York.

There are two main types of insulin therapy: ambulatory insulin therapy and insulin coma therapy.

In *ambulatory insulin therapy* the patient receives increasing insulin doses ranging from five to 40 units of U40 insulin daily (or every other day, according to the patient's need) until symptoms of hypoglycemia occur. (NOTE: With the advent of the standardized U100 insulin, the U40 or U80 insulin will be eliminated within the very near future; therefore, use prescribed dosage.) When hypoglycemia occurs (usually in two or three days of increasing from base of 5 to 10U of insulin), the dosage that triggered the hypoglycemic reaction will be maintained until the physician believes that the therapy has accomplished its goal—that of decreasing the patient's neurotic symptoms sufficiently so that he can adapt to the demands of daily living. Ambulatory insulin therapy is found to be most useful in relaxing and rejuvenating patients with varying mild conditions, such as (1) premenstrual and menopausal anxieties; (2) occasional panic attacks of hyperactive businessmen and similar personality types; (3) rundown physical conditions due to anorexia; and (4) exhaustion following one of various infectious diseases, as a protective mechanism for liver function.

The second type of insulin therapy is *insulin coma therapy*. As the name implies, the goal of this treatment is to induce an insulin coma. Deep coma therapy is used to treat patients for whom the following diagnoses have been made: (1) paranoid or catatonic active schizophrenic psychoses; (2) mild and undifferentiated forms of schizophrenia; (3) hebephrenic forms of schizophrenia; (4) schizo-affective and pseudo-neurotic forms of schizophrenia; and (5) intense neurotic anxiety and tension states. Insulin coma therapy has been used less in the United States for treatment of the above illnesses since the advent of tranquilizers.

Many physicians who administer deep coma insulin therapy feel that the depth and duration of the coma play an important role in the patient's recovery. They also believe that when insulin is combined with psychotherapy or electric shock therapy, there is a likelihood of breaking down the psychoses more readily. In addition, many physicians believe that individual and group psychotherapy in conjunction with a well-organized rehabilitation program can prevent relapses.

Ambulatory and insulin coma therapy are sometimes used alternately in the treatment of the patient. Ambulatory treatment is not considered as dangerous for the patient as the coma treatment.

General Treatment Preparation. For the ambulatory and coma treatments there must be a written consent for treatment signed by either the patient or a designated party who has the legal responsibility for the patient. A complete physical workup must be finished, including X-rays of the chest, head, and spine. An electroencephalogram and electrocardiogram are taken, and complete urine and blood studies are made prior to the first treatment. The treatment is not given when abnormal conditions that could be aggravated by an insulin coma become evident.

Pre-treatment Preparation

1. Withhold food prior to and during treatment; sips of water may be allowed.
2. Carry out personal hygiene (bath, mouth care, etc.). Remove bobby pins to prevent injury to patient if she should fall.
3. Remove dentures or bridges to prevent loss or damage during treatment.
4. Record vital signs prior to insulin injection. Report deviations. The treatment may be omitted if the physician decides that the deviations from normal range are significant.
5. Ask the patient to void prior to insulin administration (if he convulses, he may become incontinent).
6. Weigh the patient prior to the first treatment and every day during the treatment.

Ambulatory Insulin Therapy

The nurse reviews with the patient just how he will feel as a result of receiving the insulin. She describes the early symptoms (given below) and assures him that she will remain with him at all times during the treatment. His physician will be in the clinical unit and on call if he is needed at any time.

Five to 40 units of U40 (U100) insulin are given subcutaneously early in the morning. The specific dosage will be ordered by the physician and is calculated by him on the basis of kilograms of body weight of the patient. Usually within a few hours (3 or 4) after the insulin injection, early symptoms of hypoglycemia will appear. Such symptoms are:

1. Staggering gait.

2. Feeling of fatigue.

3. Mild diaphoresis.

4. Mild drowsiness or sleepiness.

5. Dilated pupils.

6. Slight tremor of the hands.

Faintness, subjective feeling of weakness, and fatigue are typical signs when the blood sugar level falls below 80. (Normal blood sugar levels range from 65 to 95 mgm/100 ml in whole blood, and 70 to 105 mgm/100 ml in serum. Slight variations occur, depending on the specific method the clinical laboratory uses. Know the normal ranges for blood sugar for your agency.) You may have experienced these symptoms yourself if you have gone a long time without eating. If the patient experiences sudden weakness of the lower limbs, he may fall and injure himself. It is therefore imperative that the nurse know where her patient is during the ambulatory insulin treatment so that he can be observed for signs of hypoglycemic shock or a seizure caused by the sudden decrease in the blood sugar level.

Once the symptoms of hypoglycemia occur, the nurse should encourage the patient to sit in a comfortable chair while she continues to observe him. The reaction intensifies to the point that the patient appears to be on the verge of a coma. During this period of time, the following symptoms may be observed:

1. Profuse diaphoresis.

2. Marked drowsiness.

3. Thickened or slurred speech.

4. Yawning.

When these four symptoms occur, the treatment should be terminated immediately. The method for terminating the treatment is simple. Merely give the patient a glass of water or orange juice to which one gram of sugar (dextrose or glycogen) is added for each unit of insulin that was administered. Add an extra 5 grams of sugar for good measure, i.e., if the patient had received 30 units of U40 regular insulin, you would give 30 grams + 5 (35 grams) of sugar added to the liquid water or orange juice. (One teaspoon = 4 grams: 35/4 = 8.75 teaspoons of sugar or, rounded off, 9 teaspoons.)

After the patient drinks the sugar solution, he will become increasingly alert and responsive. As soon as possible, he should be escorted to the breakfast area (or served his breakfast); encourage him to eat the entire meal. After his breakfast, suggest that he bathe and resume his normal ward activities.

The more numerous the insulin treatments, the greater becomes the possibility that the patient will develop resistance to the insulin. In other words, it will not act as forcefully as it once did, and the daily dosage may have to be increased in order to obtain the desired patient reaction. The dosage will be adjusted by the physician as the patient's reactions indicate.

Charting the patient's response in the ambulatory insulin treatment is vitally important to enable the doctor to determine the patient's response to treatment. Your charting should include the time of injection, the dose, route, and site. The early symptoms should be described and the time noted. The time that treatment was terminated must be recorded, along with the exact amount of sugar and liquid that was administered, an accurate account of what the patient ate for breakfast and at what time, whether any additional sugar solution was given, and the response of the patient to the sugar ingestion.

The sites of the insulin injection are rotated, starting from the right arm, then the left arm, right leg, left leg, and abdomen. The method for rotating sites of injections was described in Unit 2, "Preparation and Administration of Medications." The nurse must be alert to the patient's response during the treatment period; note particularly the following:

1. The amount of salivation, e.g., an excessive amount may indicate cerebral irritation.
2. Swallowing reflex, e.g., dysphagia may indicate a drug reaction.
3. Pupillary reaction, e.g., dilated pupils may indicate a slipping into deep coma.
4. Motor activity, e.g., localized or generalized muscle movement of the clonic or tonic type.
5. Orientation to person, place, and time.
6. Level of consciousness, e.g., alertness to environment, or sinking into a comatose state.
7. Thinking or perception difficulties, e.g., confusion, hallucinations.
8. Quality of verbal communication, e.g., patient is coherent, talkative, incoherent, has slurred speech, etc.
9. Itching around the insulin injection site may indicate a drug allergy.

It is important to note the *time* and *sequence* of reaction patterns so that you may become familiar with the typical reaction pattern for each individual patient.

Insulin Coma Therapy

The deep coma or insulin shock treatment is very serious and requires that a nurse and physician be in constant attendance during the entire treatment. In a psychiatric setting (acute or ambulatory), the patients may be treated in a special intensive care area, or a ward if a large number of patients are receiving insulin therapy, to effect the best utilization of personnel observing the patients' recovery.

The effects of insulin coma have sometimes been beneficial, and several theories have been suggested. However, no theory seems to explain the exact effect upon the patient. The two most common theories are the *regressive theory*, which holds that the patient is regressed through the successive stages of his development, and then brought back through these stages during the recovery periods. This is thought to assist the patient to work through the maturing process. A *physiologic theory* states that an inhibitive and/or repressive action takes place in that part of the patient's mind that is most active during psychosis, and thus the psychotic behavior is minimized or obliterated.

Insulin coma therapy generally consists of 50 to 60 treatments. The amount of insulin (given daily or at two- and three-day intervals) begins with a dosage of about 50 units of U40, U80, or U100 insulin and is gradually increased to as much as 200 units until a coma stage is reached. Once the coma is reached with a specific insulin dose (i.e., 60 units of U80), the patient is maintained on that dosage, or one modified to achieve the results the physician desires. It should be reiterated, however, that *coma can occur with a single insulin injection*.

There are two phases in insulin coma therapy, and each phase consists of two stages.

Pre-Coma Phase

The *pre-coma phase* is similar to that of the patient on ambulatory insulin therapy. During the first half hour after the insulin injection, there are usually no observable symptoms. However, during the *early stages*, the patient perspires profusely (diaphoresis), and there is increased salivation and a slowing of the heart rate. At the same time he may become relaxed and drowsy, with feelings of hunger and thirst.

You may make the patient more comfortable by wiping his brow with a slightly moistened, warm washcloth. You may want to "bundle" the patient by wrapping him securely in a bath blanket to absorb the perspiration. This will prevent rapid evaporation of the sweat and chilling.

The *second stage* of the pre-coma occurs during the second hour following the injection. The previous symptoms become exaggerated, the patient's speech slurs and is usually incoherent. The patient's sensorium begins to cloud and he becomes disoriented as to person, time, and place. A common response by the patient at this time may be "a return to childhood behavior."

Voluntary muscular activity is difficult and he may experience extreme restlessness and excitement. Singultus (hiccups) may occur because the oxygen and carbon dioxide balance is disturbed.

Constant attention is needed during this stage to reassure the patient and to help reduce his anxiety. Give simple commands. Do not carry on a lengthy, detailed conversation.

Coma Phase

Manifestations of the *early comatose stage* usually begin within the third hour. The patient loses contact and does not respond verbally. There will be beginning signs of muscle twitching. This is an indication that the coma is beginning. You will need to become skillful in differentiating between muscle jerking and an actual convulsion.

Keep the patient as comfortable as possible by wiping away the perspiration. It is recommended that the bed not be changed during this stage because the slightest stimulus activates his highly sensitive nervous system and may cause convulsions.

Note: If there is generalized twitching, you may have to insert the mouth gag. Any sudden stimulation can induce a generalized convulsion at this time as the body is extremely sensitive to stimuli.

Since there may also be increased salivation during this time, keep the patient's head turned to the side so that saliva can drain. A suction machine and/or bulb syringe should be ready for use in case salivation becomes excessive.

The autonomic system, which is now taking over, will present new signs to the observer: flushed face, dilated pupils, and an increased heart rate.

During the *second coma stage*, the previous symptoms disappear, the pupils contract, and the pulse rate decreases. The respirations are shallow and irregular. You must observe the patient very closely to be sure that the airway is maintained.

Spasms may occur at this point. The two types of spasms you need to be able to identify and describe are the tonic and clonic.

Tonic—sustained muscle spasms, the trunk arched and the legs rigidly extended. There is an increase in pulse rate and blood pressure, and the pupils are non-reactive. This phase lasts only a short time.

Clonic—extensor spasms begin, and arms move outward and upward during the spasms. The muscles alternately contract and relax. The pupils are dilated and the pulse increases. The skin becomes pale and cold. This period is usually considered the most dangerous, and the patient is rarely allowed to remain at this level for longer than fifteen minutes.

Coma treatment is usually terminated after the fourth hour following the insulin injection, or earlier if complications such as absence of swallowing reflex, laryngospasm, respiratory distress, or convulsions occur. The coma may be treated by gavage or intravenous injection.

If the patient's swallowing reflex is absent, a nasal gavage of approximately 400 cc of sugar solution is administered. The amount of sugar in the solution is usually 1 gram of sugar per unit of insulin given. The liquid used is either water or orange juice. Follow the gavage procedure you learned.

If complications arise, such as respiratory embarrassment, laryngospasms or convulsion, an intravenous injection of 20 to 100 cc of 50 per cent glucose is administered immediately by the physician.

When the patient awakens he will have no memory of any events from the onset of the coma until he regained consciousness.

Accurate, frequent observation of vital signs is extremely important during the recovery stage to try to pick up warning signs of shock before the actual symptoms appear.

1. An increasing pulse rate and decreasing blood pressure may indicate approaching shock.

2. An increasing pulse rate and an increasing blood pressure may indicate hypersensitivity to the drug.

3. A decreasing pulse rate and an increased blood pressure may be beginning signs of increased intracranial pressure.

4. A decreasing pulse rate and a decreased blood pressure may indicate a severe physiological reaction which could lead to a cardiac collapse.

In all of the above situations the physician must be notified to start the corrective treatment. Examples of treatment for the above symptomatology are:

1. Position change—Trendelenburg position or rocking bed; warm blankets; intravenous fluids; and transfusion.

2. Sedation; antihistamines.

3. Intravenous $MgSO_4$ (check fundi of eyes for signs of increased intracranial pressure or "choking" of optic discs) and neurological consultation. NOTE: Do *not* do spinal tap; it is contraindicated.

Upon awakening, the patient's body will be soaking wet from the profuse diaphoresis during the treatment. The gown and bedding should be changed at once. You may need to give a light warm bath to help soothe him before changing the linen. Permit him to rest for an hour or two before he returns to full ward activities. Keep him warm during the rest period. Add more blankets if necessary.

When the patient is refreshed, encourage him to eat the entire contents of the breakfast tray. This will prevent a secondary hypoglycemic reaction. Breakfast should be served within 30 minutes to an hour following the complete recovery from the coma. If he is alert, he can be assisted with personal hygiene (oral, hair, shaving, etc.). Suggest that he participate in light ward activities, e.g., reading or watching television. Only a light lunch will be served since his breakfast was so late, but the patient should eat the regular dinner and participate in evening activities.

Continue to observe the patient's full recovery; continue to reassure him and answer his questions directly.

The care of the patient receiving insulin therapy requires a nurse who is warm, understanding, and supportive. In your learning experience in the psychiatric setting, you will have an opportunity to gain insight into the therapy expectations as you participate in various staff development conferences.

The insights you acquire during this experience will help you when handling other patients, and will also help you to learn more about yourself and how you relate to others.

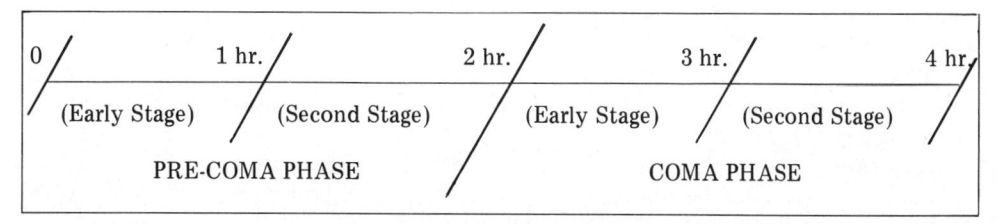

0	1 hr.	2 hr.	3 hr.	4 hr.
(Early Stage)	(Second Stage)	(Early Stage)	(Second Stage)	
PRE-COMA PHASE		COMA PHASE		

Stages of Insulin Coma Therapy.

VI. ADDITIONAL INFORMATION FOR ENRICHMENT

As you work with patients who have mental illnesses, you will need to be aware of various adaptive mechanisms. For your information, the following acceptable and unacceptable adaptive devices are briefly described. If you wish additional information, discuss with your instructor other available resources from which you may gain further knowledge and understanding. Knowledge of the following defense mechanisms will help you adapt to everyday pressures, as well as to understand the behavior patterns of others.

Personality develops through seven stages of life. These arbitrary stages are designated as:

a. Infancy period—birth to 18 months

b. Muscle-training period—1 1/2 to 2 1/2 years

c. Family triangle period—2 1/2 to 6 years

d. Latency period—6 years until puberty

e. Puberty—11 to 14 years

f. Adolescence—from end of puberty to 18 or 20 years

g. Maturity—includes parenthood, change of life, and old age

The transition from one stage to another is muted. In other words, there is no abrupt change from one stage to another, but rather an orderly progression. As the individual grows, he develops certain adaptive (defense) mechanisms, which assist him in adjusting to the daily pressures and changes of life. These adaptive mechanisms, used by everyone and considered abnormal only when used to an excessive and sustained extent, are:

Repression	Introjection	Reversal
Reaction Formation	Turning Against Self	Sublimation
Regression	Projection	
Isolation	Undoing	

Psychological *defense mechanisms* are devices employed by the Ego in order to deal with unacceptable ideas, feelings and impulses. They are interrelated and somewhat overlapping. They appear at different times in the development of the personality.

Psychoanalysts list nine general defense mechanisms (Repression, Reaction Formation, Regression, Isolation, Introjection, Projection, Undoing, Turning Against the Self, and Reversal) and one special defense, Sublimation. Defenses are, for the most part, unconscious and operate in an apparently automatic fashion.

Repression: Develops with Ego differentiation, probably as a sort of conditioned reflex. The offending affect is driven out of consciousness into the unconscious. This defense is basic in the ultimate formation of the psychoneuroses.

Reaction Formation: Conscious wishes which are acceptable to the Ego are used to *oppose* the repressed affect. Thus, an unconscious wish to play with dirt may be opposed by an *overemphasis* of the wish for cleanliness.

Regression: A retreat of the Ego from a more mature level of development to a more primitive (point of fixation) in order to avoid painful affects.

Isolation: A process of preparation of events and wishes that are related but which together might revive a painful affect; related to displacement.

Introjection: A process of taking on characteristics of another in an effort to cover helpless and submissive feelings on the one hand or hostile and aggressive ones on the other (e.g., identification with aggressor).

Turning Against the Self: Related to the above, e.g., one who has destructive feelings toward a parent who also is also loved; by *introjecting* the parent, the hostile wishes become turned against the self.

Projection: The unconscious, unacceptable wish returns to consciousness but is credited to another. There must be something in the other for the projection to be "hooked" to. (This is also a device in "normal" communication.)

Undoing: Related to Reaction Formation in that an affect is opposed by *activity*, e.g., expiation or annulment of forbidden affects or actions, such as a wish to turn on the gas is handled by a constant "turning off" motion.

Reversal: Related to denial and also like Reaction Formation into conversion to opposite, e.g., "I don't love her—I hate her." (Note how these all relate to two sets of feelings, one of which is buried; this is ambivalence.)

There are many other names for defenses and parts of them. For example, *rationalization* is a mechanism of explaining an action or affect by giving a good reason to hide a major reason; this is part of denial and isolation.

Sublimation: A special form of defense in that the original urge or wish is elaborated and extended to such a degree that the final wish has become socially acceptable. For example, a child's wish to *observe* sexual activity between his parents is gradually altered so that curiosity is diverted to other observations. The adult may develop work or a hobby such as astronomy, microscopy, art criticism, etc. It is related to substitution, rejection formation, and other defenses.

```
                    INSULIN TREATMENT RECORD (SAMPLE)

Name _____  Date _____
Insulin Type _____
     Dose _____  Time _____
     _____
     _____


STAGES OF HYPOGLYCEMIC SHOCK                TERMINATION OF TREATMENT
                                  Init.               1st   2nd   3rd
SIMPLE HYPOGLYCEMIA                         Glucose, iv _____
   1. Body feels warm, damp _____            amount  _____
   2. Slight perspiration  _____            time given _____
   3. Hunger               _____            time awake _____
   4. Thirst               _____         Glucagon, im _____
PRECOMA                                        amount  _____
   5. Fine tremors         _____            time given _____
   6. Perspiration         _____            time awake _____
   7. Salivation (slight)  _____
   8. Slight restlessness  _____         Juice or milk _____
   9. Muscular relaxation  _____         Gavage—amount ____ time ___
  10. Somnolence: slow mental activity __     reason _____
  11. Clouded consciousness
      Difficulty in orientation _____       (how given, amount, time)
  12. Excitement, sometimes violent _____  Atropine _____
  13. Loss of environmental contact _____  Adrenalin _____
GREEN STAGE COMA (Stage I)                  Thiamin HCl _____
  14. Loss of consciousness _____        Other drugs*** _____
  15. Primitive movements  _____         ECT _____
      Motor restlessness
  16. Increased response to sensory        PSYCHOLOGICAL STATUS:
      stimuli             _____          Simple stage _____
  17. Fine myotonic twitching _____
  18. Clonic spasms       _____
  19. GRAN MAL CONVULSION* _____         Precoma stage _____
  20. Dilation of pupils  _____
      (light reflex present)
  21. Tachycardia         _____          On awakening:
  22. Diaphoresis         _____          Assaultive _____
  23. Hypersalivation     _____          Crying _____
  24. Flushing (face)     _____          Dazed _____
YELLOW STAGE COMA (Stage II)                Laughing _____
  25. Less response to sensory stimuli __  Euphoric _____
      —no trigeminal pain _____          Confiding _____
      —no intercostal pain _____
  26. Tonic spasms        _____
  27. Torsion spasms      _____          Medications received previous
  28. Babinski reflex positive _____        evening or night _____
RED STAGE COMA (Stage III)
  29. Ocular motor disturbance _____
  30. Pin point pupils (no light reflex) _ ***Other drugs
  31. Loss corneal reflex _____
  32. Bradycardia         _____
  33. Slow respiration    _____
  34. Pallor              _____          Secondary reactions of
  35. Muscular flaccidity _____            previous day:
  36. Laryngeal spasm     _____          Time  Slight  Mod-  Severe  Init.
  37. Shallow, slow breathing _____                    erate
  38. Cheyne-Stokes breathing _____
  39. Cardiac arrhythmia  _____
  40. Singultus (hiccups) _____
```

UNIVERSITY OF CALIFORNIA MEDICAL CENTER, LOS ANGELES
UNIVERSITY OF CALIFORNIA HOSPITAL
MARION DAVIES CHILDREN'S CLINIC
NEUROPSYCHIATRIC INSTITUTE

DATE _____ HOUR _____

A. (I) (WE) HEREBY CONSENT TO (1) THE PERFORMING OF ELECTROSHOCK TREATMENT AND (2) THE ADMINISTERING OF ANY ANESTHETIC IN CONNECTION THEREWITH, OR FOR PURPOSES INDEPENDENT OF SUCH TREATMENT, DEEMED NECESSARY OR ADVISABLE UPON OR TO ME

_____ (NAME OF PATIENT)
STRIKE OUT WORD "ME" IF CONSENT IS NOT SIGNED BY PATIENT, BUT IN ALL CASES INSERT NAME OF PATIENT.

AND (I) (WE) DO HEREBY AUTHORIZE THE PERFORMANCE OF ANY OTHER PROCEDURE WHICH MAY BE DEEMED NECESSARY OR ADVISABLE, IN CONNECTION WITH SUCH ELECTROSHOCK TREATMENT.

(EXCEPTIONS, IF ANY) _____

_____
(PATIENT'S OR OTHER AUTHORIZED SIGNATURE)

_____ PATIENT IS A MINOR   _____ PATIENT IS UNABLE TO SIGN BECAUSE _____

_____   _____
         FATHER   GUARDIAN

_____   _____
         MOTHER   OTHER PERSON AND RELATIONSHIP

THE SIGNER(S) OF THE FOREGOING CONSENT AND AUTHORIZATION (READ AND SIGNED SAME IN MY PRESENCE) (HAD THE SAME READ ALOUD TO (HIM) (HER) (THEM) AND THEREAFTER SIGNED IT IN MY PRESENCE) ON _____ 19_____ AND THEN STATED TO ME THAT (HE) (SHE) (THEY) UNDERSTOOD THE SAME.

_____   _____
         WITNESS   WITNESS

B.   **REPORT OF EXAMINING PHYSICIAN AS TO COMPETENCY OF PATIENT**

THE UNDERSIGNED PHYSICIAN HAS EXAMINED THE PATIENT AS TO MENTAL COMPETENCY AND FOUND THAT SAID PATIENT WAS MENTALLY COMPETENT AT THE TIME OF EXECUTING PART A, AND THAT PATIENT UNDERSTOOD THE NATURE THEREOF.

_____   _____
          DATE   PHYSICIAN

ASSISTING WITH SOMATIC PSYCHIATRIC THERAPIES

POST-TEST

I. List ten items that are part of the essential equipment needed for insulin treatment:

a. _____ f. _____
b. _____ g. _____
c. _____ h. _____
d. _____ i. _____
e. _____ j. _____

II. Match the following symptoms with various stages of insulin coma.

A. Precoma Phase I
B. Precoma Phase II
C. Coma Phase, Early
D. Coma Phase, Late

1. Flushing (face) _____
2. Hypersalivation _____
3. Profuse diaphoresis _____
4. Tachycardia _____
5. Dilation of pupils (light reflex present) _____
6. Grand mal convulsion _____
7. Clonic spasms _____
8. Relaxed and drowsy _____
9. Slurred speech _____
10. Primitive movements, motor restlessness _____
11. Loss of consciousness _____
12. Thirst _____
13. Hunger _____
14. Mild perspiration _____
15. Marked drowsiness _____
16. Loss of environmental contact _____
17. Excitement, sometimes violent _____
18. Clouded consciousness, difficulty in orientation _____
19. Staggering gait _____
20. Extreme restlessness _____
21. Salivation (slight) _____
22. Incoherence _____
23. Fine tremors _____
24. Singultus (hiccups) _____
25. Cheyne-Stokes breathing _____
26. Shallow, slow breathing _____
27. Laryngeal spasm _____
28. Alternating muscle contraction and relaxation _____
29. Pallor _____
30. Bradycardia _____
31. Loss of corneal reflex _____
32. Pin-point pupils (no light reflex) _____
33. Muscle twitching _____
34. Yawning _____
35. Tonic spasms _____
36. Mild drowsiness _____
37. Increased response to stimuli _____

POST-TEST ANNOTATED ANSWER SHEET

I. a. Written consents.
    b. X-ray reports (chest, head, spine).
    c. EKG.
    d. EEG.
    e. Laboratory reports (blood urine).
    f. Report of physical exams.
    g. Insulin and other meds (sedation, antihistamines, $MgSO_4$, etc.).
    h. B.P. apparatus.
    i. Dextrose (sugar, orange juice, intravenous glucose).
    j. Suction apparatus, pp. 380–381, 382.

II.
1. D, p. 392.
2. C, p. 392.
3. A, p. 391.
4. C, D, pp. 392, 393.
5. C, p. 392.
6. D, p. 392.
7. D, p. 392.
8. A, p. 392.
9. B, p. 392.
10. B, p. 392.
11. C, p. 392.
12. A, p. 392.
13. A, p. 392.
14. D, p. 392.
15. B, p. 392.
16. B, p. 392.
17. B, p. 392.
18. B, p. 392.
19. B, p. 392.
20. B, p. 392.
21. D, p. 392.
22. B, p. 392.
23. C, p. 392.
24. B, p. 392.
25. D, p. 392.
26. D, p. 392.
27. D, p. 392.
28. D, p. 392.
29. D, p. 392.
30. D, p. 392.
31. D, p. 392.
32. D, p. 392.
33. C, p. 392.
34. B, pp. 390, 392.
35. D, p. 392.
36. A, p. 392.
37. C, p. 392.

PERFORMANCE TEST

In the clinical setting, working with an experienced nurse or your instructor, you will prepare the patient for an EST and assist with the patient during treatment and recovery as though you were solely responsible. The instructor or experienced nurse will be there merely to lend an additional hand when you ask for assistance. You will be observed with respect not only to the actual steps of the procedure, but also to how you interact with your patient.

You will not be required to assist with an insulin therapy treatment, but only to complete the written test on that section.

PERFORMANCE CHECKLIST

ELECTROCONVULSIVE THERAPY

1. Prepare consent form
2. Check for completed EEG, ECG, and routine chest X-ray (reports are available on chart).
3. Identify patient.
4. Obtain supplies and equipment.
5. Wash hands.
6. Explain procedure to patient.
7. Request patient to void.
8. Check that patient has been NPO after midnight.
9. Check hair and remove bobby pins, etc.
10. Remove dentures and other foreign matter from oral cavity.
11. Remove nail polish and jewelry and place in locked cupboard.
12. Check pre-procedure medication.
13. Prepare and administer per proper technique.
14. Record activity (1-14) appropriately on patient's chart.
15. Assist patient onto stretcher in supine position.
16. Maintain patient at low level of anxiety.
17. Cleanse bitemplar area with acetone.
18. Follow Step 17 with highly concentrated salt solution.
19. Cleanse away salt solution.
20. Apply small amount of electrode jelly to temples and rub it in.
21. Apply electrode jelly to electrodes.
22. Assist with electrode conduction; reassure patient that this was merely a test.
23. Hold electrodes firmly in place when doctor is ready to test.
24. Check that doctor plugged electrodes into shock machine to test.

25. Insert rubber mouth gag and make sure the patient's lips are on the outside of the gag.
26. Assist with the administration of oxygen while doctor administers Anectine.
27. Assist in guiding patient's movements during convulsion.
28. Assist in returning patient to his room via gurney.
29. Take patient's blood pressure every five minutes until stable.
30. Remain with patient continuously.
31. Use simple verbal commands in assessing patient's reaction time.
32. Orient patient to person, place, and time.
33. Cleanse electrode jelly from temple area.
34. Assist patient to dress.
35. Encourage patient to eat breakfast.
36. Record treatment, vital signs, and unusual behavioral conditions; time patient awoke, etc.
37. After patient is self-motivating, assist with putting away equipment.
38. Leave room neat.

Unit 14

TECHNIQUES OF FETAL AND MATERNAL MONITORING

I. DIRECTIONS TO THE STUDENT

Please read the following paragraphs carefully. They will tell you what you will be expected to do and know regarding the various techniques of fetal and maternal monitoring. Since Obstetrics has been declining in recent years because of major national efforts to restrict population growth, many of your experiences in this specialty may be only observational.

Interpreting the recordings of the newer electronic obstetrical monitoring devices is complex and usually requires a specialized course; therefore, we will not deal with interpretations of these recordings in this Unit.

Proceed through the lesson. Practice the procedures in the laboratory. After you have practiced each step of the procedures, arrange with your instructor to take the Post-test. You will, as always, be expected to perform the activities accurately.

II. GENERAL PERFORMANCE OBJECTIVES

After completing this unit, you will be able to place the external transducers so that accurate uterine activity and fetal heart rates can be obtained. You will also be able to assist with insertion of the intra-uterine catheter, the clip electrode and/or the spiral electrode, as well as the collection of a fetal blood sample.

III. SPECIFIC PERFORMANCE OBJECTIVES

When you have finished this lesson, you will be able to:

1. Apply the tocodynamometer so that an accurate recording of uterine activity may be obtained.

2. Apply an ultrasonic transducer so that an accurate fetal heart rate (FHR) can be obtained. Also, you must be able to explain the advantages and disadvantages of the indirect monitoring technique.

3. Assist with application of an intrauterine catheter while maintaining an aseptic field, providing emotional support for the mother, and assuring that she is properly grounded to prevent the possibility of an electrical burn on the skin.

4. Be able to explain the advantages and disadvantages of the direct monitoring technique.

5. Assist with the application or removal of a clip or spiral electrode while maintaining an aseptic field, providing emotional support to the mother, and assuring that she is properly grounded to prevent the possibility of an electrical burn.

6. Assist with or obtain a fetal blood sample.

IV. VOCABULARY

Read the definitions of the terms listed below. Do not attempt to memorize these definitions before proceeding with the lesson. Each term will be explained or defined again in the text. On completion of the lesson, however, you should know the correct definitions of these terms.

amnion—the inner of the fetal membranes, a thin, transparent sac which holds the fetus suspended in the amniotic fluid.

amniotic fluid ("bag of water")—the clear liquid in which the fetus floats, helping it to maintain its temperature, cushioning it from injury, and keeping it moist.

cardiotachometer—an instrument that displays the fetal ECG rate on an oscilloscope screen or records it on magnetic tape, recording paper, or computer.

cervix—neck of an organ; e.g., neck of the uterus which protrudes into the vagina.

crystals (as in a transducer)—sensitive electronic particles that pick up and transmit sounds; e.g., uterine contractions.

delivery—the act of giving birth; expulsion or extraction of the child at birth.

duration (of uterine contraction)—interval of time between contractions, from onset of one contraction to that of the subsequent contraction.

electrode—one of the conductors or terminals by which electric current enters or leaves an electrolytic cell, vacuum tube, or the like.

embryo (human)—the product of conception (fertilized ovum) from implantation of the ovum through the eighth week.

endoscope—instrument for examining cavities through natural openings, e.g., vagina.

external maternal fetal monitoring—a method of utilizing externally applied devices (on the maternal abdomen) to assess and monitor fetal condition during labor and delivery; e.g., tocodynamometer, fetoscope.

FECG—fetal electrocardiogram.

FHR—fetal heart rate.

FHT—fetal heart tone.

fertilized ovum—the stage of development from fertilization of the female egg by the male spermatozoon until implantation; usually to the end of the first week.

fetal—pertaining to the fetus.

fetal membranes—extensions from the margins of the placenta and composed of the chorion (the layer next to the placenta) and the amnion, a thin inner layer that enveloped the original egg and now covers the umbilical cord.

fetoscope—a large, moderately heavy stethoscope used to listen through the mother's abdomen to the fetal heartbeat.

fetus—the growing product of conception, from eight weeks until the completion of pregnancy.

gestation—the period of human female intrauterine fetal development, normally about 40 weeks, 280 days, or 10 lunar months.

internal maternal fetal monitoring—a system of utilizing internally applied devices (such as uterine catheters, and fetal electrodes) connected to a recording monitor to assess fetal condition during labor and delivery.

introitus—the opening or entrance into a canal, e.g., external opening of the vagina.

labor—the process during which the fetus, placenta and membranes are separated from the body of the pregnant woman and expelled (synonymous terms: **childbirth, travail, parturition, confinement, accouchement**).

monitoring—an electronic technique used in obstetrics to assess the fetal condition during labor.

obstetrics—that branch of medical science that deals with the care of a woman in pregnancy, labor, and birth and through the postnatal period.

oscilloscope—an electronic optical device that pictures changes in electric current by means of a cathode ray tube.

palpation—the act of feeling with the hand; the application of fingers with light pressure to the surfaces of the body for the purpose of determining the consistency of the parts beneath in a medical diagnosis of disease, enlarged organ, mass, or fetus.

phonocardiogram (PCG)—a electromechanical monitoring system that picks up fetal heart tones and records them graphically on a strip chart or on a cardiotachometer.
phonotransducer—an electromechanical device that incorporates a microphone to pick up fetal heart tones.
sonogram—the picture recorded on the strip chart that records the sound energy reflected from a moving object (fetal circulatory system) through a medium (the pregnant abdominal wall).
strip chart record—the permanent FHR and UC record written out on the monitor paper (similar to ECG strips obtained on the ECG machine).
tetanic contraction—a constant contraction of the uterus.
tocodynamometer—an instrument for measuring the expulsive force of the uterine contractions in labor.
transducer—a device that converts one form of energy to another (e.g., mechanical energy from sound or pressure to electrical energy), which can then be recorded, usually on an electronic monitor.
uterine contraction (UC)—contraction of the uterus during labor, the number usually increasing as labor progresses.
uterine tone—the intrauterine pressure recorded in mm Hg while the uterus is relaxed (usually 10-12 mm Hg).
uterus (womb)—the hollow muscular reproductive organ in females. It is pear-shaped, about 2 inches wide and 3 inches long, located behind the bladder and in front of the rectum. It is the place of nourishment for the embryo and fetus.
ultrasonics—that branch of physics that deals with the acoustics of echo-sounding frequencies.
xiphoid—the sword-shaped distal end of the breast bone (sternum).

V. INTRODUCTION

HISTORICAL VIEW

Palpation and Auscultation

The earliest means of monitoring both the mother and fetus during labor and delivery utilized the techniques of palpation and auscultation. Labor is a series of rhythmic contractions of the uterus, which dilate the cervix and ultimately expel the fetus and placental membranes. Palpation has been used to assess the uterine contractions as regards their strength and frequency, as a means of determining the progress of labor. Palpation is also used in the rectal or vaginal examinations to determine fetal position and presentation, as well as to assist in determining the progress of labor. This method is still used today as an adjunct to the newer monitoring methods.

The fetal heart rate (FHR) can be monitored by a fetoscope, which is a particularly sensitive stethoscope.

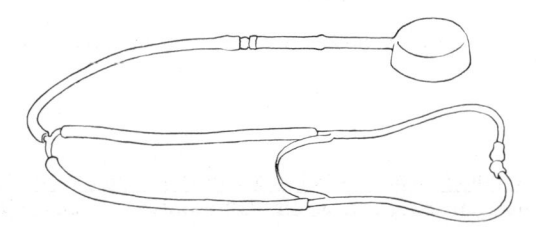

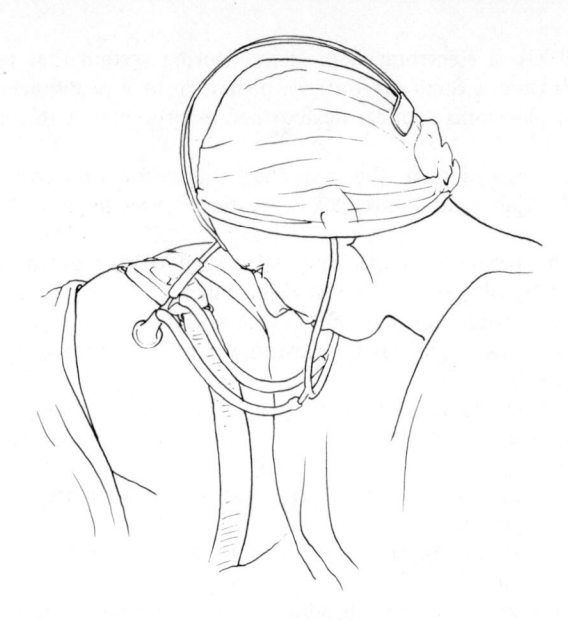

There are limitations to these two methods of monitoring: e.g., errors may occur in counting uterine contractions and fetal heart rates; vital information may be missed because readings are taken sporadically (every 15 minutes); there may be inability to obtain an instantaneous fetal heart rate, failure to detect early or slight changes until serious signs occur, difficulty in hearing an accurate FHR during the uterine contraction, and incorrect assessment of the progress of labor due to errors in the evaluating of the periodic rectal or vaginal examinations.

Although these methods are convenient and non-traumatic and are still widely used today, they require more staff members in constant attendance at the patient's side, and the data they obtain are neither precise nor very accurate.

Phonocardiography

The next stage of development of fetal monitoring techniques began with the introduction of *phonocardiography*. This technique utilizes a microphone placed on the maternal abdomen over the fundus of the uterus. The microphone amplifies the changes and picks up the fetal heartbeat. The sounds are recorded as audible tones on a speaker or as a graph on a strip chart. Phonocardiography is commonly used today because it is simple and inexpensive.

Advantages of the phonocardiograph are:

1. Its simple external application to the maternal abdomen.

2. Its ready use prior to rupture of the membranes.

3. Absence of known hazards.

Disadvantages of the fetal phonocardiograph are that:

1. It cannot be used if the patient is obese.

2. Excessive fetal movement distorts heart rate sounds.

3. Maternal movement also causes distorted sounds.

4. Environmental noises are picked up by the microphone and can become confused with the FHT.

Ultrasound

A ultrasonic technique that utilizes a scanning technique outlining tissue images was developed by a physician in Scotland, Dr. Ian Donald. He described the first obstetrical application of ultrasound early in 1962. This technique is used to some extent to diagnose early pregnancy (5 weeks). It can also be used, with reasonable accuracy, to determine the age of gestation, fetal development, ectopic pregnancies, multiple pregnancies, placenta previas, and threatened abortions, among other conditions. Sometimes it is used to determine fetal position and fetal head measurements.

Ultrasound techniques are also used in other medical specialties, such as oncology, gynecology, urology, gastroenterology, neurosurgery, and for various examinations, e.g., of the liver and gallbladder. New uses for ultrasound are continually being developed. In fact, ultrasound (sonogram) techniques are replacing many X-ray techniques, and thereby decreasing radiation hazards for patients.

A more sensitive device was introduced in 1965. A common example of this type of ultrasonic device is the *doptone*. It is also more reliable than previous techniques for listening to the FHR during the early weeks of pregnancy (up to 16 weeks). This instrument represented a major step forward in fetal monitoring beyond its precursor, the fetoscope.

The ultrasonic device is placed on the maternal abdomen, picks up the fetal heart tones by means of the Doppler principle (e.g., body tissues and fluids have specific, differing frequencies by which skilled practitioners can distinguish sounds to assist in making a diagnosis). According to the Doppler principle, a sound wave (light or radio) is projected *away from* a moving object (in this case, the fetal blood vessels or the heart), and pitch of the sound wave is converted to an audible sound via the ultrasonic device. This system has been used by the United States Navy to locate submerged submarines. For sound to be heard, three elements must be present: the *source* of the sound, the *medium* (air, water, metal, etc.) through which it is transmitted, and the *detector* (an ear, a receiver) of the wave.

Sound has three characteristics: *pitch*, *intensity*, and *quality*. If the combination of these characteristics is compatible, the sound is considered to be pleasant. However, if the combination is incompatible, the resulting sound is called noise.

Pitch is determined by the frequency of vibration of the object. Slow vibrations give off a low pitch, whereas rapid vibrations produce a high pitch.

Intensity is often mistaken for loudness. It is actually the measure of the sound's energy, while loudness is the effect of the intensity on the individual.

The *quality* of sound consists of a basic (fundamental) frequency called the first harmonic, as well as various multiples of the basic frequency.

The ultrasonic apparatus creates sound waves that can be used for scanning body tissues without apparent tissue injury. The sound waves are transmitted via a low-intensity transducer placed on the maternal abdomen. Sensitive crystals in the transducer transmit or receive the changing frequencies and record them on an audio or visual recorder.

The ultrasonic monitoring of the fetal heart rate utilizes the frequency parameter. The transducer that is monitoring the fetal heart tones is placed on the maternal abdomen, where these tones are loudest. When the sound waves encounter the moving fetus, there is a change in the sound which is recorded on a rate meter.

Biochemical Fetal Monitoring

Various techniques are used throughout pregnancy to determine physiological status, particularly in patients with a high risk of preeclampsia, eclampsia, diabetes, or who are Rh-negative.

Various tests can be utilized:

1. Amniocentesis: Withdrawal of fluid from the amnion during pregnancy. The amniotic specimens are submitted for laboratory testing to determine the sensitivity of the Rh-positive red blood cells of the fetus to the Rh-negative mother as well as other chemical determinations (creatinine, L/S ratio, orange cells, etc.).

2. Periodic fetal blood sampling: Blood may be drawn during the pregnancy as well as while the patient is on the delivery table. This test is utilized to determine the acid-base status of the fetus. If intrauterine hypoxia and/or acidosis exist, there will be variations in the fetal pH and pCO_2. A pH of less than 7.2 from at least two consecutive blood samples in the absence of maternal acidosis may suggest the need for caesarean section.

The fetal blood sampling technique will be described later in this Unit. Although usually obtained by the physician, it is possible for selected nurses who have had additional training to carry out this procedure.

Internal Electronic Monitoring

Continuing research has led to more sophisticated and reliable fetal and uterine monitoring techniques via direct (internal and external) electronic monitoring systems.

Each generation of monitoring techniques has enabled obstetrical staffs to improve their abilities with respect to accurate assessment of the condition of the fetus during active labor, the most hazardous time for the fetus.

<u>Direct electronic monitoring is now the best way to provide optimal care for the mother and fetus during the antepartum period and through the delivery.</u> Increasing numbers of labor and delivery suites are equipped with electronic monitoring devices so that every laboring patient, not only the high-risk, can be assured of accurate, continuous monitoring during the progress of labor.

It must be stated unequivocally that <u>electronic equipment cannot replace the need for direct nursing care and observation of the laboring patient.</u> It makes the skilled nurse even more necessary, since she must be in close attendance with the patient to interpret the recordings being generated by the monitoring equipment. The observant nurse can detect psychological and physiological clues, which may then be dealt with before major problems occur. The use of electronic equipment only complements the nurse's skills and knowledge; it does not replace the nurse!

Intrauterine Catheter. <u>Direct uterine monitoring is needed along with FHR to assist in determining fetal distress. A reliable method of monitoring uterine activity is via use of an intrauterine catheter. A water-filled uterine catheter is inserted through the cervix into the uterus around the presenting part to a length of approximately 18 inches. The pressure of the contracting uterus on the water-filled catheter is recorded on the strip chart in mm Hg</u> (mercury). The newest type of intrauterine catheter has a microelectronic sensor at the tip through which recordings are transmitted to a strip chart, thus providing a continuous, permanent record of uterine activity.

<u>The amniotic pressure is proportional to the tension in the uterine wall, and is an accurate measurement of uterine contractility (amniotic fluid pressure = uterine wall tension).</u>

The lowest pressure recorded between contractions while the uterus is resting is called *tone.* The average uterine tone registers 10 mm Hg, but may vary among patients.

Since the uterine tension is not felt abdominally until the uterine contraction measures at least 20 mm Hg, it is difficult to evaluate the uterine tone clinically. The peaks of contractions should reach a peak of intensity of 50 to 75 mm Hg; an intensity of 15 mm Hg above the tonus is needed to exert enough pressure on the cervix to bring about dilatation. It is at this intensity that the mother begins to feel contractions.

<u>As a general rule, the primipara requires more intensive contractions that the multigravida.</u> A multipara has lower tissue resistance and therefore requires less intense contractions, because of past pregnancies. <u>For the contractions to be most effective, they should last for 45 to 60 seconds</u>. If you evaluate the contractions clinically, they will seem shorter than the actual duration that can be recorded on the monitor, because you cannot feel the contractions until the uterus is contracting so that the tension is reading at least 20 mm Hg.

In order for labor to progress most satisfactorily, the contractions should occur every 2 1/2 to 4 minutes. If more frequent, the tone may increase and the amplitude and duration may decrease. Further, the mother would be unable to relax between contractions, and therefore may be less able to cope with them. If the fetus were in difficulty, the shorter periods between contractions would not allow sufficient time for the fetus to recover from the stress of one contraction before another was in progress.

Although the uterine catheter permits absolute frequency, duration and intensity records, the accuracy is contingent on a properly functioning catheter.

When the uterus contracts, it causes pressure on the catheter which records changes in the fluid column on the strain gauge, which in turn is recorded on the strip chart.

Advantages of intrauterine catheters are:

1. True uterine pressure is obtained.
2. There is minimal placental injury.
3. Can be used with membranes intact or ruptured.

Disadvantages of the intrauterine cathers are:

1. Possibility of rupture of the uterus.
2. Possibility of infection: amnionitis, endometritis.

Direct Electronic Fetal Monitoring

As stated above, the electronic devices for monitoring the uterine activity and fetal heart rate are only tools with which the obstetrical staff may more accurately determine the best course of action based on the presenting data. In no way do these electronic tools diminish the need for skillful, knowledgeable health personnel caring for the laboring patient.

An excellent article by Drs. Lewis A. Hamilton, Jr. and Michael J. McKeown, "Biochemical and Electronic Monitoring of the Fetus," which appeared in the *Obstetrics and Gynecology Annual*, 1973, provides an in-depth background of the subject to date.

Indirect electronic fetal heart monitoring is done by placing electrodes on the maternal abdomen. This method is complicated by the fact that the electrodes not only pick up maternal and fetal signals but also some electrical noises. Therefore, it is generally not a method of choice for obtaining a reliable fetal electrocardiogram.

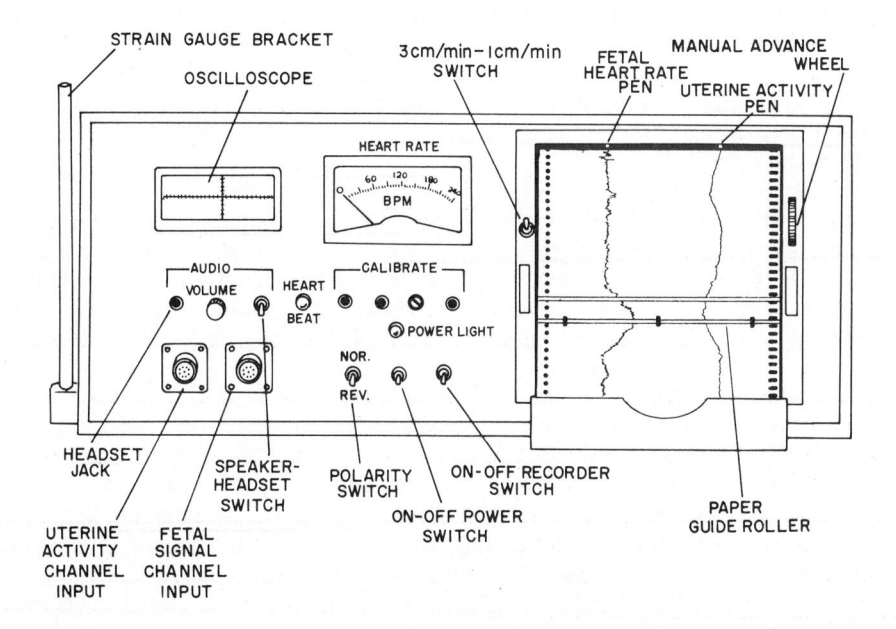

Fetal monitor

Direct fetal monitoring may be accomplished by using one of two methods: the clip electrode or the spiral electrode.

The direct methods of fetal monitoring are superior to the previous techniques and provide the clearest, most precise clinical data thus far available.

The advantages of direct fetal monitoring are that (1) a true fetal electrocardiogram may be obtained; and (2) maternal or fetal movements do not disrupt the FHR signal.

The disadvantages are that (1) the cervix must be dilated at least 2 or 3 cm.; (2) membranes must be ruptured; (3) the technique is more complex; and (4) the presenting part must be at a low station.

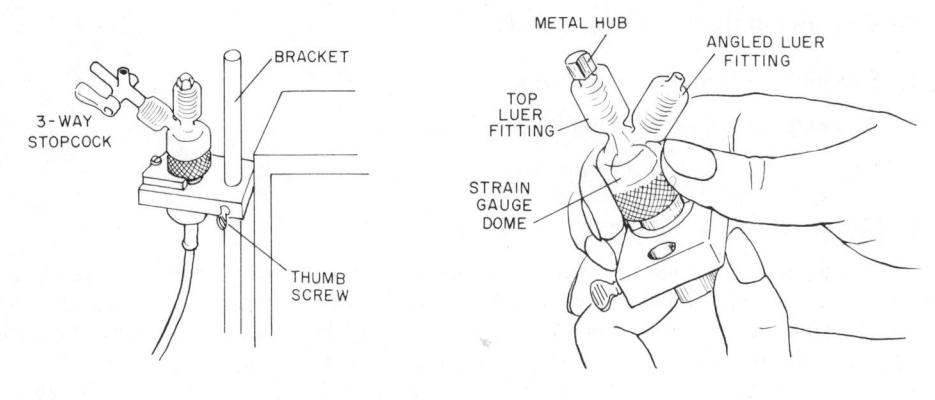

Strain gauge

PHYSIOLOGY OF UTERINE CONTRACTIONS

The uterus is a smooth muscle composed of highly excitable cells which contract when stimulated. Any group of these cells can act as a trigger, or pacemaker, to stimulate contraction. Normally, the uterine activity initiates in one or two pacemakers in the fundus, near the insertion of the fallopian tubes, with the right pacemaker predominating and usually initiating the contraction. The waves spread downward from the fundus, involving the entire uterus, within 15 to 20 seconds. Because the wave began in the upper segment, it contracts more strongly there than the lower segment. Immediately after the peak contraction, the uterus relaxes.

When contractions are initiated in locations other than the fundus, they are usually less coordinated and less efficient. For example, the wave may originate in the lower segment and spread upward; this does not dilate the cervix. Uncoordinated contractions may also occur when the right and left pacemakers initiate contractions simultaneously, producing a labor pattern in which large contractions alternate with small. Since minor contractions are inefficient and major contractions develop some cervical dilatation, the labor progress is very slow.

The assessment of labor must be considered in relation to the uterine contractions displayed on the clinical monitor. It is important to recognize that the clinical monitor is only another tool to assist in evaluating the contractions and to assess the progress of labor. It should not interfere with your continuing supportive nursing care to the patient.

A normal labor pattern is one in which the contractions are infrequent, with low amplitude, in the early stages. As labor progresses, the contractions become more intense, more frequent, and of longer duration, until they dilate the cervix and expel the fetus.

The uterine contraction must register at least 20 mm Hg on the monitor before the uterus is hard enough to palpate. The tone must increase to at least 25 mm Hg before the cervix starts to dilate and the patient feels pain. The clinical duration of contractions (the time during which it can be palpated) is shorter than the actual duration recorded on the monitor.

A uterus in which the tone remains high *(hypertonus)* between contractions is less productive than one in which the tone returns to the relaxed state, or approximately 10 mm Hg. The effectiveness of the contraction depends upon its *amplitude*, i.e., the increased amniotic fluid pressure from the resting phase to the peak of the intensity. When the tone remains high between contractions, the uterus does not completely relax, and the strength of the contractions gradually decreases, thereby losing effectiveness and failing to dilate.

There are many causes of hypertonus:

1. The catheter may not be functioning properly.
2. The patient may be on the bedpan, or in a sitting position.
3. The patient may change her position.
4. The patient may move in such a way as to change the relationship of the uterine catheter to the strain gauge.
5. The patient may be lying in the dorsal recumbent position.

Since hypertonus stemming from any of the above causes can be observed on the strip chart, the nurse must first check these activities before assuming that a true hypertonus exists. True hypertonus occurs in abruptio placentae and over stimulation of the uterus. Although the nurse must be alert to hypertonus as a forewarning of abruptio placentae, it is important to understand that hypertonus does not always indicate an abruptio placentae.

Overstimulation of the uterus may occur during the process of inducing and augmenting contractions with oxytocin. This can be dangerous because it may allow the uterus too little time to relax between contractions. Excessive stimulation of the uterine muscle will cause hypercontractility and hypertonus. If allowed to continue, the uterus can reach a state of tetanic contraction, which could lead to a possible rupture of the uterus.

Overstimulation is also dangerous to the fetus, for each contraction must be considered a stress to the fetus. Various oxytoxic agents may be given to the patient to speed up and strengthen the uterine contractions. Extreme caution must be used to monitor the patient's response to the oxytoxic agent (increase in maternal vital sign rates, tonic uterus, fetal hyperactivity). In normal labor, the placental-fetal unit has enough reserve oxygen to stand the stress of labor. However, with uterine overstimulation, the oxygen reserve is decreased and the fetus becomes hypoxic. In other words, the fetus does not have enough oxygen to meet its physiological requirements.

Past studies on the frequency of contractions indicate that when the interval between contractions is less than 2 1/2 minutes, problems may arise for the fetus. How quickly these problems will occur depends on the fetal reserve.

For example, the fetus of a normal, healthy mother will withstand a great deal more uterine activity than that of a chronically hypertensive mother. Young hypertensive mothers often have inadequate diet and rest. Plasma proteins are lowered in toxemia and the developing fetus requires proteins. Proteinuria may lead to vascular changes which are due to spasms of the glomerular vessels. If the toxemia goes untreated, convulsions may occur, leading to fetal anorexia, etc. Toxemia is a grave concern for the fetus. Toxemia patients should be maintained under close medical surveillance.

When the uterus is overstimulated so that there is almost no relaxation between contractions, the fetus becomes physiologically isolated from the mother because the oxygen supply is cut off during the tetanic contraction and during the brief or non-existent rest-periods between contractions. This creates a crisis situation for the fetus which mandates immediate corrective action. (i.e. cessation of the induction method, delivery, or caesarean section).

Overstimulation of the uterus during oxytocin induction varies with individuals. Tetanic contractions can occur even with low infusion rates. The various methods of induction will not be discussed at this time. When you take your course in Obstetrical Nursing, you will learn about these methods.

EXTERNAL INDIRECT MONITORING OF UTERINE ACTIVITY

ITEM 1: PLACEMENT OF THE TOCODYNAMOMETER FOR UTERINE CONTRACTION DETECTION

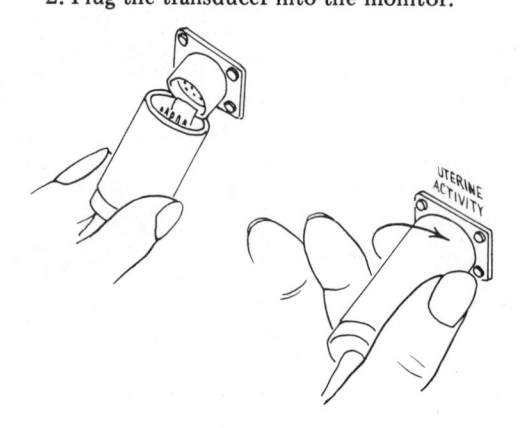

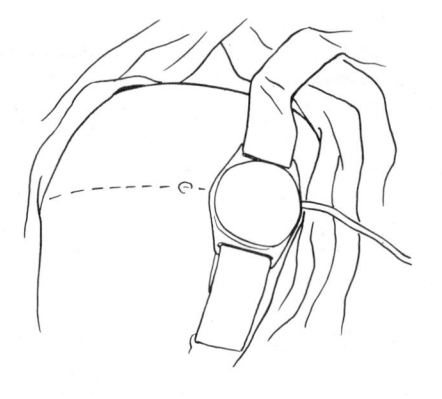

Important Steps	Key Points
1. Turn on the monitor.	Flip the "Power Switch" on.
2. Plug the transducer into the monitor.	The transducer is attached to the elastic belt that fits around the mother's abdomen. The plug is inserted into the outlet marked "Uterine Activity Input". Wash your hands.
3. Palpate the abdomen.	This enables assessment of the uterine and fetal positions, locating the head and shoulder of the fetus.
4. Place the transducer on the abdomen.	For best results, the <u>pressure sensors are placed on the *upper midline over the fundus of the uterus*</u>. In this position there is minimal maternal tissues intervening, thus providing optimal uterine activity reading.
5. Wrap the elastic belt around the abdomen.	The white discs that sense the pressure changes are located on one side of the transducer. This side is placed directly against the abdomen. Do not use gel or electrode paste. Draw the belt toward you, downward and back under the patient. It is helpful if the patient can raise her hips; if she cannot, have her roll on her side away from you so that you can put the elastic belt around her. Bring the distal end of the belt up and forward and connect it to the distal metal buckle on the transducer.
6. Adjust the belt tension.	This will secure the transducer firmly to the abdomen so that it does not slip from its desired location. The belt is tightened in a manner similar to that of an automobile seat belt—by pulling on the end until the belt fits snugly in place.
7. Locate the transducer.	Place it in the preselected spot of greatest uterine activity.

TECHNIQUES OF FETAL AND MATERNAL MONITORING

Important Steps	Key Points
8. Turn the strip recorder "ON."	
9. Adjust the pen tension.	Turn the pen set-knob (on top of the transducer) clockwise until the pen is recording the uterine activity on the lower strip chart record. Because tensions vary from patient to patient, this adjustment is necessary. NOTE: It takes several minutes for the recorder to warm up enough so that recording stabilizes.
10. Record the procedure.	Use the strip chart. Indicate time.

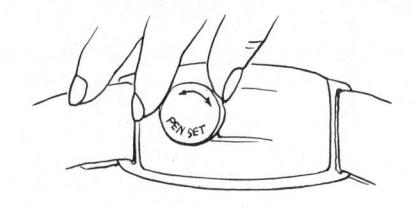

ITEM 2: PLACEMENT OF THE ULTRASONIC TRANSDUCER FOR FHR DETECTION

Important Steps	Key Points
1. Put on a head set, if available.	The headset plug is inserted into the outlet jack on the monitor. It will assist you in the placement of the transducer by locating the FHT.
2. Connect the transducer cable.	Plug it into the FHR input jack.
3. Apply conductive gel to the transducer crystals.	The sensitive transducer crystals are protected by a cap, which must be removed and put aside for safekeeping. The gel provides a firm contact point between the transducer and the skin.

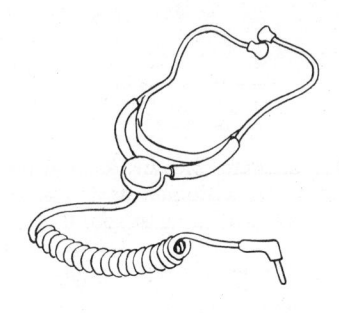

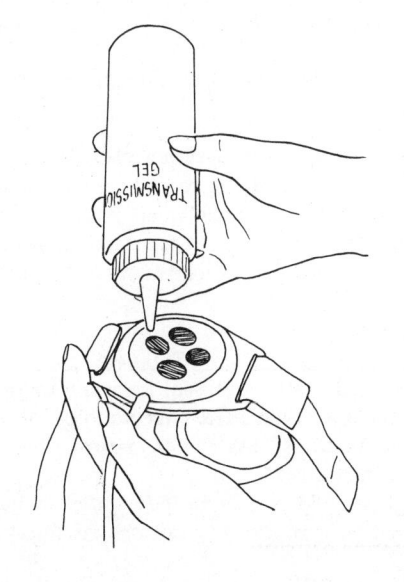

Important Steps	Key Points
4. Apply the elastic belt.	Bring the belt toward you, downward, and back underneath the patient anteriorly. Attach it to the metal buckle on the *distal* edge of the transducer.
5. Adjust the belt tension.	Secure the belt snugly around the patient's abdomen so that it does not move away from the FHT area.
6. Adjust the transducer on the abdomen.	It must be located in the area of the FHT, where the heart tone sounds like a horse galloping through water. (It takes some time to learn the specific sound; this will come with practice.) Also, here the needle will hold at a steady rate on the heart meter.
7. Adjust the volume control on the headset, if used.	Obtain the optimal FHT by moving the transducer around the abdomen until you establish the exact location of the best sounds.
8. Check monitor for correct placement of the transducer.	a) A square wave will appear on the oscilloscope. b) Beats per minute (BMP) meter will record FHR. c) Heart beat light will flash with FHR. d) FHR pen will record beats on strip chart.
9. Record the procedure.	Use the strip chart and indicate the time.

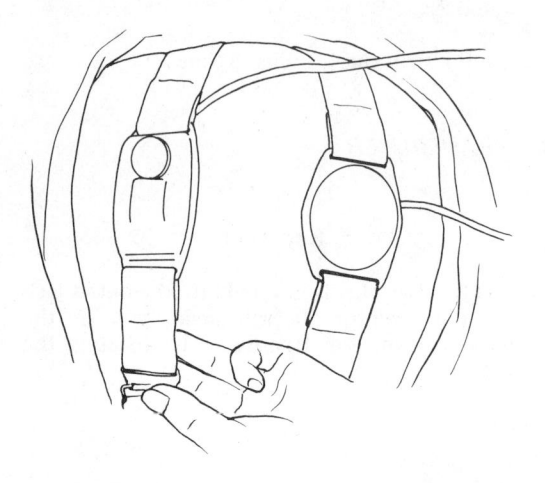

The recording paper is marked off in one-minute intervals between each heavy line (see illustration in this Unit, p. 425). Thus each major fold of the record represents four minutes of FHR or UC activity. It seems easiest to record the time between contractions by noting the distance (time) between the peaks of the contractions. However, some agencies prefer to record the time from the beginning of the contraction, when the recording begins to rise above the resting tone on the strip chart.

The numbers printed on the upper section of the paper record the fetal heart rate in beats per minute. The normal baseline FHR range is between 120 and 160 beats per minute (BPM). The baseline fetal heart rate is defined as the FHR pattern present (a) when there are no uterine contractions, or (b) in the interval between periodic FHR changes. The latter is sometimes evaluated "with the interval between contractions" but this is incorrect because late decelerations are seen in the period between contractions.

A decrease (fall) in the baseline FHR below 120 BPM is called *bradycardia*, while an increase (rise) in the baseline FHR above 160 is called *tachycardia*. The normal baseline FHR varies with each fetus. Periodic FHR increases are called accelerations, while the periodic FHR decreases are called decelerations.

The numbers printed on the lower section of the record indicate the pressure of the uterine contraction in mm Hg. The shape of the UC is usually uniform.

ITEM 3: PLACEMENT OF THE INTRAUTERINE CATHETER (DIRECT MONITORING METHOD)

This procedure is usually done at the labor bedside by the physician; the nurse may assist.

Important Steps	Key points
1. Select the equipment and place it on a sterile surface.	Intrauterine catheter, towels, long forceps (Allis) and a 10 or 20 cc syringe.
2. Approach and identify the patient; explain the procedure.	The leg plate and electrode paste are usually kept in a drawer or on a shelf on the monitor cart. The direct electrode is also placed on the sterile tray as it is inserted at the same time. Put stopcocks on the strain gauge and the monitor.
3. Apply electrode paste to the leg-plate.	The paste may be in a tube or in a bottle. Attach the leg-plate to the mother's proximal thigh. Secure the Velcro strap snugly in place. Attach the leg-plate plug to the monitor.
4. Position the patient and drape for vaginal examination.	Prep the perineal area with an antiseptic.
5. Fill the syringe.	Withdraw 10 to 20 cc of distilled water into the syringe.
6. Select the polyethylene catheter.	Attach the syringe tip to the intrauterine catheter.
7. Flush the catheter with the distilled water.	This cleans and lubricates the inside of the catheter. Approximately 5 cc of fluid is needed for this step. Hold the syringe in your non-dominant hand between the thumb and little finger.

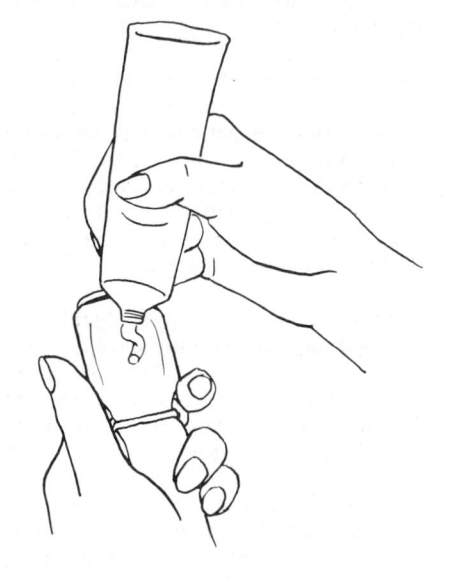

Important Steps	Key Points
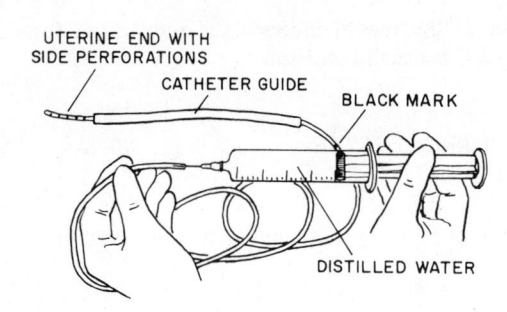 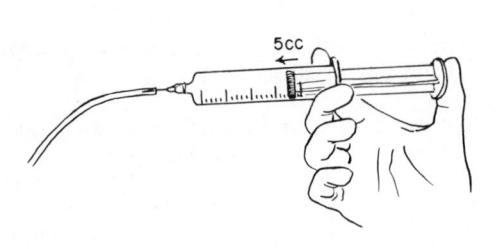	NOTE: Some physicians may hand the syringe to the nurse and she will slowly flush the catheter during the insertion. The flushing will avoid blockage of the catheter. The syringe will be kept connected to the catheter during insertion so that the sterile water can be retained in the catheter.
8. Insert your left index finger into the patient's vagina just inside the cervix.	The finger will act as a catheter guide during insertion.
9. With your right hand, insert the uterine catheter and guide.	Hold the catheter guide in place while advancing the catheter between the examining fingers. Tell the patient that some discomfort due to the pressure may occur. There is danger that the catheter may also perforate the uterus; this must be avoided at all costs. Infection may occur unless strict aseptic technique is followed during the catheter insertion.
10. Continue to advance the catheter.	Do this serially through the guide until it lies free within the amniotic cavity. The catheter insertion is complete when the black marker reaches the introitus (external opening of the vagina). The catheter should advance easily, with limited resistance.
	Do not force the catheter because it will become kinked or coiled, which in turn will cause malfunction of the system. A slight change in the angle of the catheter guide may be indicated if some obstruction is felt. Care must be taken so that the catheter is not occluded by the fetus or the uterine wall.

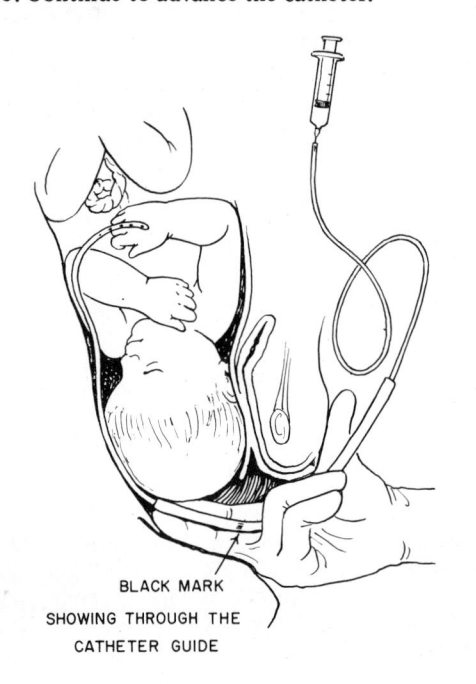

Important Steps	Key Points
11. Remove the soiled catheter guide.	a) Pull the guide back off of the catheter toward the needle adaptor. Maintain extreme caution to avoid dislodging the catheter.
	b) Temporarily remove the syringe and needle adaptor from the catheter.
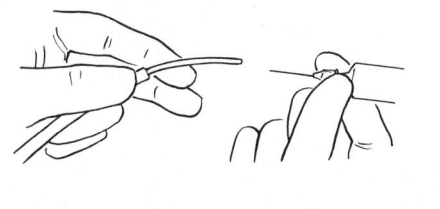	c) Remove the catheter guide from the catheter.
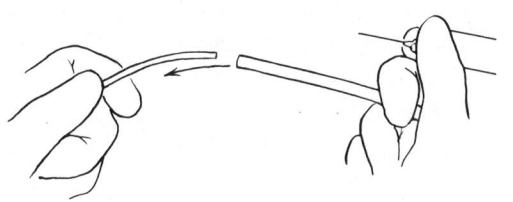	d) Reattach the catheter to the needle adaptor.
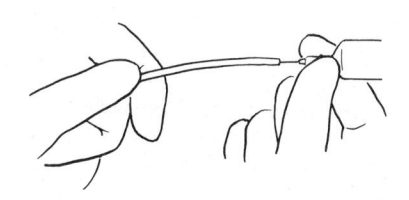	Place the guide in a designated container for cleaning; this will also keep it from being lost. Some agencies use a disposable system and therefore the guide may be discarded into a designated container.
12. Attach the needle adaptor to the 3-way stopcock on the strain gauge.	Push the adaptor into the stopcock.
13. Tape the intrauterine catheter to the inner thigh of the patient.	This will prevent dislodgement of the catheter during monitoring in case the patient should move. Refill the 20 cc syringe.

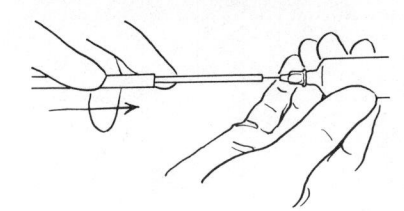

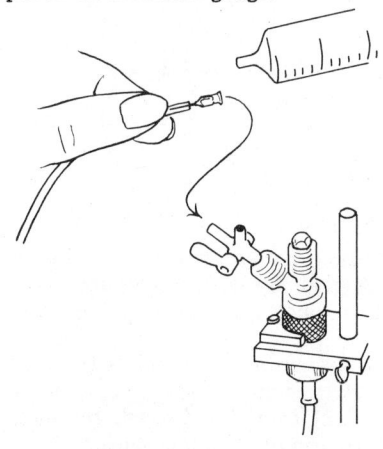

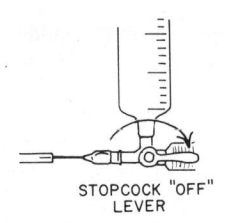

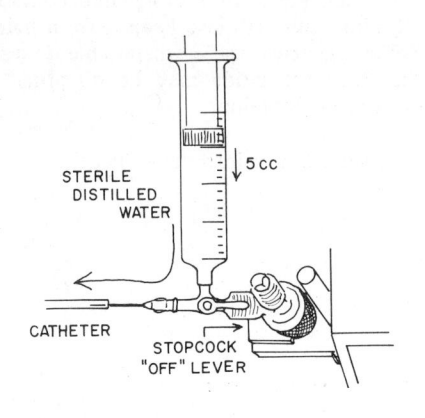

Important Steps	Key Points
14. Attach the syringe to the middle female fitting of the stopcock on the strain gauge.	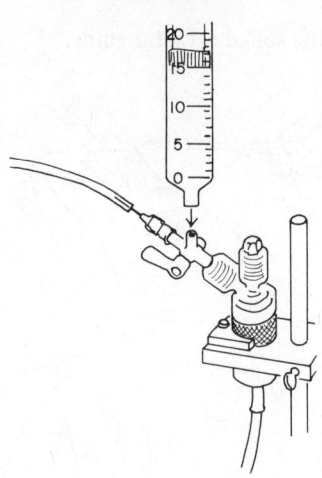
15. Turn the stopcock lever clockwise.	This will prevent the water from flowing into the dome of the strain gauge.
16. Flush the catheter.	Use at least 5 cc of distilled water to remove the air bubbles which may have collected in the catheter during insertion. Air bubbles in the catheter will cause incorrect uterine pressure readings.
17. Exclude the catheter.	By turning the top stopcock counterclockwise 180 degrees so that the lever points toward the catheter, open the syringe to the strain gauge.
18. Flush the strain gauge dome with distilled water.	This will remove all air bubbles from the system so that accurate readings can be obtained. Water will overflow through the metal screw (hub) on top of the strain gauge.
19. Tighten the screw on the strain gauge.	Turn the screw counterclockwise until it feels secure.

TECHNIQUES OF FETAL AND MATERNAL MONITORING

Important Steps	Key Points
20. Remove the syringe from the stopcock.	The uterine pressure is now open to air and should register "0" on the pressure channel on the strip chart.
21. Adjust the height of the strain gauge.	It should be set at the same height as the patient's xiphoid process.

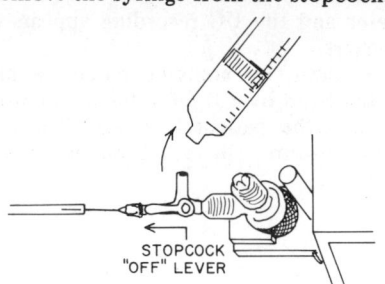

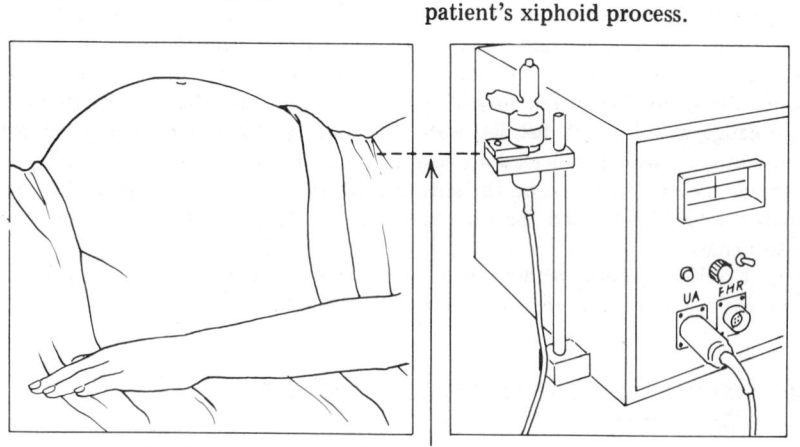

APPROXIMATE HEIGHT OF THE MATERNAL XIPHOID PROCESS

22. Turn the recorder "ON".

23. Calibrate the uterine pressure system to "0".

Insert a small screwdriver (kept on the monitor) into the zero potentiometer, adjust screw, and turn counterclockwise until "0" is recorded on the strip chart.

NOTE: When the "50" uterine calibration button is depressed, the pressure records at 50 on the strip chart. When the finger is removed from the button, the pressure again falls to "0." Changes in the recording of the uterine pressure occur when the patient moves, e.g., moving onto the bedpan, coughing, pushing. The resting uterine pressure is recorded at 5 to 15 mm Hg. The pressure may rise as much as 40 mm Hg when the patient moves. This rise does not mean a change in the uterine tone, but simply reflects the change in the relationship between the tip of the catheter and the strain gauge.

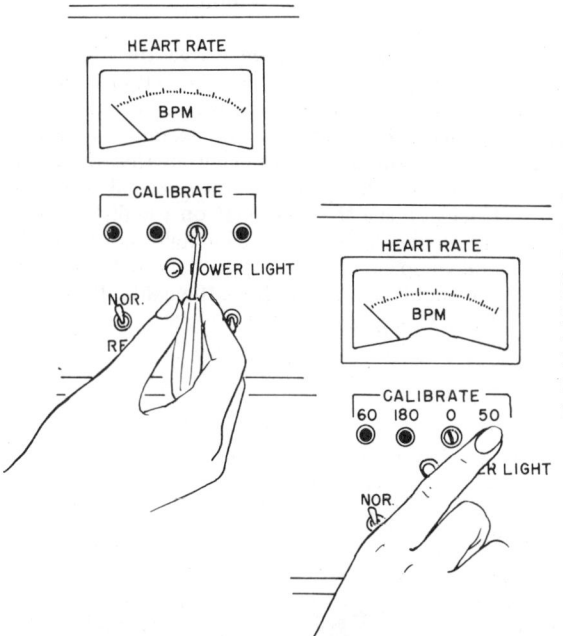

Important Steps	Key Points
24. Open the top stopcock.	This connects the strain gauge to the uterine catheter and the UC recording appears on the strip chart.
25. Take a functional recording of the uterine pressure system.	This is done by applying moderate pressure with the hand over the fundus of the uterus or by asking the patient to cough. The changed uterine pressure will record deflections on the strip chart.
26. Record the calibration on the strip chart.	

The uterine tone should be checked periodically throughout the monitoring process in order to ascertain the progress of the labor. The resting uterine pressure should be between 5 and 15 mm Hg and pressures outside this range may indicate: poor calibration, a plugged catheter, air in the strain gauge, or an incorrect strain gauge height in relation to the maternal xiphoid. The uterine pressure system should be calibrated at periodic intervals throughout the labor. To correct any of the above conditions, flush the uterine catheter and the strain gauge with 5 cc of distilled water. *Do not use saline* because it leaves salt crystals in the instrument, which will lead to corrosion of the delicate parts. Uterine contractions should show an even roundness on the strip record. If they become angulated or squared off, the catheter should be flushed. Be sure to record the flushing of the catheter and the gauge on the strip chart.

Note: Uterine pressure reading outside the 5 to 15 mm Hg range may also indicate a slowly increasing tonus of a progressive abruptio placentae.

ITEM 4: INSERTION OF THE CLIP ELECTRODE (DIRECT FHR MONITORING)

Usually this is a sterile procedure done in the labor room by the physician, with the nurse in attendance. Since the newer, more reliable spiral electrodes are now available, the clip electrode is rapidly becoming obsolete.

Important Steps	Key Points
1. Select the equipment and put it on a sterile surface.	This includes the clip electrode, the forceps for applying the electrode, the endoscope for visualizing the presenting part of the fetus, and sponges. Be sure that the examining light is placed behind the physician so that he has an unobstructed view of the vaginal opening. Check to see that the light on the distal end of the scope is working. The light cord for the endoscope is attached to a hand-battery. Turn the monitor on and check the calibration (as in Item 3, Step 23, p. 417).

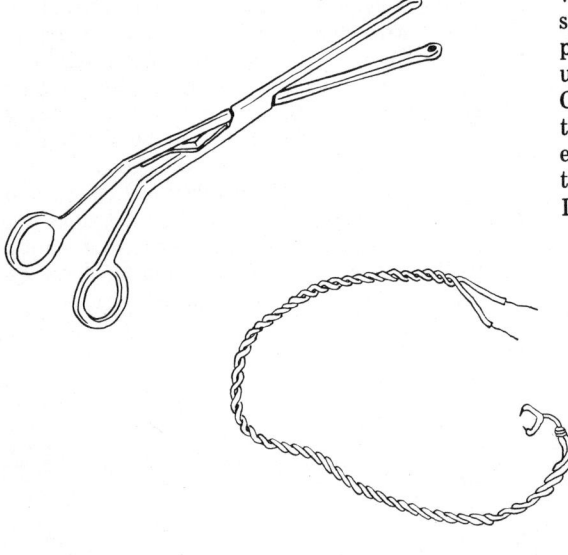

TECHNIQUES OF FETAL AND MATERNAL MONITORING 419

Important Steps | Key Points

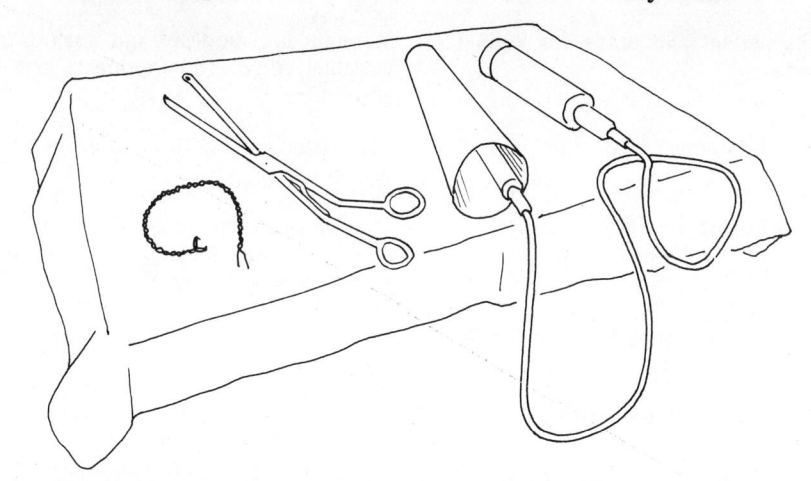

2. Approach and identify the patient.

3. Apply conductive gel to the leg-plate.

Explain the procedure.

This assures a firm skin contact for the electrical ground.

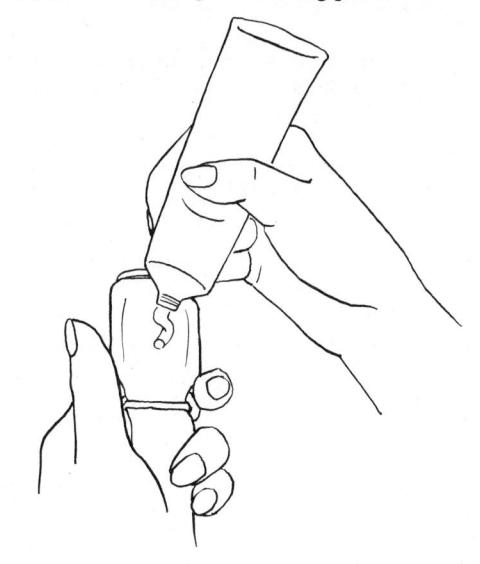

4. Place the leg-plate on the mother's thigh.

Attach the leg-plate plug to the monitor, to make certain that the patient is properly grounded.

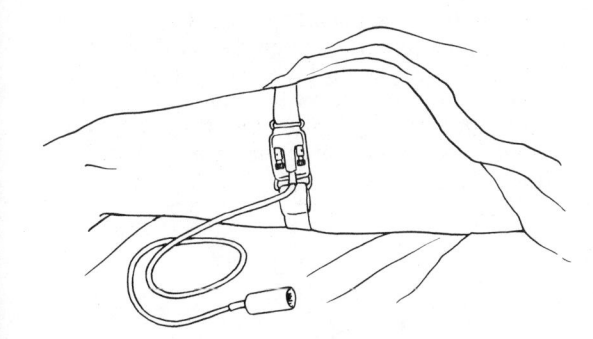

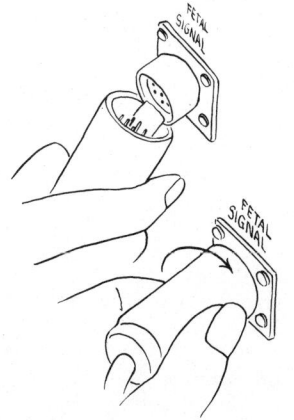

UNIT 14

Important Steps	Key Points
5. Position the patient and drape for vaginal examination.	Maintain her modesty and warmth as much as possible. Prep the perineal area with an antiseptic.
6. Insert the endoscope into the vaginal opening.	The distal end of the endoscope rests against the presenting part.
7. Wipe the attachment site.	This cleanses the blood from the site of the fetal presenting part so that the physician can see the area better.
8. Pick up the clip electrode with the special forceps.	
9. Attach the clip electrode to the fetal presenting part.	Pinch the clip together so that it has a strong hold on the presenting part. This will assure both a good connection and clear FHR signals.
10. Remove the forceps from the electrode clip.	Open the forceps by spreading the handles apart; put them aside on the sterile surface for reprocessing later.
11. Remove the endoscope.	Put it aside on the sterile tray and turn off the light on the endoscope. (This is usually done by the circulating nurse.)
12. Attach the electrode wires to the leg plate.	Fasten the green wire to the green post on the electrode plate and the red wire to the red post.

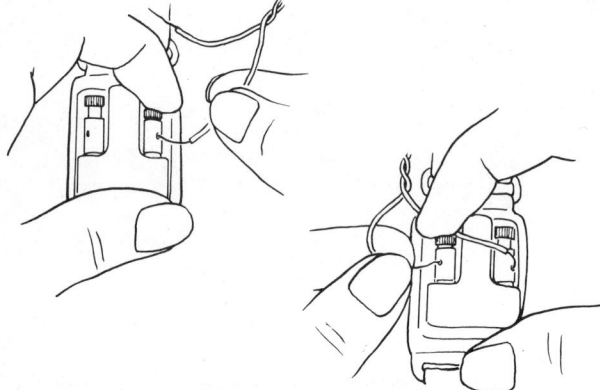

13. Turn on the monitor.	Check the FHR recording. The R wave should be in an upright position on the oscilloscope. If the R wave is downward (negative), reverse the polarity switch on the monitor. This will make the wave upright on the scope. If you fail to do this, the monitor wire will be noisy and the record unclear.

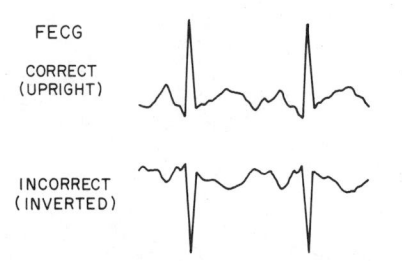

FECG
CORRECT (UPRIGHT)

INCORRECT (INVERTED)

14. Reposition the patient for comfort and safety.	
15. Record the procedure.	Write it on the strip chart and also on the nurse's notes, if required by your agency.

One of the internal mechanisms of the monitor is the Automatic Gain Control. This feature adjusts the readings for smaller fetal heart signals. Occasionally, fetal heart signals produce an electrical impulse that is too small for the machine to count. If this occurs, the pen on the heart rate recorder drops to its lowest point of 30 or below for a few seconds. When you check the oscilloscope and see that the FECG is small and increasing, it can be very alarming. However, you will be relieved to see that it is simply a temporary artifact (malfunction) of the machine.

ITEM 5: REMOVAL OF THE CLIP ELECTRODE

The removal of the electrode from the presenting part of the fetus is usually done after delivery. Therefore, continuous FHR monitoring is possible throughout the actual delivery. The patient will be in the lithotomy position, draped and prepped.

Important Steps	Key Points
1. Insert the clip remover forcep at the center of the clip electrode.	Open the clip remover forcep by spreading the prongs of the electrode apart until the clip is loosened and can be easily disengaged from the presenting part.
2. Discard the clip electrode.	Put it in the designated container.
3. Set the clip remover forcep aside on the sterile table.	
4. Cleanse the attachment site with an antiseptic.	Use a gauze sponge and inspect the site for possible tears in the skin.
	Observe the site through at least one contraction so that any unusual bleeding may be remedied at once.
	Some physicians may put a bactericidal ointment on the puncture site. Follow your agency's procedure.
	Because of the tiny puncture holes made by the clip electrode, it is often difficult to see the attachment site.
	NOTE: If the delivery is done with the clip electrode in place, then the device will be removed immediately after delivery when the infant's vital signs are stable. The electrode must be disconnected from the leg-plate. Follow Steps 1 through 4.
5. Proceed with the delivery.	
6. Record the procedure.	Write it either on the strip chart or the nurse's notes. Follow your agency's procedure.

When the leg-plate is removed from the mother, it should be unplugged from the monitor. Use warm water to wipe the coupling gel from the mother and the leg-plate. Return the clean leg-plate to its designated storage in the machine.

ITEM 6: INSERTION OF THE SPIRAL ELECTRODE (DIRECT FHR MONITORING)

The spiral electrode is made up of three parts: the introducer, the driving tube, and the locking pin. Most of the present spiral electrodes are disposable and come in a sterile package.

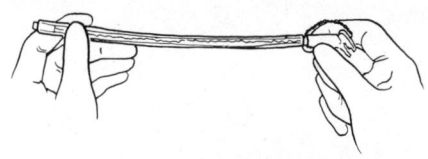

Usually this sterile procedure is done by the physician in the labor room with the nurse assisting. Be sure that the examining light is located behind the physician so that he has an unobstructed view of the vaginal opening.

Important Steps	Key Points
1. Select the equipment and put it on a sterile surface.	The spiral electrode set comes in a sterile package. Open it and drop the items on a sterile towel, along with sponges, applicator, and lubricant.
2. Turn on the monitor.	Calibrate the machine to be sure that it is functioning properly (Item 3, Step 23, p. 417).
3. Approach and identify the patient.	Explain the procedure, if the patient is awake.
4. Apply conductive gel to the leg-plate.	Spread a thin, even coat of gel with a sterile applicator. This will assure a secure contact on the skin so that the electrical grounding is complete.
5. Attach the leg-plate to the mother's thigh.	This is usually done on the side nearest the monitor. Secure it in place with the belt. Attach the leg-plate plug to the monitor.
6. Position the patient and drape for a vaginal examination.	Prep the perineal area with an antiseptic sponge.
7. Pick up the spiral electrode.	Remove the electrode wires from between the drive tube and guide tube (introducer).

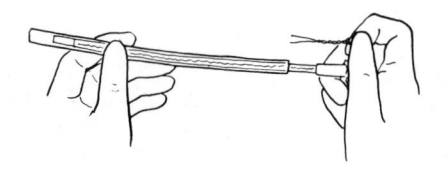

TECHNIQUES OF FETAL AND MATERNAL MONITORING

Important Steps	Key Points
8. Place the guide tube (introducer) at a right angle against the presenting part.	Retract the drive tube and electrode back inside the introducer about a half inch from the distal end of the introducer.
9. Advance the driving tube and electrode.	Simultaneously press toward the presenting part and rotate in a clockwise motion, until a slight resistance is met. A minor recoil of the driving tube can be felt when the resistance is met. The electrode is attached to the presenting part to a depth of 2 mm and a width of 6 mm. NOTE: Attachment to the face or fontanels is avoided because of possible injury to these parts.

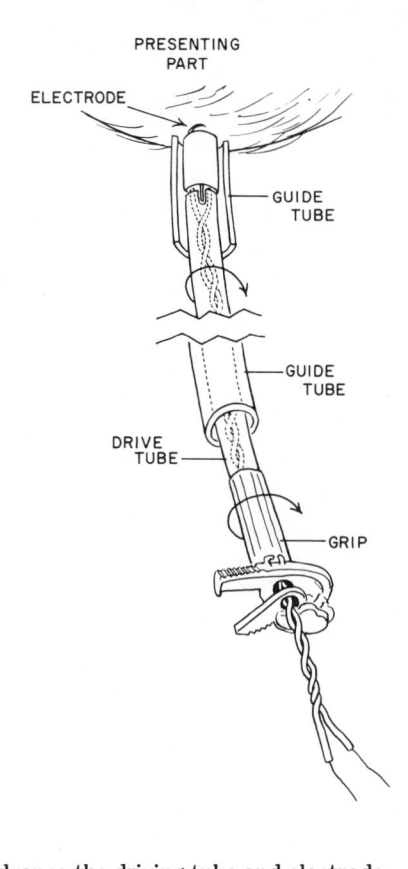

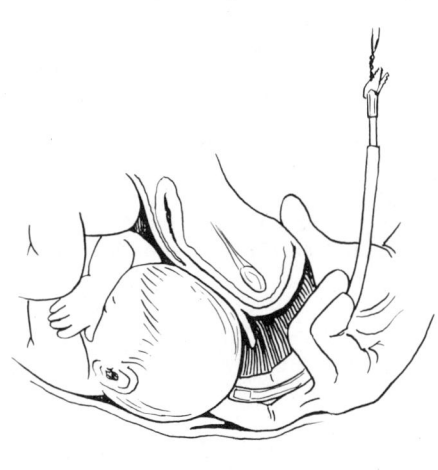

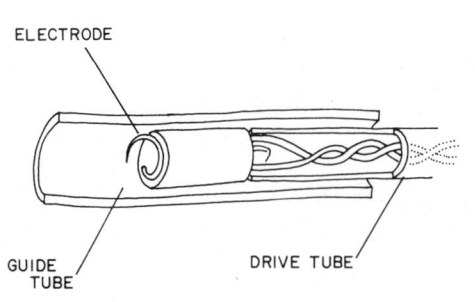

Important Steps	Key Points
10. Remove the locking pin.	Release the locking device by pressing its arms together. Slide the introducer back off of the electrode wires and place it to one side on the sterile table.
11. Attach electrode wires to the leg-plate.	Attach color-coded wires (red, green) to color-coded push-posts on the leg-plate. Turn on the recorder. The direct FHR monitoring will begin as soon as the electrodes are attached to the leg-plate.
12. Depress the calibration button.	This will cause a deflection of the needle on the strip chart and the FHR monitor-meter.
13. Calibrate the FHR.	Depress the 60-beat-per-minute (BPM) button. The calibration may be observered both on the strip chart and the FHR meter on the monitor.

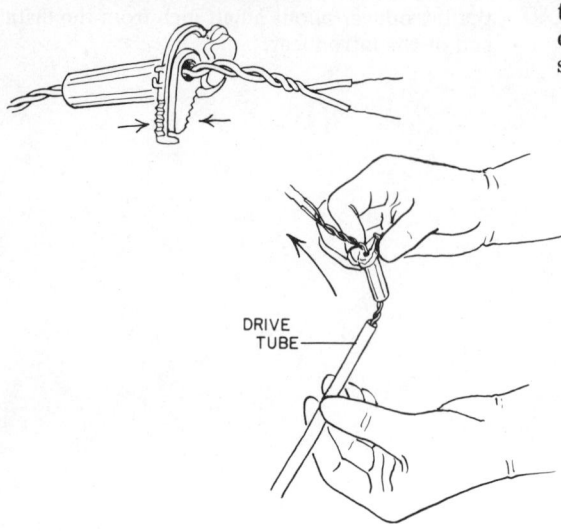

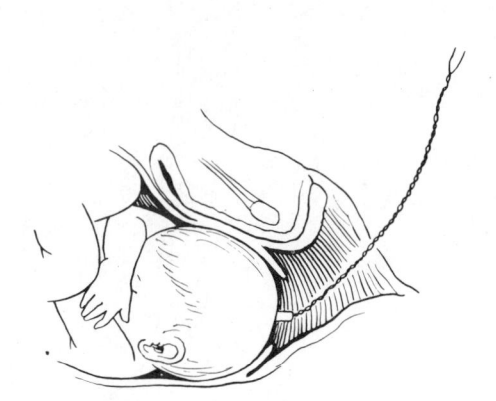

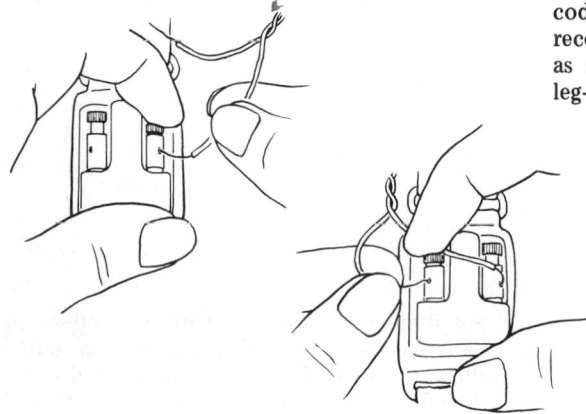

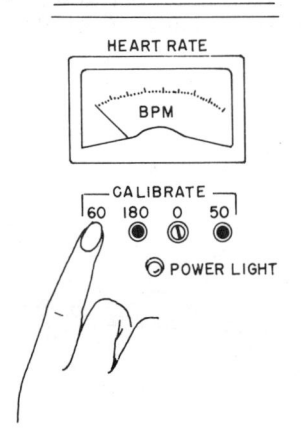

TECHNIQUES OF FETAL AND MATERNAL MONITORING

Important Steps

14. Depress the 180 BPM button.

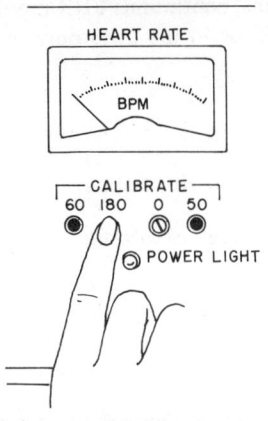

15. Record data on strip chart.

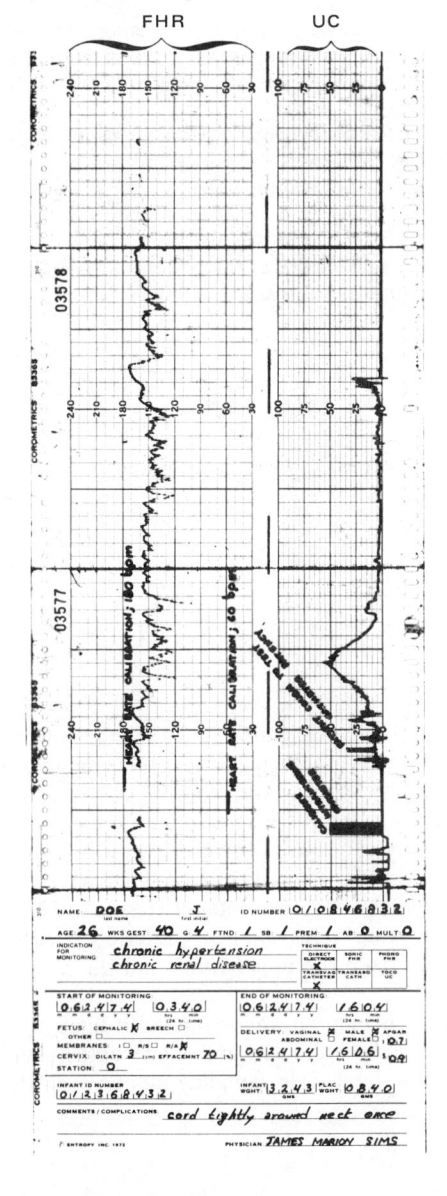

Key Points

Make sure that there is an accurate recording level.

Recording is essential to assure information retrieval.

Include the patient's name, identification number, and physician's name at the beginning of the record.

Clearly note the instrument calibration tests on the strip chart at the precise time the calibration is made.

Calibration of the FHR is done at the beginning of the record and at least hourly to assure that the system is continuing to work correctly.

NOTE: The monitoring equipment is only as good as the staff that is using it! Extreme caution must be maintained to assure that knowledgeable staff members utilize the delicate instrument without damaging the equipment.

Continue to record activities on the strip chart whenever any take place, e.g., when using the bedpan, coughing, or turning on the right or left side.

ITEM 7: REMOVAL OF THE SPIRAL ELECTRODE

This sterile procedure may be done immediately before delivery, although the delivery is usually accomplished with the electrode in place. If it remains, continuous FHR monitoring may be provided during the actual delivery. The patient will be in the lithotomy position, draped and prepped.

Important Steps	Key Points
1. Detach the electrode wire.	Twist it counterclockwise until it is free of the presenting part.
	NOTE: Do not pull the wire out of the fetus because it may tear the skin. A tear is a likely location for an infection to occur.
2. Discard the electrode.	Put it in a designated container.
3. Cleanse the attachment site.	Use an antiseptic sponge. Inspect the area for possible tears in the skin. It is often difficult to see exactly where the electrode was attached.
	NOTE: Some physicians may apply a bacteriostatic ointment to the puncture site. Follow your agency's procedure.
4. Proceed with the delivery.	NOTE: If the delivery is done with the electrode in place, then Steps 1 through 3 will be done as soon as the infant is delivered.
5. Record the procedure on the strip chart.	

After delivery, the ground plate must be removed from the mother. Unplug it from the monitor. Warm water easily removes the coupling gel from the leg-plate and the mother's leg. Return the cleansed leg-plate to its designated storage.

ITEM 8: FETAL SCALP SAMPLING

This technique was introduced in Germany by Dr. Erick Saling in 1962. It is one of various biochemical tests that assist in evaluating fetal well-being when fetal distress is suspected. It can be used as a prophylactic measure in high risk pregnancies. Fetal pH determination is an accurate indicator of fetal hypoxia; the pH is related to FHR changes. With this technique, a small blood sample from the fetal scalp is obtained for various tests: pH, blood gases, hematocrit and bilirubin. The results of these tests can assist the physician in determining if a blood exchange is needed for the Rh baby, or if fetal distress is so severe that surgical intervention may be indicated. The scalp veins are the preferred site for obtaining fetal blood sampling because blood taken from the upper trunk and the head is better oxygenated.

Instruments required to take the blood sample include an endoscope with light, long forceps, several sponges, tongue blade with silicone on it, blade and blade holder, and heparinized capillary tubes. (There are also disposable fetal scalp sampling kits now on the market.)

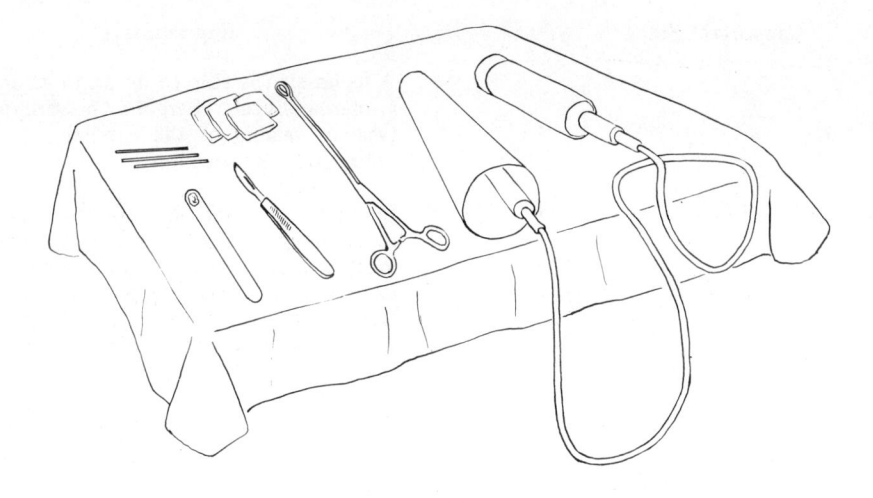

Place the patient in the lithotomy position for a vaginal examination.

Important Steps	Key Points
1. Insert the endoscope.	Be sure that the light is attached to the scope and it is working.
2. Cleanse the fetal scalp.	Pick up an antiseptic sponge with the forceps.
	The cleansing of the fetal scalp permits unobstructed visualization of the scalp.
3. Apply silicone to the scalp.	Apply a thin coating of the silicone to the fetal scalp with the tongue blade. The silicone will cause beading of the blood sample. If it is not used, the blood disperses over the scalp when the puncture is done, making it difficult to obtain a blood sample that is free of air bubbles.
4. Spray ethyl chloride (optional).	This provides local anesthesia of the vaginal canal in cases where the mother is hypersensitive. It also causes a capillary flush just before the sampling is done.
5. Insert the knife blade.	Go through the endoscope.
6. Make a small puncture in the scalp.	A 2 mm puncture is sufficient. Remove the knife and put it aside.
7. Insert a heparinized capillary tube through the endoscope.	Move it toward the point of the puncture. Do not put directly on the scalp, but only into the drop of blood on the surface of the scalp.
	The blood is withdrawn into the tube by capillary action or gentle suction on the tubing. Only a small amount of blood (50 microliters) is needed to determine the fetal pH.
8. Give the capillary tube to the laboratory technician or nurse.	The technician or nurse will cut and seal the tube to prevent loss of the blood sample from the tube. This sealer is available with the capillary equipment.

Important Steps	Key Points
	A technician is able to do an immediate pH on a microanalyzer. There may be variations in the type of sealing of the capillary tube. Follow your agency's procedure.
	If there is fetal distress, the pH can be immediately available on a blood gas machine located in the obstetric department. In other instances, the blood sample can be taken to the laboratory for processing. A laboratory requisition must accompany the specimen; be sure that it is correctly filled out.
9. Remove the endoscope.	Put the soiled scope on a designated tray to be cleaned later and returned for processing.
10. Reposition the patient for comfort and safety.	Dry the perineal area, remove the patient's legs from the stirrups, and remove the drapes. Take the patient to her bed, and leave her comfortable and safe with the light signal and bedside stand easily reachable.
11. Record the procedure.	Write it either on the strip chart or the nurse's notes.

V. ADDITIONAL INFORMATION FOR ENRICHMENT

If you are interested in further information about current fetal and maternal monitoring systems, ask your instructor for additional references or more clinical experience in the labor and delivery suite so that you can observe first-hand the various monitoring systems.

Inasmuch as the state of the art is still in its infancy (or perhaps its adolescence), you will need to keep yourself apprised of new developments by continuing to read obstetrical journals and textbooks.

In order to be able to interpret the monitoring records, you would be required to take an extensive specialized course lasting several months.

POST-TEST

1. List four indirect fetal-maternal monitoring techniques:

   Palpation, auscultation...

2. List two common biochemical fetal monitoring techniques:

3. Why are the electronic monitoring systems at present the best way to provide optimal care to the mother and fetus during the antepartum period and delivery?

4. List three common internal electronic monitoring methods:

5. List the major advantages of direct fetal monitoring:

POST-TEST ANNOTATED ANSWER SHEET

1. Palpation, auscultation, tocodynamometer, phonocardiography, ultrasound, pp. 403-405.

2. Amniocentesis, fetal blood sampling, p. 405.

3. They provide continuous, accurate monitoring of vital information (uterine activity and fetal heart rate) throughout the antepartum period and delivery, p. 406.

4. Intrauterine catheter, clip, or spiral electrode, pp. 406-407.

5. A true fetal electrocardiogram can be obtained; fetal and maternal movement do not disrupt the FHR signal, p. 408.

PERFORMANCE TEST

1. Given a patient in active labor, you will apply an external monitoring device (tocodynamometer or ultrasonic transducer).
2. Given a patient in active labor, you will assist with the introduction of a uterine catheter or the application of a clip or spiral electrode.
3. Given an antepartal patient, or one who is delivering, you will assist with obtaining a fetal scalp blood sample.

PERFORMANCE CHECKLIST

TECHNIQUES OF FETAL AND MATERNAL MONITORING

The student will demonstrate the placement of a tocodynamometer.

1. Turn on monitor and plug transducer into monitor.
2. Wash hands and palpate patient's abdomen.
3. Place transducer on upper midline of patient's abdomen over uterine fundus.
4. Apply elastic belt around patient's abdomen and attach to transducer.
5. Adjust belt tension for security and comfort.
6. Locate transducer over site of greatest uterine activity.
7. Turn on recorder and adjust pen tension.

PLACEMENT OF ULTRASONIC TRANSDUCER

1. Connect headset (optional).
2. Plug in transducer cable.
3. Apply gel to transducer crystals.
4. Apply and secure elastic belt.
5. Locate transducer on patient's abdomen for the best FHR.
6. Adjust volume control on headset (optional).

PLACEMENT OF INTRAUTERINE CATHETER

1. Assemble required equipment and place it on a sterile surface.
2. Approach and identify patient and explain procedure.
3. Apply paste to leg-plate and attach it to mother's thigh.
4. Attach leg-plate plug to monitor.
5. Position and drape the mother.
6. Fill syringe with 10 to 20 cc distilled water.
7. Select intrauterine catheter and flush catheter with the distilled water.

8. Put index finger into patient's vagina to help insert catheter.
9. Insert guide and catheter through it to the 18 inch mark.
10. Remove soiled guide; avoid dislodging catheter.
11. Discard soiled guide and tape catheter to patient's thigh.
12. Remove needle adapter and allow amniotic fluid to drain.
13. Replace needle adapter and attach catheter.
14. Remove syringe and lay it aside.
15. Attach catheter to stopcock and flush it with distilled water.
16. Adjust height of strain gauge to patient's xiphoid.
17. Exclude catheter, loosen screw on top of strain gauge, and flush dome of strain gauge.
18. Tighten screw on strain gauge and remove syringe.
19. Calibrate uterine pressure system to zero.
20. Open lower stopcock and take functional reading of uterine pressure.

INSERTION OF THE CLIP ELECTRODE

1. Select required equipment and assemble it on a sterile surface.
2. Approach and identify patient and explain procedure.
3. Apply conductive gel to leg-plate and attach it to mother's proximal thigh.
4. Attach leg-plate cord to monitor.
5. Position, drape, and prep patient for vaginal examination.
6. Insert lighted endoscope into vagina and cleanse attachment site on fetal presenting part.
7. Pick up clip electrode with forceps and attach clip to fetal presenting part.
8. Remove clip forceps without dislodging clip. Put them aside on a sterile surface.
9. Remove endoscope and turn off light. Lay aside on sterile surface.
10. Attach electrode wire to leg-plate and turn on monitor.
11. Remove drapes, reposition patient, and record the procedure.

REMOVAL OF THE CLIP ELECTRODE

1. Insert clip remover at center of clip.
2. Open clip remover and loosen clip to disengage it from the presenting part.
3. Discard used clip electrode in designated container and put it on a sterile surface.
4. Cleanse attachment site. Proceed with delivery.

INSERTION OF THE SPIRAL ELECTRODE

1. Select required equipment and arrange it on sterile surface.
2. Approach, identify, and explain procedure to patient.

3. Apply conductive gel to leg-plate, fasten leg-plate to mother's thigh, and attach leg-plate plug to monitor.
4. Position, drape, and prep patient for vaginal exam.
5. Place introducer against fetal presenting part.
6. Advance driving tube and electrode until a firm contact with the fetal presenting part is made.
7. Remove locking pin and remove introducer and driving tubes. Put aside on a sterile surface.
8. Attach electrode wires to leg-plate.
9. Calibrate the FHR by depressing first the 60, and then the 180 BPM button.
10. Record activities on strip chart.

REMOVAL OF SPIRAL ELECTRODE

1. Detach electrode wires from fetal presenting part and discard.
2. Cleanse attachment site and proceed with delivery.

FETAL SCALP SAMPLING

1. Insert lighted endoscope into patient's vagina.
2. Cleanse fetal scalp.
3. Apply silicone to the fetal scalp and apply topical anesthesia, if used.
4. Insert knife blade through the endoscope to a depth of 2 mm, remove knife and put it aside.
5. Insert heparinized capillary tube into drop of blood.
6. Give capillary tube to nurse or technician, who will seal the tube at once to prevent loss of blood sample from the tube.
7. Remove endoscope and reposition patient for comfort and safety.
8. Record procedure.

INDEX

Page numbers in *italics* indicate illustrations.
(t) following a page number indicates tabular material.

ABD (abdominal) pads, 51, *51*
Abdominal-perineal resection, 206
Abscess(es), as complication of wound, 42
Acidity, of body, 3-4
Acoustic nerve, 156
Acute pulmonary edema, 288-295, *290*, *293*, *294*
  heart disease and, 288
  symptoms of, 288
  treatment of, 288-295, *290*, *293*, *294*, 304
  with tourniquets, 289-295, *290*, *293*, *294*, 304
    electric, 293, *293*, 294
Adam's apple, 262, *263*
Adhesive ties, 52, *52*
Adolescent, injections in, 100
Adults, sites for intramuscular injections in, 98-99, *98*, *99*
Air-conditioning unit, sterile field and, 10
Air intake, physiology of, 247
Airway(s), artificial, types of, *385*
    obstruction of, causes of, 247
    signs and symptoms of, 248
Alcock catheter, 223(t), *224*
Alcohol(s), as antiseptic, 8
Alkalinity, of body, 3-4
Allergen(s), 348
  modes of transmission, *352*
  reactions to, 349
    forms of, 350
Allergic patient, nursing responsibilities for, 354
Allergy, definition of, 348
Alveolus(i), definition of, 284
Ambu resuscitator, 375
Ambulatory insulin therapy, 389-391
Ambulatory patient, draping of, 143
Amnion, definition of, 402
Amniotic fluid, definition of, 402
Ampule, 64, *82*
Amyl nitrate, 124
Analgesic, definition of, 64
Analysis, gastric, insertion of tube for, 316-318
Anaphylactic shock, 64, 348, 350, 352-353
  nursing measures in, emergency, 353
  treatment for, emergency, 350
Anesthetic(s), definition of, 64
Anodyne, definition of, 64, 156
Anoxia, 227, 263, 285
  causes of, 247
  signs and symptoms of, 248
Antalgesic, definition of, 156
Antalgic, definition of, 156
Anthelmintic, definition of, 64
Antibiotics, use in wound cleansing, 50
Antibody(ies), definition of, 1, 348
Anticoagulant(s), use, in taking blood sample, 117-118, *118*

Antidote(s), definition of, 64
Antigen, definition of, 348
Antigen-antibody complex, in allergic reaction, 349
Antipruritic(s), definition of, 64
Antipyretic(s), definition of, 64
Antiseptic(s), 8, 50
Antispasmodic(s), definition of, 64
Antitoxin(s), 351
Anxiety, 156, 376
Aphonia, definition of, 262
Apothecary measures, 64
Arteriole(s), 1, 284
Arthus reaction, 350
Asepsis, 9
  in surgery, 4
  medical vs. surgical, 3
Aseptic technique, 1-62
  anatomy and physiology in, 50
  chemistry of, 50
  historical background of, 48-49
  in changing sterile dressings, 48
  microbiology and, 50
  pharmacology and, 50
  physics of, 50
  psychology of, 51
  sociology and, 51
Asepto syringe, 158, *158*
Asphyxia, definition of, 262
Astigmatism, definition of, 196
Astringent(s), defined, 64, 156
Atomizer(s), nasal, 187
Atopy, 353
Audiometer, 193
Auscultation, 136, 139, *139*
Autoimmunity, 353
Autosensitive reaction, 349-350
Awareness, level of, 376
Ayer spatula, 330, *330*

Babinski reflex, 376
Bacille Calmette-Guérin, vaccination with, 351
Bacillus, infection by, 5
  Koch-Weeks, eye infections and, 195
Bacterium(a), 5, 7
  characteristics of, 7
  common modes of transmission of, 6
  on skin, 50
Bandage, Kling, 54, *54*
  traction, 53, *53*
  types of, 51-54, *51-54*
Bandaging, principles of physics applied to, 50
Barbiturate(s), state laws and, 67
Barrier technique, and transfer of microorganisms, 8

433

BCG vaccination, 351
Bifurcation, definition of, 262
Bini, Lucio, 379
Binocular vision, 196
Biochemical fetal maternal monitoring, 405-406
Biopsy, definition of, 325
Bitters, definition of, 64
Bladder, urinary, catheterization, in female, equipment for, 208, *208*
    procedure for, 208-212, *208-212*
    uses of, 207-208
  Escherichia coli and, 192
  evacuators of, 159, *159*
  instillation of drugs, equipment for, 164
    procedure for, 164-166, *165*, *166*, 202
  irrigation of, 160-164, *162*, *163*, 201
    irrigation of, through and through, 166-169, *167*, *168*, 202
  pathogens affecting, 207
Bladder evacuator, Ellick, 159, *159*
Blastomycin test, 348
Blood, composition of, 285
  flow in legs, inadequate, 300
    Perthes circulatory test for, 298-300, *299*, *300*, 305
    Trendelenburg test for, 295-298, *295-297*, 304
  samples of, alternate venipuncture technique for obtaining, 116-118, *117*, *118*, 134
    anticoagulants in, 117-118, *118*
    taking of, anticoagulant in, 117-118, *118*
    transfer to tube, technique for, 117-118, *117*, *118*
  Vacutainer for obtaining, 118-120, *118*
  venipuncture technique for, 116-118, *117*, *118*, 133
Blood pressure, effect of vasodilator on, 66
Blood sugar, low, 376
Body, resistance of, to infection, 1, 5
Body cavity, definition of, 156
Body reactions, to infectious agents, 4-5
Body surface, pH range of, 50
Body symmetry, definition of, 136
Body tract, definition of, 1
Breast bone, definition of, 263
Breathing, physiology of, 247
British Pharmacopoeia, 66
Bronchiole(s), definition of, 246, 262
Bronchoscope, 136
Bronchoscopy, definition of, 136
Bronchus(i), 246, 262, 264, *264*, 265, 284
Bunts catheter, 223(t), *224*
Burette, definition of, 307
Butterfly ties, on bandage, 52, *52*

Cancer, of stomach, enterostomy feeding in, 318-321, *319*, *320*, 324
Candida albicans, 6
Cannula(s), 262, 267, *267*
  inner, 267, *267*
  of tracheostomy tube, cleansing of, 269-273, *270*, *272*, 282
  outer, 267, *267*
Cantor tube, 307, 315, *315*
Capillary (ies), 1, 284
  of sin, absorption of injected medications and, 83

Capsule, definition of, 64
Cardiac fibrillation, 376
Cardiotachometer, definition of, 402
Cardiovascular system, examination of, 137
Carina, definition of, 262
Cart, emergency, definition of, 376
Cartilage, 262-263
  cricoid, 264, *264*
  thyroid, 264, *264*
Cataract, 177
Cathartic, definition of, 65
Catheter, 206
  Alcock, 223(t), *224*
  Bunts, 223(t), *224*
  Coudé, 223(t), *224*
  Councill, 224(t), *224*
  de Pezzer, 224(t), *224*
  elbowed, 223(t), *224*
  Emmett hemostatic, 223(t), *224*
  Foley, 207
  four-winged, 224(t), *224*
  French, 207
  Hendrickson, 223(t), *224*
  hollow-tip, 223(t), *224*
  intrauterine, for electronic fetal monitoring, 406-407
    placement of, 413-418, *413-417*, 431
  Malecott, 224(t), *224*
  retention, insertion of, 215-219, *217-219*
    removal of, 219-220
  Robinson, 223(t), *224*
  Trahner, 223(t), *224*
  urinary, types of, 223-224(t), *224*
Catheter guide, definition of, 206
Catheter syringe, 158, *158*
Catheterization of urinary bladder, 206-226
  history of, 222-223
  in female, 208-212, *208-212*
  in male, 212-215, *213*, *214*
  self-, by paraplegics, advantages of, 219
Caustic, definition of, 64
Cauterization, definition of, 325
Cavity, of body, definition of, 156
Cell(s), endometrial, obtaining by irrigation, equipment for, 336
    procedure for, 336-339, *337-339*, 346
  of body, pH of, 50
Cellulitis, 42
  as wound complication, 42
Cerebral functioning, examination of, 152-153
Cerletti, Ugo, 379
Cerumen, removal of, 172-176, *172-175*, 176, *176*, 203, 204
Cervix, 402
  smear and culture of, equipment for, 327, *327*
    procedure for, 327-335, *327-334*, 345
Chamberland, Charles, 49
Chemotherapy, definition of, 206
Children, sites for intramuscular injection in, 99-101, *99-101*
Chloride compounds, 8
Cilia, definition of, 263
Circadian rhythm, definition of, 64
Circulation, in legs, inadequate, treatment of, 300
  Perthes test for, 298-300, *299*, *300*, 305
  Trendelenburg test for, 295-298, *295-297*, 304
  systemic, 285

INDEX

Circulatory system, anatomy and physiology of, 285-286, *286, 287*
   examination of, 137
Cleansing, of inner cannula, of tracheostomy tube, procedure for, 269-273, *270, 272,* 282
Clip electrode, procedure for, placement of, 418-421, *418-420,* 431
   procedure for, removal, 421, 431
Clitoris, definition of, 376
Clonic convulsion, definition of, 376
Closed technique, of self-gloving, 23-26, *23-26,* 60
Clostridial infection, 5
Clostridium tetani, 5
Clostridium welchii, 5
Clysis. See *Hypodermoclysis.*
Coccal infection, 5
Coccidioidin test, 349
Coccus(i), 5, 7
Cochlea, definition of, 156
Cold, local application of, 229-230
Cold compresses, 238-241, *239, 240*
   equipment for application of, 239, *239*
   procedure for application of, 239-241, *239, 240,* 245
Cold packs, 238-241, *239, 240*
   equipment for application of, 239, *239*
   procedure for application of, 239-241, *239, 240,* 245
Colloid, definition of, 64
Color blindness, definition of, 196
Colostomy, definition of, 156
Colposcopy, definition of, 325
Coma, insulin, definition of, 376
Compresses, cold, 238-241, *239, 240*
   application of, 239-241, *239, 240,* 245
   hot, equipment for application of, 235, *235*
   application of, 235-238, *235, 236,* 244
Conduction, of heat, 227
   of electricity, 376
Conductive shoe covers, definition of, 1
Conductivity, of shoes, test for, 12, *12*
Confection, definition of, 64
Conization, definition of, 325
Consciousness, level of, 376
Consent form, for electroconvulsive therapy (sample), *396*
Contagion, definition of, 1
Containers, types of, for sterile solution injection, 82
Contamination, principles of physics in, 50
   remedying of, 9
Contents, gastric, removal for diagnostic study, insertion of tube for, 316, *316*
Contraction(s), tetanic, 403
   uterine, 403
   and oxytocin, 409
   duration of, 402
   physiology of, 408-409
Convalescent period, following infection, 4
Convulsant, definition of, 64
Convulsion(s), 376
   clonic, 376
   grand mal, 376
   petit mal, 377
   tonic, 376
Corium, 83, *83*
Coudé catheter, 223(t), *224*
Cough reflex, definition of, 246

Coughing, induction of, using external mechanical tracheal stimulation, 253-254, *253, 254*
   forceful exhalation for, 254-255, *254*
   techniques for, 253-255, *253, 254*
Councill catheter, 224(t), *224*
County of Los Angeles Health Department Recommendations for Use of Common Immunizing and Other Prophylactic Agents, 365-371
Cranial nerve, eighth, 156
Cranium, definition of, 376
Cricoid cartilage, 264, *264*
Cross-eye, definition of, 195
Crude drug, definition of, 64
Crystals, of transducer, definition of, 402
Cuff, inflated, uses in tracheostomy, 266
   tracheal, 263
   procedure for, inflation and deflation of, 277-279, *277-279,* 283
Culture(s), flow, 10
   purpose of, 326
   smear and, cervical, equipment for, 327, *327*
   cervical, procedure for taking, 327-335, *327-334,* 345
   rectal, equipment for, 327, *327*
   procedure for taking, 327-335, *327-334,* 345
   vaginal, procedure for, 327-335, *327-334,* 345
   throat, equipment for, 340
   procedure for, 340-341, *340, 341,* 346-347
   wound, equipment for, 341
   procedure for, 341-343, *342,* 347
Curettage, definition of, 325
Cyanosis, definition of, 246
Cystitis, definition of, 156
Cystocath, advantages of, 221
   insertion of, 220-221, *221, 222*
   patient with, care of, 220-222, *221, 222*
Cystoscope, 136, 206
Cystoscopy, 136, 206
Cytologic classifications, in Papanicolaou smear, 327
Cytologic specimen, obtaining of, general steps for, 326, *326*
Cytology, definition of, 325

Daltonism, 196
Decompression, of wound, definition of, 307
Defense mechanisms, 394-395
Defibrillator, definition of, 376
Deflation, and inflation, of tracheal cuff, procedure for, 277-279, *277-279,* 283
Dehiscence, as complication of wound healing, 49
   symptoms of, 49
Delayed healing of wounds, 49
Delivery, 402
   removal of clip electrode following, 421, 431
Deltoid muscle, as site for intramuscular injection, 98, *98,* 99, 100
Dementia praecox, 377
Deodorant, definition of, 64
de Pezzer catheter, 224(t), *224*
Depressant, definition of, 64
Depression, definition of, 376
Dermis, 83, *83*

Diabetic patient, sites for administering medications in, 85, *85*
Diagnosis, general physical examination in, 136
Diaphoresis, definition of, 64
Diaphoretic, definition of, 64
Dick test, definition of, 349
Dilution, 64
Diphtheria toxoid, immunization procedures for, 366(t)
Direct electronic fetal monitoring, 407-408, *407, 408*
Direct fetal monitoring, placement of clip electrode for, 418-421, *418-420*, 431
 placement of intrauterine catheter for, 413-418, *413-417*, 430-431
 placement of spiral electrode for, 422-425, *422-425*, 432
 removal of spiral electrode in, 426, 431-432
Disabled persons, self-catheterization in, advantages of, 219
Disinfection, 1, 8
Dispensatory of the United States, 66
Distention, definition of, 307
Distributive care, definition of, 349
Diuresis, definition of, 206
Diuretic, definition of, 64, 206
Donald, Ian, 404-405
Drains, gastrointestinal, 53, *53*
Drainage, intestinal, insertion of tubes for, 314-316, *314-316*
 Miller-Abbott tube for, 314-315, *314-315*
Drape, fenestrated, 207
 four-towel, in changing sterile dressings, 45
 surgical, 207
Draping, of ambulatory patient, 143
 of patient, for perineal examination, 143-144, *144*
 for physical examination, 142-144, *143, 144*
Dressing(s), spray-on, 52, *52*
 sterile. See *Sterile dressings.*
Dressing materials, common, 51-54, *51-54*
Dressing retainer, placement of, 46-47, *46-47*
Drugs. See under *Medications*, and under specific procedures.
Dust cloths, and sterile fields, 10
Dysplasia, definition of, 325
Dyspnea, definition of, 284
Dysuria, definition of, 207

Ear(s), anatomy of, 171-172, *171*, 192, *192*
 examination of, 137
 instillation of, 176, *176*, 203
 irrigation of, 172-176, *172-175*, 203
 equipment for, 172, *172*
 scientific principles relating to, 192-194, *192, 193*
Ear wax, removal of, 172-176, *172-175*, 176, *176*, 203, 204
ECG machine, portable, *386*
ECT. See *Electroconvulsive therapy; Electroshock therapy.*
Edema, 227, 263, 284
 acute pulmonary. See *Acute pulmonary edema.*
Eighth cranial nerve, 156
EKG machine, portable, 386
Elasticity, of skin, and injected medications, 83
Elbowed catheter, 223(t), *224*

Electricity, static, and conductive shoe covers, 1, 12, *12*
Electrocardiograph, portable, *386*
Electroconvulsive therapy, 376
 assisting with, 383-388, *383-387*, 399-400
 consent form for (sample), *396*
 preparation for, 379-383, *381, 382*, 399-400
 on morning of treatment, 380-383, *381, 382*, 399-400
 on night before treatment, 379-380
Electrode, 376, 402
 clip, placement of, 418-421, *418-420*, 431
 removal of, 421, 431
 insertion of, 422-425, *422-425*, 431-432
 spiral, insertion of, 422-425, *422-425*, 431-432
 removal of, 426, 432
Electrode paste, definition of, 376
Electronic monitoring, internal, of fetus, 406-407
Electroshock machine, *384, 385*
Electroshock therapy, 376
 preparation for, 379-383, *381, 382*, 399-400
 on morning of treatment, 380-383, *381, 382*, 399-400
 on night before treatment, 380-383, *381*
 procedure for, assisting with, 383-388, *383-387*, 399-400
Elixir, definition of, 64
Ellick bladder evacuator, 159, *159*
Embolism, definition of, 284
Embolus(i), definition of, 284
Embryo, definition of, 402
Emergency cart, for somatic psychiatric therapy, 378
Emetic, definition of, 64
Emmett hemostatic catheter, 223(t), *224*
Emollient, definition of, 65
Empyema, 42
Emulsion, definition of, 65
Endocrine glands, examination of, 137
Endocrine system, in general physical examination, 137
Endogenous infection, definition of, 2
Endometrial cells, irrigation for obtaining, equipment for, 336
 procedure for, 336-339, *337-339*, 346
Endoscope, 136, 402
Endoscopy, definition of, 136
Endotoxin, definition of, 2
Endotracheal tube, definition of, 263
Enterostomy, feeding via, 318-321, *319, 320*, 324
 purpose of, 307
Enuresis, definition of, 207
Epidermis, 83, *83*
Epiglottis, definition of, 246
Epilepsy, definition of, 376
Erosion, definition of, 263
Eructation, definition of, 307
Escherichia, and urinary tract infections, 192
Escherichia coli infection, 5
Esophagus, 156, 263, 307
EST. See *Electroconvulsive therapy; Electroshock therapy.*
Ethmoid bone, relation to nose, 183
Evacuators, bladder, 159, *159*
Evanescence, definition of, 349
Evisceration, as complication of wound healing, 49

INDEX

Ewald tube, 307, *316*
Examination(s), audio, 153
  general physical. See *General physical examination.*
  neurologic, 152-153
  of body systems, in general physical examination, 137
  perineal, draping for, 143-144, *144*
  physical, 135-155
    draping of patient for, 142-144, *143, 144*
    equipment for, 140, *140*
    methods of, 138-139, *138, 139*
    positioning for, 141-142, *141, 142*
    preparation of patient for, 144
  proctoscopic, procedure for, 149-151, *149, 150*
    special table for, 142, *142*
  pulmonary, 153
  rectal, equipment for, 147, *147*
  sigmoidoscopic, patient preparation for, 155
    procedure for, 149-151, *149, 150*
    special table for, 142, *142*
  special, 138
    gastroscopy as, 152
  urologic, 153
  vaginal, equipment for, 147, *147*
Examining table, for physical examination, 141, *141*
Excoriation, definition of, 2
Exhalation, forceful, to induce coughing, 254-255, *254*
Exogenous infection, definition of, 2
Exotoxin, definition of, 2
Expectorant, definition of, 65
Expectoration, definition of 246
External indirect monitoring, of uterine activity 410-428
External maternal fetal monitoring, 402
External stimulation of trachea, to induce coughing, 253-254, *253, 254*
Extract, 65
  fluid, 65
Eye(s), accommodation of, definition of, 196
  anatomy of, 177-178, *177*, 194, *194*, 195, *195*
  cataract of, 177
  examination of, 137
  infections of, 195
    prevention of, 195
  irrigation of, equipment for, 178, *178*
    procedure for, 178-180, *178, 179*, 203-204
  pH of, 196
  physiology of, 194-195, *194, 195*
  refraction in, 195-196, *195, 196*
  scientific principles relating to, 194-198, *194-196*
  treatment of, drugs in, 196-197
Eye drops, 197
  instillation of, 180-182, *181, 182*, 204
Eye tests, 196
Eyesight, changes in, sociological implications of, 197

Farsightedness, 196, *196*
Faulty injection technique, 86
  avoidance of, 86
  hazards of, 86
F.D.A., role of, 66

FECG, 402. See also *Monitoring; Fetal maternal monitoring;* and *Fetal monitoring.*
Federal Food, Drug and Cosmetic Act of 1938, 66
Feeding, via tube, equipment for, 319
  procedure for, 318-321, *319, 320*
Feelings, guilt, 156
Female urinary tract, catheterization of, equipment for, 208, *208*
  procedure for, 208-212, *208-212*
Fenestrated drape, 207
Fertilized ovum, 402
Fetal and maternal monitoring, techniques of, 401-432
  historical view of, 403-408, *403, 404, 407, 408*
  phonocardiography in, 404
  ultrasound in, 404-405
Fetal heart rate, measurement of, placement of ultrasonic transducer in, 411-413, *411, 412*, 430
  measurement of, recording paper for, 411, *425*
  palpation and auscultation for, 403-404, *403, 404*
Fetal membranes, 402
Fetal monitor, *407*
Fetal maternal monitoring, biochemical, 405-406
Fetal monitoring, direct, placement of clip electrode for, 418-421, *418-420*, 431
  placement of intrauterine catheter for, 413-418, *413-417*, 430-431
  placement of spiral electrode for, 422-425, *422-425*, 432
  removal of spiral electrode in, 426, 432
  direct electronic, 407-408, *407, 408*
Fetal scalp sampling, procedure for, 426-428, *427*, 432
Fetoscope, 402, 403-404, *403, 404*
Fetus, 402
First intention, healing by, 42
Fistula, 42
FHR, 402. See also *Fetal heart rate.*
FHT, 402
Fiberoptics, definition of, 136
Fibrillation, cardiac, 376
Flaccidity, definition of, 376
Flagellum(a), 2, 8
Flatus, definition of, 307
"Floating specks," 196
Floor cultures, 10
Fluid, amniotic, definition of, 402
Fluid extract, definition of, 65
Floor stocks, in unit-dose system, 69
Foam rubber traction bandage, 53, *53*
Foley catheter, 207, 223(t), *224*
  application of, 235-238, *235, 236*, 244
Foment, equipment for application of, 235, *235*
  vs. compress, 235
  vs. soak, 235
Fomites, 2, 7, 8
Food and Drug Administration, role of, 66
Forceful exhalation, to induce coughing, 254-255, *254*
Forceps, 2, 35
  in handling sterile equipment, 34-37, *34-37*, 62
  in handling Vaseline gauze, 37, *37*

Foreign travel, immunization for, 366
Foreskin, definition of, 207
Formaldehyde, as disinfectant, 8
Four-towel drape, in changing sterile dressings, 45
Four-winged catheter, 224(t), *224*
Fowler's position, for physical examination, 141
Franklin, Benjamin, 222
French catheter, 207
Frequency, of urination, 207
Frozen syringe, freeing of, 97, *97*
Fungal infection, 6
Furniture, in sterile field, 10

Gag reflex, definition of, 308
Galen, 48
Gamma globulin, immunization procedures using, 369(t)
Gangrene, 2
  as complication of wound, 42
  gas, 5
Gaping wound, 2
Gargle, 188-190
  vs. throat irrigation, 188
Gas gangrene, 5
Gastric analysis, insertion of tube for, equipment for, 317
  procedure for, 316-318
Gastric contents, removal for diagnostic study, insertion of tube for, 316, *316*
Gastric gavage, equipment for, 319
  procedure for, 318-321, *319, 320,* 324
Gastric intubation, for drainage, equipment for, 309
  procedure for 309-313, *310, 311*
Gastric tube, insertion for drainage, 309-313, *310, 311*
  procedure for, feeding with, 318-321, *319, 320,* 324
Gastrointestinal intubation, uses of, 308
Gastrointestinal tubes, nursing considerations for, patient with, 321
  removal of, procedure for, 313-314
Gastroscope, 136
Gastroscopy, 136
  procedure for, 152
Gastrostomy, 308
  for feeding in carcinoma, 308
Gastrostomy tube, feeding by, 318-321, *319, 320,* 324
Gauge, strain, *408*
Gauze dressing materials, 51-54, *51-54*
Gavage, 308
  gastric, equipment for, 319
    procedure for, 318-321, *319, 320,* 324
General physical examination, 136-138
  anatomic and physiologic testing in, 137-138
  assisting with, 154
  body systems in, 137
  equipment for, 145
  preparing for, 154
  procedure for, 145-148, *146, 147*
Generic name, of drug, 65, 66-67
Genitalia, 156
Genitourinary system, in general physical examination, 137

Germicide, 2
Gestation, definition of, 402
Glands, endocrine, examination of, 137
  sebaceous, 2
Glandular activity, in general physical examination, 137
Glaucoma, 195
Glottis, 246, 263
Gloves, rubber, first use of, 49
Gloving, of self, closed technique of, 23-26, *23-26,* 60-61
  open technique of, 26-28, *26-28,* 60
  of someone else, 28-31, *28-31,* 61
Gluteal muscles, as site for intramuscular injections, 98, *98*
Gonococcal infection, 5
Gonococus(i), 5
  in eye infections, 195
Goodyear, Charles, 222
Gooseneck lamp, 140, *141*
Gowns, in sterile field, 10
Gowning, of self, 19-22, *19-22*
  of someone else, 28-31, *28-31,* 61
  unsterile worker in, 20-22, *20-22*
Gowning and gloving, of someone else, 28-31, *28-31,* 61
Grand mal seizure, 376
Granulation, healing by, 42
Great saphenous vein, *287, 295*
Guide, catheter, 206
Guilt feelings, definition of, 156
Gynecologic tests, smears and cultures in, 327

"H" injections, 86-97. See also *Subcutaneous injections.*
Hair follicle, definition of, 2
Halitosis, definition of, 263
Halsted, William Stewart, 49
Hammer, percussion, 140, *140*
Handwashing, in surgical scrub, 15-17, *15-17*
Harris tube, 316, *316*
Harrison Narcotic Act of 1917, 67
Head mirror, 140, *140*
Heaf Test, for tuberculin skin testing, procedure for, 360-361, *360,* 374
Healing of wound, 42, 49
  by first intention, 42, 49
  by granulation, 42
  by second intention, 42, 49
  complications of, 49
  delayed, 49
    causes of, 49
  hemorrhage as complication of, 49
  primary, 49
  secondary, 49
Healing process, normal, 49
Hearing, sociology of, 194
  testing of, 153
Hearing loss, causes of, 193
Heart, anatomy of, 285-286, *286, 287*
  diseases of, and acute pulmonary edema, 288
  examination of, 137
Heart monitoring, direct electronic fetal, 406-407
  fetal, direct electronic, 407-408, *407, 408*
  fetal maternal, biochemical, 405-406

INDEX

Heart monitoring *(Continued)*
  fetal maternal, historical view of, 403-408, *403, 404, 407, 408*
    palpation and auscultation in, 403-404, *403, 404*
    phonocardiography in, 404
    ultrasound in, 404-405
Heart rate, fetal, placement of ultrasonic transducer for detection of, 411-413, *411, 412,* 430. See also *Fetal heart rate.*
Heat, application of, local, 229-230
  skin in regulation of, 228
  water as conductor of, 228
Heister, 222
Hemorrhage, 49
Hemostatic, definition of, 64, 65
Hendrickson catheter, 223(t), *224*
Heparin, sites for injection of, 85
Hexachlorophene, 2, 8
Hiccups, definition of, 377
Hippocrates, 48
HISG, 352
Histology, definition of, 325
Histoplasma capsulatum, 349
Histoplasmin test, definition of, 349
Hives, definition of, 349
Hollow-tip catheter, 223(t), *224*
Holmes, Oliver Wendell, 48
Hormone, definition of, 376
Host, definition of, 2
  resistance to infection of, 4-5
Hot compress, application of, 235-238, *235, 236,* 244
  equipment for application of, 235, *235*
Hot pack, application of, 235-238, *235, 236,* 244
  equipment for application of, 235, *235*
Hot soaks, application of, 230-235, *231-234,* 244
  equipment for, 231, *231*
Hubbard tank, definition of, 227
Human immune serum globulin, 352
Hydrocollator, 235, *235*
Hyoid bone, 263, 264, *264*
Hyperalimentation, vs. infusion, 108
Hypermetropia, 196, *196*
Hyperopia, 196, *196*
Hypersalivation, definition of, 376
Hypersensitivity, 376
Hypersensitivity reaction, 349
  types of, 349, 352-353
Hypertonus, in uterine contractions, 409
Hypnotic, definition of, 65
Hypodermic, definition of, 65
Hypodermic injections, 86-97, *86-96.* See also *Subcutaneous injections.*
Hypodermic needle, removal when stuck, 97, *97*
Hypodermoclysis, definition of, 65
  for administration of medications, 79, *79*
Hypoglycemia, definition of, 376
Hyposensitivity, 350
Hypospray Tuberculin Test, procedure for, 361-362, *361, 362,* 374
Hypothalamus, definition of, 227
Hypothermia, definition of, 227
Hypoxia, 263, 285
  causes of, 247
  signs and symptoms of, 248

Imferon, administration of, 105
Immune serum globulin, immunization procedures using, 369(t)
Immunity, 349
  acquired, 348
  natural, 349
  passive, 352
Immunization, definition of, 349
Immunizing agents, contraindications to use of, 366(t)-368(t)
  County of Los Angeles Health Department recommendations for, 365-371
  guidelines for, 365-371
  schedules for, 366(t)
  tuberculin skin testing and, 366
Incision, definition of, 2
Incubation, definition of, 325
Incubation period, in infection, 4
Indirect monitoring, external, of uterine activity, 410-428. See also under *Monitoring.*
Infant(s), injections in, 100-101
  intramuscular injection sites in 99-100, *99, 100*
  suctioning in, 251-252, *251, 252*
Infection(s), 2
  acute period of, 4
  bacilli, 5
  bacterial, 5-6
  Clostridium tetani, 5
  Clostridium welchii, 5
  coccal, 5
  course of, 4
  endogenous, 2
  Escherichia coli, 5
  exogenous, 2
  fungal, 6
  gonococcal, 5
  metazoal, 6
  mold, 6
  Mycobacterium tuberculosis, 5
  of eye, prevention of, 195
  of throat, 198
  poliovirus, 6
  postoperative, 2
  prodromal period of, 4
  protozoal, 6
  Pseudomonas aeruginosa, 5
  Pseudomonas pyocyanea, 5
  purulent, 2
  staphylococcal, 5
  streptococcal, 5
  tissue reactions to, 4-5
  types of, 4
  viral, 5-6
    of intestinal tract, 6
    of neurosensory organs, 5
    of respiratory tract, 5
    of skin, 5
  poliovirus, 6
  yeast, 6
Infectious agents, body reactions to, 4-5
Inflammation, course of, 349-350
Inflated cuff, uses in tracheostomy, 266
Inflation and deflation, of tracheal cuff, procedure for, 277-279, *277-279,* 283
Influenza vaccine, immunization procedure for, 367(t)
Infusion, intravenous, 108-111
  preparation of liquid additive for, 121, 133
  preparation of, 109-111, 132

Infusion *(Continued)*
  removal of, 120-121, 133
Inhalation, drug administration by, 123-124 *123-124*
Inhalers, 187
Injections, intradermal, sites for, 105
  administration of, 105-108, *106, 107*, 132
  intramuscular, 97-105, *97-105*
    administration of, 101-104, *102-104*, 131
    sites for, 99-101, *99-101*
    Z-track technique for administration of, 105, *105*, 131
  intravenous, 108-116, *111, 112, 114, 115*
    administration of, 111-116, *111, 112, 114, 115*, 132
    LPN/LVN's roles in, 108
    preparation of liquid additive for, 121
    preparation of solid additives for, 122-123, 133-134
    RN's roles in, 108
    sites for, 111-112, *111, 112*
  subcutaneous, 86-97, *86-96*
    administration of, 93-97, *93-96*, 131
    preparation of, 87-93, *87-93*, 130
    sites for, 84-85, *84, 85*
Injection sites, choice of, 84-85, *84, 85*
Injection technique, faulty, 86
  avoidance of, 86
  hazards of, 86
Inner cannula, of tracheostomy tube, 267, *267*
  cleansing of, 269-273, *270, 272*, 282
Inoculation, definition of, 325
Instillation(s), administration of, nursing guides in, 159-160
  nasal, 185-187, *186, 187*, 204-205
  of drugs, via bladder, 164-166, *165, 166*, 202
  of ear, 176, *176*, 203
  of eye drops, 180-182, *181, 182*, 204
    equipment for, 180
  of wounds, procedure for, 191-192
  vs. irrigation, 157
Insufflator, 136
Insulin, 376
  sites for injection of, 85, *85*
Insulin coma, 376
Insulin coma therapy, 391-393
  phases of, 391-392, *393*
  vs. ambulatory insulin therapy, 389
Insulin shock, definition of, 376
Insulin syringe, *81*, 82
Insulin therapy, 389-393
  ambulatory, 389-391
    nurse's role in, 390-391
    vs. insulin coma therapy, 389
  general treatment preparation for, 389
  pre-treatment preparation for, 389
Insulin treatment record (sample), *395*
Integument, 136
  examination of, in general physical examination, 137
Intercostal muscle, definition of, 376
Intercostal space, definition of, 376
Internal organs, viral infections of, 5
Internal electronic fetal monitoring, 406-407
  intrauterine catheter in, 406-407
Internal maternal fetal monitoring, 402
Intestinal tract, viral infections of, 6
Intestinal tubes, insertion for drainage purposes, 314-316, *314-316*

Intradermal injections, administration of, 78, *78*, 83, 105-108, *106, 107*, 132
  needle and syringe for, 106
  sites for, 105
Intramuscular injections, 78, *78, 83*, 97-105, *97-105*
  administration of, 101-104, *102-104*, 131
  Z-track technique of, 105, *105*, 131
  sites for, 98-101, *98-101*
Intraspinal administration of medications, 79
Intrauterine catheter, in internal electronic fetal monitoring, 406-407
  placement for direct fetal monitoring, 413-418, *413-417*, 430-431
Intravenous infusion(s), 108-111
  preparation of, 109-111, 132
  preparation of liquid additive for, 121, 133
Intravenous injections, 108-116, *111, 112, 114, 115*
  administration of, 78, *78*, 111-116, *111, 112, 114, 115*, 132
  liquid additive for, preparation, 121, 133
  preparation of solid additive for, 122-123, 133-134
Introitus, definition of, 325, 402
Introjection, as defense mechanism, 394
Intubation, gastric, for drainage, 309-313, *310, 311*
  equipment for, 309
  gastrointestinal, uses of, 308
Inunction, definition of, 65
Involutional melancholia, definition of, 376
Iodine compounds, in aseptic technique, 8
Iodophors, in aseptic technique, 8
Iron preparations, Z-track method for administration of, 66
Irrigating syringe, plastic disposable, 158
  reusable glass, 158, *159*
Irrigation(s), administration of, nursing guides in, 159-160
  for obtaining endometrial cells, 336-339, *337-339*, 346
    equipment for, 336
  nasal, 183-185, *184*, 204
    equipment for, 183
  of bladder, with catheter in place, 160-164, *162, 163*, 201
    through and through, 166-169, *167, 168*, 202
    equipment for, 167
  of ear, 172-176, *172-175*, 203
    equipment for, 172, *172*
  of eye, 178-180, *178, 179*, 203-204
    equipment for, 178, *178*
  of kidney pelvis, 169-171, *170*, 202-203
    equipment for, 169
  of throat, 188-189, 205
  of wounds, 190-191, 205
    equipment for, 190
  vs. instillation, 157
Irrigators, types of, 158-159, *158, 159*
Isolation, as defense mechanism, 394

Jawbone, relation to nose, 183
Jet Gun Test, for tuberculin skin testing, procedure for, 361-362, *361, 362*, 374
Jutte tube, 308, *316*

Kardex, in unit-dose system, 68, 69, 70
Keloid(s), 42
Kidney function tests, 153
Kidney pelvis, irrigation of, 169-171, *170*, 202-203
    equipment for, 169
Kling bandage, 54, *54*
Knee-chest position, for physical examination, 141-142, *142*
    draping for, 143
Koch, Robert, contributions to aseptic technique, 48
    contribution to tuberculin skin testing, 357

Labia majora, definition of, 156
Labia minora, definition of, 156
Labor, definition of, 402
Lamp, gooseneck, 140, *141*
Laryngeal mirror, 136, 140, *140*
Laryngopharynx, 247
Larynx, 247, 263, 264, *264*
    visualization of, 136
Lateral position, for physical examination, 141
Lavage, definition of, 157, 308
Laws regulating drugs, 66-67
    exemptions to, 67
Laxative, definition of, 65
Legs, venous system of, *287*
Lensometer, 196
Level of awareness, 376
Level of consciousness, 376
Level of perception, 376
Levin tube, 308, 309, *309, 316*
Liniment, 65
    application of, 124-125, 134
Liquid additive, preparation for intravenous infusion, 121, 133
Lister, Joseph, 48
Lithotomy position, 136, 141-142, *142*
    draping for, 143, *143*, 144, *144*
    for physical examination, 141-142, *142*
Local application, of cold, 229-230
    of heat, 229
Lotion, 65
    application of, 124-125, 134
Low blood sugar, 376
Lozenge, definition of, 65
LPN/LVN's, and administration of intravenous injections, 108
Lumen (ina), definition of, 263
Lungs, anatomy of, considerations for tracheostomy, *264*

Malaise, definition of, 2
Male urinary tract, procedure for, catheterization of, 212-215, *213, 214*
Malecott catheter, 224(t), *224*
Manic-depressive psychosis, 376
Mantoux Test, for tuberculin skin testing, advantages and disadvantages of, 364
Mask, surgical, 13-14, *13-14*
    equipment for, 362
    procedure for, 362-364, *363, 364*, 374
Materials savings, in unit-dose system, 69
Maternal-fetal monitoring. See under *Monitoring.*

Maxilla, relation to nose, 183
Measles vaccine, immunization procedure with, 367(t)
Measure, apothecary, 64
Measurements, physiological, in general physical examination, 137-138
Mechanisms, defense, 394-395
Medical personnel, duties in administering drugs, 67
Medications, administration, by inhalation, 123-124, *123, 124*
    bladder instillation of, 164-166, *165, 166*, 202
    choice of injection sites in, 84-85, *84, 85*
    faulty technique of, avoidance of, 86
    hazards of, 86
    hypodermoclysis for, 79, *79*
    intradermal, 78, *78*, 83, 132
    intramuscular, 131
        Z-track technique of, 105, 131
    intraspinal, 79
    intravenous, 78, *78*, 108-116, *111, 112, 114, 115*, 132
        liquid additives for, preparation of, 121
        solid additives, preparation of, 122-123
        technique of, 111-116, *111, 112, 114, 115*, 132
    oral, 75-77, *75*, 130
    parenteral, 77-118, 120-122
        methods of, 77-79, *78, 79*
    subcutaneous, 77, *78*, 131
        preparation for, 130
    unit-dose system and, 67-70
    duties of medical personnel in administering, 67
    injected, absorption of, 83
    intravenous, preparation of, 132
    liquid preparation of, 70-73, *71-73*
    oral, narcotic, preparation from narcotic dispenser, 73, *74*
    preparation of, 70-74, *71-74*, 130
    solid preparation of, 70-73, *71-74*
Medulla, of brain stem, definition of, 308
Melancholia, involutional, 376
Membranes, fetal, 402
Mercurials, 8
Metazoal infections, 6
Methods of physical investigation, 138-139, *138, 139*
Metric system, 65
Microbes, 2
Microbiologist, 2
Microbiology, principles in aseptic technique, 50
Microorganisms, classification of, 5-6
    contamination by, 50
    transmission of. See also *Transmission, of microorganisms.*
    and barrier technique, 8
Micturition, 157, 207
Miller-Abbott tube, 308, 314, *314*
    procedure for insertion for drainage, 314-315, *314, 315*
Miotic(s), 65, 157. See also *Eye drops.*
Mirror, head, 140, *140*
    laryngeal, 136, 140, *140*
Mold infection, 6
Moleskin, 53, *53*

Monilia albicans, 6
Monilial vaginitis, procedure for taking vaginal smear for, 335-336, 346
Monitor, fetal, *407*
Monitoring, direct fetal, placement of clip electrode for, 418-421, *418-420*, 431
  placement of intrauterine catheter for, 413-418, *413-417*, 430-431
  placement of spiral electrode for, 422-425, *422-425*, 432
  removal of spiral electrode in, 426, 432
  external indirect, of uterine activity, 410-428
  fetal, direct electronic, 407-408, *407*, *408*
  internal electronic, 406-407
  fetal-maternal, 402
    biochemical, 405-406
    external, 402
    historical view of, 403-408, *403*, *404*, *407*, *408*
    internal, 402
    palpation and auscultation in, 403-404, *403*, *404*
    phonocardiography in, 404
    ultrasound in, 404-405
Mono-vacc Test, for tuberculin skin testing, procedure for, 359, *359*, 374
Montgomery tape, 52, *52*
Mops, and sterile fields, 10
Movement, primitive, definition of, 377
Mucopurulence, definition of, 247
Mucous membranes, function of, in asepsis, 50
Mucous membrane tests, 354
Mucus, 247
  tenacious, 247
Multi-eyed catheter, 223(t), *224*
  uses of, 223(t)
Mumps vaccines, immunization procedures using, 367(t), 368(t)
Murphy drip, for special feedings, 318
Muscle(s), deltoid, as site for intramuscular injection, 98, *98*
  gluteal, as sites for intramuscular injections, 98, *98*
  intercostal, 376
Musculoskeletal system, in general physical examination, 137
Mushroom catheter, 224(t), *224*
Mycobacterium tuberculosis, 5, 349
Mydriatics, 65, 157. See also *Eye drops*.
Myopia, 196, *196*
Myotonic twitching, 377

Name, proprietary, of drug, 65
Narcotic, oral, from narcotic dispenser, 73, *74*
Naris(es), 247
Nasal atomizers, 187
Nasal instillation, equipment for, 185
  procedure for, 185-187, *186*, *187*, 204-205
Nasal irrigation, equipment for, 183
  procedure for, 183-185, *184*, 204
NAS-NRC, 66
Nasal speculum 140, *140*
Nasogastric tube, 308
Nasopharyngeal suctioning, equipment for, 248, *248*, 249, *249*
Nasopharynx, 157, 247

National Academy of Sciences-National Research Council, 66
National Formulary, 66
National Institute of Mental Health, 377
National Mental Health Act, 377
Natural immunity, 349
Nausea, 308
Nearsightedness, 196, *196*
Necrosis, 2
  as complication of wound, 42
Needles, 79-80, *79*, *80*
  for intradermal injections, 106
  hypodermic, removal when stuck, 97, *97*
  parts of, 80, *80*
Nephritis, 207
Nerve(s). See under specific name.
Nervous system, examination of, 137, 152-153
Neurologic examination, 137, 152-153
Neurologic tests, 137, 152-153
Neurological system, examination of, 137, 152-153
Neurosensory organs, viral infections of, 5
New and Nonofficial Remedies, 66
Newborns, intramuscular injection sites in, 99-100, *99*, *100*
N.N.R., 66
Nonsterile person, 9, 10
  near sterile field, 10
Nose, anatomy of, 182-183, *182*
  examination of, 137
  instillation of, equipment for, 185
    procedure for, 185-187, *186*, *187*, 204-205
  irrigation of, equipment for, 183
    procedure for, 183-185, *184*, 204
  suctioning of, 246-261
Nostril(s), 247
Nurse(s), licensed practical, duties in administration of medications, 67
  licensed vocational, duties in administration of medications, 67
  registered, and administration of intravenous injections, 108
    duties in administration of medications, 67
  role, in physical examination, 137
  student, duties in administration of medications, 67
"Nurseserver," 71
Nursing care, distributive, 349
Nursing considerations, for patients with gastrointestinal tubes, 321
Nursing measures, general, for tracheostomy patient, 268-269
Nursing responsibilities, toward allergic patient, 354
  unit-dose system and, 69

Observation, 138, *138*
Obstetrics, 207, 402
Obstetric scrub (OB scrub), 18-19
Obstruction, of airway, causes of, 247
Obturator, 263, 267, *267*
Official name, of drug, 66-67
Ointment, 65
  application of, 125-126, 134
Old sightedness, 196
Open technique, of self-gloving, 26-28, *26-28*, 60

Opening of sterile packages, 31-34, *31-34*, 61
Ophthalmologist, 157
Ophthalmoscope, 136, 140, *140*
Optometrist, 157
Oral medications, preparation and administration of, 70-77, *71-75*, 130
Organisms, pathogenic, 2
Orifice, vaginal, 157
Oropharyngeal suctioning, procedure for, 251
Oropharynx, 247
Oscilloscope, 402
Otitis media, 193
Otologist, 157
Otosclerosis, 157
Otoscope, 136, 140, *140*
Outer cannula, 267, *267*
Ovum, fertilized, 402
Oxygen lack, causes of, 247
  signs and symptoms of, 248
Oxytocin, and uterine contractions, 409
Oxytocic, definition of, 65

Pack, cold, 238-241, *239*, *240*
  equipment for application of, 239, *239*
  procedure for application of, 239-241, *239*, *240*, 245
  hot, equipment for application of, 235, *235*
  procedure for application of, 235-238, *235*, *236*, 244
  vs. compress, 235
  vs. soak, 235
Packages, sterile. See *Sterile packages.*
Pain, trigeminal, 377
Palate, relation to nose, 183
Palpation, 136, 138, *139*, 402
  in physical examination, 138, *139*
Pancreas, 377
"Pap" smear, 325
  contraindications to, 327
  uses of, 327
"Pap test," purpose of, 136
Papanicolaou smear, 136, 325
  contraindications to, 327
  purpose of, 136
  uses of, 327
Paraplegics, self-catheterization in, advantages of, 219
Parasite, 2
Parenteral route, for administering medications, 77-118, 120-122
  reasons for using, 77
Parkinson position, 186, *186*
Passive immunity, 352
Paste, electrode, 376
Pasteur, Louis, 48
Patch Test, current uses of, 354
  interpretation of results of, 355
  procedure for, 354-355, *355*, 373
Patency, 136
Pathogen, 2
  affecting urinary tract, 207
Patient(s), allergic, nursing responsibilities for, 354
  ambulatory, draping of, 143
  draping, for perineal examination, 143-144, *144*
    for physical examination, 142-144, *143*, *144*

Patient(s) *(Continued)*
  positioning, for examination, 141-142, *141*, *142*
  with Cystocath, care of, 220-222, *221*, *222*
    nursing precautions in, 222
  with gastrointestinal tubes, nursing considerations for, 321
  with tracheostomy, complications in, 269
    general nursing measures for, 268-269
Patient preparation, for physical examination, 144
  for proctoscopy, 148, *148*
  for sigmoidoscopy, 148, *148*
Patient Profile Record, in unit-dose system, 68
PCG, 403
P.D.R., 66
"P.E." See *General physical examination.*
  examination of. See also under names of various examinations.
Pelvis, of kidney, irrigation of, 169-171, *170*, 202-203
  equipment for, 169
  renal, irrigation of, 169-171, *170*, 202-203
  equipment for, 169
Penicillin, use in wound cleansing, 50
Perception, level of, 376
Percussion, 136, 139, *139*
  in physical examination, 139, *139*
Percussion hammer, 140, *140*
Perineal examination, draping for, 143-144, *144*
Perineum, 157
Peristalsis, 308
Personality development, 394
Perthes circulatory test, equipment for, 298
  procedure for, 298-300, *299*, *300*, 305
Pertussis vaccine, immunization procedures for, 366(t)
pH, 2, 3-4, 157
  of body cells, 50
  of body surface, 50
  of eyes, 196
Pharmacist, duties in administering medications, 67
Pharmacology, principles in aseptic technique, 50
Pharmacopeia Internationalis, 66
Pharyngeal and endotracheal suctioning, equipment for, 255-256, *255*, *256*
  procedure for, 255-258, *256*, *257*
Pharyngeal suctioning, 246-261
Pharynx, 157, 247
  anatomy of, 187, *187*
  visualization of, 136
Phenolics, 8
Phlebitis, 285
Phlebotomy, 285
Phlegm, 247
Phonocardiogram, 403
Phonocardiography, in fetal and maternal monitoring, 404
Phonotransducer, 403
Phosphates, precipitate of, 157
"Physical." See *General physical examination.*
"Physical exam." See *General physical examination.*
Physical examination(s), 135-155
  auscultation in, 139, *139*
  draping of patient for, 142-144, *143*, *144*

Physical examination(s) *(Continued)*
  equipment for, 140, *140*
  examining table for, 141, *141*
  general. See *General physical examination.*
Physical investigation, auscultation for, 139, *139*
  methods of, 138-139, *138*, *139*
  observation for, 138, *138*
  palpation for, 138, *139*
  percussion for, 139, *139*
Physicians, duties in administering medications, 67
Physicians' Desk Reference, 66
Physician's tray, in somatic psychiatric therapy, 378
Physics, principles in aseptic technique, 50
Physiological measurements, in general physical examination, 137-138
Physiology, of circulatory system, 285-286, *286*, *287*
  of skin, 50
  of uterine contractions, 408-409
Pikel, 222
Plastic dressing materials, 51-54, *51-54*
Poison, neutralization of, 64
Poliovirus, infection by, 6
Poliovirus vaccines, immunization procedures using, 368(t)
Pomeroy syringe, 172, *172*
Portable electrocardiograph, *386*
Position, Fowler's, 141
  knee-chest, 141-142, *142*
    draping for, 143
  lithotomy, 136, 141-142, *142*
    draping for, 143, *143*, 144, *144*
  Parkinson, 186, *186*
  Proetz, 186, *186*
  prone, 141, *142*
    draping for, 143
  semi-Fowler's, 141
  Sims', 141, *141*
    draping for, 143
  supine, 141, *141*
    draping for, 143, *143*
  Trendelenburg, 141, *142*
Positioning, of patient, for examination, 141-142, *141*, *142*
Postoperative infection, 2
Pouring of sterile solutions, 62
Powders, 65
PPD, for tuberculin skin testing, 357
Precipitate of phosphates, 157
Premature infant, gavage feeding in, procedure for, 318-321, *319*, *320*, 324
Prepuce, 207
Presbyopia, 196
Pre-school child, injections in, 100
Primitive movement, 377
Process, xiphoid, 403
Proctoscope, 136
Proctoscopy, equipment for, 148, *148*
  preparation of patient for, 148, *148*
  procedure for, 149-151, *149*, *150*
  special table for, 142, *142*
Prodromal period, of infection, 4
Proetz position, 186, *186*
Projection, as defense mechanism, 394
Prone position, 141, *142*
  draping for, 143
Prophylaxis, 349

Proprietary name, of drug, 65, 66-67
Protozoal infection, 6
Pseudomonas aeruginosa (pyocyanea), 5
Psychological defense mechanisms, 394-395
Psychiatric therapy(ies), somatic, assisting with, 375-400
  emergency cart for, 378
  general preparations for, 378-379
  history of, 377-378
  physician's tray in, 378
  treatment room in, 378
  shock treatment tray for, 379
Psychological defense mechanisms, 394-395
Psychosis, 377
  manic-depressive, 376
Publications, relating to drugs, 66
Puerperium, 207
Pulmonary edema, acute, 288-295, *290*, *293*, *294*
  heart disease and, 288
  symptoms of, 288
  tourniquet application for, 289-295, *290*, *293*, *294*, 304
Pulmonary function tests, 153
Pupillary reaction, 377
Pure drug, 65
Pure Food Act of 1906, 66
Purgative, 65
Purified protein derivative, in tuberculin skin testing, 357
Purpura, 349
Purulence, 2
Purulent infections, 2
Pus, 2
Pyelonephritis, 207

Rabies, prophylaxis of, 370(t)
Rationalization, as defense mechanism, 395
Reactions, allergic, forms of, 350
  types of, 350
  Arthus, 350
  autosensitive, 349-350
  hypersensitivity, 349
    types of, 349, 352-353
  pupillary, 377
Reaction formation, as defense mechanism, 394
"Reactor," definition of, 349
Record, insulin treatment (sample), *395*
Record, strip chart, 403
Recording paper, 412, *425*
Rectal examination, equipment for, 147, *147*
Rectal smear and culture, equipment for, 327, *327*
  procedure for taking, 327-335, *327-334*, 345
Rectus femoris muscle, as site for intramuscular injections, 99, *100*
Reflex, Babinski, 376
  cough, 246
  gag, 308
Refraction, in eye, 195-196, *195*, *196*
Region, temporal, 377
Regression, as defense mechanism, 394
Rehfuss tube, 308, *316*
Removal of gastrointestinal tubes, procedure for, 313-314
Removal of infusion, technique for, 120-121, 133

Renal pelvis, irrigation of, 169-171, *170*, 202-203
  equipment for, 169
Repair, vaginal, 207
Repression, as defense mechanism, 394
Reproductive system, examination of, 137
Resection, abdominal-perineal, 206
Respiration, physiology of, 247
Respiratory tract, anatomy of, 263-265, *264*, *265*
  examination of, 137
  in general physical examination, 137
  viral infections of, 5
Response, allergic, 349
  types of, 349
Resuscitator, Ambu, 375
Retention, of urine, 207
Retention catheter, nursing considerations with, 216-217
  procedure for insertion of, 215-219, *217-219*
  procedure for removal of, 219-220
Retraction, rib, 247
Reversal, as defense mechanism, 395
Rhythm, seasonal, 65
Rib retraction, 247
Robinson catheter, 223(t), *224*
Role of nurse, in physical examination, 137
Route, parenteral, for administering medication, 77-118, 120-122
Rubber bulb syringe, 158, *158*
Rubber gloves, first use of, 49
Rubella vaccine, immunization procedure using, 367(t)

Sakel, Manfred, 389
Saling, Erick, 426
Saliva, excessive secretion of, 376
Salve, definition of, 65
Sample, blood. See also under *Blood*.
  Vacutainer for obtaining, 118-120, *118*
Saphenous veins, 285, *287*
Scalp sampling, fetal, procedure for, 426-428, *427*, 432
Schick test, 349
Schizophrenia, definition of, 377
School-aged child, injections in, 100
Scratch Test, interpretation of results of, 357, *357*
  procedure for, 355-357, *356*, *357*, 373
  supplies needed for, 355
  uses of, 355
Scrub, surgical, handwashing procedure in, 15-17, *15-17*
Scrub, short surgical, 18
Scrub suit, 2, 11, *11*
Seasonal rhythm, definition of, 65
Sebaceous gland, 2
Second intention, healing by, 42
Secretions, removal following tracheostomy, 273-277, *274-276*, 282
  equipment for, 274
Sedatives, 65
  state laws and, 67
Sedimentation rate, definition of, 2
Seibert, Florence, 357
Seizure, grand mal, 376
  petit mal, 377

Self, turning against, as defense mechanism, 394
Self-catheterization, by paraplegics, advantages of, 219
Self-gloving, closed technique of, 23-26, *23-26*, 60
  open technique of, 26-28, *26-28*, 60
Semi-Fowler's position, for physical examination, 141
Semmelweis, Ignaz, 48
Sense organs, in general physical examination, 137
Sensorium, definition of, 247
Serum sickness, 353
Set, tracheostomy, components of, 267, *267*
Setup, in sterile field, 9
Sex organs, examination of, in general physical examination, 137
Shock, anaphylactic, 64, 348, 350, 352-353
  emergency nursing measures in, 353
  emergency treatment for, 350
  insulin, 376
Shock treatment tray, for somatic psychiatric therapy, 379
Shoes, conductive, 12-13, *12-13*
Shoe covers, conductive, 1, 12, *12*
Sigmoidoscope, 136
Sigmoidoscopy, equipment for, 148, *148*
  preparation of patient for, 148, *148*, 155
  procedure for, 149-151, *149*, *150*
  special table for, 142, *142*
Sims' position, 141, *141*
  draping for, 143
Singultus, definition of, 377
Skin, anatomy of, 50
  capillaries of, function in absorption of injected medications, 83
  elasticity of, and injected medications, 83
  examination of, in general physical examination, 137
  in regulation of temperature, 228
  physiology of, 50
  structure of, 83, *83*
  viral infections of, 5
Skin bacteria, 50
Skin tests, 349
  for tuberculosis. See *Tuberculin skin testing*; also see under names of various tests.
Skull, anatomy of, *193*, 383
Small saphenous vein, *287*, 295
Smear(s), 325
  general steps for obtaining, 326, *326*
  Papanicolaou (Pap), 136
    contraindications to, 327
    purpose of, 136
  purpose of, 326
  vaginal, for monilial vaginitis, taking of, 335-336, 346
    for trichomonas vaginitis, taking of, 335-336, 346
Smear and culture, cervical, equipment for, 327, *327*
  procedure for taking of, 327-335, *327-334*, 345
  rectal, equipment for, 327, *327*
    taking of, 327-335, *327-334*, 345
  vaginal, equipment for, 327, *327*
    taking of, 327-335, *327-334*, 345
Snellen test, for visual acuity, 196
Soaks, hot, equipment for, 231, *231*

Soaks, hot *(Continued)*
    procedure for application of, 230-235, *231-234*, 244
Soaps, germicidal, for skin, 50
Sociology, in aseptic technique, 51
    in hearing, 194
Solid additives, preparation for intravenous solutions, 122-123, 133-134
Solubility, definition of, 65
Solute, definition of, 65
Solution(s), definition of, 65
    hypodermoclysis for administration of, 79, *79*
Solution(s), intravenous, preparation of liquid additive for, 121, 133
    preparation of solid additives for, 122-123, 133-134
    sterile, containers used in injection of, *82*
    pouring of, 37-39, *37-39*, 62
    withdrawal, from vial, 39-40, *39-40*, 62
Solvent, definition of, 65
Somatic psychiatric therapy(ies), assisting with, 375-400
    emergency cart for, 378
    general preparation for, 378-379
    history of, 377-378
    physician's tray in, 378
    shock treatment tray for, 379
    treatment room in, 378
Somnolence, definition of, 377
Sonogram, definition of, 403
Sound, characteristics of, 405
Space, intercostal, 376
Spasm, torsion, 377
Spatula, Ayer, 330, *330*
Special examination(s), 138
    gastroscopy as, 152
Special table, for proctoscopic and sigmoidoscopic examinations, 142, *142*
Specimen(s), cytologic, obtaining of, general steps for, 326, *326*
    gastric, insertion of tube for collection of, 316-318
        equipment for, 317
Speculum, 136, 326
    nasal, 140, *140*
    vaginal, 140, *140*
Sphincter, definition of, 207
Spiral electrode, in direct fetal monitoring, procedure for insertion of, 422-425, *422-425*, 431-432
    procedure for removal of, 426, 432
Spirits, drug solutions of, 65
Spore, definition of, 2
Spray-on dressing, 52, *52*
Spread of microorganisms. See *Transmission, of microorganisms.*
Staphylococcal infections, 5
Staphylococcus(i), 5
    in eye infections, 195
Stenosis, definition of, 326
Sterile dressings, changing of, 41-48, *41-47*, 62
    educating patient and/or family about, 51
    four-towel drape in, 45
    placement of dressing retainers in, 46-47, *46-47*
    principles of aseptic technique in, 48
    procedure for, 42-47, *42-47*
    supplies needed for, 42, *42*

Sterile dressings *(Continued)*
    zinc oxide in, 50
Sterile equipment, handling of, using forceps, 34-37, *34-37*, 62
Sterile field, 10
Sterile forceps, use of, in handling sterile equipment, 62
Sterile items, recognition of, 9
Sterile materials, handling of, 10
Sterile packages, opening of, 31-34, *31-34*, 40-41, *40-41*, 61
Sterile person, 9, 10
    in sterile field, 10
Sterile solution(s), containers used in injection of, 82
    pouring of, 37-39, *37-39*, 62
    withdrawal from vial, 39-40, *39-40*, 62
Sterile technique, 1-62
Sterile worker, and unsterile worker, in gowning, 22, *22*
    movement in sterile field, 10
    gowning and gloving of someone else, 28-31, *28-31*
    self-gloving by, 23-25, *23-25*, 26-28, *26-28*
    self-gowning by, 19-23, *19-22*
Sterile zone, boundaries of, 10
Sterilization, 49
    by steam under pressure, first use of, 49
    methods of, 9
Steripak, 53
Sterneedle Test, for tuberculin skin testing, advantages and disadvantages of, 361
    procedure for, 360-361, *360*, 374
Sternum, 263, *265*
Stimulant, definition of, 65
Stimulation, of coughing, techniques for, 253-255, *253*, *254*
Stocks, floor, in unit-dose system 69
Stock supply, definition of, 65
Stoma, definition of, 263
Stomach, drainage of, insertion of gastric tube for, 309-313, *310*, *311*
    reasons for intubation of, 308
Stomach cancer, enterostomy feeding in patients with, 318-321, *319*, *320*, 324
Stomach tubes, procedure for removal of, 313-314
Strabismus, as visual impairment, 195
Strain gauge, *408*
Streptococcal infections, 5
Streptococcus(i), 5
Stricture, definition of, 326
Stridor, definition of, 247
Strip chart record, 403
Structure, of skin, 83, *83*
Stylet, 206
Styptic, definition of, 64
Subcutaneous injections, 77, 78, *83*, 86-97, *86-96*
    administration of, 93-97, *93-96*, 131
    preparation of, 87-93, *87-93*, 130
    sites for, 84-85, *84*, *85*
Sublimation, as defense mechanism, 395
sub q (subq). See *Subcutaneous.*
Suction, 247
Suctioning, bulb syringe, procedure for, 251-252, *251*, *252*
    in infants, procedure for, 251-252, *251*, *252*
    nasopharyngeal, equipment for, 248, *248*, *249*, *249*

Suctioning *(Continued)*
  nasopharyngeal, procedure for, 248–250, *248, 249*
  oropharyngeal, procedure for, 251
  pharyngeal, 246–261
  pharyngeal and endotracheal, equipment for, 255–256, *255, 256*
    procedure for, 255–258, *256, 257*
  tracheobronchial, equipment for, 274
    procedure for, 273–277, *274–276*, 282
Supine position, draping for, 143, *143*
  for physical examination, 141, *141*
Supplies, in changing sterile dressing, 42, *42*
  stock, 65
Suppository, 65
Suppression, kidney, 207
Suppuration, 2, 227
Surfaces, in sterile field, 10
Surgery, asepsis in, 3
Surgical drape, 207
Surgical mask, 13–14, *13, 14*
Surgical sound, 326
Surgical scrub, 11–18, *11–17*, 60
  handwashing in, 15–17, *15–17*
  short, 18
Symmetry of body, 136
Syringe(s), 80–82, *80–82*
  Asepto, 158, *158*
  catheter, 158, *158*
  for intradermal injections, 106
  frozen, freeing of, 97, *97*
  insulin, *81*, 82
  Pomeroy, 172, *172*
  rubber bulb, 158, *158*
  tuberculin, 82
  types of, 80–82, *80–82*
  U100, 82
Syrup, definition of, 65
Systemic circulation, 285

Table, special, for proctoscopic and sigmoidoscopic examination, 142, *142*
Tablets, definition of, 65
Technique(s), alternate venipuncture, for obtaining blood samples, 133
  aseptic. See *Aseptic technique.*
  of physical examination, 138–139, *138, 139*
Technologists, duties in administering medications, 67
Telfa, 51, *51*
Temperature, for compresses, packs, and soaks, factors affecting choice of, 228
  skin in regulation of, 228
Temporal region, 377
Tenaculum, 326
Test(s), blastomycin, 348
  coccidioidin, 349
  Dick, 349
  histoplasmin, 349
  kidney function, 153
  mucous membrane, 354
  neurologic, 153
  Schick, 349
  tuberculin skin, 357–364, 374
Tetanic contraction, 403
Tetanus, 5

Tetanus toxoid, immunization procedures for, 366(t)
Therapy(ies), ambulatory insulin, 390–391
  electroshock, 376
  insulin shock, 391–393
  somatic psychiatric, assisting with, 375–400
    emergency cart for, 378
    general preparations for, 378–379
    physician's tray for, 379
    treatment room in, 378
Throat, anatomy of, 187, *187*, 198
  examination of, 137
  infections of, 198
  scientific principles relating to, 198
  suctioning of, 246–261
Throat culture, equipment for, 340
  obtaining of, 340–341, *340, 341*, 346–347
Throat gargle, 188–190
Throat irrigation, 188–189, 205
Thrombophlebitis, 285
Thrombosis, 285
Thrombus(i), 284
Through and through bladder irrigation, 166–169, *167, 168*, 202
  equipment for, 167
Thyroid cartilage, 264, *264*
Tincture, definition of, 66
Tine Test, for tuberculin skin testing, advantages and disadvantages of, 359
  procedure for, 358, *358*, 374
Tissue erosion, 263
Tissue reaction, to infection, 4–5
Tocodynamometer, 403
  procedure for placement of, 410–411, *410, 411*, 430
Toddler, intramuscular injections in, 100
Tone, uterine, 403
Tongs, 2, 35
Tonic, definition of, 66
Tonic convulsion, 376
Toomey bladder evacuator, 159, *159*
Topical drugs, 124
  application of, 124–126, 134
Torsion spasm, 377
Tourniquet(s), 285
  acute pulmonary edema, 289–295, *290, 293, 294*, 304
  application of, 284–305
Toxin, 2
Trachea, 247, 263, *264*
  stimulation to induce coughing, 253–254, *253, 254*
  suctioning of, 246–261
Tracheal cuff, inflation and deflation of, 277–279, *277–279*, 283
Tracheal stimulation, external mechanical, procedure for, 253–254, *253, 254*
Trachelotomy, 263
Tracheobronchial suctioning, equipment for, 274
  procedure for, 273–277, *274–276*, 282
Tracheostomy, 263
  care of, 262–283
  complications following, 269
  equipment, for emergency care, 268
    for routine care, 268
  indications for, 265
  inflated cuff in, 266
  patient with, general nursing measures for, 268–269

Tracheostomy *(Continued)*
  removal of secretions following, 273-277, *274-276*, 282
    equipment for, 274
  site for, 264-265, *264, 265*
  uses of, 265
Tracheostomy set, components of, 267, *267*
Tracheostomy tube(s), 266, 266(t)
  cleansing inner cannula of, 269-273, *270, 272*, 282
  cuffed, inflation and deflation of, 277-279, *277-279*, 283
  metal, 266, 266(t)
  plastic, 266, 266(t)
  rubber, 266, 266(t)
Traction bandage, foam rubber, 53, *53*
Trade name, of drug, 66-67
Trahner catheter, 223(t), *224*
Tranquilizer, 377
Transducer, 403
  crystals of, 402
  ultrasonic, placement for detection of fetal heart rate, 411-413, *411, 412*, 430
Transfer of blood sample to tube, 117-118, *117, 118*
Transfer forceps, for handling sterile equipment, 34-37, *34-37*
  for handling Vaseline gauze, 37, *37*
Transmission, of allergens, modes of, *352*
  of bacteria, 3
  of disease, 2
    methods of, 6-7
  of microorganisms, 6-7
    disinfectants in prevention of, 8
    modes of, 6, 8
Travel, foreign, immunization for, 366
Treatment room, in somatic psychiatric therapy, 378
Trendelenburg circulatory test, 295-298, *295-297*, 304
  equipment for, 296
  interpretation of, 297, *297*, 297(t)
  procedure for, 296-298, *296, 297*, 304
Trendelenburg position, 141, *142*
Treponemata, and ear infection, 193
Trichomonas vaginitis, procedure for taking vaginal smear for, 335-336, 346
Trocar, 263
Troche, 65
Tube(s), endotracheal, 263
  gastrointestinal, procedure for removal of, 313-314
Tuberculin, 349
Tuberculin skin testing, and immunizing agents, 366
  Heaf Test for, procedure for, 360-361, *360*, 374
  Hypospray Test for, procedure for, 361-362, *361, 362*, 374
  Jet Gun Test for, procedure for, 361-362, *361, 362*, 374
  Mantoux Test for, equipment for, 362
    procedure for, 362-364, *363, 364*, 374
    methods of, 357-364, *358-364*, 374
  Mono-vacc Test for, procedure for, 359, *359*
  Sterneedle Test for, advantages and disadvantages of, 362
    procedure for, 360-361, *360*, 374
  Tine Test for, procedure for, 358, *358*, 374
Tuberculin syringe, *82*
  for intradermal injections, 106

Tuberculosis, diagnosis of. See under *Tuberculin skin testing;* also see under names of various skin tests.
  immunization against, 351
  skin testing for. See *Tuberculin skin testing;* also see under names of various skin tests.
Turban, 2, 12, *12*
Turning against the self, 394
Twitching, myotonic, 377
Typhoid vaccines, immunization procedures using, 368(t)

U100 syringe, 82
Ultrasonics, definition of, 403
Ultrasonic transducer, placement for detection of fetal heart rate, 411-413, *411, 412*, 430
Ultrasound, in fetal and maternal monitoring, 404-405
Undoing, as defense mechanism, 395
Unguent, definition of, 65
Unit-dose system of administering medications, 66, 67-70
  advantages of, 67-69
  difficulties in, 68
  floor stocks in, 69
  Kardex in, 68-70
  materials savings in, 69
  Patient Profile Record in, 68
  nursing responsibilities in, 69
  safety precautions in, 69-70
United States Pharmacopeia, 66
Unsterile worker, in gowning, 20-22, *20-22*
Unused drugs, in unit-dose system, 68
Urgency, of micturition, 207
Urinary bladder, catheterization of, uses of, 207-208
  Escherichia and, 192
  instillation of medications in, 164-166, *165, 166*, 202
    equipment for, 164
  irrigation of, through and through, 166-169, *167, 168*, 202
    with catheter in place, 201
  scientific principles relating to, 192
Urinary catheters, types of, 223-224(t), *224*
Urinary catheterization, 206-226
  history of, 222-223
Urinary tract, examination of, 137
  in general physical examination, 137
  pathogens affecting, 207
Urination, 157, 207
  frequency of, 207
Urine retention, 207
Urologic examinations, 153
Urticaria, 349
U.S.P., 66
Uterine activity, external indirect monitoring of, 410-428
Uterine contractions, 403
  and oxytocin, 409
  duration of, 402
  hypertonus in, 409
  physiology of, 408-409
  placement of tocodynamometer for detection of, 410-411, *410, 411*, 430
Uterine tone, 403
Uterus, 403

INDEX

Vaccination, with Bacille Calmette-Guérin, 351
Vaccine(s), 349, 351–352
 different, simultaneous administration of, 366
Vaccinia virus vaccines, immunization procedures using, 368(t)
Vacoliter, 82
Vacutainer, obtaining blood sample using, 118–120, *118*
Vaginal examination, equipment for, 147, *147*
Vaginal orifice, 157
Vaginal repair, 207
Vaginal smear, for monilial vaginitis, procedure for taking, 335–336, 346
 for trichomonas vaginitis, procedure for taking, 335–336, 346
Vaginal smear and culture, equipment for, 327, *327*
 procedure for taking, 327–335, *327–334*, 345
Vaginal speculum, 140, *140*
Vaginitis, monilial, procedure for taking vaginal smear for, 335–336, 346
 trichomonas, procedure for taking vaginal smear for, 335–336, 346
Vaseline gauze, handling with forceps, 37, *37*
Vasoconstriction, 227
Vasoconstrictor, 66
Vasodilation, 227
Vasodilator, 66
Vasomotor, 227
Vastus lateralis muscle, as site for intramuscular injections, 99, *99*
Veins, of legs, tests for patency of, 295–300, *295–297, 299, 300*, 304–305
 saphenous, 285
 valves of, 286, *286*
Venesection, 285
Venipuncture, 285
Venipuncture technique, alternate for obtaining blood samples, 116–118, *117, 118*, 133
Ventrogluteal area, as site for intramuscular injections, 99, *99*
Venules, 1, 284
Vermifuge, 64
Vesalius, 48
Vescettes, 66
Vesicant, 66
Vestibule, 157
Vial, 82
 withdrawing solution from 39–40, *39–40*, 62
Viral infections, 5
Virulence, of organism, 2
 in body resistance, 4
Virus(es) 5–6
 characteristics of, 7
Viscosity, 227, 263
Vision, binocular, 196
Visual acuity, tests for, 196
Visual defects, sociological implications of, 197

Voice box, 247
Voiding, 157, 207
von Hochstetter's site, for intramuscular injections, 99, *99*

Water, vs. air, as conductor of heat, 228
Wheal, 349
Whistle-tip catheter, 223(t)
Wick effect, in gowning, 19
Windpipe, 247
 suctioning of, 246–261
Womb, 403
Worker, sterile. See *Sterile worker.*
 unsterile, in gowning, 20–22, *20–22*
World Health Organization, and Pharmacopeia Internationalis, 66
Wound(s), 190–192
 classification of, 42
 disruption of, 49
 gaping, 2
 healing of, 42, 49
  by first intention, 42, 49
  by granulation, 42
  by second intention, 42, 49
 complications of, 49
  dehiscence as complication of, 49
  delayed, 49
  evisceration as complication of, 49
  hemorrhage as complication of, 49
  primary, 49
  secondary, 49
Wound cleansing, use of antibiotics in, 50
 use of antiseptics in, 50
Wound culture, equipment for, 341–343, *342*
 procedure for, 341–343, *342*, 347
Wound dressings, principles of physics in, 50
 properly applied, psychological effect on patient, 51
Wound instillation, procedure for, 191–192
Wound irrigation, equipment for, 190
 procedure for, 190–191, 205
Wound management, using tetanus toxoid, 369(t)

Xiphoid process, 403

Yeast, infections, 6

Z-track technique of administering intramuscular injections, 66, 105, *105*, 131
Zinc oxide, use in changing sterile dressings, 50